FIRST AID FOR THE® MEDICINE CLERKSHIP

NOTICE

Medicine is an ever-changing science. As new research and clinical experience broaden our knowledge, changes in treatment and drug therapy are required. The authors and the publisher of this work have checked with sources believed to be reliable in their efforts to provide information that is complete and generally in accord with the standards accepted at the time of publication. However, in view of the possibility of human error or changes in medical sciences, neither the authors nor the publisher nor any other party who has been involved in the preparation or publication of this work warrants that the information contained herein is in every respect accurate or complete, and they disclaim all responsibility for any errors or omissions or for the results obtained from use of the information contained in this work. Readers are encouraged to confirm the information contained herein with other sources. For example, and in particular, readers are advised to check the product information sheet included in the package of each drug they plan to administer to be certain that the information contained in this work is accurate and that changes have not been made in the recommended dose or in the contraindications for administration. This recommendation is of particular importance in connection with new or infrequently used drugs.

FIRST AID FOR THE® MEDICINE CLERKSHIP

4th Edition

Editors

Matthew S. Kaufman, MD, FACEP
Department of Emergency Medicine
Jersey City Medical Center
Jersey City, New Jersey

Latha Ganti, MD, MS, MBA, FACEP, FAHA
Vice Chair for Research and Academic Affairs
UCF HCA Emergency Medicine Residency Program of Greater Orlando
Associate Medical Director, Polk County Fire Rescue
Professor of Emergency Medicine and Neurology
University of Central Florida College of Medicine
Editor-in-Chief, International Journal of Emergency Medicine
Orlando, Florida

Dennis Chang, MD, FHM
Associate Professor
Interprofessional Education Thread Director (MD Curriculum)
Hospital Medicine, Department of Medicine
Washington University School of Medicine
St. Louis, Missouri

Alfredo J. Mena Lora, MD, FACP
Assistant Professor of Clinical Medicine
Program Director, Infectious Diseases Fellowship
Associate Program Director, Internal Medicine Residency
Assistant Director, M3 Medicine Clerkship
Division of Infectious Diseases | Department of Medicine
University of Illinois at Chicago
Chicago, Illinois

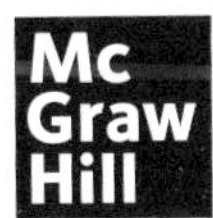

New York Chicago San Francisco Athens London Madrid Mexico City
New Delhi Milan Singapore Sydney Toronto

First Aid for the® Medicine Clerkship, Fourth Edition

1 2 3 4 5 6 7 8 9 DSS 25 24 23 22 21 20

ISBN 978-1-260-46062-9
MHID 1-260-46062-2

This book was set in MinionPro by MPS Limited.
The editors were Bob Boehringer and Kim J. Davis.
The production supervisor was Catherine Saggese.
Project management was provided by Ishan Chaudhary and Jyoti Shaw, MPS Limited.

This book is printed on acid-free paper.

Library of Congress Cataloging-in-Publication Data

Names: Kaufman, Matthew S., editor. | Ganti, Latha, editor. | Chang, Dennis, editor. | Mena Lora, Alfredo J., editor. | Kaufman, Matthew S. First aid for the medicine clerkship.
Title: First aid for the medicine clerkship / editors, Matthew Kaufman, Latha Ganti, Dennis Chang, Alfredo J. Mena Lora.
Description: 4th edition. | New York : McGraw Hill, [2021] | Preceded by First aid for the medicine clerkship / Matthew S. Kaufman, Latha G. Stead, Arthur Rusovici. 3rd ed. 2010. | Includes bibliographical references and index. | Summary: "First Aid for the Medicine Clerkship is a high-yield review of the clerkship's core competencies presented in the trusted First Aid format"—Provided by publisher.
Identifiers: LCCN 2020024470 (print) | LCCN 2020024471 (ebook) | ISBN 9781260460629 (paperback ; alk. paper) | ISBN 9781260460636 (ebook)
Subjects: MESH: Clinical Clerkship | Career Choice | Fellowships and Scholarships | First Aid | Handbook
Classification: LCC R839 (print) | LCC R839 (ebook) | NLM W 49 | DDC 610.71/1—dc23
LC record available at https://lccn.loc.gov/2020024470
LC ebook record available at https://lccn.loc.gov/2020024471

CONTENTS

CONTRIBUTORS

Eric Barna, MD, MPH
Associate Professor
Department of Internal Medicine
Mount Sinai Medical Center
New York, New York
18 Inpatient Emergencies

Stephen Berns, MD, FAAHPM
Associate Professor
Division of Palliative Medicine
Department of Family Medicine
The Larner College of Medicine
University of Vermont
Burlington, Vermont
19 Palliative Care

Scott Borgetti, MD
Assistant Professor of Clinical Medicine
Department of Internal Medicine
Division of Infectious Diseases
University of Illinois-Chicago College of Medicine
Chicago, Illinois
9 Infectious Diseases

Daniel Bunker, MD
Assistant Professor of Medicine
Georgetown University School of Medicine
Washington, DC
15 Rheumatology

Miriam Chung, MD
Associate Professor
Department of Internal Medicine
Division of Nephrology
Icahn School of Medicine at Mount Sinai
New York, New York
14 Nephrology

Andrew Coyle, MD
Assistant Professor of Medicine and Medical Education
Associate Program Director for Ambulatory Care
Internal Medicine Residency Program
Icahn School of Medicine at Mount Sinai
New York, New York
17 Ambulatory Medicine

John Cummins, MD
Pyschiatry Fellow
University of Illinois at Chicago
Chicago, Illinois
12 Psychiatry

Lindsay A. Dow, MD, MS
Assistant Professor
Associate Director of Non-Fellowship Education
Brookdale Department of Geriatrics and Palliative Medicine
Icahn School of Medicine at Mount Sinai
New York, New York
19 Palliative Care

Richard J. Doyle, MD, PhD
Attending Physician
Department of Emergency Medicine
Jesse Brown VA Hospital
Chicago, Illinois
11 Dermatology

Yuval Eisenberg, MD
Assistant Professor of Clinical Medicine
Department of Medicine
Division of Endocrinology
Diabetes and Metabolism
University of Illinois at Chicago
Chicago, Illinois
7 Endocrinology

Michelle T. Fabian, MD
Assistant Professor
Corinne Goldsmith Dickinson Center for Multiple Sclerosis
Director
Neurology Residency Program
Icahn School of Medicine at Mount Sinai
New York, New York
16 Neurology

Samira S. Farouk, MD, MS, FASN
Assistant Professor
Department of Medicine
Division of Nephrology
Assistant Professor Medical Education
Icahn School of Medicine at Mount Sinai
New York, New York
14 Nephrology /Acid–Base Disorders

Christopher P. Gans, MD, FACC, FASE
Assistant Professor of Clinical Medicine
Division of Cardiology
University of Illinois at Chicago
Chicago, Illinois
6 Cardiology

Michael Herscher, MD, MA
Assistant Professor
Division of Hospital Medicine
Icahn School of Medicine at Mount Sinai
New York, New York
2 Physical Examination Pearls

Horatio (Teddy) Holzer, MD
Assistant Professor
Inpatient Medicine Clerkship Director
Department of Medicine
Icahn School of Medicine at Mount Sinai
New York, New York
4 Electrocardiogram

Peter H. Jin, MD
Assistant Professor
Department of Neurology
University of Maryland School of Medicine
Baltimore, Maryland
16 Neurology

Tonia Kim, MD
Associate Professor
Department of Internal Medicine
Division of Nephrology
Icahn School of Medicine at Mount Sinai
New York, New York
14 Nephrology

Katie Mena, MD
Assistant Professor
Internal Medicine & Pediatrics
University of Illinois at Chicago
Chicago, Illinois
11 Dermatology
12 Psychiatry

Vinh-Tung Nguyen, MD
Assistant Professor
Department of Internal Medicine
Icahn School of Medicine at Mount Sinai
New York, New York
Chapter 3 Chest X-ray

Mahesh C. Patel, MD
Associate Professor
Internal Medicine-Infectious Diseases
University of Illinois at Chicago College of Medicine
Chicago, Illinois
9 Infectious Diseases

Kamron Pourmand, MD
Assistant Professor, Division of Liver Diseases
Recanati/Miller Transplantation Institute
Icahn School of Medicine at Mount Sinai
New York, New York
13 Gastroenterology and Hepatology

Ardaman Shergill, MD, MSPH
Assistant Professor of Medicine in Oncology
The University of Chicago
Chicago, Illinois
8 Hematology/Oncology

Melissa Wagner, MD, PhD
Clinical Assistant Professor of Psychiatry and Pediatrics
Medical Director of Inpatient Psychiatry
Associate Medical Director
Women's Mental Health
Department of Psychiatry
University of Illinois College of Medicine
Chicago, Illinois
12 Psychiatry

Travis Yamanaka, MD
Physician
Section of Pulmonary and Critical Care
Mercy Hospital and Medical Center
Chicago, Illinois
10 Pulmonology

Maryam Zia, MD
John H. Stroger Hospital of Cook County
Chicago, Illinois
8 Hematology/Oncology

STUDENT CONTRIBUTORS

Deepa Chellappa, MD
Internal Medicine Resident
Hospital of the University of Pennsylvania
Philadelphia, Pennsylvania

Claire Eden, MD
General Surgery Resident
New York Presbyterian Queens Hospital
Queens, New York

Sean Llewellyn, MD, PhD
Family Medicine Resident
University of Colorado
Anschutz Medical Campus
Aurora, Colorado

Jamilur Reja, MD
Internal Medicine Resident
Mount Sinai Beth Israel Hospital
New York, New York

Emily Tixier, MD
Internal Medicine Resident
Massachusetts General Hospital
Boston, Massachusetts

PREFACE

As current and former medicine clerkship directors, we know firsthand how difficult and stressful the Internal Medicine Clerkship is for medical students. But it doesn't have to be that way. The skills and knowledge to succeed in IM clerkships can be mastered. And in the process, you can enjoy yourself and grow to become the best physician you can be.

This 2020 updated *First Aid for the® Medicine Clerkship* is a complete and thorough revision. In this revision we have made major changes in response to in-depth reviews and feedback from current and former medical students and internal medicine residents. We give deep thanks to these outstanding students and residents for their thoughtful and brilliant suggestions.

We have gone away from bullet points to a more narrative format with more tables, figures, pictures, and color. We have also added three new boxes to each chapter to emphasize important points:

1. **Conquer the Boards**
   These boxes highlight facts and knowledge that will be tested on your IM shelf exam.
2. **Conquer the Wards**
   These boxes highlight facts and knowledge important to take great care of patients and that your team will ask about.
3. **High- Yield Literature**
   These boxes will give you the high-yield literature that every physician should know about on a given topic.

We have also added a new section entitled Skills for the Medicine Clerkship. In this section we cover the basic skills needed to enjoy and succeed on the IM clerkship:

1. **Basics** – Tips from former and current clerkship directors on how to succeed on the IM clerkship and basic tips on what to do on pre-rounds, rounds, and after rounds. We also give pointers on how to present your patients and write a SOAP note.
2. **Physical Examination Pearls** – High-yield physical exam facts and explanations to impress your teams. ECG – Electrocardiogram (ECG) reading basics and example ECGs with thorough explanations.
3. **ECG** – Electrocardiogram (ECG) reading basics and example ECGs with thorough explanations.
4. **Chest Radiograph** – Chest x-ray reading basics and example chest X-rays with detailed readings.
5. **Inpatient Floor Emergencies** – Learn how experienced physicians approach common inpatient floor emergencies like chest pain, dyspnea, and so much more.
6. **Evidence**- Based Medicine – This is a succinct review of how you approach a medical question and appraise the literature, as well as basic medical statistics
7. **Palliative Care and Pain Management** – In addition to diagnosing and treating our patients, critical tasks of IM doctors are communicating with and helping patients through times of pain and severe illness. As Hippocrates once said, "Cure sometimes, treat often, and comfort always." This section reviews basic concepts and communication tools in end-of-life care and pain management from palliative care experts.

We hope this book helps you enjoy and learn during the IM clerkship. And as Sir William Osler once said, "Live neither in the past nor in the future, but let each day's work absorb your entire energies and satisfy your widest ambition." Good luck!

Dennis Chang, MD, FHM
Alfredo J. Mena Lora, MD, FACP

SECTION I

SKILLS FOR THE MEDICINE CLERKSHIP

CHAPTER 1 BASICS

OVERVIEW OF HIGH-YIELD TOPICS IN BASICS OF THE MEDICINE CLERKSHIP

INTRODUCTION

During the Internal Medicine (IM) clerkship, you will learn and be tested on both knowledge and skills. This chapter will give you tips for success on the IM clerkship.

TIPS FOR SUCCESS

At the beginning of the IM clerkship, you will be given a list of objectives that you need to meet. No matter how long this list is for your clerkship, these 5 tips will help you meet and hopefully exceed that list of objectives.

1. DO EVERYTHING FOR YOUR PATIENTS

During the IM clerkship, you will be asked to help take care of patients along with an intern. Successful students do 3 things for all their patients:

1. Perform daily tasks
2. Contribute to creating the medical plan of care (see number 4 later)
3. Teach about what they have learned from their patient

Daily Tasks

After rounds there will be a "To Do List" of things that need to get done for the patient. Your role as a student is to *proactively* volunteer to do these things for your patient and go above and beyond to accomplish these daily tasks. You should also constantly communicate with your team the status of those tasks, and once you have completed your tasks, ask your team if there is anything else you can do to help.

Common tasks are:

- Calling consults to other services (surgery, pulmonology, cardiology, etc.)
- Reaching out to consult services to clarify plans of care
- Ensuring radiology tests and procedures are done in a timely manner
- Getting medical records from outside hospitals
- Calling primary care providers and other doctors who take care of the patient as an outpatient
- Speaking to and educating patients and families
- Helping perform procedures (lumbar punctures, paracentesis, thoracentesis)

This is just to name a few. At first, it may not be possible to accomplish these tasks on your own, so *proactively* ask your team if they can help or teach you how to do them. Your goal by the end of the clerkship is to be able to accomplish these tasks on your own.

Teaching and Extra Tasks

It will impress your team if you do more than what is asked. Here are some examples of extra tasks that impress IM teams:

- Visiting your patients several times a day to get to know them better and educate them about their disease and medical plan
- Calling patients to see how they are doing after discharge
- Looking up journal articles that help the team make decisions (see Chapter 5 on evidence-based medicine)

- Creating short (less than 5 minutes) topic presentations on diseases your patient is being treated for

2. TALK TO YOUR PATIENTS

At the center of your IM clerkship will always be the patients. They will be your greatest teachers and will be the reason you want to come to work. As a medical student, you are in a unique and amazing position. You have access to all the patient care information, are present for every physician discussion about your teams' patients, and have time to spend with your patients. Make sure you are the best ambassador between your patient and the medical team.

The information you gather from your patients is the most comprehensive and accurate history in the hospital, and medical students often have the closest and most meaningful relationships with patients and their families. These relationships and information truly make a positive difference in the care patients receive. Every year, I have a medical student who uncovers a key piece of history that completely alters our plan of care.

Talk to your patients as much as possible, advocate for them to your medical team, and make sure they understand their plan of care. It will help them receive better care and help you become a better doctor.

3. READ AND ASK QUESTIONS

All students go home and read about the diseases their patients have. However, many students do not show that they are reading on rounds. Unfortunately with clinical clerkships, unless you show what you know, people will assume you don't know it. For many students, speaking out on rounds is challenging and intimidating. Here are 2 tips:

1. Practice patient presentations: This is your time to shine, so own it and practice your presentations so they have a smooth flow without ums or pauses. And this only comes with practicing your presentations at night and in the morning. Make sure, when you practice, you do the following (see Soap Notes and Presentations later):
   - **Build in questions** you had and/or journal articles or facts you looked up the night before.
   - **Work on efficiency:** Teams expect a great, efficient presentation and expect you to bring in your knowledge. When students stumble during their presentation, teams assume you are unprepared and will quickly jump in before you get to your questions and reading.
   - **Make time to discuss the assessment and plan with your team:** When it comes to your assessment and plan, build in time in the morning to discuss this with your intern and resident so you can confidently tell the plan to your attending. Your resident's success is tied to yours, and when you present, you are representing the team – so make them proud.
2. Pay attention: Even though you may not be primarily following all the patients on the team, pay attention to every discussion. Take notes. There is nothing more impressive than when students ask questions about patients they are not following or suggest a possible diagnosis. Obviously, this will not be possible for every patient, but a few questions here and there show you are engaged and interested. Make it a goal to ask 1 to 2 questions about patients that are not yours each day. Teachers love questions, and your questions help

them know what to teach you. Each question shows how you are applying your knowledge to clinical care, and this is an objective of every clerkship.

4. STATE YOUR ASSESSMENT AND PLAN

For every patient presentation you give, you must have an assessment and plan. And do not worry if it is right or wrong. This is not what your team is looking for. They just want you to try, and it shows how much you are applying your knowledge to clinical care (see SOAP Notes and Presentations later). It is also important to always prioritize your differential diagnoses and to have a reason why you think that is or is not the diagnosis. The same thing goes for your plan – have a reason or logic behind why you are suggesting that plan.

5. GOALS, EXPECTATIONS, AND FEEDBACK

As a student on clerkships, you will be evaluated by your interns, residents, and attendings. And as much as medical schools try to standardize their faculty and house staff expectations, each individual person and team may have very different expectations. So the only way to know is to ask.

Before you ask, *it is important to think about what your goals are for the rotation.* Do you want to work on your patient presentations, physical exam, assessment and plan, procedures, etc.? "Everything" is too broad of an answer, as we are all trying to improve, but pinpoint a specific area that you want to improve.

On day 1 or 2, you *must* sit down with your intern and resident and attending and get their expectations. And don't be satisfied with just "work hard and take good care of patients." Ask them specifically about the following:

1. Presentations: How should patients be presented in the morning? Do they want a classic subjective, objective, and assessment plan (SOAP) format or just pertinent events overnight? Do they want you to state your assessment and plan by problem?
2. Write-ups: What are the expectations on writing your own history and physical and daily progress notes in the chart? What format is preferred: problem list or by organ system?
3. Presenting topic presentations: What format is preferred? How long should they be?
4. Feedback: Let them know that you would like feedback at the midpoint of your rotation, as well as at the end.
5. Communication: Ask your residents and interns how they like to communicate: text message, paging, phone, etc.

Lastly, enjoy your time on the IM clerkship – it is a transformative year that you will look back on fondly for the rest of your career.

WHAT TO DO EACH DAY

Here is a blueprint of what you will be doing each day.

PRE-ROUNDS

Table 1-1 provides a to do list for you when you pre-round. When you first start, pre-rounds may take you more time than you think so leave plenty of time. When you start out I would give yourself at least 30 minutes per patient.

TABLE 1-1. Pre-Rounds		
		Tips and Tricks
1	Get signout	The intern covering your patients will meet with the day intern every morning. Make sure you are there to also hear what happened to your patient overnight. (This is called signout.)
2	Read all notes for the last 24 hours	A multitude of people will be seeing your patients (physical therapist, social worker, case manager, nurses). Read their notes. Look out for any event notes, which are notes from the covering intern describing significant events that happened overnight such as hypotension or chest pain.
3	Vital signs 1. Temperature 2. Blood pressure (BP) 3. Pulse (P) 4. Respiratory rate (RR) 5. O_2 sat 6. Pain score 7. Input and output 8. Weight	• **Write a range of vital signs** that your patient had, including the lowest and highest and most recent vitals. For example, BP: 111–150/55–85 (122/75). • Look for **overnight fevers**. • Don't forget to look at oxygen saturation (O_2), pain score, weight, and input (IV fluids, oral intake) and output (urine output, stool, drains, etc.).
4	Medications	• **As-needed medications:** Did the patient take any pain medications or antinausea medications, for example? These are also known as PRN (*pro re nata*, Latin for "as needed"). • How many days has a patient been on an antibiotic (e.g., ceftriaxone day 5)?
5	Labs	Don't forget to look at: • **culture results** (blood, urine, drains) • **pending lab tests** Know how labs have changed, especially white count, hemoglobin, platelets, and creatinine.
6	Radiology	Remember to look at all actual images even if you don't know what you are looking at. It is good practice.
7	See and examine patient	
8	Discuss with intern or resident assessment and plan	Set this up with your intern the day before.

*** Leave time to practice your presentation before rounds.***

ROUNDS

TABLE 1-2. Rounds		
1	**Present**	This is your show. Take it and own it. Bring in what you've read or literature that supports your ideas.
2	**Stay involved**	Ask questions about other people's patients. Not on all of them, but a few questions that come up.
3	**Take notes on all patients**	You will likely get asked to do something for other patients, and it helps if you know something about them.
4	**Write questions**	Write down questions you have to look up later or ask later.

AFTER ROUNDS

1. Accomplish your **"to do list"** from rounds. (see Table 1-2)
2. **Communicate** constantly your progress on the "to do list" with your residents.
3. **See your patients** several times a day to update them.
4. **Help:** After you are done with your tasks, ask the interns and resident if there is anything else you can do to help. If they say no, there is no need to continue to ask them. Remember to be proactive. If you know there is a task to do, tell them that you will take care of it. Interns will often default to just taking care of it themselves.
5. **Read:** As with many rotations, there is definitely downtime; make sure you have reading material or questions you can study.
6. **When should I go home?** Try to stay until the team does, but if they insist on you leaving that is OK.

ADMISSIONS

A couple of tips on admissions include the following:

1. **Try to see patients on your own**: This is the best way to learn and start to build independent history taking, as well as assessment and plan creation. However, due to time constraints you will often see patients with your resident and/or intern. As you become more comfortable with your teams, ask if you can lead the interview.
2. **Time:** Remember to give yourself time after interviewing the patient to read and think about the assessment and plan. Your team may ask you questions right after interviewing the patient or tell you what the plan is. Ask them if you could have 30 minutes or an hour to collect your thoughts and notes and then discuss the plan with them. This time for solo thinking is invaluable in your progress toward independently creating assessments and plans.
3. **Return visit:** It's OK to come back and speak to your patient to get more information. Residents and attending physicians do this all the time.

DISCHARGES

Approximately 1 in 5 patients is readmitted to the hospital within 30 days after discharge. Your role in their discharge can help prevent this.

1. **Teach:** The discharge process is a complex and challenging time for your patients. The time you spend with your patients communicating to them the plan and explaining medications can make all the difference.
2. **Coordinate discharge:** Make sure patients have follow-up appointments with their primary care provider within 2 weeks of discharge, and make sure they have all their other follow-ups with surgeons or other medicine specialties prior to discharge.
3. **Follow up**: Give your patients a call after discharge to see how they are doing. Your team will love hearing any updates on patients they have sent home.

WHAT TO DO AT NIGHT

Many times you will come back after a day on the wards feeling physically exhausted and emotionally spent. As one of the most important clerkships, the IM clerkship is one where you must use your time efficiently and wisely. One of the challenges as a medical student on clerkships is finding a way to motivate yourself to continue to study when you get home while maintaining your well-being. First, find something to do that you like or that helps you clear your head, even if it's for only 10 or 20 minutes. You need to give yourself time to unwind. Second, set realistic goals that you can accomplish each night.

We've all been there where you are excited to read an entire chapter at night and because it's unrealistic to read 20 pages in 1 hour, you just end up watching videos and streaming your favorite show. Instead, set up realistic and attainable goals, like doing 10 practice questions and looking up one literature review or one clinical trial about the patient you are taking care of. If you do this every day, in the course of a 2- or 3-month clerkship, you will have done 600 to 1000 questions and read on 60 or 80 different topics. Question banks prepare you for the medicine shelf exam, and reading on topics helps you build habits to continue to learn and improve throughout your career. As far as which question banks to use, ask higher-level classmates what they used – they are the best resource.

SOAP NOTES AND PRESENTATIONS

From the beginning of medical school, you have practiced writing and presenting a full history and physical. One of the new skills on the clerkship is presenting and writing follow-up notes on patients for each day they are in the hospital. These are called SOAP notes, and following is an explanation of how you should write one. Presentations are a simplified and more succinct version of your SOAP note. For example, in your SOAP note you will write a full physical, but during your presentation you would only include the pertinent negative and positive findings.

S – SUBJECTIVE

This is any history you get from the patient that day. When you present this information, you want it to be pertinent to the patient's main diagnosis. If they are here for asthma, then do not go into a long discussion about their issue with the breakfast they were served.

O – OBJECTIVE

This is for data. And during your presentation, *do not interpret* that information. This is for irrefutable facts. The data you need to include in this order is:

1. Vital Signs – Temperature (and mention any fevers), pulse, blood pressure, respiratory rate, oxygen saturation
2. Input and Output
3. Physical Exam – When you present, only include pertinent negative and positive physical exam findings (e.g., if the patient is here for asthma, the normal abdominal exam is not pertinent)
4. Labs and Radiology
   - If a lab is abnormal, it is always good to mention what it was the day before and/or what their baseline lab value is (e.g., creatinine is 2 , but yesterday it was 2.6 and their baseline is 1.5)
5. Current Medications (if this is what your team wants – some teams do not want the list of medications, as it is on their patient lists)

A/P – ASSESSMENT AND PLAN

The beginning of this section should always have a **summary statement**. A summary statement, or "one-liner," is a succinct sentence that summarizes the patient's past medical history and the reason for their admission. Each word in this statement must be pertinent to their diagnoses. Example: 55-year-old male with a history of diabetes mellitus, hypertension, former smoker who presented with chest pain and now found to a have non-ST-elevation MI.

Then list their problems by acuity, meaning list the main reason they are still in the hospital or their chief complaint first and then each subsequent problem in order of importance. For each problem, there should be an **assessment and plan**. Following is a formula for discussing assessments and plans:

Known Diagnosis

Assessment: Status with supporting evidence (e.g., for a patient with pneumonia – Assessment: Overall improving. Cough improved and white count down)

Plan: Discuss the plan and *why* you are deciding on that plan (e.g., change to oral antibiotics, as now tolerating PO and anticipate discharge in 1 day)

Unknown Diagnosis

Assessment: List your differential diagnosis from what you think is most likely to least likely. Explain why you think this is the diagnosis or why it isn't the diagnosis. A simple format to provide supporting evidence is anything in the history, physical, labs, or radiology that supports or disproves that diagnosis.

Plan: Discuss the plan and why you decided on it.

CONQUER THE WARDS!

The most likely diagnosis is often the most common diagnosis. However, it is OK to include zebras in your differential, just not as the most likely. If you don't go looking for zebras, then you will never find one.

CONCLUSION

We hope this will help jump-start your experience and maximize your learning on the IM clerkship. We leave you with one last thought:

"Observe, record, tabulate, communicate. Use your five senses. Learn to see, learn to hear, learn to feel, learn to smell, and know that by practice alone you can become [an] expert." – William Osler

CHAPTER 2 PHYSICAL EXAM PEARLS

OVERVIEW OF HIGH-YIELD TOPICS IN PHYSICAL EXAMINATION PEARLS

LUNG EXAM

BREATH SOUNDS

There are 2 main types of breath sounds that you should know: vesicular and bronchial breath sounds.

- **Vesicular breath sounds:** These are the soft breath sounds that are best heard at the periphery in normal, healthy lungs, most prominently during inspiration. This is what you hear when you describe the lungs as "clear to auscultation."
- **Bronchial breath sounds:** Also known as **tubular** breath sounds or **tracheal** breath sounds, these are more coarse-sounding breath sounds. These can normally be appreciated by auscultating with the stethoscope placed directly over the trachea; however, they are abnormal when heard over other parts of the lung. Bronchial breath sounds are heard when a consolidation or collapsed lung tissue transmits sound from the trachea or central airway to the periphery (thus "tracheal" breath sounds). They are 96% specific for pneumonia but only 14% sensitive.

Adventitious sounds: The main three extra, or "adventitious," sounds are crackles, wheezing, and rhonchi.

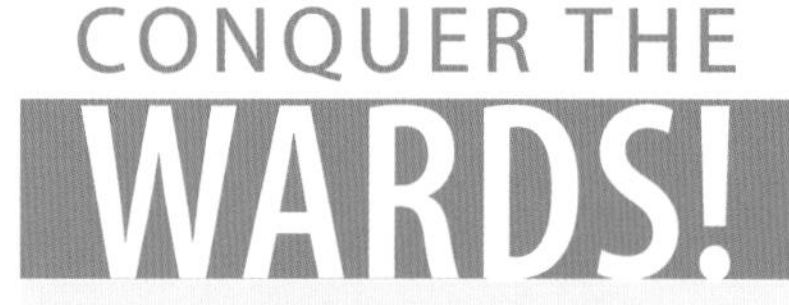

It is often said that "all that wheezes is not asthma." Also consider CHF.

- **Crackles:** Also known as "rales," these discontinuous sounds represent alveoli snapping open and therefore are predominantly inspiratory. Crackles can be further subdivided into course and fine crackles.
  - Coarse crackles: These sound coarser because of a lower frequency (i.e., fewer crackles per second). Most commonly caused by pulmonary edema, pneumonia, or atelectasis.
  - Fine crackles: Often heard in interstitial lung disease. "Velcro" rales are characteristic of interstitial pulmonary fibrosis.
- **Wheezing:** High pitched and continuous, can be only expiratory or both inspiratory and expiratory. Wheezing represents airway obstruction – the sound is made by the vibrations of the walls of the narrowed airway. Classic for asthma and chronic obstructive pulmonary disease (COPD), it can also be heard in other diseases such as congestive heart failure (CHF), sometimes referred to as "cardiac asthma."
- **Rhonchi:** Low pitched and continuous. The pathophysiology is thought to be similar to wheezing; however, secretions may also play a role. Often heard in COPD, can also be present in asthma.

Stridor: One other extra sound to know is stridor, which is caused by upper airway obstruction. This sound is similar to wheezing in that it is high pitched and continuous. However, stridor is inspiratory, whereas wheezing is either expiratory or both inspiratory and expiratory, and stridor is louder over the neck than over the lungs.

PHYSICAL FINDINGS OF COMMON PULMONARY DIAGNOSES

- **Pneumonia:** The physical exam for pneumonia should include evaluation for egophony, pectoriloquy, and tactile fremitus. Also, asymmetric chest expansion, while insensitive, has a positive likelihood ratio (LR) of 44 for pneumonia when present.

- **Egophony:** The "E to A change" was first described as resembling the sound of a goat ("ego" comes from a Greek root meaning "goat"). The easiest way to do it is ask the patient to say "ee" while you are auscultating the usual lung fields. If egophony is present, you will hear "ay" overlying the area of consolidation. The pathophysiology is that low-frequency sounds are normally transmitted by the lung, but a consolidation can also transmit high-frequency sounds to the periphery, which changes the timbre of E to the characteristic A sound heard when pneumonia is present. This test is 96% to 99% specific but has very low sensitivity.
- **Pectoriloquy:** When the patient speaks or whispers (for example, ask them to say "1, 2, 3"), the words can be heard clearly while auscultating the lung. Although pectoriloquy can be spoken or whispered, whispered pectoriloquy is used most in practice. The consolidated lung transmits the words, allowing them to be heard through the stethoscope.
- **Tactile fremitus:** To elicit this, use the ulnar aspects of your hands to feel the vibrations overlying the patient's lung fields while they repeat a phrase such as "99" or "toy boat." Increased vibration can be felt over an area of consolidation; however, the finding is only considered abnormal if asymmetric. Consolidation will increase fremitus, while air (e.g., pneumothorax), fluid (e.g., effusion), or tumor will decrease it.

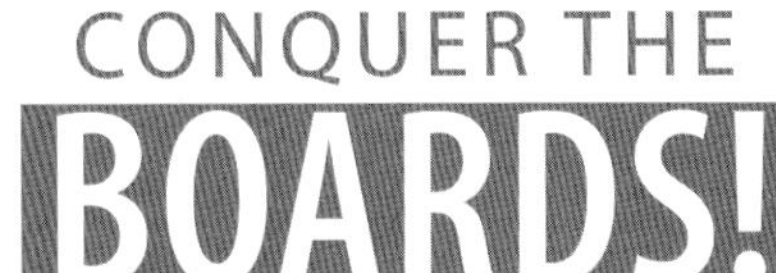

Legionella typically happens in summer, when water towers are active.

- **COPD:** In addition to the characteristic lung findings, decreased breath sounds, wheezing, and rhonchi, a number of findings of COPD can be appreciated by inspection alone.
  - Patients often appear barrel chested and have an increased anteroposterior (AP) diameter due to lung hyperinflation.
  - They often have hypertrophied sternocleidomastoid muscles but generalized muscle wasting from using their energy to breathe.
  - They often sit in a tripod position with their elbows on their thighs and can develop a dermatitis known as Dahl sign or Thinker's sign (see Figure 2-1).
  - Harrison groove or sulcus is a groove between the lower ribs caused by the pull of the flattened diaphragm.

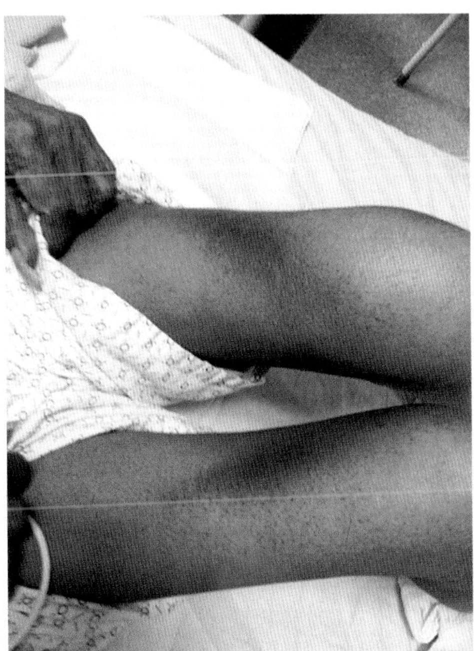

FIGURE 2-1. Dahl sign or Thinker's sign.

CONQUER THE WARDS!

Clubbing is usually absent in COPD, even if hypoxia is present, and should make you consider an alternative explanation (e.g., idiopathic pulmonary fibrosis [IPF] lung cancer).

- The flattened diaphragm can also cause paradoxical inward movement of the rib cage during inspiration, known as Hoover sign.
- **Pleural effusions:** Effusions can be detected by decreased breath sounds (+LR 5.2, –LR 0.1), decreased tactile fremitus (+LR 5.7, –LR 0.2), and dullness to percussion, although consolidations can also cause dullness to percussion. You can occasionally hear a pleural friction rub, a loud rubbing sound associated with pleural disease.

CARDIAC EXAM

STETHOSCOPE BASICS

Most stethoscopes have a diaphragm (larger diameter) and a bell (smaller diameter). The diaphragm is best for hearing higher-frequency sounds, while the bell is best for lower-frequency sounds. Many newer stethoscopes (e.g., Littman stethoscopes) have a combined bell/diaphragm that is sensitive to the amount of pressure applied. When firm pressure is applied, they function as a diaphragm, whereas when light pressure is applied, they function as a bell (think "hard high, light low"). The most important cardiac sounds are high frequency and best heard with the diaphragm or with firm pressure on the combined bell/diaphragm models. Some exceptions that are lower frequency and better heard with the bell (or light pressure) include S3 and S4 gallops and the low diastolic rumble of mitral stenosis.

HEART SOUNDS

S1 is caused by the closing of the mitral and tricuspid valves, with the mitral valve contributing more due to higher pressures on the left side. It is loudest at the apex.

Abnormalities of S1 tend to relate to its **intensity**. Two factors determine its intensity: the position of the mitral valve at the beginning of systole (if the valve is more open, it will slam shut more forcefully and S1 will be louder) and the strength of ventricular contractions (which also cause the mitral valve to close more forcefully).

a. Loud S1
    i. Due to vigorous ventricular contractions (e.g., sepsis, albuterol, hyperthyroidism)
    ii. Due to an open mitral valve at the beginning of systole (e.g., mitral stenosis or a short PR interval, which decreases the time between atrial and ventricular contractions)
b. Soft S1
    i. Due to weak ventricular contractions (e.g., myocardial infarction)
    ii. Due to partially closed mitral valve at beginning of systole (e.g., long PR interval)

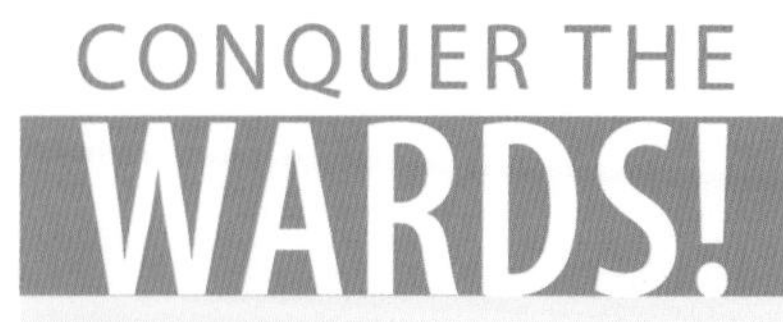

S2 splitting during expiration is always abnormal.

S2 is caused by the closing of the pulmonic and aortic valves and is often auscultated in the pulmonic area, second intercostal space, and left sternal border.

Abnormalities of S2 are generally related to its **splitting** (see Figure 2-2):

- Physiologic splitting: A normal finding. When breathing in, decreasing intrathoracic pressure causes a pressure gradient that leads to increased

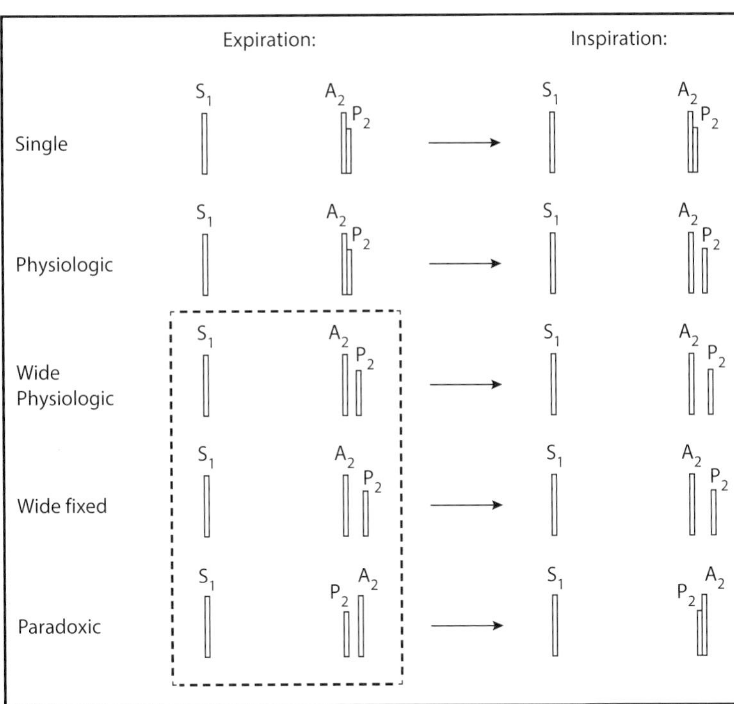

FIGURE 2-2. S2 splitting. Note that splitting during expiration is always abnormal.

venous return to the heart. The increased blood flow to the right heart causes the pulmonic valve to close a bit after the aortic valve, resulting in physiologic splitting.

- Wide physiologic splitting: If something causes the pulmonic valve to close later than normal or the aortic valve to close earlier, the split can be appreciated during both inspiration and expiration. Then, during inspiration, the increased venous return described earlier widens the split even more.
  - Late pulmonic valve closure (e.g., pulmonic stenosis or right bundle branch block [RBBB])
  - Early aortic valve closure (e.g., mitral regurgitation causing shortening of LV systole)
- Wide fixed: This occurs when there is an equal amount of splitting during both expiration and inspiration. For example, in RV dysfunction of any cause, the splitting does not get wider with the increased venous return during inspiration because right ventricular congestion is already present. In other words, more venous return when breathing in doesn't further delay pulmonic valve closure, since there is already an excess of blood in the ventricle to begin with. Another cause of wide fixed splitting is atrial septal defect with a left-to-right shunt.
- Paradoxical: In paradoxical splitting, the aortic valve closes *after* the pulmonic valve. However, with the increased venous return during inspiration, the pulmonic valve becomes late enough to catch up with the aortic valve and causes a single S2. Therefore, splitting is heard during expiration but not during inspiration. Causes of delayed aortic valve closure include conditions that delay LV contraction (e.g., left bundle branch block [LBBB], myocardial dysfunction, or aortic stenosis), as well as conditions that cause early RV contraction (e.g., ectopic beats originating in the RV or RV pacing).

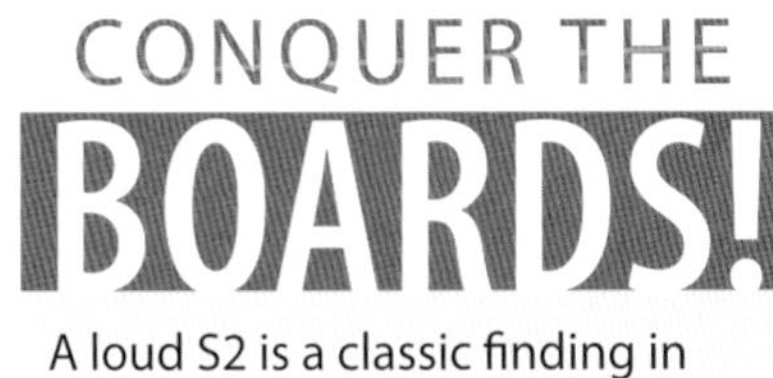

A loud S2 is a classic finding in pulmonary hypertension.

CONQUER THE WARDS!

On their own, crackles or edema are not statistically significantly associated with CHF, so always check for an S3 gallop and elevated neck veins.

Both S3 and S4 have similar pathophysiology; they are caused by rapid deceleration of blood going from the left atrium to the left ventricle.

In the case of S3, the blood decelerates due to a congested LV from CHF, whereas in S4 it decelerates due to a hypertrophied LV. They are both **low-pitched** sounds that are therefore best heard with the bell while listening at the apex. S3 is heard immediately after S2, whereas S4 is heard immediately prior to S1. S3 comes and goes with changes in volume status and is therefore an important tool for evaluating volume overload (positive LR 3.9 for elevated left heart pressures), whereas S4 generally does not come and go.

SYSTOLIC MURMURS

a. When reporting murmurs, try your best to include the following; it will be challenging at first:
   i. Intensity (see later)
   ii. Location – aortic area, pulmonic area, tricuspid or mitral area
   iii. Radiation – aortic stenosis murmur radiates to carotids
   iv. Pitch – high or low pitch
   v. Quality – harsh, blowing, rumbling
   vi. Shape – crescendo-decrescendo, holosystolic
   vii. Timing – early, mid, or late systole
b. Intensity is rated 1/6 to 6/6
   i. 1/6 very faint, quieter than S1/S2
   ii. 2/6 faint, same as S1/S2
   iii. 3/6 louder than S1/S2, no palpable thrill
   iv. 4/6 loud and with palpable thrill
   v. 5/6 palpable thrill and can hear with stethoscope partially off the chest
   vi. 6/6 palpable thrill and can hear with stethoscope completely off the chest
c. There are many systolic murmurs, but the following are the most common and most important to know for your wards and boards:
   i. **Aortic stenosis (AS)**
      - Best heard at the aortic area (second intercostal space at the right sternal border)
      - Radiates to carotids (can hear while auscultating over carotids)
      - Crescendo-decrescendo murmur
      - **Special exam finding:**
        - "Parvus et tardus" – A slow and late pulse compared to the point of maximal impulse (PMI) of the heart. Can appreciate by feeling the carotid pulse and comparing with the PMI.
        - Single S2 or paradoxical splitting – Due to delayed closure of the aortic valve (see S2 splitting, earlier).
   ii. **Mitral regurgitation** (MR)
      - Best heard at the apex (fifth intercostal space, midclavicular line)
      - Radiates to axilla or inferior left scapula
      - Holosystolic
   iii. **Tricuspid regurgitation** (TR)
      - Best heard in the tricuspid area (fifth intercostal space [ICS], left sternal border)
      - Usually does not radiate
      - Holosystolic
      - **Special exam findings**: Becomes louder with inspiration (see later), known as Caravallo sign

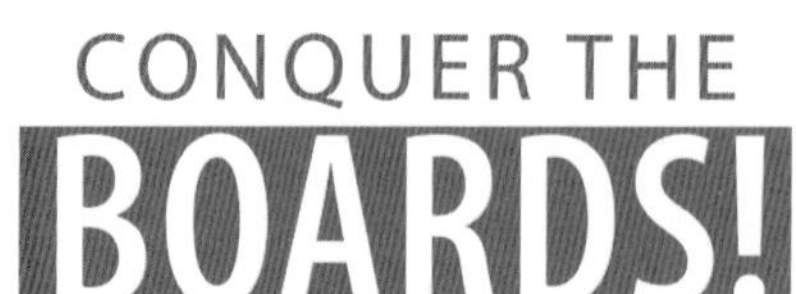

AS = crescendo-decrescendo,
TR/MR = holosystolic

iv. One other murmur that deserves mention is the "flow" murmur resulting from increased blood flow through a normal valve, as can be heard in anemia, thyrotoxicosis, or sepsis. This is usually a crescendo-decrescendo murmur that can be heard well over the pulmonic area.
v. Other systolic murmurs that are less commonly encountered include pulmonic stenosis and ventricular septal defect.

d. Several maneuvers can be useful for isolating systolic murmurs:
   i. **Inspiration:** Distinguishes left-sided vs. right-sided murmurs. As discussed earlier, when breathing in, decreased intrathoracic pressure leads to increased venous return, thereby making right-sided murmurs louder by increasing flow through the valves (+LR 7.8). However, increased capacitance of the pulmonary veins during inspiration causes blood to pool in the pulmonary veins and therefore *decreased* blood to the left heart, so left-sided murmurs generally become softer.
   ii. **Valsalva:** For distinguishing AS vs. hypertrophic cardiomyopathy (HCM). The Valsalva maneuver causes increased intrathoracic pressure, which **decreases** venous return to **both** right and left sides, thereby decreasing most murmurs. HCM is an exception; blood flow props open the dynamic obstruction of HCM and decrease the murmur. Therefore, decreasing blood flow with the Valsalva maneuver will increase HCM murmur intensity (+LR 14.0). AS murmurs will be decreased by the Valsalva maneuver.
   iii. **Hand grip:** To distinguish between AS and MR, ask the patient to maintain their grip for 20 to 30 seconds. If blood is in the LV, it can either travel through to the aorta or regurgitate back to the left atrium. Hand grip increases afterload and increases pressure in the aorta. More blood will therefore go down the path of least resistance and increase flow over a regurgitant mitral valve, therefore making MR louder, and will decrease flow through a stenosed aortic valve, making AS quieter.

CONQUER THE **BOARDS!**

Murmurs that get louder with inspiration are likely to be right sided.

CONQUER THE **WARDS!**

A good way to do the Valsalva maneuver is ask your patient to put their thumb in their mouth and blow.

DIASTOLIC MURMURS

The 2 diastolic murmurs we encounter most frequently are mitral stenosis (MS) and aortic insufficiency (AI).

- **Mitral stenosis**
  - Best heard at the mitral area (fifth intercostal space, left sternal border)
  - Low-pitched rumble
  - **Special exam findings:**
    - Left lateral decubitus position can help with hearing MS murmur
    - Associated with a loud S1
    - Often has a "presystolic accentuation" (louder at the end of diastole)
- **Aortic insufficiency**
  - Best heard at the aortic area
  - Decrescendo murmur
  - **Special exam findings:**
    AI results in a wide pulse pressure that causes a number of interesting physical exam findings:
    - Water-hammer pulse (Corrigan pulse) – Rapidly rising and falling pulse.
    - Quincke pulse – Pulsation of the nailbed of the fingers.
    - Müller sign – Pulsation of the uvula.
    - Pistol shot pulse – Audible pulse over the femoral, brachial, or radial arteries with auscultation. Resembles the thumping sounds (Korotkoff sounds) heard when taking blood pressure with a manual cuff.

- **Pericardial friction rub:** Rubbing or scratching murmur; classically has 3 components, 2 systolic and 1 during early diastole, though they can have only 1 or 2 components. Thought to correspond to the rubbing of the inflamed layers of the pericardium. Can increase intensity when patient leans forward. Can come and go over hours, though when present has high specificity for acute pericarditis. Can have patient hold their breath, and if rub continues this will help distinguish pericardial from pleural rubs.

NECK VEINS

a. Technique
   i. Preferred to assess veins on the right side as the right internal jugular (IJ) is in a more direct line to the right heart; however, the left side can be used as well if needed.
   ii. IJ is preferred but external jugular (EJ) is also acceptable.
   iii. There is no "correct" angle for viewing neck veins; the correct angle is the angle where you can see the top of the column of fluid.
   iv. It can often be helpful to use tangential light (e.g., a pen light).
   v. Distinguishing vein from artery:
      - Try to observe the **dual pulsations** representing A and V waves of the vein, whereas the artery will have only a single pulsation.
      - Can look for respiratory variation that will be present in the venous pulsation but not arterial.
      - An increase in venous distention occurs with abdominal pressure, known as the **abdominojugular test**.
      - The artery will have a palpable pulse, whereas the vein generally does not.

> CONQUER THE WARDS!
> Identify the dual pulsations of the venous waveform to distinguish the vein from the artery.

b. Interpretation
   i. Determine the height of venous distention – you should report jugular venous distention (JVD) in centimeters rather than anatomically (e.g., "up to the mandible"). To quantify, measure vertically from the sternal angle of Louis (the notch where the manubrium and the sternum meet) to the highest point of visualized pulsation (see Figure 2-3). Add 5 cm to approximate the distance from the sternal angle to the right heart. If the total is >8 cm, this is elevated and has positive LR 3.9 for increased left-heart filling pressure (i.e., volume overload).

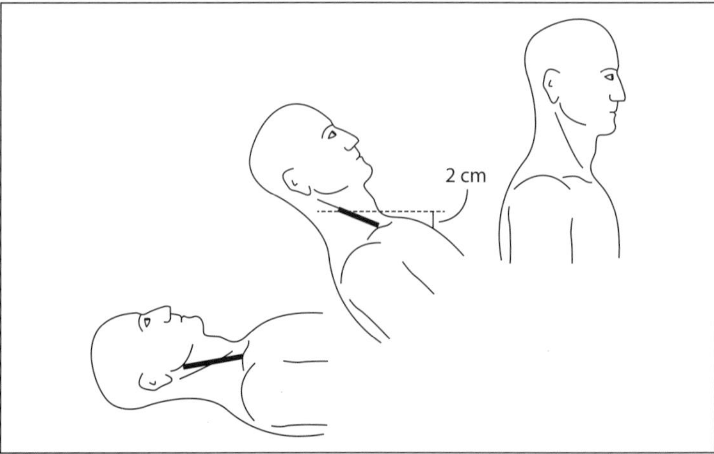

FIGURE 2-3. Measuring jugular venous distention. The height should be measured vertically from the sternal angle. Five centimeters are then added to this to approximate the distance to the right heart.

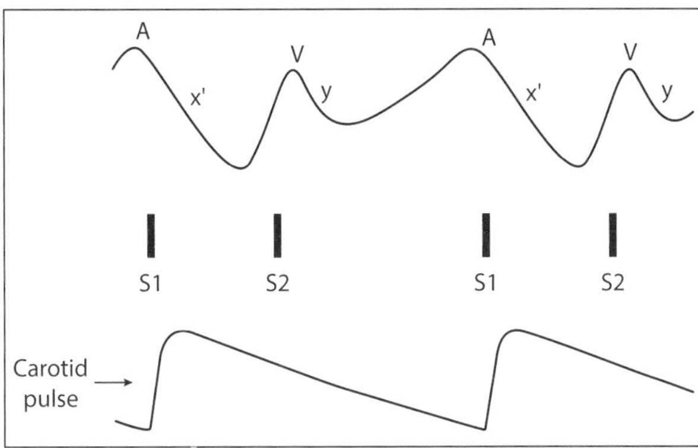

FIGURE 2-4. Jugular venous pulsations.

ii. Understanding the venous waveforms – The **right heart tracing represents pressures in the right atrium** that are conducted to the neck veins (Figure 2-4). The "c" wave (corresponding to tricuspid bulging into the right atrium during ventricular systole) is visible during a right-heart catheterization but not on simple inspection of the neck; therefore, only 2 positive waves are seen on physical exam, the A and V waves.
   - A wave corresponds to **A**trial contraction.
   - V wave corresponds to **V**enous filling (of the right atrium).
   - After atrial contraction comes atrial rela**X**ation.
   - After venous filling comes venous empt**Y**ing (from the right atrium to the right ventricle).
   - The A wave occurs mostly during diastole (the tricuspid valve needs to be open during atrial contraction).
   - The V wave occurs mostly during systole (venous filling of the right atrium with closed tricuspid valve).

iii. Now that you understand what causes the different waveforms, you can understand what will cause abnormalities of the waveforms.
   - **Cause of absent A wave:** Atrial fibrillation (no atrial contraction)
   - **Cause of large A wave:** Tricuspid stenosis (atrium contracts against a stenosed tricuspid valve, thereby increasing right atrial pressure)
   - **"Canon" A wave:** Atrium contracts against a closed tricuspid valve, classically in complete heart block
   - **Cause of large V wave:** Tricuspid regurgitation (Lancisi sign). The V wave occurs mostly during systole; therefore, significant regurgitant flow over the tricuspid valve will increase the V wave.
   - **Kussmaul sign:** Increased JVD with inspiration. Due to severe RV dysfunction (or classically constrictive pericarditis), the RV cannot handle the increased venous return during inspiration and therefore JVD increases.

ABDOMINAL EXAM

1. **Abdominal inspection:** In addition to assessing shape**,** distention, prior surgical scars, striae (e.g., from Cushing disease), caput medusa (from cirrhosis), and hernias, there are several eponymous exam findings that are often mentioned on the wards.
   a. **Grey Turner sign (flank ecchymosis)** in pancreatitis. Reflects retroperitoneal hemorrhage.
   b. **Cullen sign (periumbilical ecchymosis)** also seen in pancreatitis. Seen in <3% of cases of pancreatitis but often asked on the wards. Keep these

straight by remembering that Grey Turner is 2 words and we have 2 flanks, whereas Cullen is 1 word and we have 1 umbilicus.

   c. **Sister Mary Joseph nodule** – Hard umbilical nodule, associated with abdominal malignancy.

2. **Carnett sign:** A test for an abdominal wall cause of abdominal pain. Ask the patient to fold the arms on the chest and lift the head and shoulders as if doing a sit-up, while at the same time palpating the area of tenderness. Increased tenderness is more likely due to abdominal wall pain rather than visceral pain.

CONQUER THE WARDS!

It is not necessarily abnormal to be able to palpate the liver below the costal margin, though in adults it is generally abnormal to have a palpable spleen.

3. **Liver exam:** Consists of 2 parts, palpation to evaluate consistency and shape, and percussion to estimate size.
   a. Palpation – Starting well below the costal margin, ascend 1 to 2 cm at a time, feeling for the liver's descent as the patient breathes in. The goal is to feel for tenderness (e.g., hepatitis or heart failure) or nodularity (e.g., cirrhosis or cancer).
   b. Percussion – Percuss in descending intercostal spaces starting around the third intercostal space in the midclavicular line. Note where the resonance changes to dullness—this is the superior border of the liver. Next percuss ascending from below the umbilicus until the tympani of the abdomen changes to dullness, corresponding to the inferior border. The normal liver span in the midclavicular line is 6 to 12 cm. *Note:* Clinicians generally underestimate the liver span by several centimeters.
4. Ascites – Can be detected either by fluid wave or shifting dullness. Fluid wave is more specific; LR 5.0 for ascites when present.
   a. Fluid wave – Have either patient or assistant put a hand on the abdominal wall to limit the motion of subcutaneous tissue, which can cause a false positive. A tap on one lateral wall of the abdomen is transmitted and can be felt on the other side if ascites is present.
   b. Shifting dullness – The horizontal border where dullness changes to resonance, which represents the interface of dependent ascites with overlying gas-filled bowel, will move as the patient changes position. If the patient is supine, mark the border with your hand and then ask the patient to move on to their side. Then percuss again. The border where dullness changes to resonance should change in ascites.
5. **Spleen exam:** There are a number of techniques for palpating the spleen, and none have been shown to be superior. One technique is described here:
   a. An enlarged spleen can descend inferiorly to the pelvis and can cross the midline to the right lower quadrant (RLQ). Therefore, it is important to start palpating inferiorly and right of the midline to ensure that the spleen border is not missed.
   b. While gently palpating, feel for the spleen with inspiration; it may only be palpable as it descends at end inspiration.
   c. A palpable spleen is generally abnormal in adults (LR 8.5 for splenomegaly).
   d. Some clinicians feel the exam is enhanced when the patient is in the right lateral decubitus position, though this has not been confirmed in trials.
   e. An advanced technique: Splenomegaly can cause dullness to percussion of Traube space – the area overlying the gastric bubble that is normally resonant. This is formed by the triangle above the costal margin, medial to the anterior axillary line and inferior to the cardiac dullness, which connotes the inferior border of the heart.
6. **Gallbladder abnormalities**
   a. Murphy sign – For acute cholecystitis. When the patient inspires, the inflamed gallbladder descends against the examiner's fingers, causing pain and an abrupt cessation of the breath, "as though it had been shut off" per Murphy's original description.

b. Courvoisier sign – A painless, palpable gallbladder, classically described in patients with jaundice and associated with malignancy causing biliary obstruction (e.g., pancreatic cancer). It is now recognized that this can be caused by any extrahepatic biliary obstruction (LR 26 for biliary obstruction when present).

7. **Cirrhosis exam:** Many of the findings of cirrhosis are actually appreciated on inspection:
   a. Jaundice – Subtle jaundice can begin to be seen at bilirubin 2.5 to 3. Often noted in the frenulum of the tongue.
   b. Scleral icterus – A misnomer, the pigment is actually deposited in the conjunctiva.
   c. Spider telangiectasias – Small, blanching, spider shaped, often on the trunk.
   d. Fetor hepaticus – Sulfurous breath.
   e. Caput medusae – See Figure 2-5.
   f. Asterixis – Flapping of hands when arms are outstretched with wrists extended. Related to difficulty in maintaining a fixed posture. It is a form of "negative myoclonus," meaning the muscle relaxes and then there is a compensatory flap.
   g. Palmar erythema – Over the thenar and hypothenar eminences.
   h. Gynecomastia – Due to increased estrogen.
   i. Testicular atrophy.
   j. Terry nails – Cloudy nails with a dark distal band and loss of the lunula (Figure 2-6).

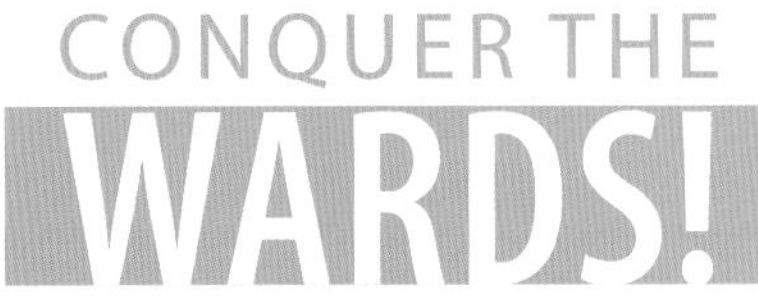

Asterixis is present in other causes of encephalopathy besides hepatic (e.g., uremic or hypercarbic encephalopathy).

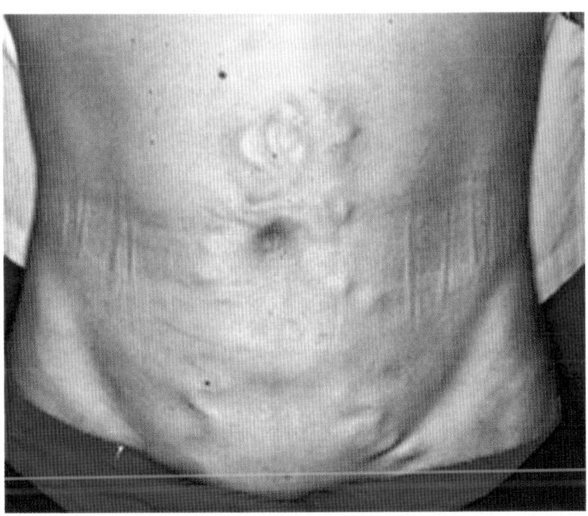

FIGURE 2-5. Caput medusae.

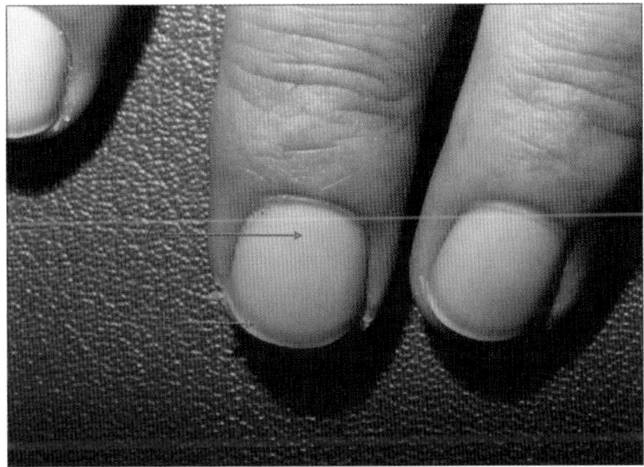

FIGURE 2-6. Terry nails. Loss of lanula (A) and Dark distal band (B).

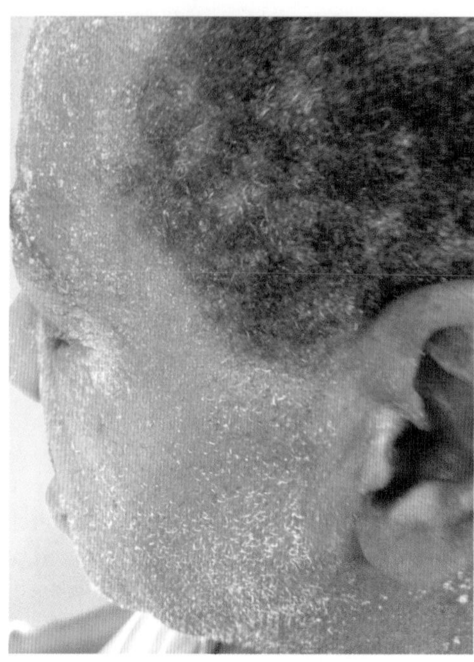

FIGURE 2-7. Uremic frost.

DERMATOLOGIC PHYSICAL EXAM PEARLS

- **ESRD:** There are a number of skin manifestations with end-stage renal disease (ESRD). Nonspecific findings include excoriations from scratching, pallor from anemia, or Lindsay nails ("half and half" nails – distal half is darkened, proximal half is lighter). More specific findings include uremic frost (a white frost on the skin due to precipitation of urea; see Figure 2-7) and calciphylaxis (calcium deposition into blood vessels causing skin changes and necrosis).
- **Cellulitis:** A very common internal medicine diagnosis, characterized by warmth, erythema, and edema.
  - If there is purulence such as drainage or an abscess, then it is most likely caused by *Staphylococcus aureus*, whereas if there is no purulence, the most likely cause is strep, so this is an important distinction to make.
  - Cellulitis is very rarely bilateral, so if you see bilateral redness, consider other diagnoses such as stasis dermatitis. Studies show that we frequently misdiagnose other conditions as cellulitis.
  - Deep vein thrombosis (DVT) should also be in your differential diagnosis for a red, warm leg.
- **Stevens–Johnson syndrome (SJS) and toxic epidermal necrolysis (TEN):** Both are severe skin reactions most often to medications. They cause necrosis and detachment of the epidermis. If <10% of the skin is involved, it is defined as SJS; if >30%, then TEN; if between 10% and 30%, then defined as SJS/TEN overlap.
- **Erythema nodosum:** Erythematous, tender nodules on the shins (Figure 2-8). Biopsy will yield panniculitis. Can have many causes (e.g., sarcoid, irritable bowel syndrome [IBD], drugs, malignancy).

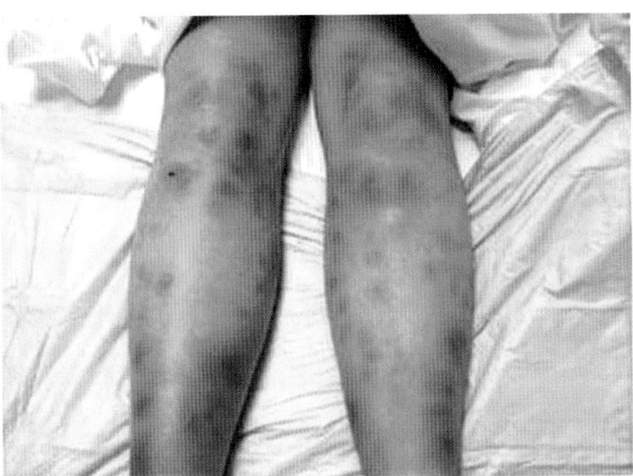

FIGURE 2-8 Erythema nodosum.

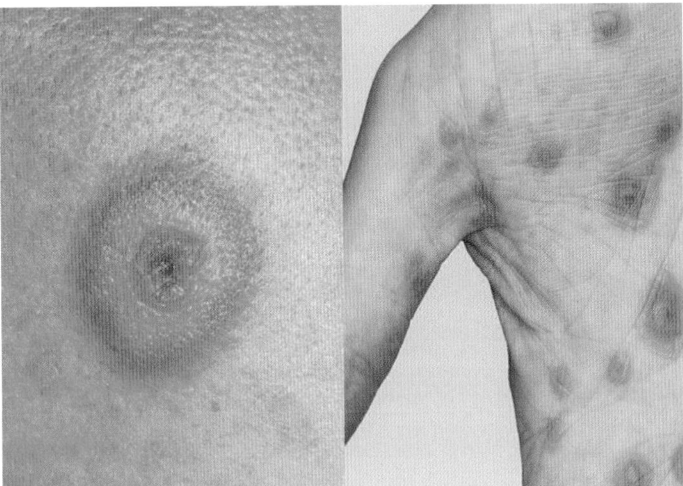

FIGURE 2-9 Erythema multiforme.

- **Erythema multiforme:** Target-shaped lesions, starting on extensor surfaces of extremities (Figure 2-9). Many causes, though infections, especially herpes simplex virus, are the most common cause by far.
- **DRESS syndrome:** Drug reaction with eosinophilia and systemic symptoms. Occurs several weeks after starting the offending medication. Patients have fevers, a "morbilliform" (measles-like) rash that is erythematous and often covers >50% of the body, and can develop organ failure.

CHAPTER 3 CHEST X-RAY

OVERVIEW OF HIGH-YIELD TOPICS IN CHEST X-RAY

BASIC APPROACH TO READING A CHEST X-RAY

There are many approaches to reading a chest x-ray. The "ABCDEF" method described here will take you through a systematic way to read a chest x-ray, accounting for all the different elements. In this method, the lung fields are examined last to ensure that all the elements of the x-ray are accounted for before interpreting the largest field of the chest x-ray.

1. **Type of Chest X-ray:** The first step in interpreting a chest x-ray is to identify what type it is: **posteroanterior (PA)** or **anteroposterior (AP)**. Generally this is printed on the x-ray itself. PA chest x-rays are typically done in radiology with the patient standing and are paired with a lateral x-ray. This is the most accurate and highest-quality film. AP chest x-rays are done as portable x-rays when a patient is unable to stand and go to radiology. It gives generally accurate information, but sizes of structures are difficult to interpret.
2. **Quality:** For accurate interpretation of a chest x-ray, we must consider the technical aspects that can affect image interpretation:
    - **Inspiration:** Seven to nine posterior ribs should be identified on a chest x-ray with adequate inspiratory effort. Poor inspiratory effort can make the image more difficult to interpret, for instance, making the hilar structures appear more prominent. Fewer than 7 ribs visible may also be suggestive of conditions such as restrictive lung disease. More than 9 ribs visible may suggest hyperinflated lungs in conditions including obstructive pulmonary disease.
    - **Rotation:** High-quality chest x-rays are captured when the x-ray beams are perpendicular to the patient. Any deviation from the perpendicular will result in a rotated x-ray and some distortion of the image. In an image that is captured straight, the medial heads of the clavicles should be equidistant from the spinous processes of the upper thorax. Deviation from this pattern indicates that the patient is rotated obliquely relative to the x-ray.
    - **Penetration:** Penetration refers to the exposure of the film to the x-rays. Optimal penetration allows readers to distinguish between adjacent structures of various densities. The intervertebral disk spaces of the thoracic spine (behind the heart) should be barely visible on a film with adequate penetration. With an overpenetrated film, the thoracic spine will look very distinct and the lung markings be darker to the point that they are decreased or absent. In contrast to an underpenetrated film, where the thoracic spine will not be visible at all, there will be an abundance of white in the lung fields.

      If there is a question about the quality of a film, the chest x-ray should be repeated.
3. **ABCDEF**
    - **Airway:** Examine the trachea for size and deviation, tracing inferiorly to the carina. The bifurcation of the right and left main bronchi is usually at an angle of 60 to 100 degrees (an increased angle can indicate left atrial enlargement, lymph node enlargement, or mass). Check the mediastinum for any widening (beyond 8 cm), which can indicate masses or dissection.
    - **Bones:** Check the bones for fractures, dislocations, masses, or lytic lesions. Attention should be given to the clavicles, ribs, spine, and humerus. Look for hardware, including wires, staples, and pins. Note deformities (e.g., curvature of the spine).
    - **Cardiac:** Examine the shape of the heart and the size, which should be half the hemithorax. A larger heart size is suggestive of cardiomegaly.

CONQUER THE WARDS!

Read as many chest x-rays as you can, and use the same systemic approach every time.

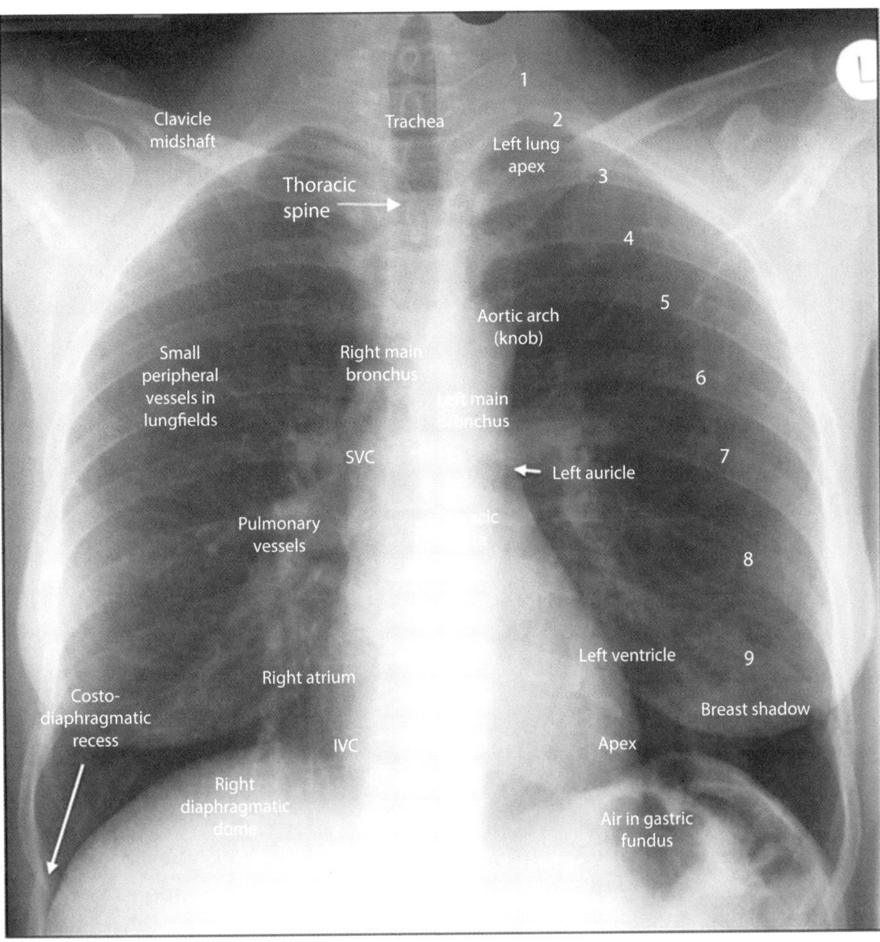

FIGURE 3-1. Anatomy as shown in a chest x-ray

Examine the heart borders to make sure they are sharp and distinct; examine the aorta for widening or tortuosity. Note any devices, including mechanical valves and pacemakers.

- **Diaphragm:** The diaphragm and the costophrenic angles should be sharp. Obscuration of the diaphragmatic line or blunting of the angle can indicate effusion, infiltrates, or masses. Note whether there is flattening or elevation of the diaphragms. Examine the area underneath the diaphragm for free air or bowel abnormalities.
- **Everything else:** Look for hardware including chest tubes, wires, and defibrillators. Confirm the position of devices, including nasogastric tubes (the tip should be below the diaphragm), central lines (the tip should be in the cavoatrial junction), and endotracheal tubes (the tip should be 2 to 4 cm superior to the carina).
- **Lung Fields:** Look for radiolucencies, which indicate air (e.g., emphysema or pneumothorax). Examine shapes of the lung, which can be affected by masses, pneumothorax, effusions, and fibrosis. Look at the lung fields for radiodensities or opacities. Within the clinical context, the shape and pattern of the opacities may suggest the underlying pathology. Opacities can be described by their location, size, shape, and pattern. Table 3-1 lists some descriptive terms you might encounter when describing an opacity.

Next, we will go through some case examples and test your ability to read chest x-rays. One major clinical point here is that chest x-rays are another data point

CONQUER THE WARDS!

Under the left hemidiaphragm, air can be normally seen as a gastric bubble. However, air under the right hemidiaphragm is not normal and should raise suspicion for bowel perforation or obstruction.

Table 3-1. Common Descriptive Terms for Chest X-ray		
Description	**Definition**	**Example Pathology**
Consolidation	Radiodensity within the lung fields that indicates the alveoli are filled with fluid.	Fluid causing consolidation may be blood (alveolar hemorrhage), "water" (transudate), purulence (exudate), cells, or protein (malignancy, chronic inflammation)
Focal, patchy, or diffuse	Refers to location and distribution of a consolidation.	Focal: pneumonia, malignancy, infarct, atelectasis Patchy: hemorrhage, edema, pneumonia Diffuse: edema, vasculitides, interstitial lung disease
Reticular or nodular	Refers to shape and pattern of a consolidation. Both terms indicate involvement of the interstitial tissues. Reticular means lines or lacey patterns. Nodular patterns mean discrete small dots. Pathologic processes involving the interstitium may have both patterns (reticulonodular).	Atypical or viral pneumonia, pulmonary fibrosis, pulmonary edema, Langerhans cell histiocytosis, sarcoidosis

along with laboratories, your history, and physical exam. Your chest x-ray findings must correlate with your other clinical workup. For example, a chest x-ray may reveal a consolidation but the patient has no fever and no respiratory symptoms. This patient does not have pneumonia, and you may consider other diagnoses such as a mass or scarring from previous infection or surgery.

As you work through these cases, first read the clinical story and in your mind think of your top 3 differentials. Then read the chest x-ray and decide on a diagnosis.

CASE EXAMPLES

CASE 1

A 55-year-old man with a past medical history of hypertension and chronic obstructive pulmonary disease (COPD) is admitted with 2 days of shortness of breath and cough. He is found to have a temperature of 38.3°C, blood pressure of 110/75, and heart rate of 121. Oxygen saturation is noted to be 87% on room air. Physical examination is notable for crackles on his right lung base and diffuse wheezing throughout. His bloodwork reveals a white blood cell count of 16,000 cells. Chest x-ray (Figure 3-2) is obtained.

CXR Finding

The main finding of this chest x-ray is a focal consolidation in the right lower lung field. The radiographic differential for a focal consolidation includes pneumonia, infarct, and malignancy.

Sample Reading

If you were asked to read this chest x-ray on rounds, this is a sample of how you would read this using the ABCDEF technique: "The **A**irway is midline, there are no **B**one fractures, **C**ardiomediastinal silhouette is normal, **D**iaphragms

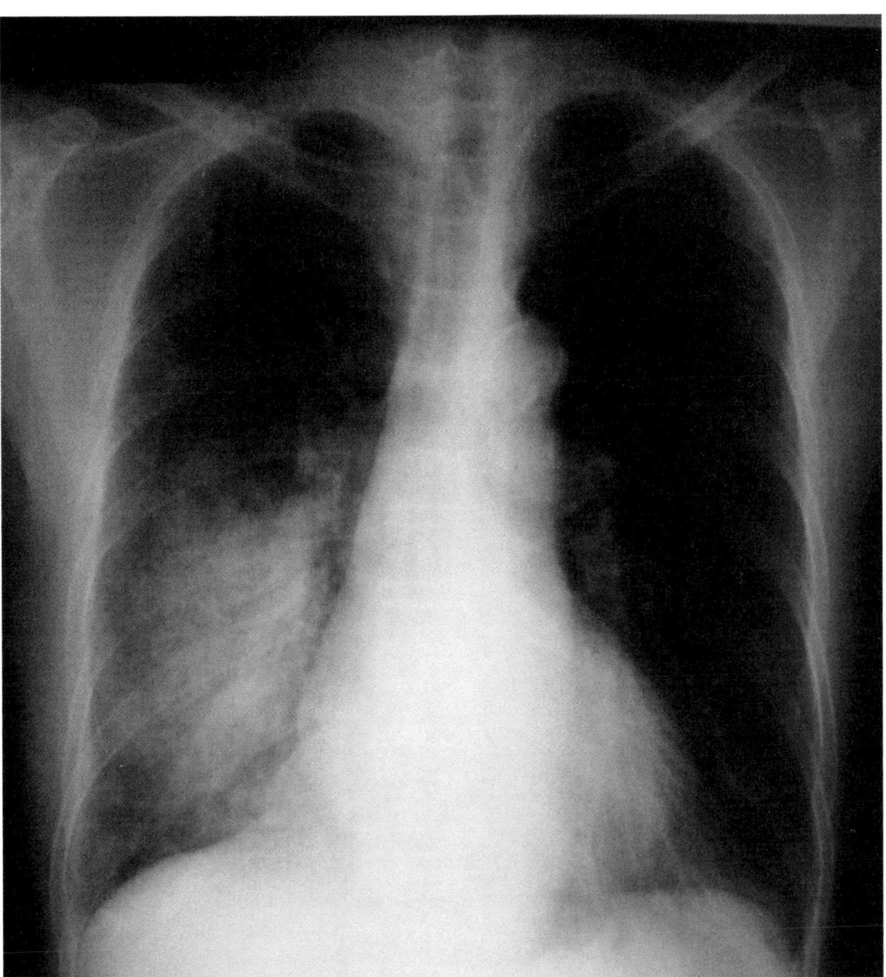

FIGURE 3-2. (Reproduced, with permission, from Jameson JL, Fauci AF, Kasper DL, et al, eds: *Harrison's Principles of Internal Medicine*, 20th ed. www.accessmedicine.com. Copyright © McGraw-Hill Education. All rights reserved.)

appear slightly flattened (consistent with COPD) but costophrenic angles are sharp, lung fields have a focal consolidation in the RLL (right lower lobe)."

Clinical Diagnosis

Given the symptoms of shortness of breath and cough with the systemic inflammatory response syndrome (SIRS), this patient has a RLL pneumonia.

CONQUER THE WARDS!

It is a right lower lobe pneumonia because you can make out the right heart border. If the right heart border is obscured, it is a right middle lobe pneumonia because the right middle lobe and right heart border are anterior.

CASE 2

A 76-year-old woman with a past medical history of hypertension, diabetes mellitus, coronary artery disease, and congestive heart disease is admitted with 2 weeks of shortness of breath and cough. Her vital signs reveal temperature of 37.1°C, blood pressure of 191/98, and heart rate of 84. Her oxygen saturation is 88% on room air. On physical examination, she is noted to have an S4 gallop, crackles diffusely throughout both lung fields, jugular venous distention, and bilateral lower extremity edema. Laboratory work demonstrates normal white blood cell count at 8000. Chest x-ray (Figure 3-3) is obtained.

CXR Finding

This chest x-ray demonstrates diffuse reticular opacities in both lung fields. The arrows point to horizontal, radiodense lines in the periphery of the lung fields,

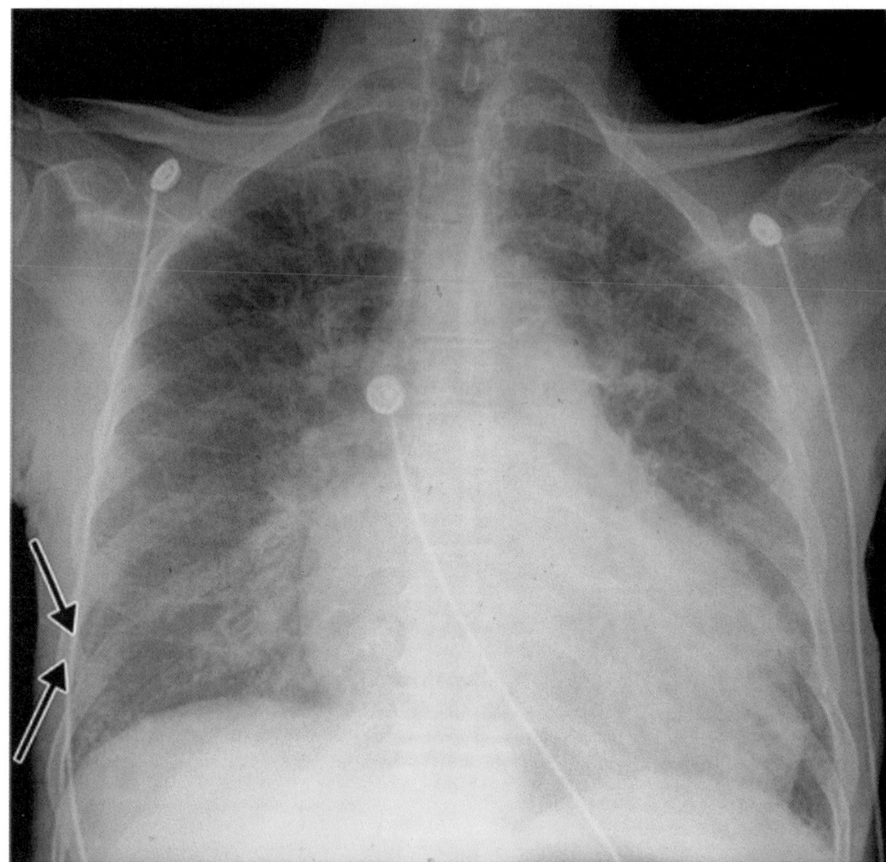

FIGURE 3-3. (Reproduced, with permission, from Elsayes KM, Oldham SAA: *Introduction of Diagnostic Radiology*. www.accessmedicine.com. Copyright © McGraw-Hill Education. All rights reserved.)

called Kerley B lines. Additional findings include an enlarged cardiac silhouette and electrocardiogram (ECG) leads. The radiographic differential includes pulmonary edema, acute lung injury, acute respiratory distress syndrome, interstitial lung disease (ILD), and atypical pneumonia.

CONQUER THE WARDS!

The radiographic findings can represent a number of different disease states. Correlate the chest x-ray findings to the clinical findings to help you get the diagnosis!

Clinical Diagnosis

Given the clinical context of a history of heart failure and volume overload on physical examination, the findings are consistent with pulmonary edema. The Kerley B lines represent distended pulmonary lymphatic channels in the interlobular septae due to pulmonary edema.

CASE 3

A 48-year-old woman with a history of colon cancer currently undergoing chemotherapy with metastases to bone and lungs is admitted for progressive shortness of breath over the last month. Her vital signs reveal a temperature of 36.9°C, blood pressure of 114/73, and heart rate of 75. Oxygen saturation is 88% on room air. Physical examination is notable for temporal wasting and cachexia and decreased breath sounds in the right lung field. Bloodwork reveals a white blood cell count of 24,000. Chest x-ray (Figure 3-4) is obtained.

CXR Finding

The chest x-ray demonstrates a large opacity that fills the right lung field and obliterates the right diaphragmatic line and right heart border (arrows). The radiographic differential includes malignancy, pneumonia, hemorrhage, or

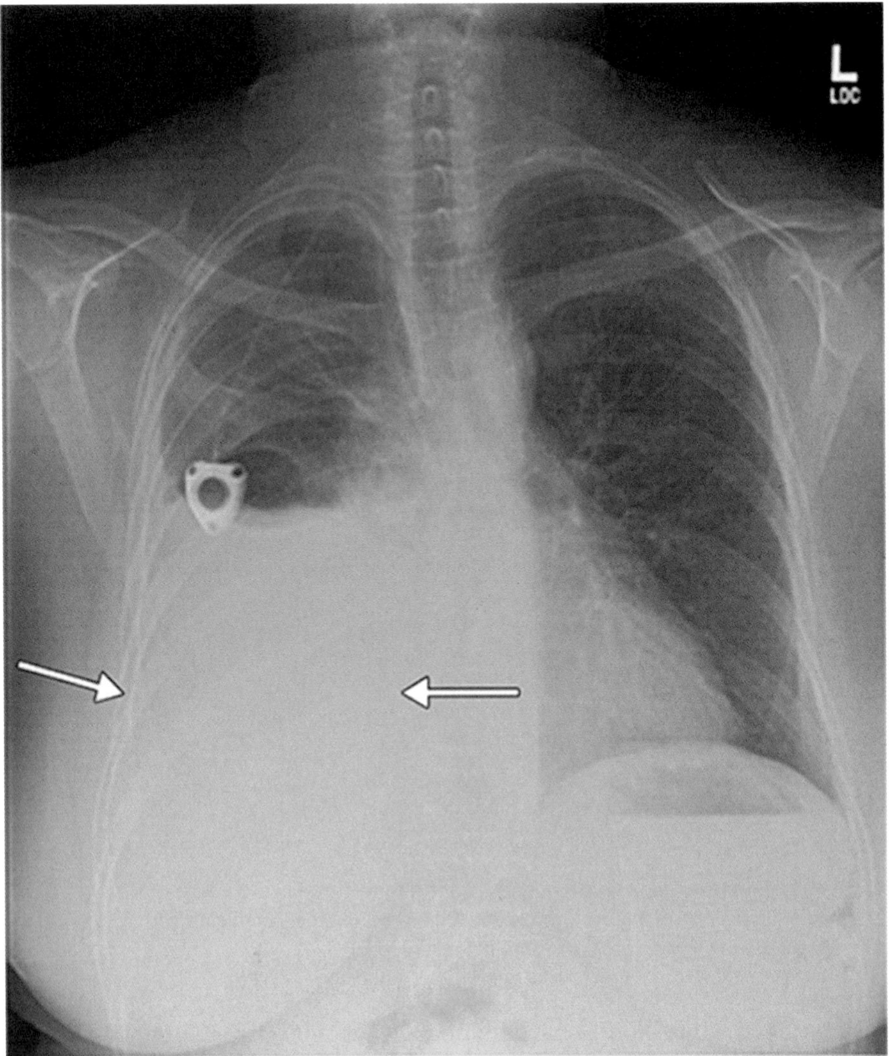

FIGURE 3-4. (Reproduced, with permission, from Elsayes KM, Oldham SAA: *Introduction of Diagnostic Radiology*. www.accessmedicine.com. Copyright © McGraw-Hill Education. All rights reserved.)

effusion. The x-ray is also notable for the presence of a right-sided central venous catheter (chemo port), with the tip terminating in the superior vena cava. The gastric bubble is visible below the left hemidiaphragm.

Clinical Diagnosis

The slowly progressive nature of the patient's symptoms, along with the history of cancer, suggests a malignant pleural effusion. The meniscus in the opacity indicates fluid layering and is more consistent with an effusion rather than a mass.

CASE 4

A 64-year-old man with a history of rheumatoid arthritis and hypertension is admitted for progressive shortness of breath over the last 8 months. His vital signs show a temperature of 37.6°C, blood pressure of 146/72, and heart rate of 81. Oxygen saturation is 87% on room air. Physical examination is notable for normal heart sounds and diffuse fine crackles throughout both lung fields. He has no jugular venous distention and no peripheral edema. Laboratory work

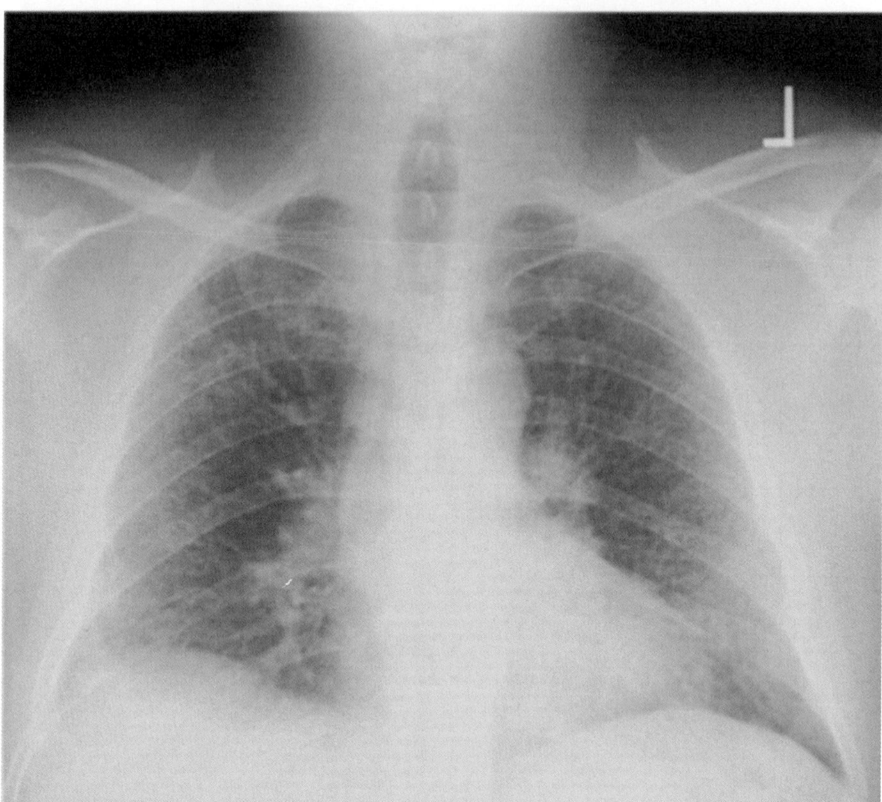

FIGURE 3-5. (Reproduced, with permission, from Jameson JL, Fauci AF, Kasper DL, et al, eds: *Harrison's Principles of Internal Medicine*, 20th ed. www.accessmedicine.com. Copyright © McGraw-Hill Education. All rights reserved.)

demonstrates a white blood cell count of 4000 and a brain natriuretic peptide (BNP) of 88 pg/mL. Chest x-ray (Figure 3-5) is obtained.

CXR Finding

The chest x-ray is notable for opacities with a diffuse reticulonodular pattern (fine lines and small nodules in a lacelike pattern) throughout both lung fields. The hilar structures are prominent in this chest x-ray as well. The radiographic differential includes congestive heart failure, ILD, acute lung injury, atypical pneumonia, and sarcoidosis.

Clinical Diagnosis

This patient's findings are most consistent with ILD, the most common pulmonary manifestation of rheumatoid arthritis. There is no fever, tachycardia, or leukocytosis to suggest pneumonia. The indolent onset of the symptoms also argue against pneumonia. The patient is not volume overloaded and has a normal BNP, making congestive heart failure unlikely.

CASE 5

A 60-year-old woman with a history of hypertension, diabetes mellitus, and congestive heart disease presents with 3 months of cough and progressive weight loss. The patient endorses a 20 pack-year smoking history as well. Her temperature is 37.5°C, blood pressure is 155/90, and heart rate is 98. Oxygen saturation is 99% on room air. On examination she is thin, coughing

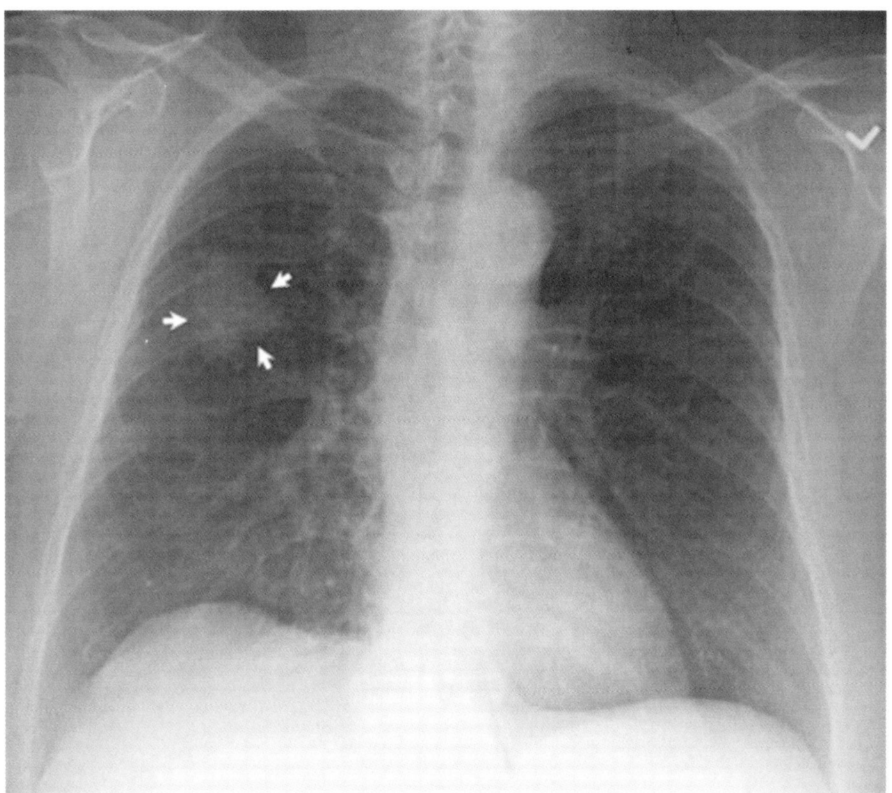

FIGURE 3-6. (Reproduced, with permission, from Lechner AJ, Matuschak GM, Brink DS: *Respiratory: An Integrated Approach to Disease*. www.accessmedicine.com.

but otherwise in no apparent distress, with normal heart sounds and normal breath sounds on lung auscultation without crackles or wheezing. Chest x-ray (Figure 3-6) is obtained.

CXR Finding

This chest x-ray reveals a large, well-defined, focal consolidation in the right upper lung field. The radiographic differential includes pneumonia, infectious or noninfectious granuloma, pulmonary arteriovenous malformation, malignancy, or benign tumor such as hamartoma.

Clinical Diagnosis

Given the clinical context of significant smoking history and cough with progressive weight loss, there is high suspicion that this consolidation is lung cancer. The subacute onset of symptoms and the lack of SIRS argue against an infectious etiology.

CASE 6

A 43-year-old man with a history of HIV is admitted for progressive shortness of breath and cough for 6 months. He has also noted intermittent fevers and night sweats. He reports being off antiretroviral medications for over a year now. Vital signs reveal temperature of 37.8°C, blood pressure of 109/67, and heart rate of 105. His oxygen saturation is 94% on room air. On examination he appears cachectic, heart sounds are regular, and he has decreased breath sounds on the right upper lobe. His bloodwork reveals a white blood cell count of 2000, viral load over 1 million copies/mL, and CD4 count of 183 cells/mm^3. Chest x-ray (Figure 3-7) is obtained.

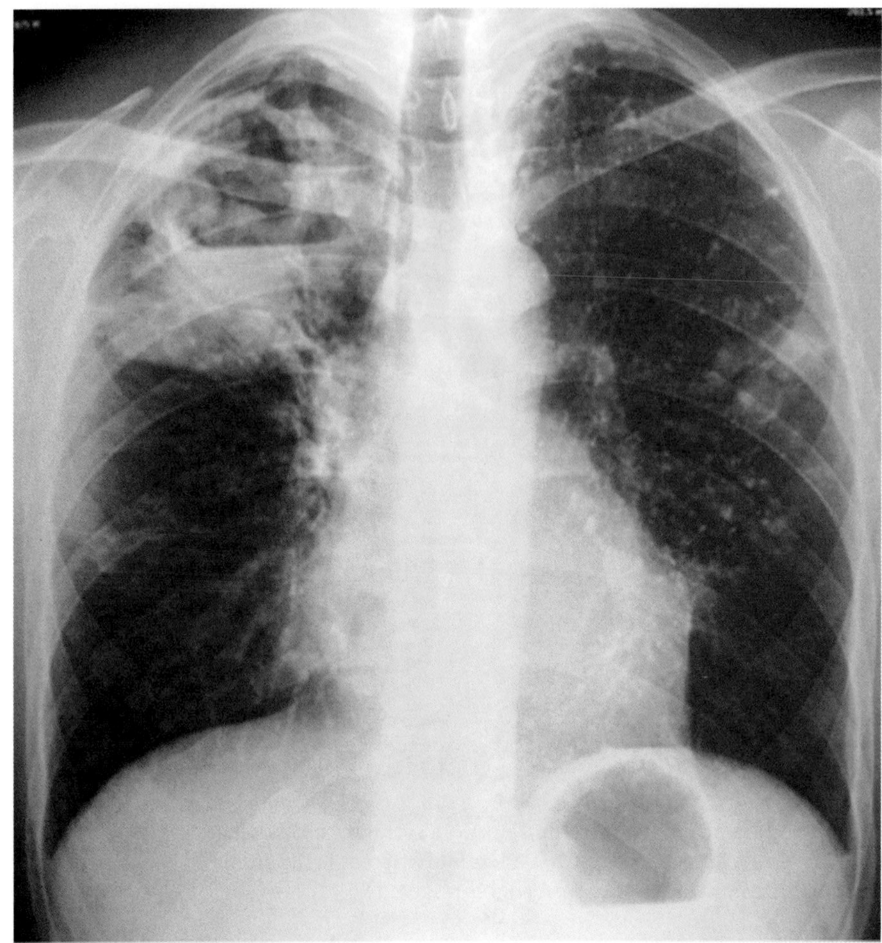

FIGURE 3-7. (From Jameson JL, Fauci AF, Kasper DL, et al, eds: *Harrison's Principles of Internal Medicine*, 20th ed. www.accessmedicine.com. Copyright © McGraw-Hill Education. All rights reserved. Used with permission from Dr. Andrea Gori, Department of Infectious Diseases, S. Paolo University Hospital, Milan, Italy.)

CXR Finding

This chest x-ray is notable for a large, well-defined opacity on the right upper lobe. The upper part of the opacity is radiolucent (air-filled), and the bottom is radiodense with a meniscus (fluid-filled), suggestive of a fluid-filled cavity. The x-ray is also notable for small nodular densities scattered throughout both lung fields. The radiographic differential for cavitary lesions include pulmonary abscess, tuberculosis (TB), nontuberculous *Mycobacterium* infection, sarcoidosis, granulomatosis with polyangiitis, and malignancies.

Clinical Diagnosis

The patient's high viral load and low CD4 count make him susceptible to opportunistic infections, and the presenting symptoms with leukopenia and tachycardia support this diagnosis. The right lung opacity's cavitary appearance and the location in the upper part are suggestive of TB. The small radiodensities in both lungs suggest miliary hematogenous spread of TB. Malignancies may also cause cavitary lesions, and patients with AIDS are at higher risk of malignancy. They may similarly present with weight loss and night sweats. The milia make TB more likely in this case.

CASE 7

A 71-year-old man with a history of emphysema is admitted for sudden shortness of breath at home. His vital signs indicate temperature of 37.3°C, blood

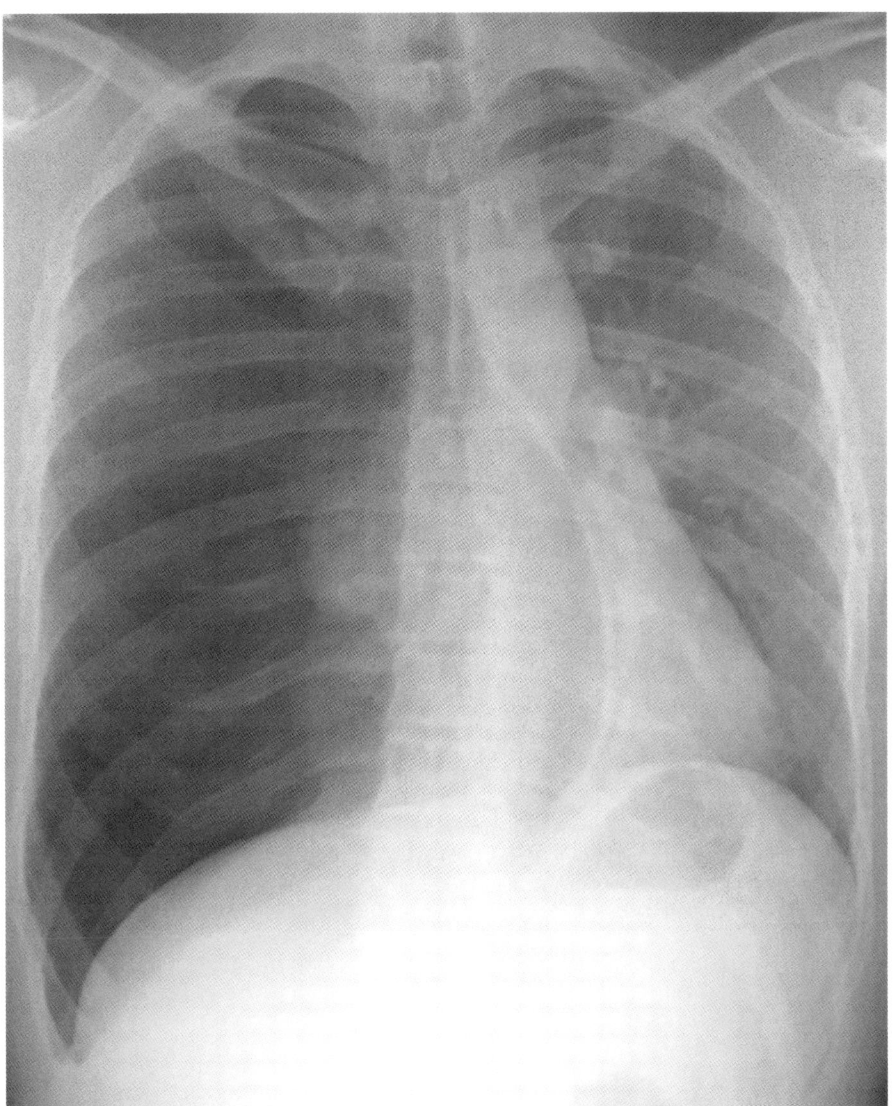

FIGURE 3-8. (Reproduced, with permission, from McKean S, Ross JJ, Dressler DD, Scheurer DB, eds. *Principles and Practice of Hospital Medicine*, 2nd ed. www.accessmedicine.com. Copyright © McGraw-Hill Education. All rights reserved.)

pressure of 97/54, and heart rate of 111. Oxygen saturation is 82%, and respiratory rate is 31. On examination, he is in extremis. Heart sounds are tachycardic and decreased. Breath sounds are absent on the right side. Chest x-ray (Figure 3-8) is rapidly obtained.

CXR Finding and Clinical Diagnosis

The chest x-ray is notable for radiolucency throughout the entire right lung field and complete lack of lung markings on the right side. This chest x-ray is indicative of pneumothorax. Collapsed right lung is visible in the midline. Additionally the midline is pushed toward the left, indicating a tension pneumothorax.

CASE 8

A 73-year-old woman with a history of hypertension and chronic kidney disease is admitted for worsening abdominal pain of 5 days' duration. Her temperature is 38.5°C, blood pressure is 89/53, and heart rate is 121. Oxygen saturation is 97% on room air. On physical examination, her abdomen is distended,

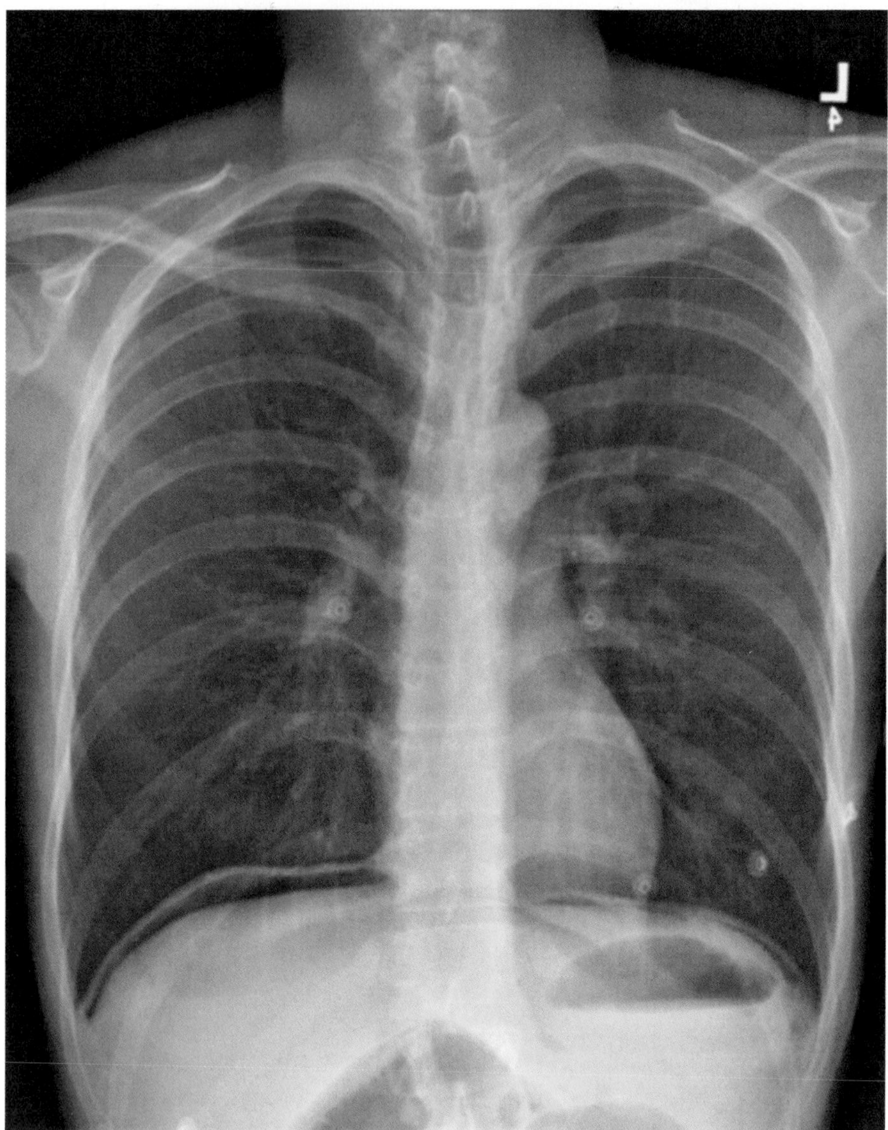

FIGURE 3-9. (From Jameson JL, Fauci AF, Kasper DL, et al, eds: *Harrison's Principles of Internal Medicine*, 20th ed. www.accessmedicine.com. Copyright © McGraw-Hill Education. All rights reserved. Image courtesy of Dr. John Braver; with permission.)

tympanic on percussion, and tender to palpation diffusely. Heart sounds are regular and breath sounds are clear without wheezing or crackles. Laboratory work reveals a white blood cell count of 28,000. She is found to have dilated loops of small bowel on abdominal x-ray. She undergoes a chest x-ray concurrently for shortness of breath, demonstrated in Figure 3-9.

CXR Finding and Clinical Diagnosis

This chest x-ray is notable for radiolucencies under the diaphragm. The liver should be abutting the right hemidiaphragm, and the stomach normally abuts the left hemidiaphragm. Radiolucencies underneath both hemidiaphragms are suggestive of free air. Given the clinical context, this patient likely has bowel perforation and requires urgent surgical consult.

CHAPTER 4
ELECTROCARDIOGRAM

OVERVIEW OF HIGH-YIELD TOPICS IN ELECTROCARDIOGRAM

CONQUER THE WARDS!

Read every ECG, even normal ones, and do it the same way every time.

SYSTEMATIC ANALYSIS

The electrocardiogram (ECG) is the most common test patients receive and is important in the workup of suspected arrhythmia, myocardial ischemia, cardiomyopathy, pericarditis, and hypertension and in detecting and monitoring metabolic derangements. Because the ECG can detect many of these conditions in the preclinical stage, a systematic and consistent approach to analyzing ECGs is essential to avoid overlooking abnormalities.

1. **Rate:** Heart rate can most easily be calculated by counting the number of R waves in the 10-second "rhythm" strip (Figure 4-1) and multiplying by 6. Another method for calculating heart rate in *regular rhythms only* is to divide 300 by the number of large squares between QRS complexes.
2. **Rhythm:** The rhythm is "normal sinus" if 1) P waves are present, 2) there is a P wave before every QRS, 3) there is a QRS after every P, 3) the QRS complexes are spaced at regular intervals, and 4) the PR intervals are constant.
3. **Axis:** Leads I and aVF are most helpful. Assess whether each is positive (R > S), isoelectric (R = S), or negative (R < S). See Table 4-1 and Figure 4-1 (which also shows a quadrant map).
4. **Intervals:** Measure the PR, QRS, and QT intervals. A long PR interval (>200 ms or 1 large box) suggests conduction delay. A long QRS interval (>120 ms or 3 small boxes) suggests a bundle branch block or a ventricular origin of depolarization. The QT interval does not have the exact parameters of what is normal or abnormal because the QT interval is dependent on heart rate. The most clinically relevant parameter to screen for prolonged QT is if the QT is less than half the RR interval, the QTc is probably normal. If it is more than half the RR interval, then the QTc is abnormal.
5. **P wave**: Analyze in leads II, aVF, and V1, where the P wave is most prominent. A normal P-wave axis is upright in leads I and II and inverted in aVR. If the P-wave axis deviates, this suggests an ectopic origin of the atrial beat. In lead II, a "wide" P wave (>120 ms or 3 little boxes) suggests left atrial enlargement; a "tall" P wave (>2.5 mm) suggests right atrial enlargement.
6. **QRS complex:** Assess for left ventricular hypertrophy using one of several validated methods, for example, the Sokolov-Lyon criteria: S wave in V1 + tallest R wave in V5 or V6 > 35 mm (7 big boxes). Assess for pathologic Q waves that indicate previous myocardial infarction. There is debate over what constitutes a pathologic Q wave, but the simplest explanation is any

TABLE 4-1. QRS Axis Determination by the "Quadrant" Method

QRS Deflection		Axis	Common Differential
Lead I	**Lead aVF**		
Positive	Positive	NORMAL (–30 to +90°)	Normal
Positive*	Negative*	LEFT* (–30 to –90°)	LVH, inferior MI, LBBB, VT
Negative	Positive	RIGHT (+90 to 180°)	RVH, cor pulmonale, lateral MI, RBBB, VT
Negative	Negative	EXTREME (–90 to 180°)	Rare – assess for ventricular arrhythmia

LBBB, left bundle branch block; *LVH*, left ventricular hypertrophy; *MI*, myocardial infarction; *RBBB*, right bundle branch block; *RVH*, right ventricular hypertrophy; *VT*, ventricular tachycardia.
*Note that if lead I is positive and lead aVF is negative, there is *possible* left axis deviation; however, you *must* confirm this by looking at lead II. If lead II is negative, there is indeed left axis deviation. If lead II is positive, the axis is normal.

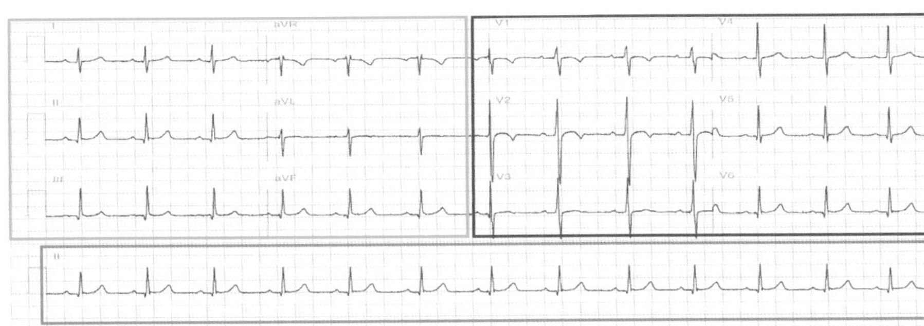

FIGURE 4-1. Components of a typical 10-second ECG showing limb leads (green box), precordial leads (red box), and a rhythm strip (blue box). (Reproduced, with permission, from Jameson JL, Fauci AF, Kasper DL, et al, eds: *Harrison's Principles of Internal Medicine*, 20th ed. www.accessmedicine.com. Copyright © McGraw-Hill Education. All rights reserved.)

Q wave deeper than 1 small box in any 2 leads of a **contiguous lead grouping** (I, aVL,V6—indicating lateral ischemia; II, III, and aVF—indicating inferior ischemia; V4 to V6—indicating anterior ischemia).

7. **ST segment and T wave:** Assess for ST depressions or elevations or T-wave inversions, which can suggest myocardial ischemia, cardiomyopathy, or metabolic derangements. These will be further explained under myocardial ischemia later in this chapter.
8. **Summary:** Only after systematically progressing through the previous steps should you summarize the key findings in one sentence (see the cases later for examples of ECG summary statements).

HIGH-YIELD ECG FINDINGS

TACHYCARDIA

If the heart rate is elevated, you will always get an ECG. Figure 4-2 shows the algorithm for the differential.

1. **QRS width:** A *narrow* QRS is suggestive of a *supraventricular tachycardia (SVT) (origin above* the ventricles). A *wide* QRS complex suggests either a *ventricular* tachycardia or, rarely, an SVT with another reason for a wide QRS, such as a baseline bundle branch block (this is termed SVT with aberrancy). Table 4-2 shows the common differential for narrow vs. wide tachycardia.
2. **R-R interval:** Is the R-R interval regular or irregular? True irregular rhythms (see Table 4-2) typically have no identifiable R-R pattern. So-called "regular" rhythms (see Table 4-2) can sometimes appear irregular if there is a *variable atrioventricular (AV) block* (e.g., the AV refractory period is not constant from beat to beat). Typically, there will still be an identifiable pattern, and these rhythms are sometimes termed "regularly irregular." This situation most classically arises in atrial flutter.
3. **P wave:** The P-wave rate, rhythm, and appearance provide important clues to the etiology (see Table 4-2).

> **CONQUER THE WARDS!**
>
> Ventricular arrhythmias are extremely high risk. Assume that all wide complex tachycardias are ventricular in origin until you can prove otherwise.

Sinus tachycardia: This is exhibited by a narrow complex tachycardia with uniform P waves before every QRS, QRS complexes after every P wave, and the R-R interval is regular (Figure 4-3). Important causes to rule out with history and exam are fever, dehydration, hypoxia, uncontrolled pain, and sepsis.

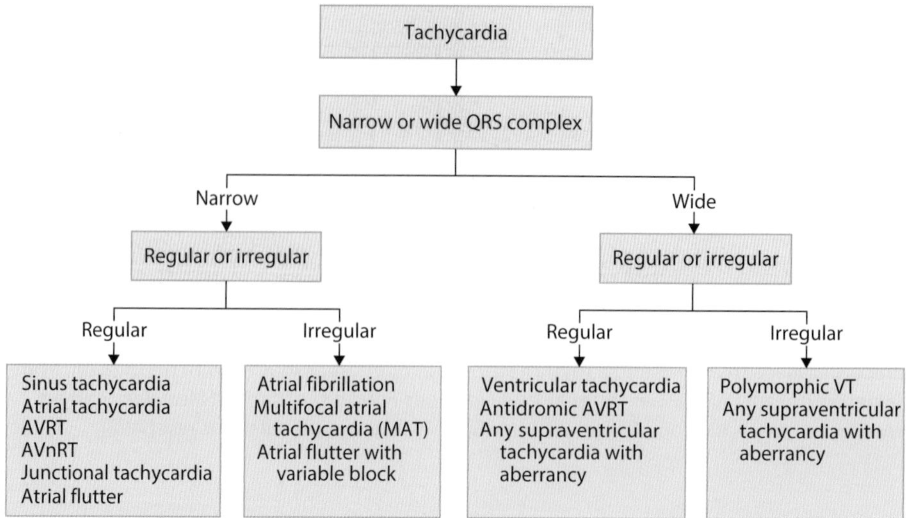

FIGURE 4-2. Algorithm for tachycardia. (Reproduced, with permission, from Tintinalli JE, Stapczynski JS, Ma OJ, Yealy DM, Meckler GD, Cline DM: *Tintinalli's Emergency Medicine: A Comprehensive Guide*, 8th ed. www.accessmedicine.com. Copyright © McGraw-Hill Education. All rights reserved.)

TABLE 4-2. Approach to Tachycardia on ECG

	NARROW						WIDE	
	IRREGULAR		REGULAR*				REGULAR IRREGULAR	
	Atrial fibrillation	MAT	Atrial flutter	Atrial tachycardia	Junctional tachycardia	AVRT AVnRT	VT	VF
Atrial rate	N/A	Variable	250–300	150–200	150–200		AV dissociation	
P wave	None	3+ distinct P waves	Flutter/ sawtooth	Ectopic	Retrograde	Retrograde P wave in QRS or T wave	AV dissociation	
Beat origin	Many atrial foci	Multiple atrial foci	Single atrial focus	Single atrial focus	AV node/ HIS bundle	Single atrial focus	Ventricle	

AV, atrioventricular; *MAT*, multifocal atrial tachycardia; VF, ventricular fibrillation; *VT*, ventricular tachycardia.
*Note that any "regular" rhythm can appear irregular on an ECG if there is variable AV block.

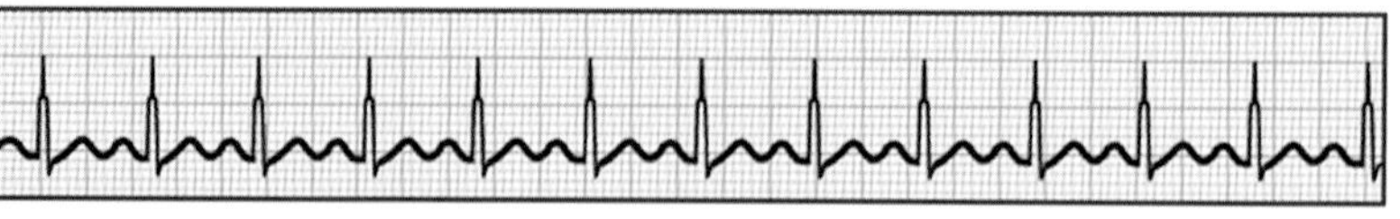

FIGURE 4-3. Sinus tachycardia. (Reproduced, with permission, from Elmoselhi A. *Cardiology: An Integrated Approach*. Copyright © McGraw-Hill Education. All rights reserved.)

Atrial tachycardia: This is exhibited by a narrow complex tachycardia with uniform P waves and regular R-R intervals (Figure 4-4). The key electrocardiographic difference from sinus tachycardia is that the P waves originate outside the sinoatrial (SA) node and will have a morphology that differs from the baseline sinus P waves.

Atrial fibrillation: This is exhibited by narrow complex tachycardia with an irregular ventricular response and there are no discernable P waves (Figure 4-5).

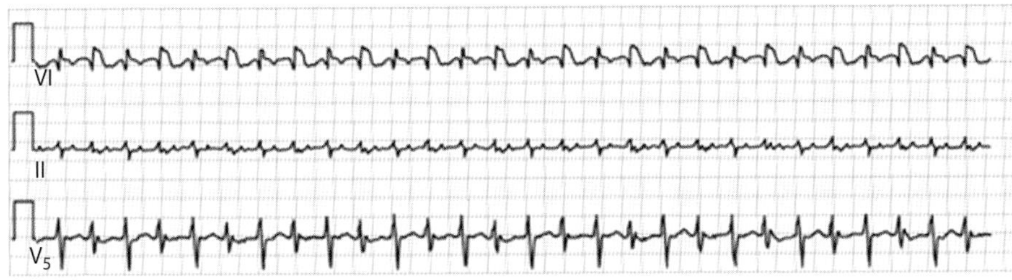

FIGURE 4-4. Atrial tachycardia. (Reproduced, with permission, from McKean S, Ross JJ, Dressler DD, Scheurer DB, eds. *Principles and Practice of Hospital Medicine*, 2nd ed. www.accessmedicine.com. Copyright © McGraw-Hill Education. All rights reserved.)

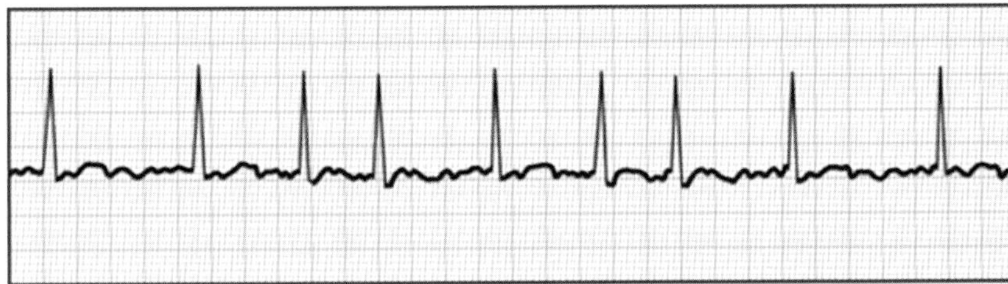

FIGURE 4-5. Atrial fibrillation. (Reproduced, with permission, from Elmoselhi A. *Cardiology: An Integrated Approach*. Copyright © McGraw-Hill Education. All rights reserved.)

In atrial fibrillation, the AV node is continually bombarded by high-frequency (well over 300 beats per minute [bpm]), irregular atrial depolarizations. The ventricular rate, in turn, is determined by the minimum refractory period of the AV node and conducting system.

Atrial flutter: This is exhibited by a narrow complex tachycardia distinguished by the rapid (200 to 300 bpm) atrial reentrant rhythm with the stereotypical "sawtooth" pattern of P waves on ECG (Figure 4-6). The R-R interval is regular, but can appear "regularly" irregular when there is variable AV block.

CONQUER THE WARDS!

It is important to differentiate atrial fibrillation from flutter, as the latter is less likely to respond to "rate control" and more likely to require cardioversion or ablation.

Multifocal atrial tachycardia (MAT): This is exhibited by an irregular narrow complex tachycardia with at least 3 *morphologically distinct* P waves (Figure 4-7). MAT results from atrial overexcitability with multiple origins of ectopic atrial beats. It is commonly associated with acute pulmonary conditions such as chronic obstructive pulmonary disease (COPD). Note that when this rhythm is noted at a heart rate of 60 to 100 bpm, the term **wandering atrial pacemaker** is used instead.

Atrioventricular reentrant tachycardia (AVRT) and AV nodal RT (AVnRT): Both involve an accessory pathway that leads to a reentrant loop through the AV node and the accessory pathway. The difference is that **AVRT** is an

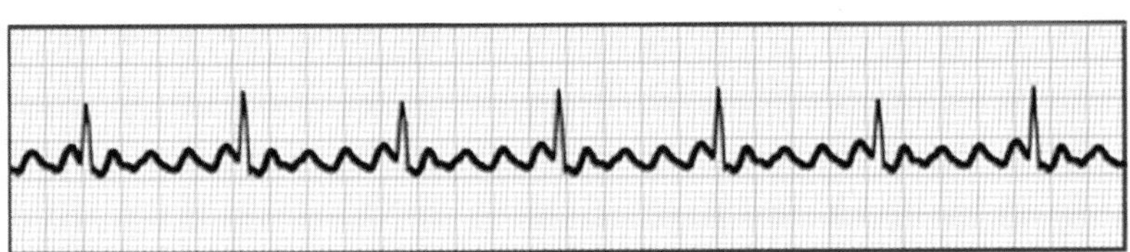

FIGURE 4-6. Atrial flutter. (Reproduced, with permission, from Elmoselhi A. *Cardiology: An Integrated Approach*. Copyright © McGraw-Hill Education. All rights reserved.)

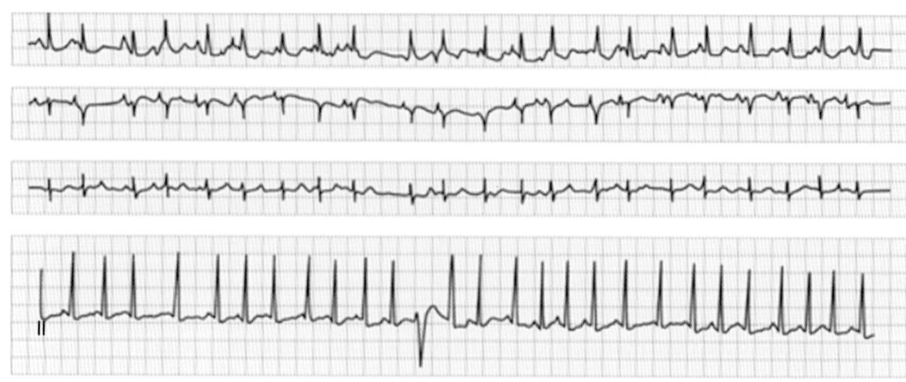

FIGURE 4-7. Multifocal atrial tachycardia. (Reproduced, with permission, from McKean S, Ross JJ, Dressler DD, Scheurer DB, eds. *Principles and Practice of Hospital Medicine*, 2nd ed. www.accessmedicine.com.)

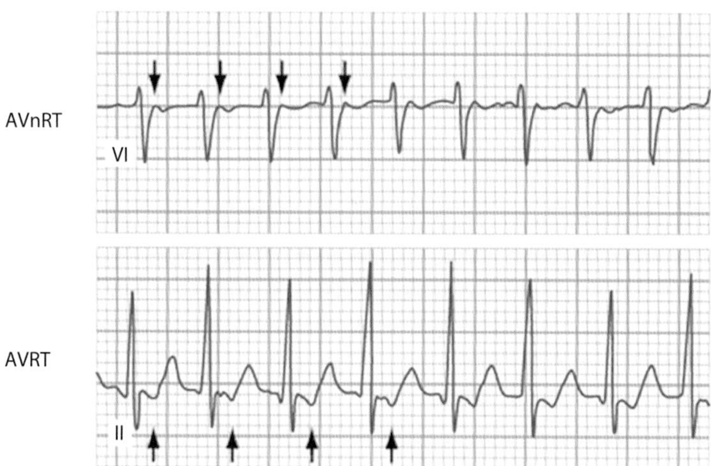

FIGURE 4-8. AVnRT and AVRT. (Reproduced, with permission, from Nicoll D, Lu CM, McPhee SJ: *Guide to Diagnostic Tests*, 7th ed. www.accessmedicine.com.)

accessory pathway outside of the AV node, whereas the accessory pathway in **AVnRT** is next to or inside the AV node. *Note:* AVnRT is a form of junctional tachycardia. **Wolff-Parkinson-White syndrome (WPW)** is a form of AVRT. On ECG you will often see no P wave or a P wave buried in the QRS or T wave (see Figure 4-8). This P wave is a retrograde P wave, since it is occurring because of the signal going down the AV node and then coming back up through the accessory pathway or vice versa (Figure 4-8). The QRS is usually regular, since it's a reentrant loop but can be difficult to diagnose if the heart rate is extremely fast. Use of adenosine will often unveil these buried P waves.

CONQUER THE WARDS!

If present in a wide complex tachycardia, AV dissociation, capture beats, and fusion beats are all pathognomonic for ventricular tachycardia.

Ventricular tachycardia: This is a wide complex tachycardia with a ventricular origin of depolarization (Figure 4-9). The differential includes a supraventricular arrhythmia in the setting of aberrant conduction (e.g., a bundle branch block). Ventricular tachycardia (VT) is generally of much higher clinical concern, and a wide complex tachycardia is thus presumed to be ventricular until proven otherwise (especially in a patient with risk

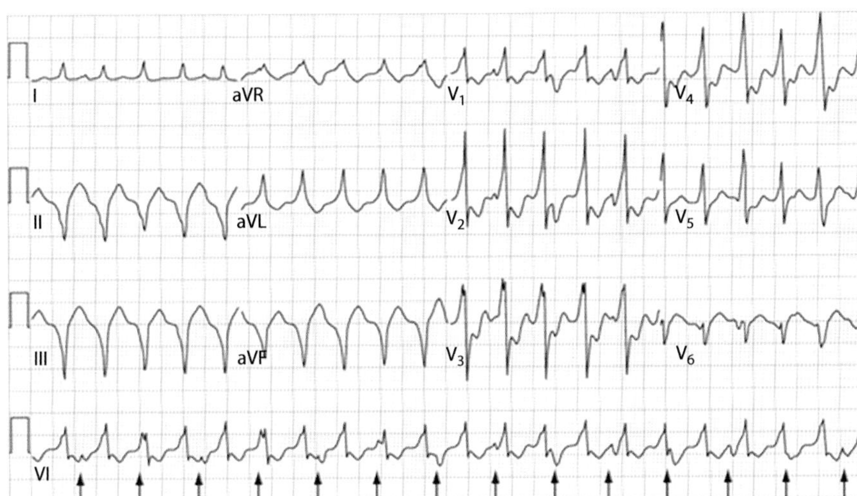

FIGURE 4-9. Ventricular tachycardia. (Reproduced, with permission, from Fauci AS, Braunwald E, Kasper DL, et al, eds: *Harrison's Principles of Internal Medicine,* 17th ed. New York: McGraw-Hill, 2008, Fig. 226-10, p. 1437.)

factors for VT, such as cardiac ischemia). ECG findings suggestive of a ventricular origin of depolarization are summarized in Table 4-3.

Ventricular fibrillation and polymorphic ventricular tachycardia: The ventricles are activated in a chaotic fashion – this is a life-threatening condition that requires immediate defibrillation. The distinction between the two is based on QRS amplitude (Figure 4-10).

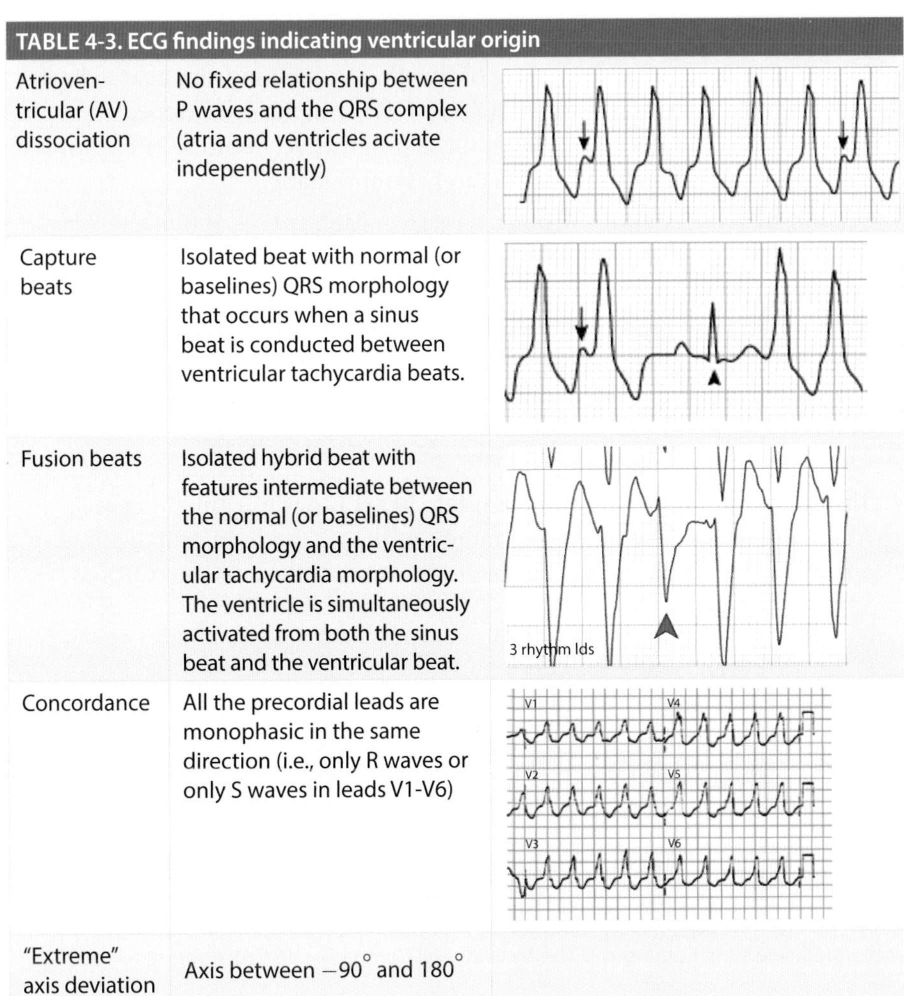

TABLE 4-3. ECG findings indicating ventricular origin

Atrioventricular (AV) dissociation	No fixed relationship between P waves and the QRS complex (atria and ventricles acivate independently)	
Capture beats	Isolated beat with normal (or baselines) QRS morphology that occurs when a sinus beat is conducted between ventricular tachycardia beats.	
Fusion beats	Isolated hybrid beat with features intermediate between the normal (or baselines) QRS morphology and the ventricular tachycardia morphology. The ventricle is simultaneously activated from both the sinus beat and the ventricular beat.	3 rhythm lds
Concordance	All the precordial leads are monophasic in the same direction (i.e., only R waves or only S waves in leads V1-V6)	V1 V4 V2 V5 V3 V6
"Extreme" axis deviation	Axis between -90° and 180°	

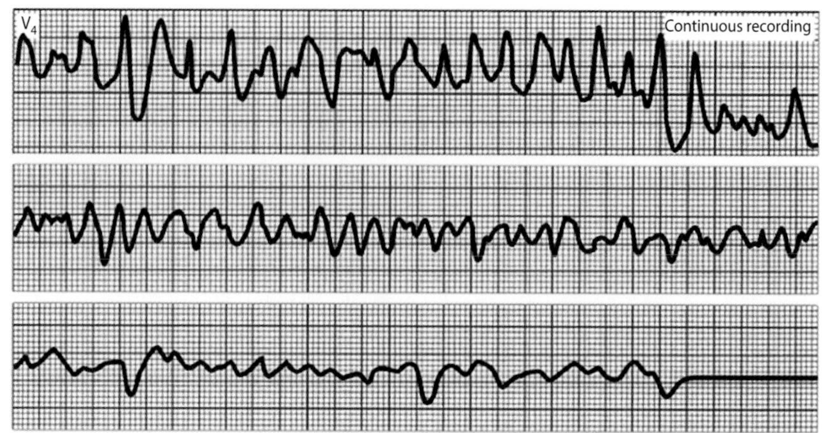

FIGURE 4-10. Ventricular fibrillation. (Goldschlager N, Goldman MJ. *Principles of Clinical Electrocardiography*, 13th ed. Originally published by Appleton & Lange. Copyright © 1989 by The McGraw-Hill Companies, Inc. p. 230, Fig 13-28.)

ATRIOVENTRICULAR BLOCK

An AV block can manifest as a prolonged PR interval (first-degree AV block), occasional nonconducted P waves (second-degree AV block), or complete dissociation of the P wave and QRS complexes (third-degree AV block).

1. **First-degree AV block:** This is exhibited by a prolonged PR interval on the ECG. It is rarely symptomatic on its own, though it can progress to a higher grade block over time.
2. **Second-degree AV block Mobitz type I (aka Wenckebach):** Mobitz type I results from progressive slowing of the AV conduction from beat to beat until the AV node fails to conduct and a QRS complex is "dropped" (Figure 4-11). The PR interval lengthens progressively until a QRS complex is dropped. Mobitz type I block is rarely symptomatic.
3. **Second-degree AV block Mobitz type II:** A Mobitz type II block results from instability of the conducting system *just below the AV node*, causing episodic and irregular "dropped" QRS complexes. The PR interval remains constant (Figure 4-12). In contrast to Mobitz type I, the pathology in Mobitz type II is lower in the conduction system and thus carries a higher risk of progression to complete heart block. Unless there is a reversible etiology, Mobitz type II is an indication for permanent pacemaker placement.
4. **Third-degree AV block (aka complete heart block):** A third-degree AV block results from complete failure of the AV node in propagating atrial impulses. There is complete dissociation of P waves and QRS

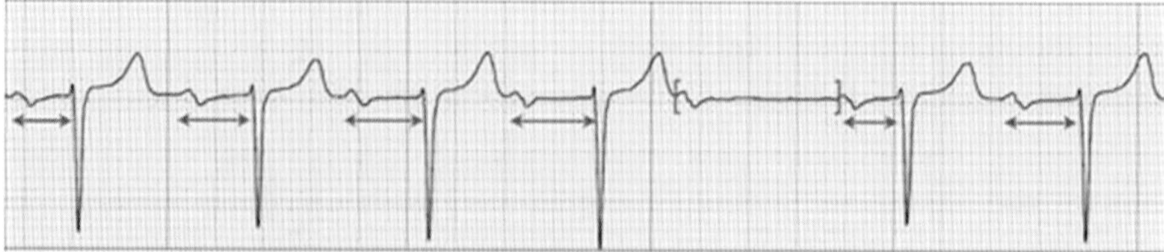

FIGURE 4-11. Second-degree AV block Mobitz type I. (Reproduced, with permission, from Knoop KJ, Stack LB, Storrow AB, Thurman RJ: *The Atlas of Emergency Medicine*, 3rd ed. www.accessmedicine.com. Copyright © The McGraw-Hill Companies, Inc. All rights reserved.)

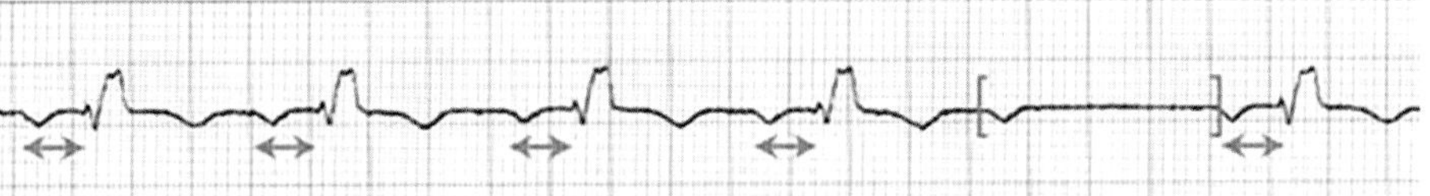

FIGURE 4-12. Second-degree AV block Mobitz type II. (Reproduced, with permission, from Knoop KJ, Stack LB, Storrow AB, Thurman RJ: *The Atlas of Emergency Medicine*, 3rd ed. www.accessmedicine.com. Copyright © The McGraw-Hill Companies, Inc. All rights reserved.)

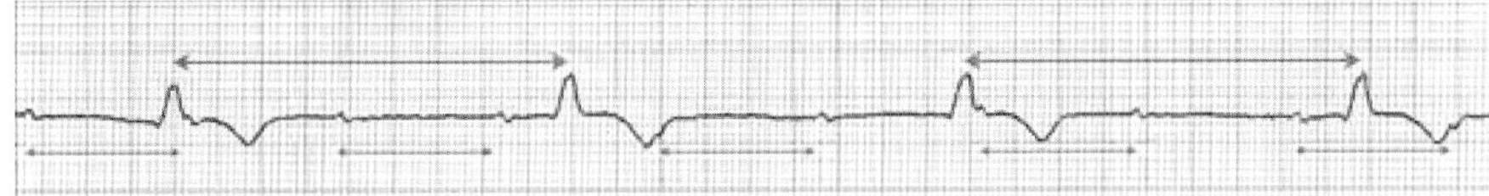

FIGURE 4-13. Third-degree AV block. (Reproduced, with permission, from Knoop KJ, Stack LB, Storrow AB, Thurman RJ: *The Atlas of Emergency Medicine*, 3rd ed. www.accessmedicine.com. Copyright © The McGraw-Hill Companies, Inc. All rights reserved.)

complexes (Figure 4-13). Ventricular depolarization occurs due to an escape rhythm originating below the AV node. The rate and width of the QRS complex are determined by the level of origin of the escape rhythm. Higher escape rhythms (often called "junctional" because they originate at the AV junction) occur at a rate between 40 and 60 bpm; junctional QRS complexes are narrow because conduction through the left and right Purkinje systems occurs simultaneously. Lower escape rhythms originate after bifurcation of the left and right bundle branches; the rate is slower and the QRS complexes are wider. Lower escape rhythms are less stable with a higher risk of cardiac arrest. A third-degree AV block is an emergency and is an indication for emergent pacemaker placement, unless a reversible etiology is present.

CARDIAC ISCHEMIA

Acute myocardial ischemia can result in both abnormal ventricular repolarization and abnormal conduction (via damage to the SA node, AV node, and Purkinje system). ECG changes consistent with abnormal repolarization have greater specificity for ischemia compared to changes in conduction and are more commonly used to diagnose acute coronary syndromes.

ECG changes consistent with abnormal repolarization include T-wave inversions, ST-segment depression, and ST-segment elevation.

T-wave inversions are defined as >0.1 mV (1 small box) inflections in 2 contiguous leads. During acute ischemic events, T-wave inversions are commonly associated with ST-segment changes in the ECG (Figure 4-14). T-wave inversions can indicate myocardial ischemia if they are in a **contiguous lead grouping (see systematic analysis # 6: QRS Complex)** or if they change over time.

ST-segment depressions are defined as >0.05 mV (0.5 little boxes) horizontal or downsloping depressions in the ST segment compared to the baseline TP segment. The depressions must occur in 2 contiguous leads. Downsloping depressions have the strongest correlation with ischemia, followed by horizontal depressions. Upsloping depressions have a much weaker association and

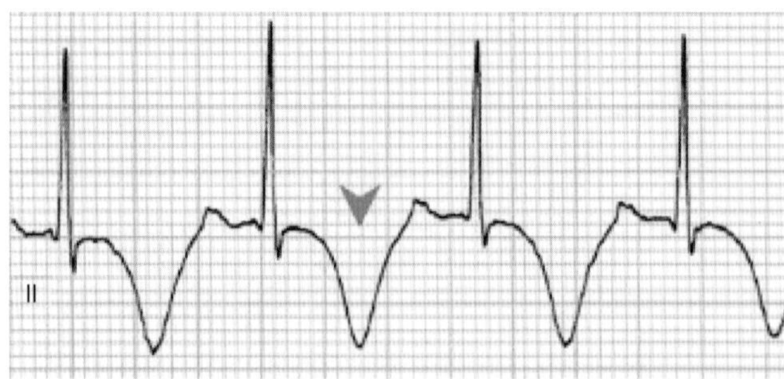

FIGURE 4-14. T-wave inversions. (Reproduced, with permission, from Knoop KJ, Stack LB, Storrow AB, Thurman RJ: *The Atlas of Emergency Medicine*, 3rd ed. www.accessmedicine.com. Copyright © The McGraw-Hill Companies, Inc. All rights reserved.)

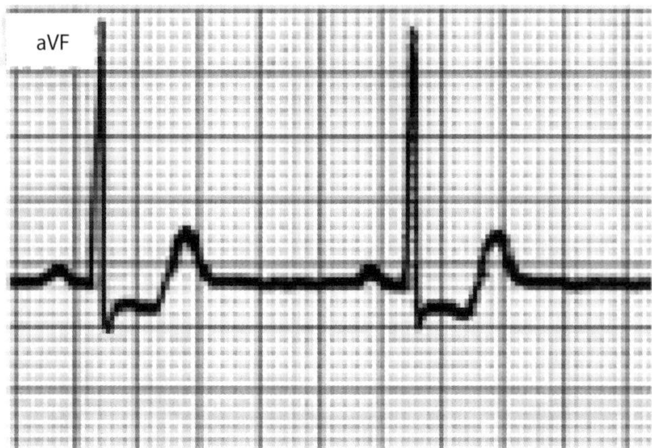

FIGURE 4-15. ST-segment depressions.

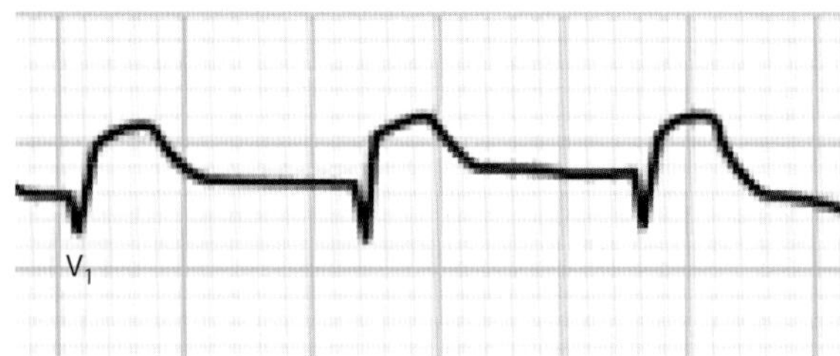

FIGURE 4-16. ST-segment elevations.

can often be a normal variant or artifact due to poor skin contact with the lead. (See Figure 4-15.)

ST-segment elevations are defined as >0.1 mV changes in the ST segment, except in V2 and V3, where the change must be >0.2 mV in men and >0.15 mV in women (Figure 4-16). ST-segment elevation is relatively specific for transmural ischemia, and the location of the elevations can be used to anatomically localize the ischemia.

A **Q wave** is any negative deflection that *precedes* an R wave; however, not all Q waves are pathologic. *Pathologic* Q waves are generally wider than 40 ms (1 little box) and have an amplitude greater than 25% of that of the entire QRS complex. It is important to identify pathologic Q waves, which suggest subacute or chronic infarction. Figure 4-17 shows pathologic Q waves in leads V4 and V5. It is tempting to label Q waves in leads V2 and V3. However, the downward deflections in these leads are preceded by a small upward deflection (i.e., an R wave) and thus are not Q waves at all (technically these are S waves)!

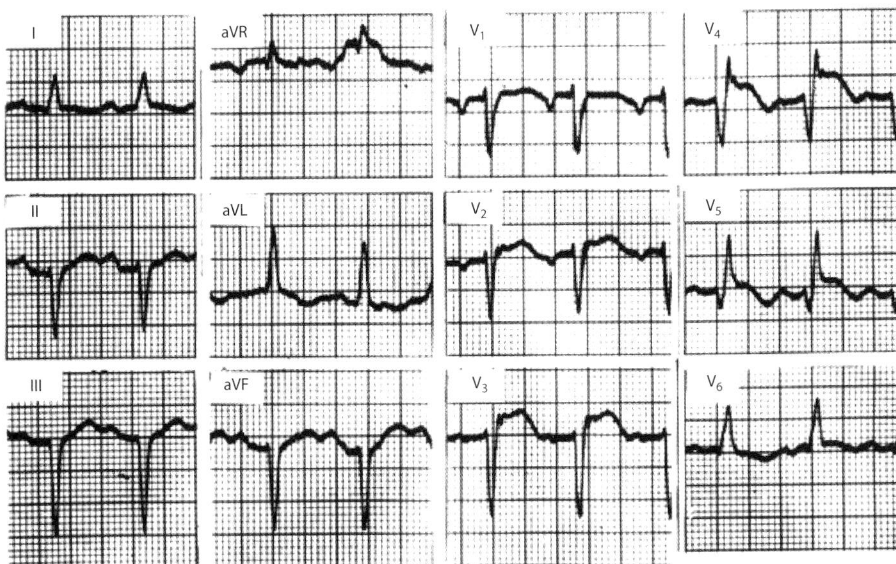

FIGURE 4-17. Q waves. (Reproduced, with permission, from Goldschlager N, Goldman MJ. *Principles of Clinical Electrocardiography,* 13th ed. Originally published by Appleton & Lange. Copyright © 1989 by The McGraw-Hill Companies, Inc., p. 124, Fig 9-25.)

BUNDLE BRANCH BLOCK

A bundle branch block arises when the normal conduction through either the left or right branch of the His–Purkinje system is interrupted. There is delayed depolarization of the associated myocardium, resulting in a widened QRS, with a characteristic pattern depending on the location of the block.

Left bundle branch block (LBBB): In LBBB, the right side of the heart depolarizes first. This results in a deep (sometimes notched) S wave in V_1 and a prominent R wave (sometimes notched) in V_6. See Figure 4-18.

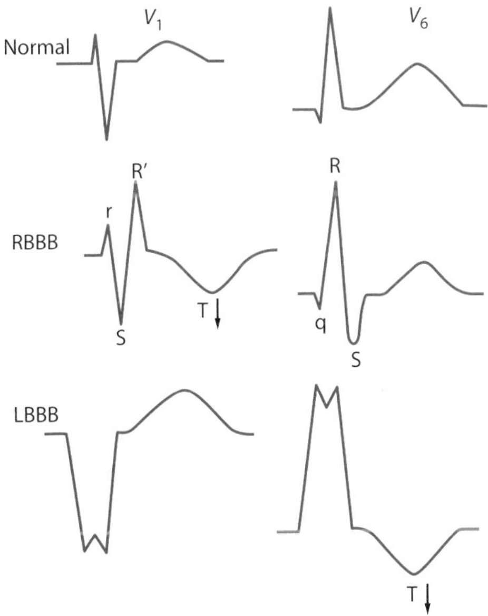

FIGURE 4-18. Left and right bundle branch block. (Reproduced, with permission, from Jameson JL, Fauci AF, Kasper DL, et al, eds: *Harrison's Principles of Internal Medicine*, 20th ed. www.accessmedicine.com. Copyright © McGraw-Hill Education. All rights reserved.)

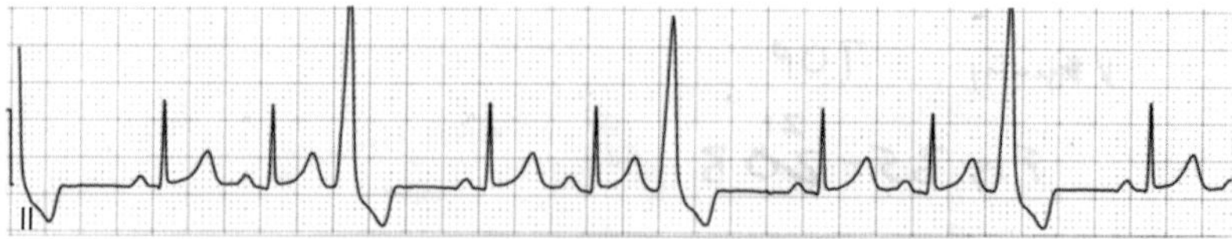

FIGURE 4-19. Premature ventricular complexes. (Reproduced, with permission, from Stone CK, Humphries RL. *Current Diagnosis & Treatment: Emergency Medicine*, 8th ed. Copyright © McGraw-Hill Education. All rights reserved.)

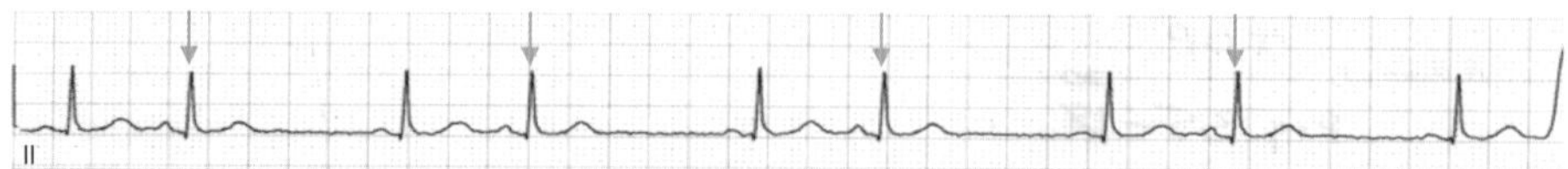

FIGURE 4-20. Premature atrial complexes. (Reproduced, with permission, from Stone CK, Humphries RL. *Current Diagnosis & Treatment: Emergency Medicine*, 8th ed. Copyright © McGraw-Hill Education. All rights reserved.)

Right bundle branch block (RBBB): In RBBB, the left side of the heart depolarizes first. This results in a second R wave (called R′ or R prime) in V1 and a slurred S wave in lead V6. See Figure 4-18.

Premature ventricular complex (PVC): Ectopic (premature) firing of a ventricular pacemaker cell results in depolarization from the "bottom" to the "top" of the heart. Because the His–Purkinje system is bypassed, the right and left sides of the heart depolarize asynchronously, resulting in an isolated wide complex QRS (Figure 4-19).

Premature atrial complex (PAC or APC): Usually an ectopic (premature) firing of a supraventricular pacemaker cell is suppressed by the more rapidly depolarizing SA node. If the ectopic focus depolarizes early enough, however, it can propagate through the AV node and "capture" the ventricles, resulting in a premature narrow QRS complex. In Figure 4-20, the PACs are highlighted with blue arrows. Note that the P-wave morphology of the PACs are different from that of the sinus beats because the atria is depolarizing from a different focus.

CASE EXAMPLES

The following cases serve to highlight common clinical scenarios in which the ECG is essential. For each case, read the relevant clinical information, systematically analyze the ECG using the earlier approach (or another systematic method), write down your own ECG summary statement, and then refer to the ECG and case discussion.

CASE 1

A 65-year-old man with long-standing, poorly controlled hypertension presents to the emergency department with acute-onset dyspnea and palpitations. The ECG is shown in Figure 4-21.

Rate – 96 bpm (16 beats in 10-second strip multiplied by 6).

Rhythm – There are QRS complexes after each P wave, but there are P waves that are not followed by QRS complexes. The rhythm is not sinus. The R-R interval is not regular, but there appears to be a pattern. It is "regularly irregular."

Axis – Positive in lead I, slightly negative in lead II. The axis is leftward.

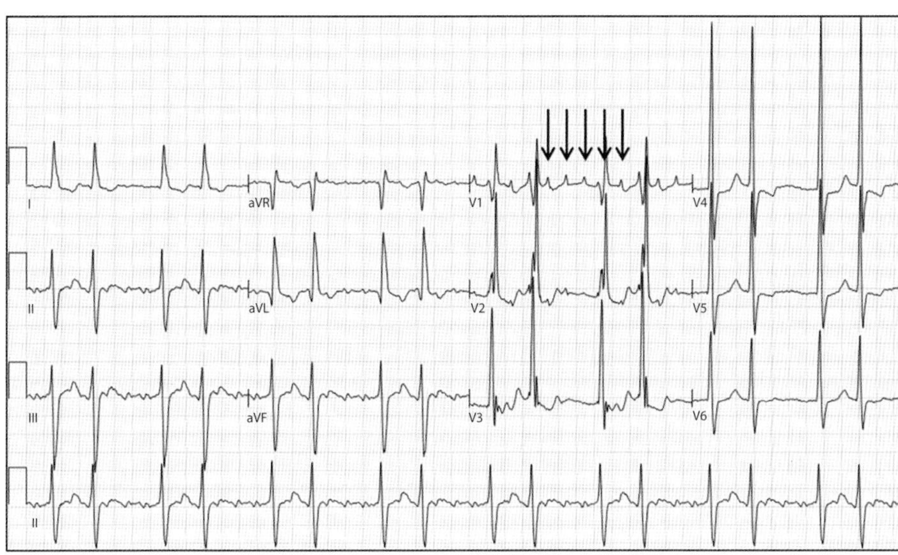

FIGURE 4-21. ECG for case 1

Intervals – PR interval is less than 200 ms, QRS complex is narrow, QT interval is less than half the R-R interval (probably normal).

P wave – P-P interval is approximately 1 large box – the atrial rate is about 300 bpm. The P wave is flat in lead I and upright in aVR – the P wave is nonsinus (and likely ectopic).

QRS complex – S wave in V1 + R wave in V5 > 35 mm consistent with left ventricular hypertrophy.

ST segment and T wave – ST depressions and T-wave inversions in leads V5 and V6.

ECG summary – Atrial tachycardia with variable AV block, left axis deviation, left ventricular hypertrophy (LVH), and left ventricular strain pattern.

The findings on this ECG that support atrial tachycardia include a narrow complex tachycardia (suggests a supraventricular arrhythmia), P-wave axis deviation (suggests ectopic origin of P wave), and regular and fast P waves. The ventricular response is often regular in atrial tachycardia, but can be regularly irregular (as in this case) if the conduction through the AV node is variable. The ST changes in this ECG are located in leads with very large R waves, a finding that is consistent with abnormal repolarization due to LVH and does not necessarily indicate ischemia.

Answer: Atrial tachycardia with variable AV block, left axis deviation, left ventricular hypertrophy (LVH), and left ventricular strain pattern.

CASE 2

A 65-year-old woman with long-standing, poorly controlled hypertension presents to the emergency department with acute-onset dyspnea and palpitations. The ECG is shown in Figure 4-22.

Rate – 78 bpm (13 beats per 10-second strip × 6 = 78).

Rhythm – There is a P wave before every QRS and a QRS after every P wave.

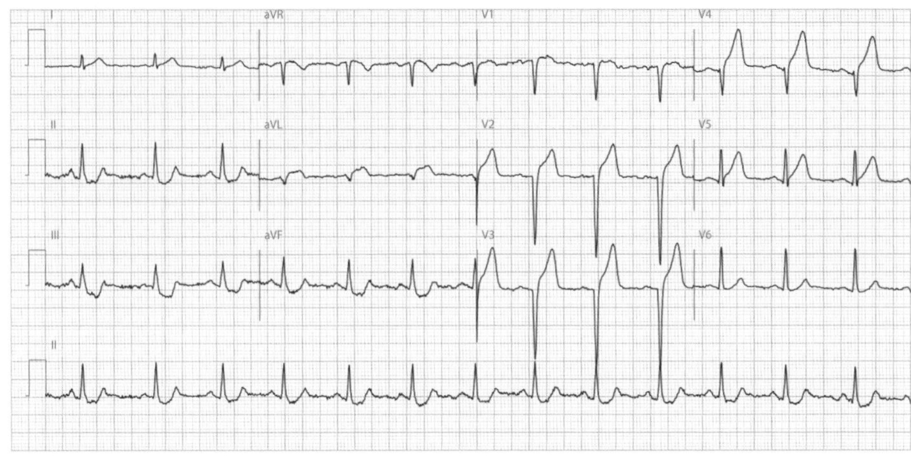

FIGURE 4-22. ECG for case 2 (From Jameson JL, Fauci AF, Kasper DL, et al, eds: *Harrison's Principles of Internal Medicine,* 20th ed. www.accessmedicine.com. Used with permission from ECG Wave-Maven, Copyright 2001 -2016, Beth Israel Deaconess Medical Center, ttp://ecg.bidmc.harvard.edu.)

R-R intervals are regular*. This is sinus rhythm.

Axis – Positive in lead I and aVF, the axis is normal

Intervals – PR interval is less than 200 ms, QRS complex is narrow, and QT interval is less than half the R-R interval.

P wave – Positive in leads I (only just positive) and II and negative in aVR; P axis is normal.

QRS complex – S wave in V1 + R wave in V5 is less than 35 mm. There are deep pathologic Q waves in leads V2 through V4.

ST segment and T wave – ST elevations >1 mm in leads V1 to V4 and aVL. There are deep, downsloping ST depressions in leads II, III, and aVF.

ECG summary – Acute anterior ST elevation myocardial infarction with pathologic Q waves and reciprocal ST depressions. This ECG suggests transmural infarction (transmural because there are ST elevations) in the anatomic region supplied by the left anterior descending artery: there is anterior injury (V3 to V4), septal injury (V1 to V2), and probably lateral injury given the ST elevation in aVL (see Chapter 6). The ST depressions in the inferior leads (II, III, and aVF) are reciprocal changes from the anterior injury; reciprocal changes are the same ST changes seen from the opposite direction. The deep pathologic Q waves suggest that the event has progressed to infarction in this territory.

Answer: Acute myocardial infarction (MI)

CASE 3

A 65-year-old woman with long-standing, poorly controlled hypertension and diabetes presents to the emergency department with lightheadedness. The ECG is shown in Figure 4-23.

Rate – 60 bpm (10 beats per 10-second strip multiplied by 6).

* Note there is actually very slight variation in the R-R interval, which may be due to small changes in vagal tone through the respiratory cycle; this beat-to-beat variability with respiration is termed sinus arrhythmia and is usually normal.

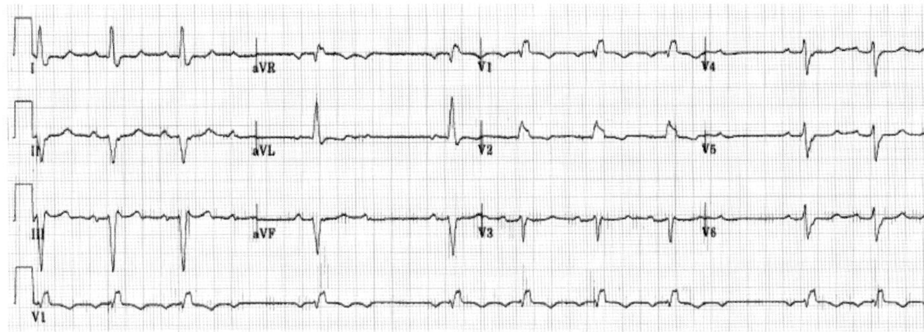

FIGURE 4-23. ECG for case 3 (Reproduced, with permission, from Knoop KJ, Stack LB, Storrow AB, Thurman RJ: The Atlas of Emergency Medicine, 3rd ed. www.accessmedicine.com. Copyright © The McGraw-Hill Companies, Inc. All rights reserved.)

Rhythm – There is a P wave before every QRS, but there are P waves that are not followed by QRS complexes. Because of the "dropped" QRS complexes, the rhythm is not sinus. The R-R interval is not regular, but there appears to be a pattern. It is "regularly irregular." The PR intervals are constant in the lead-up to dropped QRS complexes. This is Mobitz type II second-degree AV block.

Axis – Positive in lead I but negative in leads II and aVF. There is left axis deviation.

Intervals – The PR interval is just over 200 ms (1 big box), the QRS complex is wide (see later), and the QT interval is less than half the R-R interval (probably normal).

P wave – Positive in leads I and II and negative in aVR; P-axis is normal. P-wave height and width are normal in lead II. There is no atrial enlargement.

QRS complex – QRS is wide (greater than 120 ms). There are "bunny ears" (RSR′ pattern) in lead V1 and a prolonged S wave in leads I + V5 to V6. This is a right bundle branch pattern. There is no LVH.

ST segment and T wave – There are no ST elevations or depressions. There is an isolated inverted T wave in lead V2.

ECG summary – Mobitz type II second-degree AV block with concomitant first-degree AV block, left axis deviation, and an RBBB.

A Mobitz type II AV block has a high risk of progression to complete heart block. Especially when associated with symptoms (e.g., lightheadedness or syncope), this block is usually an indication for pacemaker placement. This patient has risk factors for conduction disease (age, hypertension), though cardiac ischemia is another common cause, and a thorough history should be performed to uncover any history of angina.

Incidentally, this ECG is also notable for trifascicular block (first-degree AV block + left anterior fascicular block + RBBB) (see Chapter 6). Patients with trifascicular block also have some risk of progression to complete heart block, and if symptoms are present (e.g., lightheadedness), a cardiologist should be consulted to decide if the patient needs a pacemaker.

Answer: Type II Mobitz block

CASE 4

A 65-year-old woman with hypertension and diabetes is sent to the emergency department for evaluation of acute kidney insufficiency. The ECG is shown in Figure 4-24.

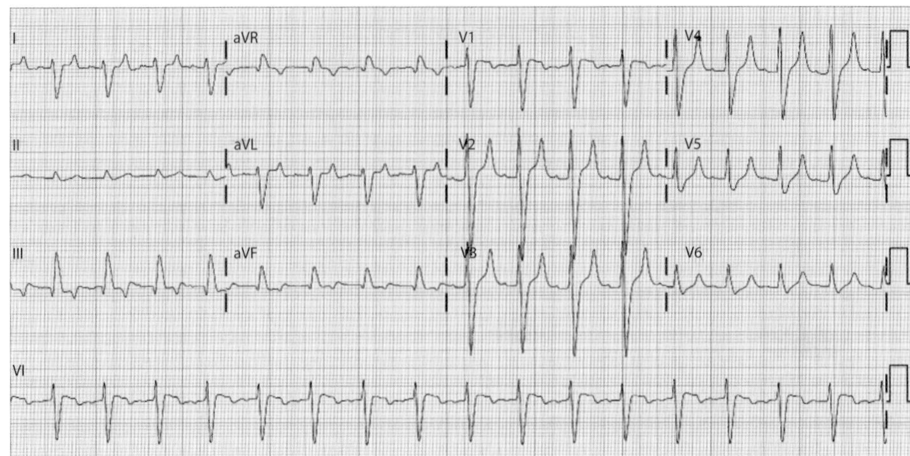

FIGURE 4-24. (Reproduced, with permission, from Knoop KJ, Stack LB, Storrow AB, Thurman RJ: *The Atlas of Emergency Medicine*, 3rd ed. www.accessmedicine.com. Copyright © The McGraw-Hill Companies, Inc. All rights reserved.)

Rate – 96 bpm (16 beats per 10-second strip multiplied by 6).

Rhythm – There is a P wave before every QRS and a QRS after every P wave.

Axis – Negative in lead I and positive in lead aVF. There is *right* axis deviation.

Intervals – PR interval is normal. QRS complex is wide (approximately 4 small boxes, or 160 ms), and the QT interval is less than half the R-R interval.

P wave – Positive in lead I; flat in leads II and aVR; negative in aVR; P axis is abnormal. The P-wave amplitude is abnormally small in lead II.

QRS complex – QRS is wide (greater than 120 ms). The QRS pattern does not fit neatly into a left or right bundle branch pattern. There is no LVH. There are no pathologic Q waves.

ST segment and T wave – There are tall, peaked (look "uncomfortable to sit on") T-waves in many of the precordial leads (V1 to V4).

ECG summary – Normal sinus rhythm with subtle flattening of the P waves, widened QRS, and tall, peaked T-waves.

This patient had a serum potassium concentration of 8 mEq/L. The findings of hyperkalemia on ECG often start with tall, peaked T waves and a shortened QT interval, though it is important to note that these findings are nonspecific and can be found in other acute conditions such as myocardial ischemia. As the cardiotoxicity from hyperkalemia progresses, ECG findings can include lengthening of the PR interval and QRS duration, flattening and disappearance of the P wave, and eventually further widening of the QRS interval to a sine wave pattern, which portends imminent cardiopulmonary arrest. Importantly, some or all of these ECG findings can be absent despite severe hyperkalemia, and a normal ECG should not be used to rule out electrolyte abnormality.

Answer: Hyperkalemia

CASE 5

A 65-year-old man admitted to the hospital with a COPD exacerbation develops acute-onset palpitations. The ECG is shown in Figure 4-25.

Rate – 96 bpm (16 beats per 10-second strip multiplied by 6).

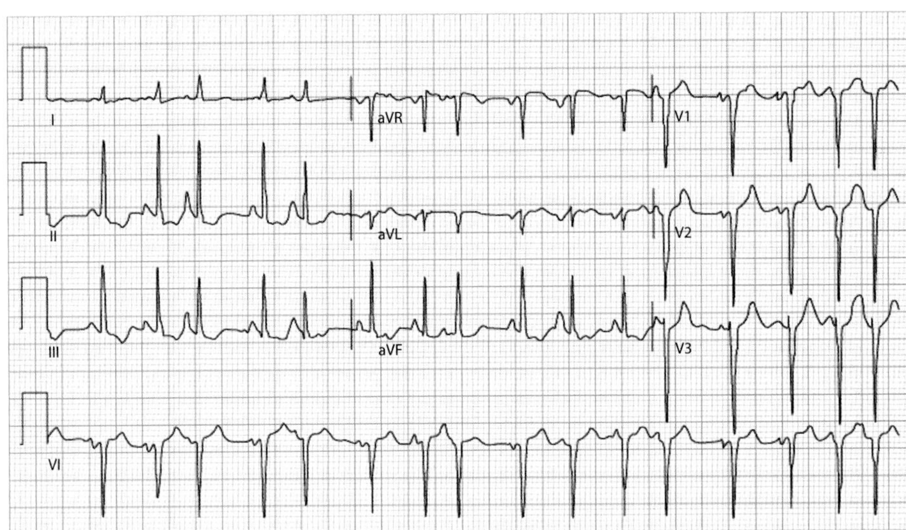

FIGURE 4-25. ECG for Case 5 (Reproduced, with permission, from McKean S, Ross JJ, Dressler DD, Scheurer DB, eds. Principles and Practice of Hospital Medicine, 2nd ed. www.accessmedicine.com. Copyright © McGraw-Hill Education. All rights reserved.)

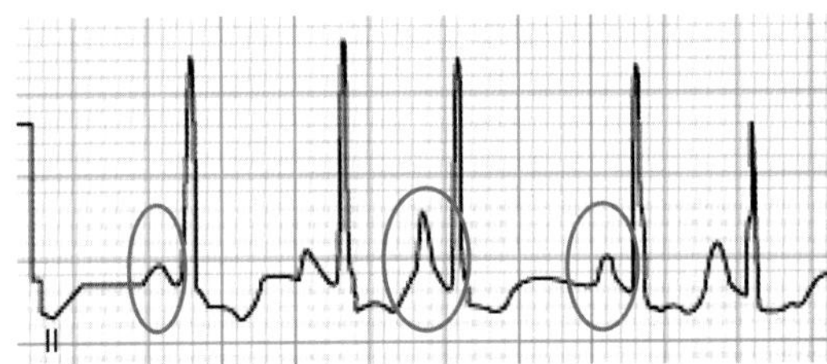

FIGURE 4-26. P-waves in Multifocal atrial tachycardia

Rhythm – There is a P wave before every QRS and a QRS after every P wave. There are at least 3 distinct P-wave morphologies (see the P waves circled in Figure 4-26). Note that the R-R interval (and the P-P interval!) is irregularly irregular.

Axis – Positive in leads I and aVF. The axis is normal.

Intervals – PR interval is less than 200 ms. QRS complex is narrow. QT interval is less than half the R-R interval.

P wave – The P-wave axis and morphology differ from beat to beat.

QRS complex – QRS is narrow. There are Q waves in lead V1 and V2 (Q waves in lead V1 – and sometimes V2 – are more often than not normal variants). The Q waves in this ECG are likely not "pathologic" Q waves.

ST segment and T wave – There are no ST elevations or depressions. T-wave inversions are present in leads II, III, and aVF.

ECG summary – Irregularly irregular, narrow, complex tachycardia with at least 3 distinct P-wave morphologies consistent with MAT. Also noted are inferior T-wave inversions.

Aside from the distinct P-wave morphologies, MAT is distinguished from other narrow complex tachycardias by the irregular P-P interval (compared to sinus tachycardia and atrial tachycardia, which both exhibit regular P-P intervals). Also note that patients with 3 or more P-wave morphologies but a normal heart rate are said to have wandering atrial pacemaker (WAP). Classically, the threshold to distinguish MAT from WAP was 100 bpm, though recent studies have suggested that a cutoff of 90 bpm is more clinically useful. Treatment of MAT is focused on addressing the underlying pathology (most commonly an acute cardiac or pulmonary condition), though AV nodal blockers (e.g., beta blockers) can be used to treat symptoms related to the tachycardia. In this patient, consideration should be given to rate-related inferior ischemia (due to the T-wave inversions).

Answer: MAT

CASE 6

A 65-year-old woman presents to the emergency department with acute-onset dyspnea and palpitations. The ECG is shown in Figure 4-27.

Rate – 102 bpm (17 beats per 10-second strip multiplied by 6).

Rhythm – There are no discernable P waves. The R-R intervals are irregularly irregular.

Axis – Positive in lead I and isoelectric in lead aVF. We can use the fact that lead II is net positive as a "tiebreaker" to show that the axis is normal (see Table 4-1).

Intervals – There is no discernable PR interval because there are no P waves. The QRS complex is narrow. The QT interval is less than half the R-R interval.

P wave – There are no discernable P waves.

QRS complex – QRS is narrow (less than 120 ms). S wave in V1 + R wave in V5 is less than 35 mm; there is no LVH. There are no pathologic Q waves.

ST segment and T wave – There are no ST elevations, ST depressions, or T-wave inversions.

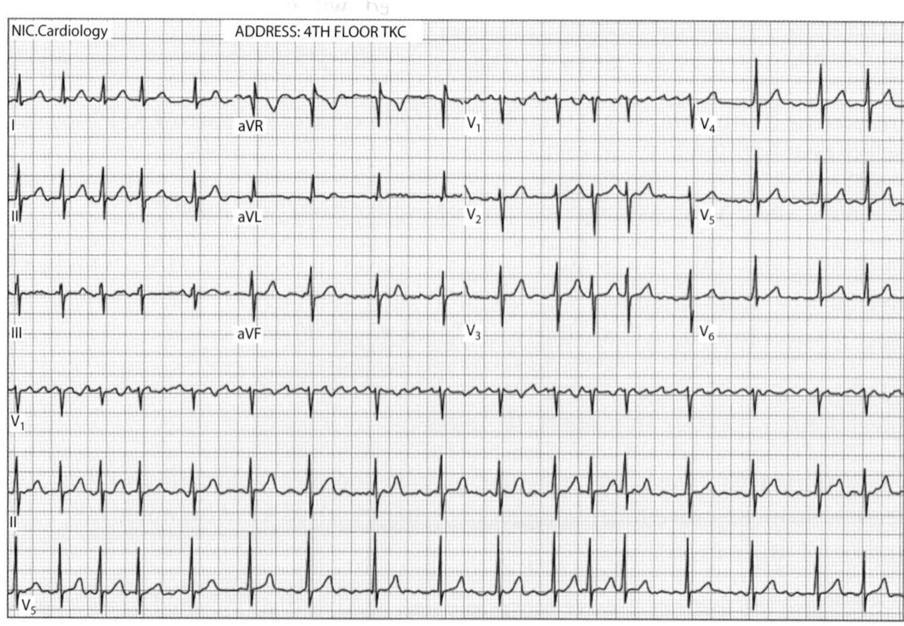

FIGURE 4-27. ECG for case 6 (Reproduced, with permission, from Fuster V, Harrington RA, Narula J, Eapen ZJ. *Hurst's The Heart*, 14th ed. www.accessmedicine.com. Copyright © McGraw-Hill Education. All rights reserved.)

ECG summary – Irregularly irregular narrow complex tachycardia without discernable P waves; this is atrial fibrillation with rapid ventricular response (> 100 bpm).

The differential diagnosis for an irregular narrow complex tachycardia includes MAT and atrial flutter with variable AV block. This ECG is distinguished from both atrial flutter and MAT by the lack of discernable P waves. You may have noted that the higher-amplitude atrial waves in lead V1 look confusingly similar to the stereotypical 200 to 300 bpm atrial reentrant rhythm ("sawtooth") of atrial flutter. The key difference is that the atrial waves in V1 here are disorganized and irregular, in contrast to the organized and regular atrial impulses found in flutter. Interestingly, high-amplitude (>2 mm) fibrillatory waves are more commonly found in new-onset atrial fibrillation and are sometimes referred to as "coarse A-fib" (though please note that the amplitude in V1 here is in fact less than 2 mm).

Answer: Atrial fibrillation

CASE 7

A 35-year-old woman presents to the emergency department with syncope 1 month after a camping trip during which she had noted onset of an erythematous rash with central clearing. The ECG is shown in Figure 4-28.

Rate – 42 bpm (7 beats per 10-second strip multiplied by 6).

Rhythm – There is no consistent relationship between the P wave and the QRS complex. This is AV dissociation.

Axis – Positive in lead I and aVF. The axis is normal.

Intervals – There is no consistent PR interval due to AV dissociation. The QRS complex is narrow. The QT interval is less than half the R-R interval.

P wave – Positive in leads I and II, negative in aVR; P axis is normal. You can actually calculate the "atrial" rate as 60 bpm (10 P waves per 10-second strip multiplied by 6). Note that one P wave is "buried" within the third QRS complex.

QRS complex – QRS is narrow (less than 120 ms). S wave in V1 + R wave in V5 is less than 35 mm. There are no pathologic Q waves.

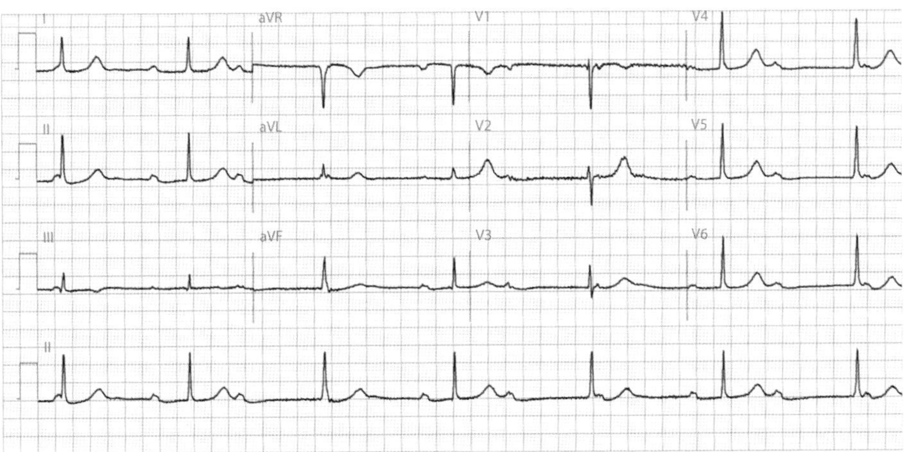

FIGURE 4-28. (Reproduced, with permission, from Jameson JL, Fauci AF, Kasper DL, et al, eds: *Harrison's Principles of Internal Medicine*, 20th ed. www.accessmedicine.com. Copyright © McGraw-Hill Education. All rights reserved.)

ST segment and T wave – There are no ST elevations or depressions. There is an isolated T-wave inversion in lead III.

ECG summary – Third-degree (complete) heart block with an atrial (sinus) rate of approximately 60 bpm and an effective heart rate of 40 bpm. The narrow QRS complex indicates an AV junctional source of the escape rhythm. Third-degree AV block is a clinical emergency that typically requires permanent pacemaker placement unless a reversible etiology is present. This patient has Lyme-related carditis, and her conduction disorder is likely to resolve with intravenous (IV) antibiotics and close monitoring (with or without temporary cardiac pacing).

Answer: Complete heart block

CASE 8

A 65-year-old woman presents to the emergency department with pneumonia. The ECG is shown in Figure 4-29.

Rate – 48 bpm (8 beats per 10-second strip multiplied by 6).

Rhythm – There is a P wave before every QRS, but there is not a QRS after every P wave (there are "dropped" beats). The PR intervals progressively lengthen prior to the dropped beat.

Axis – Positive in lead I aVF. The axis is normal.

Intervals – PR intervals progressively lengthen prior to the dropped beat. The QRS complex is narrow. The QT interval is less than half the R-R interval.

P wave – Positive in lead II, negative in aVR; P axis is probably normal. There is no evidence of atrial enlargement.

QRS complex – QRS is narrow (less than 120 ms). S wave in V1 + R wave in V5 is greater than 35 mm; there is LVH. There are no pathologic Q waves.

ST segment and T wave – There are no ST elevations. There are T-wave inversions in the inferior leads (II, III, aVF), as well as the precordial leads V2 to V5.

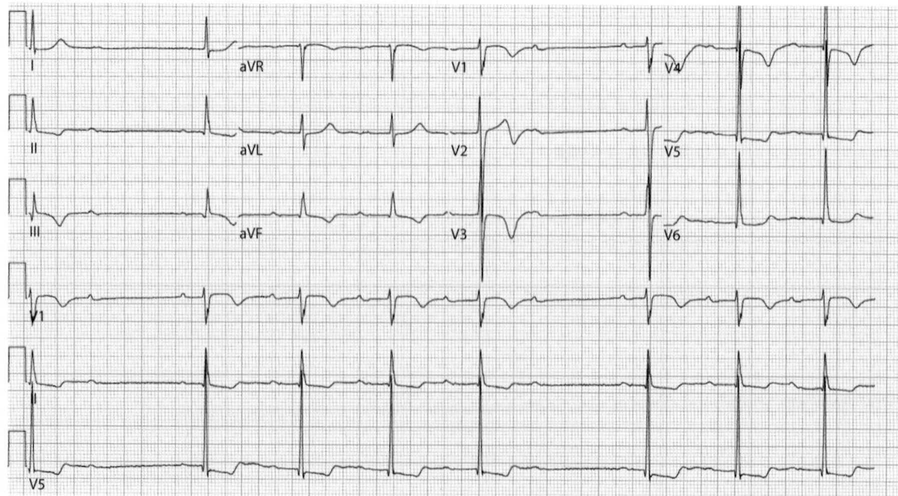

FIGURE 4-29. (From Papadakis MA, McPhee SJ, Rabow MW. *Current Medical Diagnosis & Treatment 2020*. Copyright © McGraw-Hill Education. All rights reserved. Used, with permission, from Jose Sanchez, MD.)

ECG summary – This is type I second-degree AV block (aka Mobitz I or Wenckebach) because the PR interval progressively lengthens prior to the dropped beat. The T-wave inversions and depressions should be compared to a baseline ECG. If the T waves are stable from prior and there are no clinical signs of acute coronary syndrome, these findings may indicate repolarization abnormalities due to LVH.

Answer: Type I Mobitz

CASE 9

A 65-year-old woman with a history of coronary artery disease presents to the emergency department with chest pain. The ECG is shown in Figure 4-30.

Rate – 214 bpm (300 divided by 1.4 large boxes between each R wave). You could also count 36 QRS complexes in one 10-second strip and multiply by 6 with a similar result.

Rhythm – There is no consistent relationship between P waves and QRS complexes, indicating AV dissociation. In the enlarged tracing from lead II (Figure 4-31), the P waves are highlighted with arrows.

Axis – Negative in lead I, positive in aVF. This is right axis deviation.

Intervals – Unable to determine a PR interval. The QRS complex is wide (>120 ms).

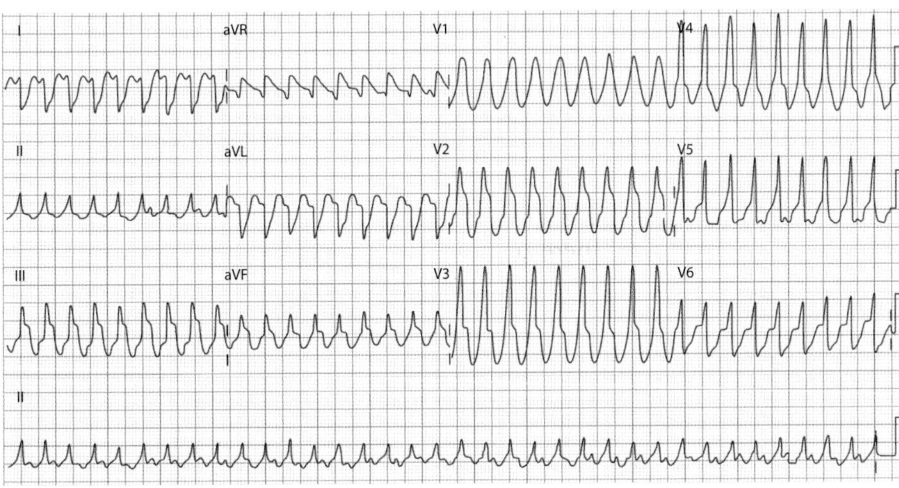

FIGURE 4-30. (Reproduced, with permission, from Klamen DL, Hingle ST. *Resident Readiness™: Internal Medicine*. www.accessmedicine.com. Copyright © The McGraw-Hill Companies, Inc. All rights reserved.)

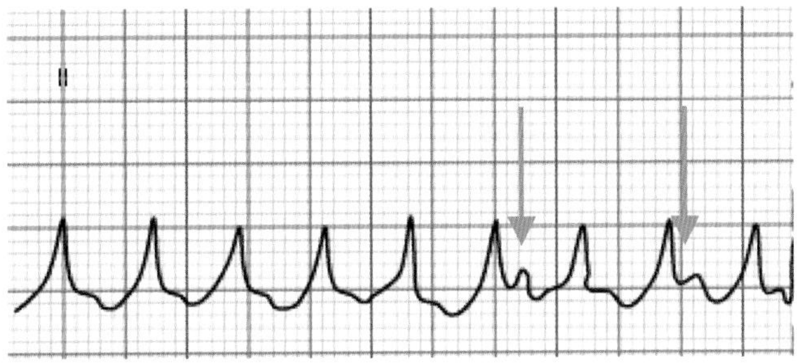

FIGURE 4-31. P-waves in AV dissociation

P wave – It is difficult to comment on P wave morphology because the observed P waves occur during repolarization.

QRS complex – QRS is wide.

ST segment and T wave – It is nearly impossible to assess for ST-segment and T-wave changes in the setting of this wide complex tachycardia.

ECG summary – Wide complex tachycardia with AV dissociation and right axis deviation consistent with ventricular tachycardia (VT). The observed AV dissociation effectively rules out SVT; indeed, in the setting of wide complex tachycardia, AV dissociation (as well as capture or fusion beats) is pathognomonic for VT. Importantly, AV dissociation, capture beats, and fusion beats all have low sensitivity for the detection of VT (many patients with VT will not show any of these signs on ECG). A wide complex tachycardia is thus presumed to be VT until proven otherwise.

Answer: Ventricular tachycardia

CASE 10

A 65-year-old man presents to the emergency department with palpitations and lightheadedness. The ECG is shown in Figure 4-32.

Rate – 188 bpm (300 divided by 1.6 large boxes between each R wave). You could also count 30 QRS complexes in one 10-second strip and multiply by 6 with a similar result.

Rhythm – The R-R interval is regular. On first glance, there are no observable P waves. On close inspection, there are "retrograde" P waves immediately after the QRS complex, best visualized in lead aVR (the first 3 retrograde P waves are highlighted with arrows in Figure 4-33).

Axis – Positive in lead I, negative in aVF. Lead II is also negative, indicating left axis deviation.

Intervals – Unable to determine a PR interval. The QRS complex is narrow (<120 ms).

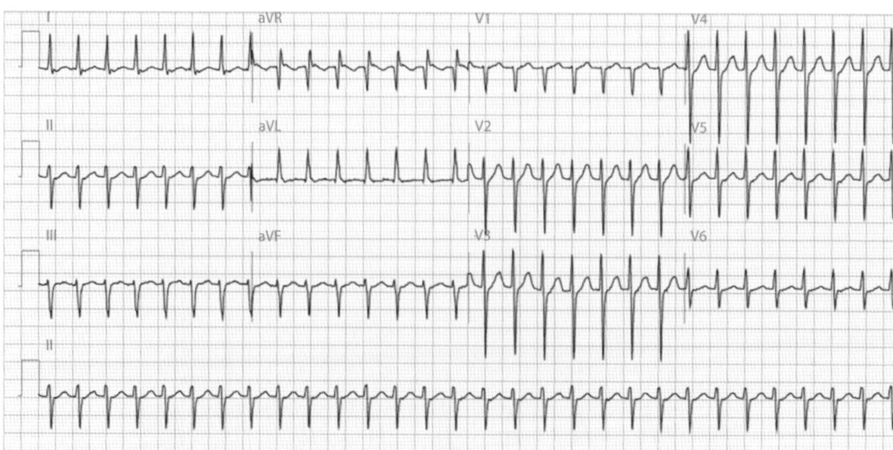

FIGURE 4-32. (Reproduced, with permission, from Jameson JL, Fauci AF, Kasper DL, et al, eds: *Harrison's Principles of Internal Medicine*, 20th ed. www.accessmedicine.com. Copyright © McGraw-Hill Education. All rights reserved.)

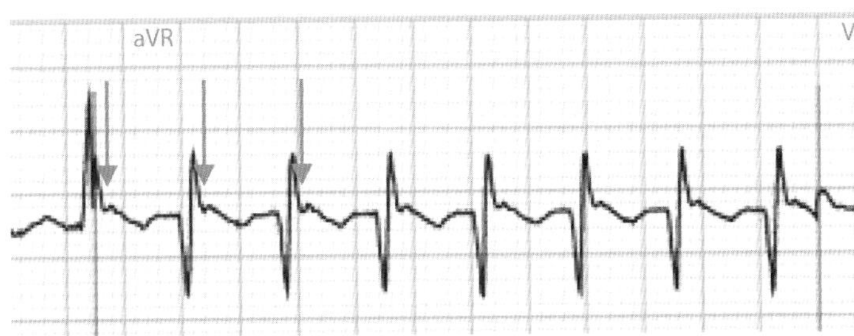

FIGURE 4-33. Retrograde P waves in Ventricular Tachycardia

P wave – The retrograde P wave in lead aVR is positive.

QRS complex – QRS is narrow (less than 120 ms). S wave in V1 + R wave in V5 is less than 35 mm. There are no pathologic Q waves (note the small upward R wave in leads II, III, and aVF; the subsequent downward deflection is therefore an S wave and not a Q wave).

ST segment and T wave – There are no ST elevations, ST depressions, or T-wave inversions.

ECG summary – Regular narrow complex tachycardia with retrograde P waves consistent with AVnRT. In AVnRT or AVRT, there is a reentrant loop through the AV node that simultaneously excites the ventricles and the atria. The resultant "retrograde" P waves are sometimes buried within, or observed just after, the QRS complex. Retrograde P waves typically have an opposite axis from a "sinus" P wave originating from the SA node (because the depolarization starts from the opposite side of the atria). Indeed, in this ECG, the retrograde P wave in aVR is positive, while a "sinus" P wave should be negative in aVR. In both AVnRT and AVRT, the P waves are often entirely hidden, and adenosine is required to unveil them.

Answer: AVnRT

CHAPTER 5 EVIDENCE-BASED MEDICINE

OVERVIEW OF HIGH-YIELD TOPICS IN EVIDENCE-BASED MEDICINE

INTRODUCTION TO EVIDENCE-BASED MEDICINE

"Evidence-based medicine is the conscientious and judicious use of current best evidence from clinical care research into the management of individual patients."[1]

KEY ASPECTS OF EVIDENCE BASED MEDICINE

- Evidence-based medicine (EBM) involves the synthesis of the best available external evidence with your existing clinical expertise to craft data-driven plans that are in keeping with the patient's values and expectations.
- Developing a comfort level with appraising and applying evidence from the literature is essential for excellent clinical care and leadership in medicine.
- We generally think of the EBM cycle as having four key steps: ASK (asking a searchable question), ACQUIRE (acquiring the best study from the literature), APPRAISE (appraising the quality of the study), and APPLY (applying the study results to specific patients). See Figure 5-1.

RELEVANCE TO THE INTERNAL MEDICINE CLERKSHIP/WARDS

- **Developing and maintaining clinical skills**: We have data that suggest that there is a consistently negative relationship between years of experience and clinical knowledge (that is, the longer you are in practice, the lower you score on medical knowledge–based examinations). EBM gives you the skills to build and maintain your clinical knowledge base by incorporating new evidence into practice.

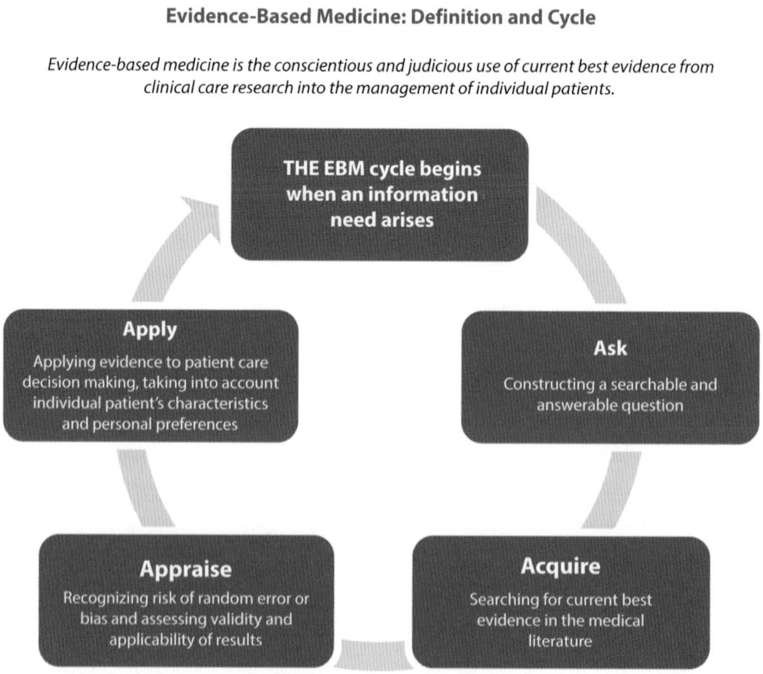

FIGURE 5-1. EBM cycle. (Figure created using data from Sackett DL, Rosenberg WM, Gray JA, Haynes RB, Richardson WS. Evidence based medicine: what it is and what it isn't. *BMJ.* 1996; 312(7023): 71-72 and Guyatt G, Drummond R, Meade MO, Cook DJ. *Users' Guides to the Medical Literature: A Manual for Evidence-Based Clinical Practice*, 3rd ed. McGraw-Hill Professional; 2014.)

- **Excellent clinical care**: EBM principles enable you to take data from the literature and, after careful consideration, choose (or not) to apply it to individual patients you are seeing on the wards.
- **Teaching your colleagues**: As a student, you are often expected to present about topics on rounds (attendings will often ask you: "tell us about [X] on rounds tomorrow"), which can sometimes feel stressful as the most junior member of the medical team. In addition to reviewing the basics of clinical manifestations, diagnosis, and treatment of chosen conditions, bringing current evidence to your presentations to the team is an outstanding way to ensure that everyone is engaged and learning.
- **Success on the wards**: Internal medicine (IM) is a very evidence-driven field, and IM will likely be one of the rotations where data are cited most often on rounds. Being comfortable with bringing evidence to the care of your patients, and using data to support your diagnostic and therapeutic strategies, is an important way to stand apart from your peers and succeed on the clerkship.

FOUR KEY STEPS TO EBM

ASK

Background Vs. Foreground Questions

Asking clear and searchable clinical questions is the first step in applying evidence to the care of your patients. It can be helpful to divide these into background vs. foreground questions.

- **Background questions**: These are questions on general knowledge about conditions, illnesses, patterns of disease, and pathophysiology (e.g., **ASK:** What microbial organism most commonly causes community acquired pneumonia (CAP)? **ASK:** What findings on chest x-ray [CXR] establish a diagnosis of CAP?)
- **Foreground questions:** These are questions on specific knowledge to inform clinical decisions or actions and tend to be more complex and specific than background questions. They often relate to a specific patient or particular population. (e.g., **ASK:** In patients with CAP, do clinical features predict outcome well enough that low-risk patients can be treated as outpatients?). You can use the PICO(T)(T) format (see next) to structure your foreground questions.

Pico(T)(T) Format Questions

PICO(T)(T) Format:

P: Patient/Population

I: Intervention/Exposure

C: Comparison/Control

O: Outcome(s)

(T): Type of Question (Therapy vs. Diagnosis vs. Prognosis vs. Etiology)

(T): Type of Study

- **Example #1:** You are wondering about what blood pressure to target for a patient with hypertension and type 2 diabetes. This might lead to the searchable question: In patients with hypertension and diabetes (P), does tight control with a systolic blood pressure (SBP) target of 120 (I) vs. typical control with SBP target of <140 (C) result in superior cardiovascular outcomes (O)? This is a Therapy question, and as such, our ideal study would be either a randomized controlled trial (RCT) or a meta-analysis.
- **Example #2:** You have a patient admitted for a chronic obstructive pulmonary disease (COPD) exacerbation, and your resident suggests treating the patient with steroids for only 5 days; you are wondering about the evidence for duration of therapy in COPD exacerbations. This might lead to the searchable question: In patients with COPD exacerbations (P), does a 5-day course of steroids (I) vs. longer courses of steroids (C) result in equivalent respiratory outcomes with regard to symptom burden, readmission risk, and mortality (O)? This is a Therapy question, and as such, our ideal study would be either an RCT or a meta-analysis.

ACQUIRE

Levels of Evidence

How to search through the various search engines is beyond the scope of this book. But it is important to understand what the types of studies are and to know the hierarchy of study types. This hierarchy does not always hold true (e.g., a really well-done cohort study may have better validity and applicability than a very poorly performed randomized controlled trial). In general, studies can be ordered in terms of strength of evidence as follows:

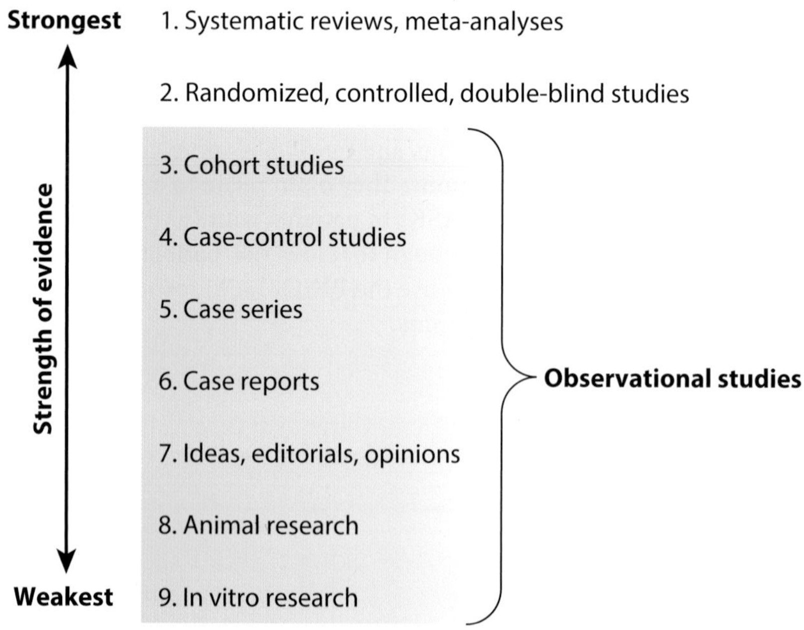

FIGURE 5-2. Hierarchy of evidence.

Study Types

1. **RCT**: Patients are randomly assigned to either the group receiving the intervention or to a group serving as a control (receiving either the standard of care or a placebo).
2. **Meta-analysis**: A statistical analysis combining the results of multiple studies. May include a systematic review (finding all studies fitting a set of inclusion criteria through a systematic search process) or the investigators may be just combining a few nonsystematically chosen studies together.
3. **Cross-sectional study**: Also known as an observational study, this uses population-level data at one point in time. Often very large studies from health systems or national health systems are used. The sample size is often the main advantage, but as data only reflect one point in time, you can only show associations (correlations) and cannot show causation.
4. **Case-control study**: This is also an observational study. The first step is to choose the disease of interest and a carefully selected control population. Then look backwards in time for an exposure. The main validity issue is recall bias. Studies will rely on odds ratios to show statistical significance. When the disease in question is rare, the odds ratio will approximate the relative risk (rare diseases assumption).

- **Cohort study**: This is also an observational study. The first step is to choose the exposure or risk factor of interest and find a cohort of patients with the exposure (and one without as a control). Then you will either look backwards in time (retrospective cohort) or forward in time (prospective cohort) for the outcome of interest. These tend to be the highest-quality observational studies with the potential ability to draw causal inferences. As with other observational studies, however, there are limitations in the ability to control for unknown confounders.

APPRAISAL

How you appraise and apply a study depend on what kind of study it is. Generally, studies for appraisal and application are grouped into the following categories: diagnostic, therapy, prognosis, and etiology studies. The vast majority of articles are therapy or diagnostic studies, so we will focus on how to appraise and apply these types of studies.

Evaluating Diagnostic Studies

1. **Bias in diagnostic studies:** You should evaluate all diagnostic studies for:
    - **Spectrum bias:** A type of sampling bias that can affect sensitivity and specificity of a test. It occurs when a test is studied in a different population than it would be applied in (e.g., a study looking at brain natriuretic peptide [BNP] where they compare results in patients in cardiogenic shock with healthy volunteers in order to calculate sensitivity and specificity, when the actual test would be performed in undifferentiated patients with shortness of breath [SOB]). When looking at initial data for a new diagnostic test, the main question to ask is if the test is being used in an appropriate clinical setting where real diagnostic uncertainty exists.
    - **Verification bias**: A type of measurement bias that can affect sensitivity and specificity. It occurs when the gold standard is not given to all patients in a diagnostic study. For example, in the original PIOPED

study[2] looking at the use of ventilation/perfusion (V/Q) scanning in the diagnosis of pulmonary embolism (PE), patients whose V/Q scans were interpreted as normal and had negative lower extremity ultrasound did not need to undergo pulmonary angiography per the protocol (only ~70% did get angiography to formally exclude PE); however, those with abnormalities on V/Q scans did generally get pulmonary angiography (>90% with abnormal V/Q scans had a pulmonary angiogram). By not performing the gold standard (pulmonary angiography) on all patients, you potentially exclude patients from analysis (since they didn't have a final diagnosis) or mistakenly misclassify patients, thereby affecting sensitivity and specificity.

2. **Considerations in application of results from diagnostic studies**
   - **Population studied:** In the study being examined, was the test performed on a similar population as the patient you are considering using the test on?
   - **Description of methods**: Was the use of the test described in sufficient detail to allow use in other settings?

Evaluating Therapy Studies

Steps in the appraisal of therapy articles include assessment of 1) internal validity, 2) results, and 3) external validity. Then decisions must be individualized to specific patients for application.

1. **Internal validity**: Do the results of the study apply to the patients in the study itself? Or were there such significant methodologic flaws that the results were rendered uninterpretable?
   - **Randomization:** The goal is to create a prognostic balance between the 2 groups to limit the impact of known and unknown confounders. Can assess success by the balance of demographics and known confounders (Table 1 of a therapeutic study).
   - **Allocation concealment:** Steps taken to conceal what group patients will be assigned to when randomized in the study. Usually done via centralized computing. The concern is that if the person randomizing the patients knows what group they will be assigned to, it may affect their decision to enroll the patient.
   - **Blinding:** Preventing study participants from knowing what group they are in, ideally, by double-blinding the study (patient and investigators). Prevents expectancy bias (preserves placebo effect).
   - **Study follow-up and attrition**: You need to make sure all patients are accounted for and that dropout rates are low (high rates can lead to attrition bias, a type of selection bias). Can confirm tracking of patients via CONSORT flow diagram (usually labeled as Figure 1 in the paper).
   - **Intention-to-treat analysis**: Results are based on the initial treatment assigned during randomization and not on what was received. This preserves the prognostic balance generated via randomization.

2. **Results**: Are the results statistically significant (as assessed by p-values)? Are they clinically significant (is the magnitude of benefit sufficiently large as to be clinically meaningful)? See Treatment: Application later.

3. **External validity**: Can the results of the study be applied to patients outside the study population? The key question is: Are there compelling reasons why the study doesn't apply to my patient? Considerations may include:
   - **Patient population:** Would my patient have been included in the study? Are patients in the study similar to my patient in terms of comorbid conditions, current therapies, and severity of disease?
   - **Comparator:** Is the intervention in the study being compared against the appropriate thing? Does the choice in the study reflect real-world choices? For example, the National Lung Screening Trial (NLST)[3] established the benefit of computed tomography (CT) screening for lung cancer. The study compared CT screening for lung cancer with annual CXR screening; however, during the entirety of the study period, most guidelines explicitly recommended against using CXR as a screening modality for lung cancer.
   - **Replicability:** Is the trial protocol something I could apply in real practice? For example, the interventions in some studies may not be realistic, depending on clinic hospital staffing (e.g., symptom-based treatment of alcohol withdrawal using the Clinical Institute Withdrawal Assessment (CIWA) protocol, or many sepsis treatment protocols).
   - **Outcome measures:** Is the outcome evaluated in the study the main outcome I would care about with my patient? Was the duration of follow-up sufficiently long? Were adverse events reported sufficiently well to assess the potential benefits and harms to my patient?

APPLICATION

Diagnosis and Clinical Reasoning: Application

The results of studies are often reported in different ways. Following are definitions of commonly used terms that are helpful when applying study results to diagnosis and clinical reasoning. After the definitions, we describe a stepwise approach to using the results in diagnosis and clinical reasoning.

Prevalence and Incidence

- **Prevalence:** Proportion of a population with the condition in question. Calculated as the number of cases divided by the number in the total population. Indicates how widespread a disease is.
- **Incidence:** Risk of occurrence of a condition in a population within a specific time period. Calculated as the number of new cases divided by the population size, divided by the time period (e.g., 17 cases per 1,000,000 persons per year). Indicates the risk of contracting the disease.

	Disease Present (+)	Disease Absent (−)
Positive Test Result	True Positive (TP)	False Positive (FP)
Negative Test Result	False Negative (FN)	True Negative (TN)

Sensitivity and Specificity

We care about sensitivity and specificity before we order a test. They are characteristics of the test itself and are not affected by changes in prevalence.

- **Sensitivity**: Of all the patients who have the disease, the proportion that will test positive. Calculated as: TP / (TP + FN). Only looks at those who have disease. Screening tests should be sensitive. A highly sensitive test means that there is a low false-negative rate.

- **Specificity**: Of all the patients who are disease free, the proportion that will test negative. Calculated as: TN / (TN + FP). Only looks at those who are disease free. Confirmatory tests should be specific. A highly specific test means there is a low false-positive rate.

Positive and Negative Predictive Values

Rarely used or discussed in actual practice, as they are very dependent on disease prevalence. In practice, we generally use likelihood ratios instead.

- **Positive predictive value**: Of all patients who test positive, the proportion who actually has the disease. Calculated as: TP / (TP + FP).
- **Negative predictive value**: Of all patients who test negative, the proportion who does not have the disease. Calculated as: TN / (TN + FN).

Positive and Negative Likelihood Ratios

Used to interpret the results of tests once they come back. As they are derived from sensitivity and specificity alone, they are not dependent on disease prevalence. You can look up the sensitivity/specificity and likelihood ratios (LR) for most physical examination maneuvers and laboratory/imaging tests.

- **Positive likelihood ratio**: Calculated as Sens / (1 – Spec) = (Proportion of patients who have disease who will test positive) / (Proportion of patients who do not have the disease who test positive). A positive LR of 10 means that a positive result is 10 times more likely to be a true positive result than a false positive result.
- **Negative likelihood ratio**: Calculated as (1 – Sens) / Spec = (Proportion of patients who have the disease who will test negative) / (Proportion of patients who have the disease who will test negative). A negative LR of 0.1 means that a negative result is one-tenth as likely to be a false negative than a true negative (or 10 times more likely to be a true negative than a false negative).

Clinical Reasoning Using Evidence

- **Step #1:** Using your clinical expertise (history and physical examination) or prediction tools (e.g., Wells criteria for outpatient deep vein thrombosis [DVT]), determine the pretest probabilities for items on your differential.
- **Step #2:** Consider your possible diagnostic tests and their associated sensitivity/specificity and LRs. Tests with high positive LRs (at least greater than 5.0) are good at confirming the diagnosis, as they will significantly increase the probability of disease with a positive result. Tests with very low negative LRs (at least less than 0.2) are good at excluding the diagnosis, as they will significantly decrease the probability of disease with a negative result.
- **Step #3:** Depending on your posttest probability of disease after initial testing, you may elect to empirically treat (if very high probability), consider further diagnostic options (if intermediate probability), or move onto other diagnostic possibilities (if very low probability).
- For the mathematically inclined, you can use Fagan nomograms or online LR calculators to model exact posttest probabilities based on your assessment of pretest probabilities and the diagnostic maneuver or to test LRs.

TREATMENT: APPLICATION

	Outcome (+)	No Outcome (−)
Intervention or Exposure	A	B
Control	C	D

The results of studies are often reported in different ways. Following are definitions of commonly used terms that are helpful when applying study results to treatment.

MEASURES OF ASSOCIATION (RELATIVE RISK, HAZARD RATIOS)

The following measure how likely an event will occur in an exposed group.

- **Relative risk (RR)**: Risk of developing a disease in the exposed group divided by the risk in the unexposed group. Calculated as: [A / A + B] / [C / C + D]. Measured at one particular point in time (e.g., 1 year into therapy).
- **Hazard ratio**: Much more commonly seen in journals. Hazard ratios are cumulative over time and reflect the "hazard" of the event at any point in time. Cannot be calculated by hand, since they are the sum of the risk at any given point. Interpreted similarly to RR.

RELATIVE RISK REDUCTION

- Tells how much the treatment reduced the risk of bad outcomes relative to the control group who did not have the treatment.
- To calculate relative risk reduction (RRR), either need the RR or need to know the control event rate (CER = C / C + D) and the experimental event rate (EER = A / A + B).
- Calculated as either 1 – RR or (CER – EER) / CER
- Commonly cited in studies, but can tend to overstate the magnitude of the effect.

ABSOLUTE RISK REDUCTION AND NUMBER NEEDED TO TREAT

- The absolute risk reduction (ARR) is the difference in event rates between the control and the intervention and gives you the absolute benefit of the therapy. Calculated as: ARR = CER – EER
- The number needed to treat (NNT) is calculated as 1 / ARR and reflects the number of patients you would need to treat to have one patient not have the outcome in question (e.g., If a new medication X caused an ARR of death of 2%, the NNT would be 1 / 0.02 = 50. This would be interpreted as: "If I treat 50 patients with medication X, I will prevent one death").
- There is no universal consensus about what number makes for a "good" NNT. The main considerations would include the duration of therapy required to achieve the outcome in question and the clinical significance of the outcome. In general, a NNT of less than 100 for a clinically significant outcome (e.g., reduction in myocardial infarctions, reduction in

hospitalizations, reduction in mortality), if achieved over a relatively short period (e.g., a few years or shorter), would indicate that a therapy is worth considering.

ATTRIBUTABLE RISK AND NUMBER NEEDED TO HARM

- **Attributable risk (AR)**: Difference in risk between exposed and unexposed groups. Typically used in cohort studies, but can be used to determine risk of adverse events in therapy trials. Calculated as the adverse event rate in the experimental arm minus the adverse event rate in the control arm.
- The number needed to harm (NNH) can be calculated as 1 / AR and reflects the number of patients who need to be treated with a therapy to have one patient be harmed by an adverse event. For example, if a new medication for pneumonia caused nausea, with 10% in the intervention arm having the side effect and 5% in the control arm having the side effect in the study in question, the AR would be 5% (10% – 5%) and the NNH would be 20 (1 / 0.05). This would mean that if we treat 20 patients with the new medication, 1 patient would develop nausea as a consequence of the medication.
- Comparing the NNT and NNH is often a useful way to see if a therapy's benefits outweigh the risks.

EBM WORKED EXAMPLE: PRIMARY PREVENTION WITH STATINS

CLINICAL CASE: You are seeing a 55-year-old male patient in clinic for routine follow-up. He is a current smoker (1 pack per day [PPD]) who is not interested in quitting but otherwise has no past medical history. You checked a screening lipid panel at the last visit, which came back with total cholesterol 252, low-density lipoprotein (LDL) 147, high-density lipoprotein (HDL) 48, and triglycerides 164. You calculate the patient's atherosclerotic cardiovascular disease (ASCVD) risk as 10.5%, so according to the guidelines would recommend statin therapy, but you are curious about the magnitude of benefit in this patient.

ASK: Our unfocused question is about the benefit of primary prevention with statin therapy (treatment of patients to prevent risk of cardiovascular events in patients without prior history of coronary artery disease [CAD]).

P: In adults without CAD
I: Does statin therapy
C: As compared to no intervention
O: Reduce risk of cardiovascular death
T (Type of Question): Therapy
T (Type of Study): RCT or Meta-analysis

ACQUIRE: You find the WOSCOPS study while searching the literature.[4]

APPRAISE
Inclusion/Exclusion Criteria: Patients aged 45 to 64 years old with total cholesterol of at least 252 with no prior history of myocardial infarction. Patients were excluded if they had known CAD, prior history of arrhythmias, or other serious illnesses.

1. **Internal validity:** *The study has good internal validity, meaning the results are interpretable.*
    - **Randomization:** Randomized to pravastatin or placebo via blocked randomization (stratified by trial site). On review of table below, there is no statistically significant differences between the 2 groups (indicating prognostic balance on known confounders and, we might assume, unknown confounders).
    - **Allocation concealment:** Centralized call center
    - **Blinding:** Double-blind (patient, doctors/investigators). No formal assessment of success of blinding, though they did note that there was no significant difference in withdrawal rates between the 2 groups (and if placebo patients knew they were taking a placebo, we would expect them to drop out at higher rates).
    - **Study follow-up and attrition:** Similar rates of dropout between the 2 groups, around 30% dropout rate at 5 years.
    - **Intention-to-treat (ITT) analysis:** All clinical end points analyzed using ITT analysis. However, in Figure 1 of the paper they did include LDL-lowering results for both an ITT analysis and an actual treatment analysis, but we would only be interested in the ITT.

2. **Results:** *The study has results that are statistically significant and potentially clinically meaningful.*
    - **Primary outcome:** Occurrence of nonfatal myocardial infarction or death from coronary heart disease as a first event.
    - **Other outcomes:** Death from coronary heart disease or nonfatal myocardial infarctions.

	Cardiac Death (+)	Cardiac Survival (−)
Pravastatin	50	3252
Placebo	73	3220

- Control event rate (CER): 73 / (73 + 3220) = 0.0222 = 2.22%
- Experimental event rate (EER): 50 / (50 + 3252) = 0.0151 = 1.51%
- Relative risk (EER / CER): 0.0151 / 0.0222 = 0.68
- Relative risk reduction (1 − RR or [CER − EER] / CER) = 32%
- Absolute risk reduction (CER − EER) = 0.71%
- Number needed to treat (1 / ARR) = 140 (would need to treat 140 patients for 4.9 years [the average duration of patient enrollment in study] to prevent one cardiac death)

3. **External validity:** Though the patients were all from one particular location (Scotland), the study has fairly general inclusion criteria reflecting a primary prevention population with elevated lipids. The study had long follow-up with clinically relevant end points. The intervention could easily be replicated in other settings. There is no clear and compelling reason why the results of this study would not apply to a more general population.

APPLY: Returning to the study design, the patient would have met criteria for inclusion in the trial. In Table 1 in the paper we can see that the patient is similar to the patients in the study – our patient is 55, which is the average age of the study. Our patient has a total cholesterol of 252, which is slightly lower than the average cholesterol in the study (272). Our patient is a smoker, as are 44% of the patients in the study. As such, we may expect our patient to derive a similar benefit to patients in the study. Based on our ARR of less than 1% and our NNT of 160 (×4.9 years), we know the magnitude of the benefit is somewhat small, but it is a reduction in the risk of death, and adverse events in the study were minimal. Therefore, we would recommend the therapy for the patient with some degree of confidence.

REFERENCES

1. Sackett DL, Rosenberg WMC, Gray JAM, Haynes RB, Richardson WS. Evidence based medicine: What it is and what it isn't. *BMJ*. 1996;312:71-72.

2. PIOPED Investigators. Value of the ventilation/perfusion scan in acute pulmonary embolism. Results of the prospective investigation of pulmonary embolism diagnosis (PIOPED). *JAMA*. 1990;263:2753.

3. National Lung Screening Trial Research Team, Aberle DR, Adams AM, et al. Reduced lung-cancer mortality with low-dose computed tomographic screening. *N Engl J Med*. 2011;365:395.

SECTION II

KNOWLEDGE FOR THE MEDICINE CLERKSHIP

CHAPTER 6 CARDIOLOGY

OVERVIEW OF HIGH-YIELD TOPICS IN CARDIOLOGY

CONQUER THE BOARDS!

Maximum predicted heart rate is 220 bpm minus the patient's age.

CONQUER THE WARDS!

Dobutamine is a vasodilator. Hypotension during exercise is a positive stress test; hypotension with dobutamine is not.

CARDIAC TESTING

STRESS TESTING

A stress test is a noninvasive test to assess for possible coronary artery disease (CAD) or risk of myocardial infarction (MI). The test is indicated to diagnose CAD or when patients have symptoms consistent with angina. Three different modalities can be used to measure risks for ischemia (myocardial perfusion, electrocardiogram, and echocardiogram). For each of these modalities, there are 2 ways to induce stress to the heart: excercise and pharmacologic. See table 6-1.

Types of Stress

1. Exercise stress test:
   - This is the preferred way to stress patients, as it is physiologic and offers the best sensitivity and specificity for stress tests.
   - Patients walk on a treadmill at increased levels of speed and incline to reach a heart rate that is 85% of predicted maximum for age.
   - Patients should not be taking medications that prevent the heart rate from increasing (beta blockers or digoxin).
2. Pharmacologic stress test:
   - Dobutamine is used for echocardiogram stress tests.
   - Adenosine or dipyridamole is used for myocardial perfusion stress tests. They both dilate the coronary arteries.
   - There is no pharmacologic stress test that uses an ECG.

Three Stress Test Modalities

1. ECG monitoring during stress test detects changes.
   - A test is considered positive for CAD if the patient develops ECG changes (ST elevation or depression), decrease in blood pressure, or failure to exercise more than 2 minutes due to cardiac symptoms.
     a. You cannot perform a pharmacologic stress test.
     b. This is the preferred test as long as there are no contraindications to the test.

TABLE 6-1. Stress Test Modalities

	ECG Stress Test	Myocardial Perfusion Stress Test	Echocardiography Stress Test
Exercise	Sensitivity: 68% Specificity: 77%	Sensitivity: 87% Specificity: 73%	Sensitivity: 86% Specificity: 81%
Pharmacologic		Dobutamine	Adenosine or Dipyridamole
Contraindications	ECG abnormalities, such as: 1. LBBB 2. ST depression 3. WPW 4. LVH repolarization 5. Digoxin	Side effects from the pharmacologic stress agent: 1. Asthma 2. Hypotension 3. Conduction disease	Abnormal echo at baseline: 1. LV outflow obstruction 2. Wall motion abnormalities

LBBB, Left bundle branch block; *LV,* left ventricular; *LVH,* left ventricular hypertrophy; *WPW,* Wolff-Parkinson-White.

2. Stress myocardial perfusion imaging
    - Nuclear imaging allows the visualization of the amount of blood perfusion in the myocardium using radioactive isotopes. Technetium is the most commonly used isotope.
    - "Defects" indicate that the blood is not getting to a part of the myocardial tissue (fixed defects = infarct; reversible = inducible ischemia). Reversible defects are ones that look normal at rest, but with exercise or stress, the flow becomes less. These are lesions that usually are amenable to an intervention, like angioplasty or stent, to improve blood flow. Fixed defects indicate an old scar, and interventions will not change the overall function of the heart.
3. Echocardiography
    - Wall motion abnormalities that were not present at rest but appear after exercise or dobutamine are considered a positive stress test.

ECHOCARDIOGRAM

- Using ultrasound technology, an echocardiogram provides a picture of the heart and can evaluate its function. It is used to evaluate many different types of heart disease, from valvular defects to the strength of the heart muscle. It can demonstrate an MI (either acute or old) by showing a defect in the movement of one of the walls (called "wall motion abnormality").
- There are two types of echocardiograms:
    1. Transthoracic echocardiography (TTE), where the probe is placed on the chest wall, is most commonly ordered because it is noninvasive.
    2. Transesophageal echocardiography (TEE) is a more invasive test where the ultrasound probe is placed into the esophagus, which requires some mild anesthesia. However, because of the probe's proximity to the heart, it can clearly see heart valves and clots in the heart. It is often obtained to rule out endocarditis to ensure there is no clot in the heart prior to cardioversion.
- For atrial fibrillation and to take a better look at the aorta.
- For specific uses of echocardiography, see Table 6-2.

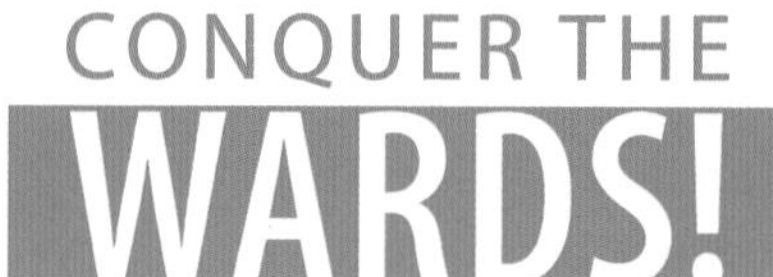

Transesophageal echo is the most common method to visualize the left atrial appendage.

TABLE 6-2. Uses of Echocardiography

Disorder	Use of Echo
Myocardial infarction	Assess wall motion abnormalities, or new valve abnormalities induced by the MI.
Heart failure	Assess ventricular function, ejection fraction.
Heart murmur	Identify and evaluate valvular disease.
Pericardial effusion	Assess volume of effusion and tamponade.
Aortic dissection	Identify presence of tear (especially TEE).
Pulmonary embolism	Identify saddle emboli or evidence of ↑ right-sided heart pressure caused by the PE.
Patent foramen ovale	Assess bubbles traversing PFO (air administered through peripheral IV).
Endocarditis	Identify vegetation, abscess (sensitivity TEE > TTE).
Congenital heart disease	Identify coarctation of the aorta, pulmonary stenosis, tetralogy of Fallot, ventricular septal defect (VSD), and atrial septal defect (ASD).

CONQUER THE **WARDS!**

MI can be silent, particularly in people with diabetes, due to neuropathy or transplanted hearts, due to denervation.

CONQUER THE **BOARDS!**

Chest pain isn't the only presentation of MI—women often only complain of nausea or dizziness as their "anginal equivalent."

TABLE 6-3. Uses of Cardiac Catheterization

Disorder	Therapy
Myocardial infarction and unstable angina	Coronary artery angiography (visualize the blockage); also can intervene with balloon dilatation of stenoses, stent placement (percutaneous transluminal coronary angioplasty [PTCA]), or laser techniques.
Valvular heart disease	"Balloon valvuloplasty": Dilatation of valves with a balloon. This can be used for mitral stenosis, pulmonary stenosis, and aortic stenosis.
Dysrhythmias	When a patient has an arrhythmia, the cause can be located and removed. This is called "electrophysiologic mapping" and radiofrequency ablation.
Myocardial disease	Biopsy of myocardium for cardiomyopathies.
Congenital heart disease	Can diagnose valvular disorder and correct in some cases (ASDs, VSDs, PFOs).
Pericardial disease	Simultaneous left and right heart catheterization will measure heart pressures and diagnose a pericardial abnormality such as restriction.

CARDIAC CATHETERIZATION

Cardiac catheterization is used for the diagnosis and treatment of many different types of heart disease.

- In *left heart catheterization*, a hollow tube is inserted through a vessel (usually the radial or femoral artery) and threaded up to the coronary vessels. Dye is injected into the coronary vessels (angiogram), and stenosis (narrowing) or blockage can be visualized and interventions such as angioplasty or stenting can be performed (see later).
- A *right heart catheterization* passes a catheter through a peripheral vein to the right atrium, ventricle, and pulmonary artery to measure pressures inside the chambers and is often used in patients with suspected pulmonary hypertension.
- For other uses of cardiac catheterization, see Table 6-3.

COMMON CAUSES OF CHEST PAIN

Chest pain is one of the most common complaints of adult patients and has a broad differential. Here we list the most common causes of chest pain and their common associated symptoms.

- **MI/angina:** Substernal or left-sided chest heaviness, pressure, or pain, typically radiating to the left arm, shoulder, or jaw. Often described as "an elephant sitting on my chest." Commonly accompanied by diaphoresis or dyspnea. *A key question* to ask is does the chest pain worsen with exertion and get better with rest.
- **Pericarditis:** Chest pain radiating to the shoulder, neck, or back; worse with deep breathing or cough (pleuritic); *relieved by sitting up and leaning forward.*
- **Aortic dissection:** Severe chest pain radiating to the back, can be associated with unequal pulses or unequal blood pressure in right and left arms. Often described as a "tearing" pain.
- **Thoracic abscess or mass:** Often sharp, localized pain; can be pleuritic.
- **Pulmonary embolism:** Often pleuritic. Frequently associated with tachypnea and tachycardia.

- **Pneumonia:** Pleuritic, frequently associated with cough, sputum, and hypoxia if severe.
- **Gastroesophageal reflux disease (GERD)/esophageal spasm/tear:** Burning pain, midline, substernal; may be associated with dysphagia. Pain made worse with lying flat, certain foods, accompanied by a bitter taste in the mouth known as "water brash." May be similar to pain of MI.
- **Costochondritis/musculoskeletal:** Sharp, localized pain with *reproducible tenderness* (touch chest wall and feel the pain); often exacerbated by exercise (second or third costochondral junction inflammation, aka Tietze syndrome).
- **Other common causes:** Peptic ulcer disease, biliary disease, herpes zoster, anxiety, pneumothorax, pleuritis (infection, systemic lupus erythematosus [SLE]).

ANGINA

Typically left-sided chest pain caused by temporary myocardial ischemia.

- **Stable angina:** A chronic, episodic, predictable pain syndrome due to temporary myocardial ischemia. The pattern of pain is similar to that of acute MI, but resolves with rest or medication. Doesn't change (i.e., it's stable). **Treatment:** Beta blocker (reduces myocardial oxygen demand), aspirin, nitroglycerin.
- **Unstable angina** (further discussed in the next section; a type of acute coronary syndrome): Defined as 1) new onset of anginal pain, 2) anginal pain that accelerates or changes in pattern location or severity, 3) anginal pain at rest. **Treatment:** See "Acute Coronary Syndromes" section.
- **Prinzmetal angina (variant angina):** Angina due to coronary vasospasm, not linked to exertion. Distinguished from unstable angina by chronic, intermittent nature. Pain usually occurs at a specific hour in the early morning. Coronary vessels are normal (no stenosis or plaques). ECG may show transient ST elevations. **Treatment:** Calcium channel blockers and nitrates to reduce vasospasm.

CONQUER THE WARDS!

Patients with angina can benefit from long-acting nitrates such as isosorbide mononitrate to help control symptoms.

CONQUER THE BOARDS!

The first step in evaluating a patient presenting with chest pain is a 12-lead ECG to look for ST segment elevation.

A 62-year-old smoker presents complaining of 3 episodes of severe chest heaviness this morning. Each episode lasted 3 to 5 minutes, but he has no pain now. He has never had this type of pain before. *Think: Unstable angina.*

CONQUER THE WARDS!

Coronary vasospasm can be seen in oncology patients being treated with 5-fluorouracil.

A middle-aged woman comes to the emergency room (ER) with severe chest pain and ST elevations on ECG. She is rushed for a cardiac catheterization, which shows no obstruction in her coronary arteries. *Think: Variant angina (aka Prinzmetal angina/vasospasm).*

HIGH-YIELD LITERATURE

Gans, C. In patients with stable angina, percutaneous coronary intervention (PCI) is as effective as placebo:

Percutaneous coronary intervention in stable angina (ORBITA): A double-blind, randomised controlled trial. *Lancet.* 2018;391(10115): 31-40.

CONQUER THE **BOARDS!**

Family history for coronary artery disease is a first-degree relative with an MI before age 40 in men, and before age 55 in women.

ACUTE CORONARY SYNDROMES

Definition: Acute coronary syndrome (ACS) refers to patients in whom there is suspicion of confirmation of acute myocardial ischemia (lack of blood flow to the heart) or MI (which is ischemia lasting long enough or severe enough that it leads to heart muscle damage).

ACS events are classified according to changes on the ECG:

1. **Non-ST-elevation changes:** This category includes *non-ST-elevation myocardial infarction (NSTEMI)* and *unstable angina.* Both NSTEMI and unstable angina have chest pain and ECG changes, but unstable angina has *no troponin elevation.* Unstable angina is associated with increased frequency and/or severity of symptoms, symptoms at rest, or new onset of symptoms compared to stable angina, which has stable chronic symptoms.
2. **ST-elevation changes** (STEMI: ST-elevation MI).

SERUM MARKERS FOR MI

If you suspect ACS in patients, all patients should have "serial enzymes" drawn, which consists of sending cardiac biomarkers every 6 to 8 hours for a 24-hour period. With the advent of highly sensitive troponins, most institutions only use troponin as a cardiac biomarker. However, it continues to be important to understand the other serum markers that can be sent (Table 6-4).

CONQUER THE **WARDS!**

Troponin I is the cardiac biomarker most commonly used clinically given its specificity for myocardium.

- **Myoglobin:** Elevated within 1 hour of MI; peak 6 hours; nonspecific.
- **Creatinine phosphokinase (CPK):** This is nonspecific but is elevated within 4 to 8 hours; peak 18 to 24 hours after an MI.
- **Creatinine kinase-MB (CK-MB):** CK-MB isoenzyme is the subgroup of CPK specific for myocardial tissue damage. The extent of elevation correlates with the amount of cardiac damage. Its onset and peak are similar to troponin but it clears in 3 to 4 days as opposed to 7 to 10 seconds with troponin. Therefore, it is extremely useful in patients where reinfarction after an MI occurs or for restent thrombosis.
- Troponin T or I: Very sensitive and specific markers for cardiac muscle injury. Elevated within 3 hours and can stay elevated for more than a week. Troponin may also be slightly chronically elevated in congestive heart failure (CHF). Troponin is renally cleared, so levels may be elevated in the setting of renal insufficiency.

A 47-year-old man presents to the ER with left-sided chest pain at rest. He is a chronic smoker with a family history of diabetes and hypertension. On examination, he is found to have stable vitals. ECG showed new ST depressions in II, III, and aVF. ASA, Plavix, and nitrate were given, and the patient still complained of pain. *Next step: Start heparin drip and send patient for cardiac catheterization.*

TABLE 6-4. Cardiac Biomarkers

Enzyme	Onset (hr)	Peak (hr)	Duration
Myoglobin	1–4	6–8	24 hr
Troponin T/I	3–12	18–24	7–10 days
Creatinine kinase (total and CK-MB)	3–12	18–24	3–4 days

WHAT DO YOU DO WITH A PATIENT SUSPECTED OF ACS?

- **Focused history and physical:** The history should focus on whether this chest pain is due to ACS. Ischemia has a number of characteristics that separate it from nonischemic causes. The symptoms associated with chest pain that have the highest relative risk for MI are *radiation to upper extremity and association with diaphoresis, nausea, or vomiting.* Following are typical symptoms for angina, but not all of these symptoms need be present to call it typical.
  - **Typical symptoms for any angina/MI:** Left-sided/substernal chest pressure (not usually pain) with radiation to the left shoulder, arm, or jaw. The patient may characterize this by putting a closed fist over the chest (Levine sign), shortness of breath, diaphoresis, nausea, or vomiting. Chest pressure is worse with activity and improves with rest or nitroglycerin sublingually.
  - **Atypical presentation**: These patients have no chest pain or no symptoms on presentation. Up to one-third of patients with MI have no chest pain on presentation. Other symptoms patients will complain about are dyspnea, weakness, nausea, epigastric pain, palpitations, or syncope. Patients at risk for atypical presentations are diabetics (they may have a neuropathy that blunts the sensation of pain; many diabetics have "silent MIs" where the MI has no symptoms) and women.
- **Initial tests:** All patients suspected of having ACS should have the following tests:
  - ECG
  - Serial troponins q6 times 3
  - Complete blood count to look for anemia or signs of infection, which can precipitate ACS
  - Electrolytes to look for any abnormalities that could precipitate arrhythmias
  - Creatinine, since patients will receive contrast if they receive cardiac catheterization, which may worsen acute kidney injury

INITIAL MANAGEMENT FOR ALL ACS

- **Telemetry:** Patients should also be placed on a cardiac monitor (telemetry) because during ischemia they are at high risk for arrhythmias.
- **Antiplatelet and anticoagulation**:
  - Aspirin 325 mg (chewable preferred) should be immediately given. Clopidogrel is an alternative for those with true aspirin allergy.
  - P2Y12 inhibitors (e.g., clopidogrel 300 mg or ticagrelor 180 mg) loading doses should be given.
  - Either unfractionated heparin or low-molecular-weight heparin can be used. The rationale behind using both aspirin and heparin is that they act at different sites.
- **High-intensity statin therapy:** The most well-studied is atorvastatin 80 mg, and this should be given prior to thrombolytics or cardiac catheterization. If a patient is on low- to moderate-intensity statin they should be switched to high intensity.
- **Pain control:** Morphine helps with pain control but does not affect outcome.
- **Oxygen:** It does not need to be given to all patients, but any patient with a low oxygen saturation should have supplemental oxygen.
- **Beta blockers:** See note under Conquer the Boards.
- *Note:* Thrombolytics are not used in unstable angina or NSTEMI because 60% to 80% of the time the infarcted artery is not occluded.

Patients presenting with ACS should be given SNAP (unless contraindicated):

Statin – high-intensity statin
Nitrate – sublingual or IV to control pain
Aspirin – non-enteric-coated, preferably chewed, 162 to 325 mg
P2Y12 inhibitors – clopidogrel or ticagrelor
Morphine

Note: Morphine should be the last medication given. It may mask angina and should only be given when a diagnosis of ACS is certain and the patient still has severe pain.

CONQUER THE **WARDS!**

Supplemental oxygen will not affect outcomes in nonhypoxic patients with ACS.

CONQUER THE **WARDS!**

Heparin does not dissolve already-present clots; rather, it prevents future ones from forming.

CONQUER THE **BOARDS!**

Beta blockers do not need to be given immediately, but rather, within the first 24 hours of ACS presentation, and only after contraindications are ruled out, including acute heart failure, cardiogenic shock, and right ventricular MI.

CONQUER THE **WARDS!**

Patients with ST elevations have better outcomes when revascularization happens within 60 minutes of arrival. This is known as door-to-balloon (DTB) time.

CONQUER THE **BOARDS!**

Patients treated with thrombolytics should still be transferred to a PCI-capable hospital, for angiography and in case the thrombus reforms!

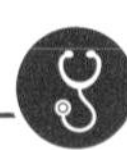

What is a TIMI score?

A scoring system used to evaluate the risks of patients with NSTEMI and determine if early invasive management (i.e., cardiac catheterization) is warranted. Each item is worth a point:

- Age > 65
- ≥ 3 CAD risk factors
- Prior coronary stenosis $> 50\%$
- ST changes on ECG
- ≥ 2 anginal episodes in 24 hours
- Use of aspirin in prior week
- Positive serum markers

TIMI > 4: Patient should get invasive management.

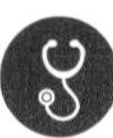

Causes of ST elevation:

- MI
- Pericarditis
- Left ventricular (LV) aneurysm
- Early repolarization (young people)

ACS is divided into 2 major types:

1. **STEMI:** This is the most dangerous type of ACS. (This group also includes those with a new left bundle branch block [LBBB] on ECG.) STEMI is typically caused by complete occlusion of a coronary artery.
   - **Treatment:** These patients need urgent opening of the blockage in the coronary artery (revascularization). This can be done with 1) thrombolytics (medicines that break up clots) and/or 2) cardiac catheterization and stenting (PCI) (see earlier). Cardiac catheterization with PCI is superior to thrombolytics in STEMI. Examples of thrombolytics include tenecteplase, alteplase, and reteplase. Contraindications are risks of bleeding, particularly in the brain, prior intracranial hemorrhage, stroke within 1 year, brain tumor, active internal bleeding, or suspected aortic dissection.
2. **Unstable angina** and **NSTEMI:** These 2 have similar pathogenesis, typically due to an incomplete occlusion of a coronary artery. NSTEMI differs from unstable angina in that the lack of oxygen is severe enough to cause myocardial damage and enzyme leakage (unlike unstable angina, where there is no enzyme leakage).
   - **Treatment:** SNAP as described earlier. Can treat with invasive treatment (cardiac catheterization) or conservatively (medications) based on risk factors (see "What is a TIMI score?" on the left margin of this page.) Ongoing chest pain and signs of cardiac dysfunction should prompt intervention.
3. Special situations:
   - **Cocaine** can cause ECG changes with elevated cardiac enzymes and chest pain due to severe vasoconstriction without plaque rupture or thrombus formation. This vasoconstriction, in addition to tachycardia and hypertension, can lead to a mismatch between oxygen supply and myocardial demand (do a urine drug screen if suspicious).
   - **Right ventricular (RV) MI—a special case:** Right ventricular MI can produce acute RV dysfunction. Dysfunctional right ventricles are very preload sensitive, and treatment must maintain preload with aggressive fluids and *avoid nitrates* (will drop preload). RV MI is most commonly seen with inferior wall MI, so in patients with ST elevations in II, III, and aVF, look for ST elevations in V1 or ST elevations greater in lead III than in lead II. If you suspect RV infarction, get right-sided ECG leads to look for ST elevation over the right ventricle.

TYPICAL ECG FINDINGS IN MI

Location of ECG abnormalities tells which vessel in the heart is affected.

- **Inferior wall MI:** ST elevation in II, III, and aVF (cor pulmonale: ST *depression* in II, III, and aVF) (see Figure 6-1).
- **Anteroseptal MI:** ST elevation in V_1, V_2, and V_3 (see Figure 6-2).

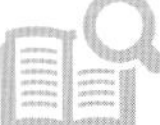

HIGH-YIELD LITERATURE

Amsterdam EA, Wenger NK, Brindis RG, et al. 2014 AHA/ACC guideline for the management of patients with non-ST-elevation acute coronary syndromes:
A report of the American College of Cardiology/American Heart Association Task Force on Practice Guidelines. *J Am Coll Cardiol.* 2014;64:e139-228.
Hofmann R, James SK, Jernberg T, Lindahl B, Erlinge D, Witt N. Patients suspected of having an acute MI don't need supplemental oxygen unless they are hypoxic:
Oxygen therapy in suspected acute myocardial infarction. *N Engl J Med.* 2017; 377:1240-1249.

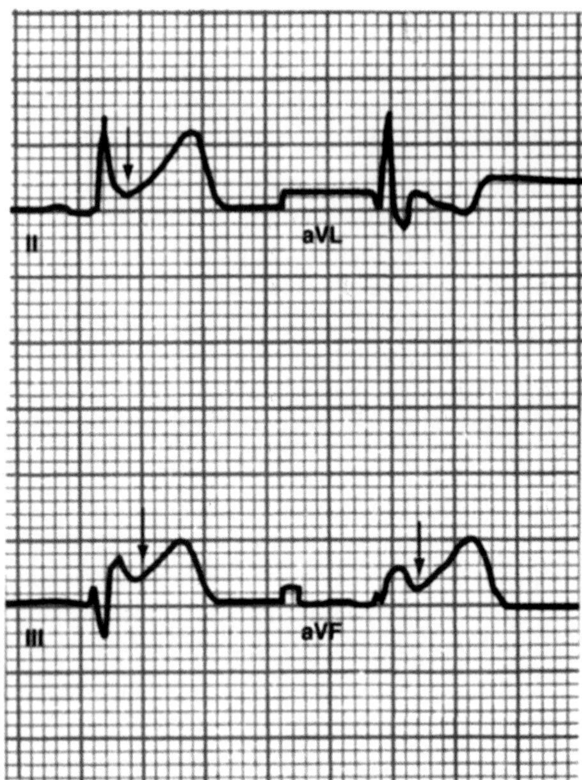

FIGURE 6-1. ECG of inferior wall MI demonstrating ST elevation in leads II, III, and aVF.

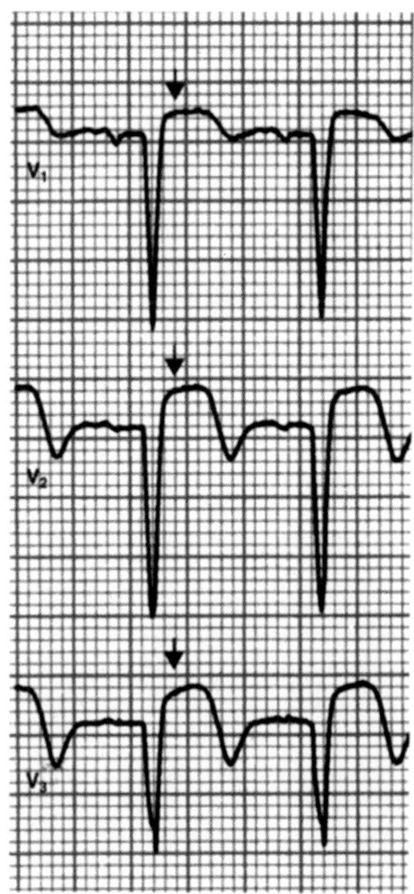

FIGURE 6-2. ECG of anteroseptal MI demonstrating ST elevation in leads V_1, V_2, and V_3.

CONQUER THE WARDS!

Lead V1 is predominantly negative in a normal ECG. A tall R wave in V1 has its own differential:

- Right bundle branch block
- Posterior MI
- Dextrocardia
- Wolff-Parkinson-White
- Duchenne muscular dystrophy
- Right ventricular hypertrophy
- And, of course, a normal variant

CONQUER THE WARDS!

Lead V1 is the only standard ECG lead that looks directly at the right ventricle.

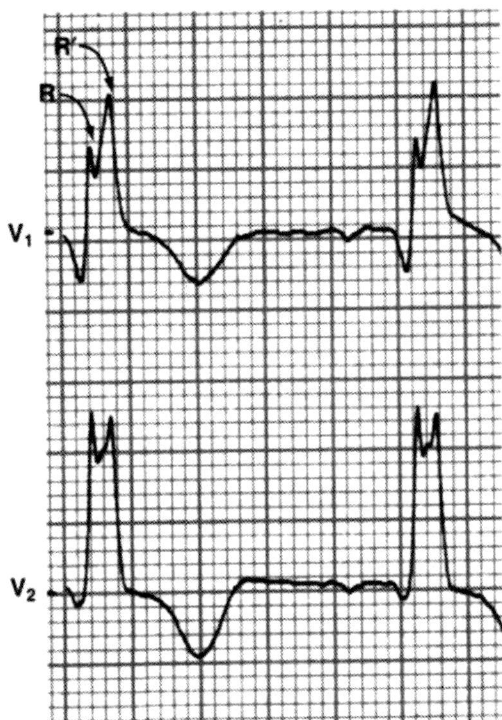

FIGURE 6-3. Right bundle branch block.

- **Lateral wall MI:** ST elevation in V_5, V_6, I, and aVL.
- **Posterior wall MI:** Tall ST elevation in II, III, and AVF; tall R with ST depression in V1 and V2; and ST elevation in V4R.
- A tall R wave in V1 has its own differential that can include a right bundle branch block (Figure 6-3), posterior MI, Wolff-Parkinson-White, and other conditions.

MEDICATIONS AT DISCHARGE FOR PATIENTS WITH ACS

It is important to carefully review and consider medications at discharge for patients with ACS. (see table 6-22 for common cardiac medications) The following medications should be continued indefinitely:

- Aspirin
- Beta blocker
- Angiotensin-converting enzyme (ACE) inhibitor in patients with resulting low cardiac function (decreased left ventricular ejection fraction [LVEF]).
- High-intensity statin (hydroxymethylglutaryl coenzyme A [HMG CoA] reductase inhibitor).
- Clopidogrel, prasugrel, or ticagrelor if a stent was placed. Clopidogrel or ticagrelor for 12 months if no stent was placed.
- **Secondary prevention of MI:** Don't forget to ensure that other risk factors are adequately managed, such as smoking cessation, hypertension, hyperlipidemia, and diabetes mellitus.

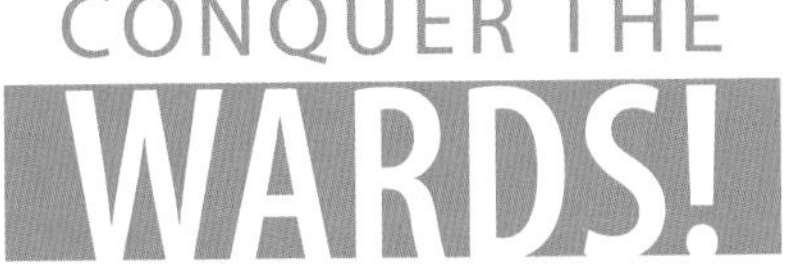

Aspirin with a P2Y12 inhibitor is commonly referred to as dual antiplatelet therapy (DAPT). The duration of DAPT after ACS is still being investigated.

A 65-year-old woman with a history of CAD and drug-eluting stent (DES) placed 6 months ago presents with acute crushing chest pain. She says that she had stopped taking her Plavix 1 week ago for a dental procedure. *Think: Acute in-stent thrombosis.*

Next step: ECG (may show ST elevation; send for urgent cardiac catheterization).

POSTINFARCTION COMPLICATIONS

- **Ruptures** (usually occur within 4 to 5 days of a large MI). These can be in the free wall of the heart, the intraventricular septum, or the papillary muscle, which causes acute mitral regurgitation. These are very rare in the era of angiography with PCI.
- **Arrhythmias:** Ventricular tachycardia (VT, usually within 48 hours, when the myocardium reperfuses), bradycardia (usually from inferior wall MI), atrioventricular block (can be from anterior wall or inferior wall MI).
- **Dressler syndrome:** Usually occurs 1 or 2 weeks after cardiac injury (MI or cardiac surgery). It is associated with fever, pericarditis, and sometimes pericardial or pleural effusions; likely a hypersensitivity process. Treat with nonsteroidal antiinflammatory drugs (NSAIDs) and steroids.

A 58-year-old man who was discharged from the hospital after an MI 2 weeks ago presents with fever, chest pain, and generalized malaise. ECG shows diffuse ST-T wave changes. *Think: Dressler syndrome.* Treat with NSAIDs.

HEART FAILURE

General Facts

CHF is the failure of the heart to pump blood effectively to the tissues. Left heart failure (LHF) causes pulmonary venous congestion (blood flow back up into the lungs) and compromised systemic circulation. Right heart failure (RHF) causes systemic venous congestion. CHF is also known as heart failure with reduced ejection fraction (HFrEF), as opposed to heart failure with preserved ejection fraction (HFpEF).

Clinical Features

Left Heart Failure

- **Symptoms include** dyspnea, orthopnea (dyspnea that worsens when lying down), paroxysmal nocturnal dyspnea (dyspnea that wakes patient from sleep), cough (usually nonproductive), nocturia, and weight gain from fluid retention.
- **Signs include** rales, S3 gallop, jugular venous distention (JVD), tachycardia, and peripheral edema.

Right Heart Failure

- **Symptoms include** right upper quadrant (RUQ) pain (due to hepatic congestion), dyspnea, abdominal swelling (ascites), and weight gain (fluid retention).
- **Signs include** hepatomegaly, hepatojugular reflex, JVD, ascites, cirrhosis, abnormal liver function tests (LFTs) (congestive hepatopathy), and peripheral edema.

Diagnostic Workup

In all patients suspected of having CHF, the workup consists of finding the underlying causes that may lead to congestion and volume overload. Causes can vary by type and side of heart failure, with right- and left-sided causes (Table 6-5).

Diagnosis:

- **Chest x-ray** can show enlargement of cardiac silhouette, pulmonary vascular congestion with redistribution to upper lobes, and effusion.

CONQUER THE BOARDS!

Acute mitral regurgitation often lacks the telltale cardiac murmur, as the orifice is nonrestrictive. The acute pulmonary edema is life threatening and requires urgent surgical repair.

CONQUER THE WARDS!

The most common cause of right heart failure is chronic left heart failure.

Congestive Heart Failure with Preserved Ejection Fraction (HFpEF; Formerly Known as Diastolic Dysfunction)

CHF with a normal ejection fraction; the problem occurs during filling (diastole) due to cardiac wall stiffness. HFpEF is a poorly understood condition. Most therapies with proven benefit for HFrEF have not been proven to have a mortality benefit in HFpEF.

- Accounts for 40% to 60% of heart failure.
- Signs/symptoms of heart failure with normal ejection fraction (>50%).
- More common in women.
- Associated with hypertension, left ventricular hypertrophy (LVH), dilated cardiomyopathy, and ischemia.
- Treat hypertension, use diuretics for congestion, and control heart rate if in atrial fibrillation.

CONQUER THE BOARDS!

The initial evaluation of left-sided heart failure should include an evaluation of ischemia as the cause: angiography or perfusion imaging.

CONQUER THE WARDS!

Orthopnea is the most specific symptom of heart failure. S3 is the most specific sign.

CONQUER THE WARDS!

Decreased LVEF is a sign of a cardiomyopathy; symptoms are necessary to diagnose the syndrome of heart failure.

CONQUER THE BOARDS!

Heart failure with a normal ejection fraction still requires evidence of ventricular dysfunction.

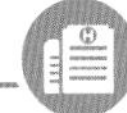

New York Heart Association (NYHA) Functional Classification of Heart Failure

Class I: No limitation

Class II: Slight limitations (symptoms with ordinary efforts)

Class III: Marked limitation (comfortable at rest, symptoms with minimal efforts)

CONQUER THE WARDS!

Pulmonary embolism can cause acute right ventricular failure by producing an acute increase in afterload.

CONQUER THE BOARDS!

ACE inhibitors are the only drug indicated in patients with a decreased LVEF without symptoms of heart failure.

CONQUER THE WARDS!

It's not enough to start medications in heart failure; they should be increased to the doses shown to be effective, or goal dose medical therapy (GDMT).

TABLE 6-5. Most Common Causes of Right- and Left-Sided Heart Failure

Right Heart Failure	Left Heart Failure
CAD (MI that has damaged the right ventricle)	CAD (MI that has damaged the left ventricle)
Second degree to LHF (then further "backup" of blood)	Hypertension
Pulmonary hypertension (right ventricle has to push against a high afterload), usually caused by any pulmonary disease such as COPD, interstitial lung disease	Mitral and aortic valve disease
VSD	Viral myocarditis
	Dilated cardiomyopathy

CAD, coronary artery disease; *COPD*, chronic obstructive pulmonary disease; *LHF*, left heart failure; *MI*, myocardial infarction; *VSD*, ventricular septal defect.

- **Brain natriuretic peptide (BNP)** is elevated in CHF with fluid retention. The most commonly used cutoff is >100 pg/mL, but this can vary among laboratories.
- **Echocardiogram** is the gold standard for diagnosing right or left heart failure.

Underlying Cause: Virtually all patients with new-onset heart failure should have a workup for CAD because of its high prevalence and because it is possibly reversible. This workup includes stress testing and usually a cardiac catheterization. If this is negative, then workup for other causes is initiated (see Table 6-5 for common causes and then the following for other types of cardiomyopathy).

Management of HFrEF

- **Lifestyle changes:** Sodium and water restriction, exercise, education, and avoidance of alcohol.
- **First-line therapy:**
  - **ACE inhibitors:** Decrease afterload and preload. They also decrease symptoms, *improve survival,* and decrease hospitalization. They decrease ventricular fibrosis and reverse the "remodeling" of the left ventricle.
  - **Diuretics:** Use in NHYA class II to IV for fluid retention. Helps to reduce preload, improve symptoms, but does *not change mortality.* Use loop diuretics like furosemide or bumetanide to produce natriuresis and diuresis, not thiazide diuretics.
  - **Beta blockers:** For NYHA class II to III (decrease symptoms, *improve survival*). Only metoprolol succinate, carvedilol, or bisoprolol are approved for heart failure in the United States.
  - **Spironolactone (potassium-sparing diuretics):** Low dose, use in NYHA class III to IV because it *improves survival.* Concomitant use of ACE inhibitors can make potassium go very high, so monitor closely.
  - **Eplerenone:** Similar to spironolactone, but fewer side effects (namely gynecomastia).
  - **Implantable cardioverter-defibrillator (ICD):** Should be implanted in any patient who has had VT or fibrillation. As primary prevention in patients with CHF, ICD has been shown to improve survival in select patients. First, pharmacologic therapy must be maximized prior to consideration for ICD. Then ICD should be considered in the patients.

- **Second-line therapy:**
  - **Neprilysin inhibition (sacubitril) with angiotensin receptor neprilysin blocker (ARNI):** Shown to improve symptoms, reduce hospitalizations, and improve survival in patients who remain symptomatic on ACE inhibitors or can't tolerate them.
  - **Angiotensin receptor blockers (ARBs):** If ACE inhibitors are not well tolerated (e.g., cough).
  - **Nitrate–hydralazine combination:** Improves symptoms and *survival.* High rate of intolerance and lower effect on mortality make this therapy a second line to ACE inhibitors. It is often used in patients who cannot tolerate an ACE inhibitor or ARB.
  - **Cardiac resynchronization therapy:** Reserved for patients who are in class III heart failure despite maximal therapy. Essentially a pacemaker that times the contractions of both ventricles for maximum efficiency and has to been shown to *improve survival.*
  - **Digoxin:** Add for NYHA class III to IV in patients in atrial fibrillation (for symptomatic relief only; *does not* improve survival but reduces hospitalization).

CONQUER THE BOARDS!

Cardiac resynchronization is effective for patients with LV dysfunction and a wide QRS complex on ECG (>150 ms with a left bundle branch morphology).

Management of HFpEF

Unlike HFrEF, there is limited evidence to support a specific drug regimen, as no drugs have been proven to change mortality. Treatment focuses on the following to help reduce symptoms:

1. **Diuresis:** Generally done with loop diuretics, with some limited evidence that spironolactone should be added in patients with high BNP. However, it is important to remember that HFpEF patients with stiff, small left ventricles are preload dependent, so it is important to avoid overdiuresis.
2. **Control of hypertension:** There is no particular regimen that has shown benefit.
3. Heart rate control in patients with atrial fibrillation.

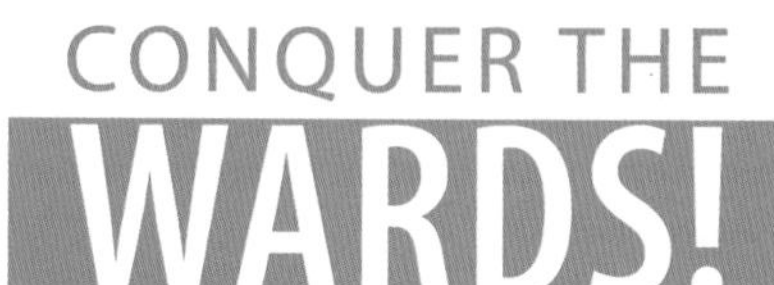

ICD implantation in heart failure patients may not prevent sudden cardiac death.

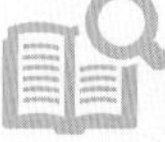

HIGH-YIELD LITERATURE

Defibrillator implantation in patients with nonischemic systolic heart failure. *N Engl J Med.* 2016;375:1221-1230.

ACUTE DECOMPENSATED HEART FAILURE

General Facts

An acute worsening of hemodynamics and tissue perfusion due to an alteration in cardiac output. Typically characterized by a combination of the consequences of venous congestion and decreased tissue perfusion.

Clinical Features

- **Pulmonary edema** is characterized by dyspnea with hypoxia as it progresses. Chest roentgenogram shows pulmonary congestion.
- **Congestive hepatopathy** is low-level hepatic ischemia and consequent dysfunction from impaired venous outflow. Traditionally described as mild transaminitis without significant bilirubinemia.

- **Renal dysfunction** typically as a result of impaired venous outflow, or the "cardiorenal" syndrome. This type of renal impairment improves as the heart failure improves, but may be a consequence of impaired tissue perfusion as well.

Diagnostic Workup

- Acute decompensated heart failure (ADHF) is primarily a clinical diagnosis and supported by the following, which should be obtained: *chest imaging, BNP,* and chemistries (looking for worsening renal and/or liver failure).
- A search for the underlying cause of the decompensation is also important. ADHF is commonly caused by myocardial ischemia, arrhythmias (VT, supraventricular tachycardia [SVT] with fast ventricular rates), infection, valvular disease, and medication and dietary noncompliance.
  - Thorough history and physical exam are important.
  - ECG and telemetry should be obtained to look for any myocardial ischemia or arrhythmias.
  - Echocardiogram can be obtained if there is concern for valvular disease based on history and physical.

CONQUER THE WARDS!

Patients not responding to loop diuretics may benefit from IV nitrates to increase venous capacitance and improve renal function.

CONQUER THE WARDS!

Hold beta blockers when using inotropes and watch for arrhythmias.

CONQUER THE WARDS!

Dilatation of the ventricle often leads to poor coaptation of the atrioventricular valve leaflets. It can be difficult to know if the resulting regurgitation is the cause of the cardiomyopathy or the effect.

Management

- **Initial Management:**
  - **Oxygen:** Supplemental oxygen should be provided to improve hypoxia, and in cases of severe respiratory distress, bilevel positive airway pressure (BiPAP) can be used and even intubation if needed.
  - **Diuretics:** Must be given immediately. They both relieve congestion and reduce afterload. Commonly used diuretics are furosemide, torsemide, and bumetanide. Higher doses are required in patients who have renal dysfunction or are already on diuretics at home.
  - **Afterload reduction:** In patients with normal or elevated blood pressure who are not responding initially to diuretics, further afterload reduction may be needed. Nitroglycerin infusions are often used. Is the patient's tissue perfusion impaired? Are they cold or warm?
  - **Inotropes:** In patients with signs of cardiogenic shock (e.g., cold extremities) ADHF will often require an inotrope to augment myocardial contractility. Commonly used inotropes for ADHF include:
    a. Dobutamine – increases contractility with vasodilation.
    b. Norepinephrine – increases contractility with vasoconstriction.
    c. Milrinone – similar to dobutamine, but expensive; useful in patients chronically on a beta blocker.

CARDIOMYOPATHIES

DILATED CARDIOMYOPATHY

Left or right ventricular enlargement with loss of contractile function.

Etiology

- Infectious: Viral myocarditis (one-third improve, one-third stay the same, one-third get worse).
- Toxic: Reversible—prolonged alcohol abuse, anthracyclines.
- Endocrine: Reversible—thyroid disease (hypo- or hyper-). Irreversible—acromegaly, pheochromocytoma.

- **M**etabolic:
  - Reversible–hypocalcemia, hypophosphatemia, thiamine deficiency (wet beriberi), selenium deficiency.
  - Irreversible–genetic: 20% of cases have positive family histories, pregnancy (postpartum cardiomyopathy, 1 to 9 months after delivery–similar prognosis as viral); neuromuscular, idiopathic.
- **M**echanical: Dysrhythmias (tachycardia-induced cardiomyopathy), valvular disease.

A 26-year-old man presents with shortness of breath (SOB), paroxysmal nocturnal dyspnea (PND), orthopnea, and pleuritic chest pain for 1 week. He had an upper respiratory infection (URI) 1 week prior to onset of symptoms. *Think: Viral myocarditis.* **Next step:** ECG shows diffuse ST-segment elevation and PR-segment depression. Treat with NSAIDs. Steroids have not been shown to change outcomes.

Diagnostic Workup

Echocardiogram shows diffusely dilated ventricles, regurgitant valves, and low ejection fraction.

Treatment

- Address any reversible causes (e.g., discontinue toxic agent).
- Medical management of heart failure (see earlier and remember ACE inhibitors and beta blockers reduce mortality).
- Implanted automatic defibrillator for patients with life-threatening dysrhythmias or ejection fraction (EF) <30% despite maximal therapy at 3 months.
- Heart transplant or left ventricular assist device (LVAD).

RESTRICTIVE CARDIOMYOPATHY

Scarring and infiltration of the myocardium causing decreased ventricular filling. Typically hypertrophy is absent. It is much less common than the other cardiomyopathies outside the tropics but has a high incidence in Africa, India, Asia, and South and Central America due to endomyocardial fibrosis.

Etiology

1. Amyloidosis – sometimes can have increased LV wall thickness.
2. Endomyocardial fibrosis – occurs mainly in children and adolescents in the tropics. Its cause is unknown but likely is due to genetics, infection, and environmental exposures.
3. Hemochromatosis.
4. Sarcoidosis.
5. Carcinoid heart disease.
6. Congenital (Gaucher disease, Hurler disease, glycogen storage disease).

CONQUER THE **WARDS!**

AL or "senile" amyloidosis occurs in the sixth decade or later and commonly spares the myocardium. Transthyretin amyloid occurs in younger patients and frequently has cardiac involvement.

A patient with multiple myeloma has SOB and a chest x-ray showing pulmonary edema. Echo shows a "speckled" appearance with biatrial enlargement. *Diagnosis: Cardiac amyloidosis. Type of cardiomyopathy: Restrictive.*

CONQUER THE WARDS!

Modern echocardiography uses harmonic imaging, making the "speckled" appearance of the myocardium a less specific finding.

CONQUER THE WARDS!

Hypertrophic cardiomyopathy used to be called idiopathic hypertrophic subaortic stenosis (IHSS). Don't get this confused with ventricular hypertrophy.

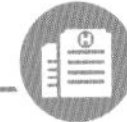

In hypertrophic cardiomyopathy (HCM), symptoms prior to 30 years of age correlate with increased risk of sudden death, but severity of symptoms (whenever they occur) does not correlate with risk of death.

CONQUER THE WARDS!

Very few murmurs decrease with squatting. HCM does.

CONQUER THE BOARDS!

Left ventricular septal thickness >1.9 mm is specific for hypertrophic cardiomyopathy.

CONQUER THE BOARDS!

Causes of paradoxical splitting of S2:
- HCM
- Aortic stenosis
- LBBB

Diagnostic Workup

- **Echocardiography**—normal-sized ventricles with *normal systolic function*, large atria (secondary to elevated atrial pressures pushing against stiff ventricles), nonthickened ventricular walls, and mitral/tricuspid regurgitation.
- **Other studies:** *Cardiac MR* can be helpful in establishing a cause, and *endomyocardial biopsy* may detect eosinophilic infiltration or myocardial fibrosis or amyloid.
- **Other findings:**
  - **Auscultation:** S3 and/or S4 gallop murmurs, occasional (generally mild) mitral or tricuspid regurgitation.
  - **ECG:** Low voltages, conduction abnormalities, nonspecific ST-segment/T-wave changes, LBBB.
  - **Chest x-ray:** Normal cardiac silhouette or enlarged atria, pulmonary venous congestion.

Management

- Address any reversible causes (treat the underlying disease).
- **Medical management:** There are very little data on optimal treatment for restrictive cardiomyopathies, but most treatment is similar to other heart failures: ACE inhibitor, beta blocker, and loop diuretics. Unlike in other cardiomyopathies, calcium channel blockers may have some benefit. Cardiac transplant is the only definitive treatment.

HYPERTROPHIC CARDIOMYOPATHY

General Facts

- Hypertrophy of the interventricular septum narrows the LV outflow tract. High-velocity systolic flow draws the anterior leaflet of the mitral valve into the tract (via the Bernoulli effect), causing a dynamic LV outflow tract obstruction.
- Disorganized myocardial fibrils can predispose patients to arrhythmias, increasing the chance of sudden cardiac death. Patients can experience sudden cardiac death from arrhythmia but also from cardiovascular collapse.
- Dehydration can lead to decreased preload, which will worsen outflow tract obstruction. When combined with tachycardia to shorten LV diastolic filling time, the decrease in stroke volume may be too severe to sustain myocardial perfusion. This leads to myocardial ischemia and ventricular arrhythmias, leading to death.
- ~50% idiopathic, ~50% familial (autosomal dominant, with variable penetrance).

Clinical Features

- Most patients have no symptoms, and the diagnosis is found on routine examinations. Some patients have dyspnea or fatigue.
- **Murmur changes with position** – systolic ejection murmur heard best along the left sternal border.
  - **Murmur** decreased with increased LV blood volume or venous return (rapidly squatting from a standing position).
  - **Murmur** increased with decreased venous return: Valsalva, squatting to standing (blood pools in the legs) volume (Valsalva) and standing.
- **Paradoxical splitting of S2**

Diagnostic Workup

- **Echocardiography**: Septal hypertrophy with significant LVH and systolic anterior motion (SAM) of the mitral leaflet.
- **ECG**: Shows left ventricular hypertrophy and large septal Q waves in the inferior and lateral leads. Atrial fibrillation can be seen, as the outflow tract obstruction often leads to mitral regurgitation, which leads to left atrial enlargement.

Management

- If patients are asymptomatic, close clinical observation is the preferred approach and counseling on refraining from vigorous exercise.
- If patients are symptomatic, beta blockers are considered first-line because they reduce heart rate, increase LV filling time, and decrease inotropy. Calcium channel blockers are considered second-line agents.
- **Medications to avoid:** Anything that decreases preload (vasodilators [e.g., nitrates], diuretics, volume depletion), as this will worsen obstruction.
- **Other treatments:**
  - Surgical septal myectomy can reduce obstruction but is not always effective.
  - ICD for primary prevention in high-risk patients.

A 25-year-old man becomes severely dyspneic and collapses while running laps. His father died suddenly at an early age. *Think: Hypertrophic cardiomyopathy.*

STRESS-INDUCED CARDIOMYOPATHY (TAKOTSUBO CARDIOMYOPATHY)

Etiology

- Rare form of cardiomyopathy that is precipitated by emotional or physical stress. More commonly seen in female patients in the postmenopausal age group.
- Commonly happens in situations with sudden sympathetic surge (death of a loved one).
- Pathophysiology thought to be a combination of sympathetic overactivation, coronary microcirculation dysregulation, and hormonal effects.

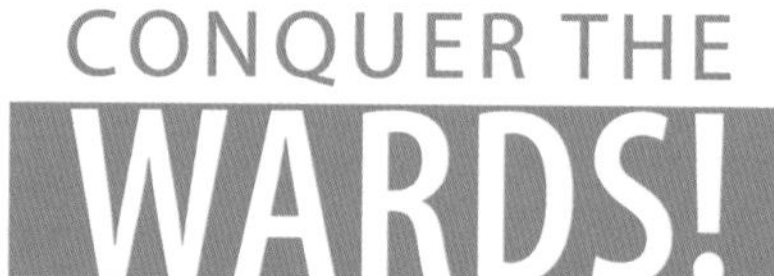

Takotsubo is a Japanese word for an octopus trap, which resembles the shape of the ventricle in stress-induced cardiomyopathy.

Diagnostic Workup

- **Echocardiography** – apical ballooning with hyperdynamic basal segments.
- **Other findings:**
  - **ECG:** Diffuse ST elevations, which can be very difficult to distinguish from the ST elevations of a STEMI.

Management

- Medical management of heart failure (ACE inhibitors and beta blockers reduce mortality).

Prognosis

Usually good, with recovery within 1 to 3 months.

HIGH-YIELD LITERATURE

Neurohumoral features of myocardial stunning due to sudden emotional stress. *N Engl J Med.* 2005;352:539-548.

MYOCARDITIS

General Facts

- Inflammation of the myocardium that can be caused by viral, bacterial, parasitic, or noninfectious systemic diseases (Table 6-6).

Clinical Features

- Spectrum of disease ranges from asymptomatic to fulminant cardiac failure and death.
- Findings may include chest pain, fever, recent URI, fatigue, signs of CHF.
- On physical examination: S3/S4, mitral or tricuspid regurgitation, friction rub (if pericardium involved).

Diagnostic Workup

- Echocardiography shows hypokinetic walls, dilated ventricles/atria, and sometimes pericardial effusion.
- Myocardial biopsy can confirm diagnosis but is rarely necessary.
- **Other findings:**
  - **ECG:** Nonspecific changes, dysrhythmias.
  - **Labs:** Leukocytosis, elevated erythrocyte sedimentation rate (ESR), elevated cardiac enzymes (slower rise and fall than acute MI; troponin I is most sensitive).

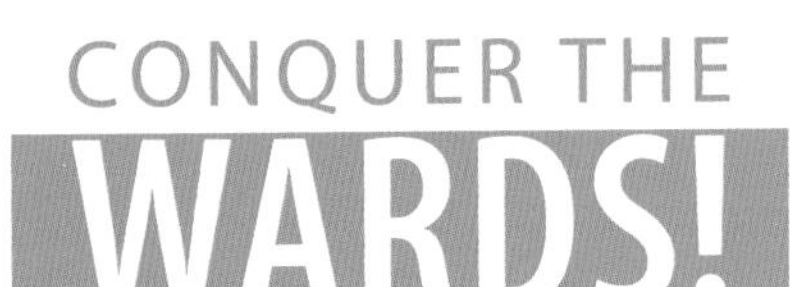

Myocarditis transiently increases the risk of ventricular arrhythmias.

Management

- Primarily supportive, limiting activities and managing any associated heart failure or dysrhythmias.
- Address etiology if known/applicable (e.g., antivirals, antibiotics, diphtheria antitoxin, discontinue drug use); intravenous immunoglobulin G (IVIG) may be of benefit.

PERICARDITIS

General Facts

- Inflammation of the pericardium that can be caused by viral, bacterial, parasitic, or noninfectious systemic diseases.
- Has a benign course and relatively low yield in finding the underlying cause. Most are presumed to be due to a viral etiology. Other causes to consider are the following:
  - **Bacterial:** Tuberculosis (TB), streptococci, staphylococci (rheumatic fever causes pericarditis).

CONQUER THE WARDS!

Coxsackie B is the most common viral cause of myocarditis.

TABLE 6-6. Infectious Causes of Myocarditis

Viral	Bacterial	Parasites	Systemic Disease
Coxsackie A or B Echovirus	Group A β-hemolytic streptococcus	*Trypanosoma cruzi* *Toxoplasma*	Kawasaki Systemic lupus erythematosus (SLE)
HIV	*Corynebacterium*	*Trichinella*	Sarcoidosis
Cytomegalovirus	Meningococcus	*Echinococcus*	
Influenza	*Borrelia burgdorferi*		
Epstein–Barr	*Mycoplasma*		
Hepatitis B virus	*pneumoniae*		
Adenovirus			

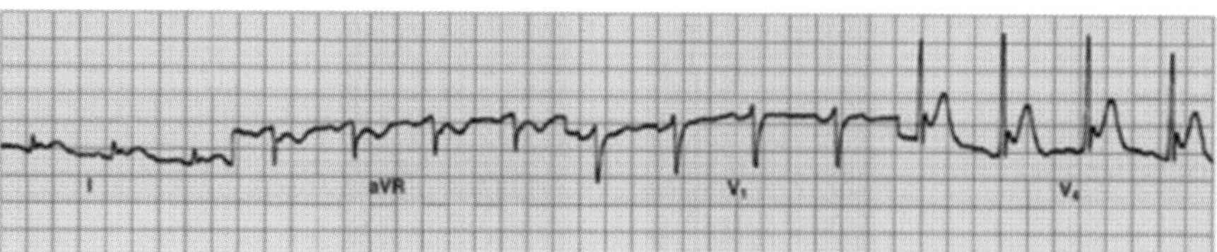

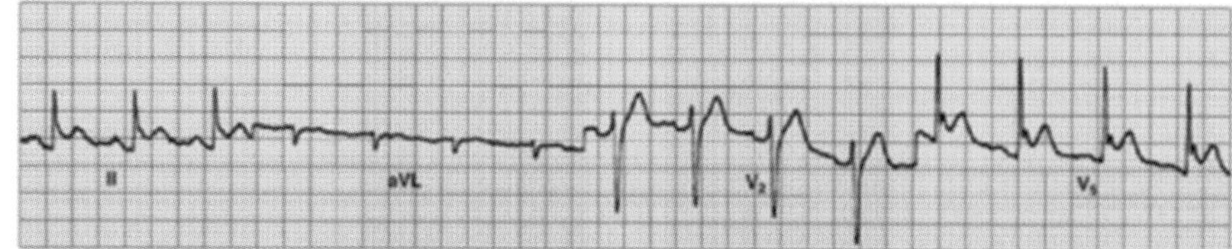

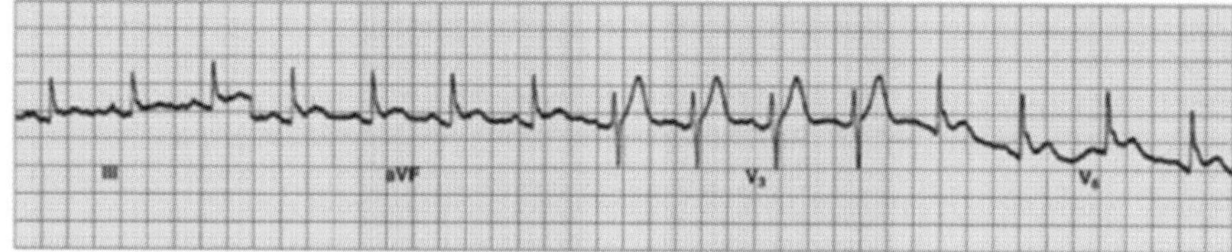

FIGURE 6-4. Pericarditis.

- **Metastases:** First-degree tumors usually breast, lung, or melanoma.
- **Immediate post-MI:** Pericarditis occurs within 24 hours of a *transmural* infarction due to direct pericardial irritation from injured myocardium.
- **Dressler syndrome:** Pericarditis occurring 1 week to months after an MI due to an autoimmune response to infarcted myocardium.
- Systemic causes such as **uremia**, rheumatologic condition (SLE, scleroderma), drug reaction, myxedema, and trauma.

Clinical Features

- **Chest pain**: Classically it is pleuritic and relieved by leaving forward. It often radiates to the left shoulder and does not respond to nitroglycerin.
- On **auscultation**, a pericardial friction rub can be heard on expiration. This is a pathognomonic finding, but variably present.

Diagnostic Workup

- **ECG:** *Diffuse* ST elevations and PR depressions (no discreet pattern of infarction) (see Figure 6-4).

Management

- Address **underlying cause** if known/applicable (e.g., hemodialysis for uremia).
- **Ibuprofen or indomethacin PLUS colchicine** is the preferred treatment to relieve pain and reduce inflammation.
- **Steroids** are generally not recommended anymore, as they have a high rate of recurrence, but can be used in combination with colchicine if patients cannot tolerate NSAIDs or have failed treatment.

PERICARDIAL TAMPONADE

General Facts

- Tamponade is the physiologic result of rapid accumulation of fluid within the relatively inelastic pericardial sac. Pericardial tamponade impairs cardiac filling and reduces cardiac output.

- Can be caused by a pericardial effusion, trauma (accidental or iatrogenic), ruptured ventricular wall (post-MI), aortic dissection with rupture into pericardium, or malignancy.

Clinical Features

In addition to dyspnea and tachycardia:

- **Beck triad:** 1) Hypotension, 2) muffled heart sounds, 3) JVD.
- **Pulsus paradoxus:** Systolic blood pressure decreases by >10 mm Hg with inspiration. It is measured by checking blood pressure and calculating the difference between the blood pressure when the first pulse is heard to when the pulse is heard regularly.
- **Narrow pulse pressure:** Only a small difference between systolic and diastolic blood pressure.
- On auscultation you will find distant heart sounds.

Diagnostic Workup

- **Echocardiogram** will show pericardial effusion and decreased filling with an engorged inferior vena cava.
- ECG: May show low voltage or electrical alternans.
- Chest x-ray (CXR): Enlarged cardiac silhouette.

Management

- Immediate pericardiocentesis for unstable patients. Placement of a pericardial drain to remove all fluid possible.
- Pericardial window (surgery) for stable patients and recurrent effusions.
- Fluids can be also infused to expand volume and is a temporizing measure only.

CONSTRICTIVE PERICARDITIS

General Facts

Granulation and scarring of the pericardium secondary to chronic or recurrent pericarditis. Cardiac output is diminished.

Clinical Features

- The presentation is usually due to fluid overload: dyspnea, fatigue, tachycardia, peripheral edema, and JVD when upright are common.
- Look for **Kussmaul sign**, a paradoxical rise in JVD during inspiration.
- Auscultation may demonstrate distant heart sounds. Pericardial "knock" may be heard.

Diagnostic Workup

- **Echocardiogram** will show *normal left ventricular function* and may show pericardial thickening.
- **Other findings:**
  - **CXR** may show pericardial calcification.
  - **ECG** may show low voltage, T wave flattening or inversion in V_1 and V_2, and notched P waves.

Management

- In stable patients, treatment is similar to pericarditis (NSAIDs plus colchicine).
- In unstable patients or patients with persistent symptoms, surgical pericardiectomy should be performed.

CONQUER THE BOARDS!

It's not the size of the pericardial effusion, but rather the rapidity at which it accumulates that correlates to the incidence of tamponade physiology. Tamponade can happen with small effusions!

CONQUER THE WARDS!

Pulsus paradoxus occurs because Inspiration leads to Increased venous return. The Increase In right ventricular volume pushes the septum Into the left ventricle, reducing Its volume and thus stroke volume

CONQUER THE WARDS!

Pericardiocentesis yielding clotted blood probably came from the right ventricle, not the pericardial sac. Fluid in the pericardium usually is not entirely blood and therefore won't clot.

CONQUER THE WARDS!

Constrictive pericarditis leads to a similar physiology as tamponade, but the impaired filling is due to the stiffness of the pericardium, not increased pressure of accumulated fluid.

VALVULAR HEART DISEASES

MITRAL STENOSIS

General Facts

- Rheumatic heart disease is the most common cause, and congenital causes are rare.
- Most cases occur in women.

Clinical Features

- Symptoms are due to the left atrium incompletely emptying, which leads to extra volume in the atrium and increased left atrial pressure. Blood then backs up into the lungs and the right heart. Symptoms of CHF and right-sided failure will ensue (dyspnea on exertion, rales, cough, JVD).
- The heart tries over time to compensate for increased left atrial pressure by dilating. See Table 6-7 for classic signs and symptoms of valvular diseases.

CONQUER THE WARDS!

Left atrial enlargement increases the risk of developing atrial fibrillation, which can be the presenting complaint of patients with mitral stenosis.

TABLE 6-7. Classic Signs and Symptoms of Valvular Diseases

	Etiology	Symptoms	Signs/Murmur
Mitral stenosis	■ Rheumatic heart disease ■ Congenital ■ Degenerative	■ Right heart failure ■ SOB (orthopnea, PND) ■ Cough/hemoptysis ■ Atrial fibrillation	■ Loud S2/tapping apex ■ Opening snap followed by mid-diastolic rumbling murmur
Mitral regurgitation	■ Rheumatic heart disease ■ Papillary muscle rupture (post MI) ■ Physiologic ■ Dilated cardiomyopathy ■ Ischemia ■ Endocarditis	■ SOB, orthopnea, PND ■ Pulmonary edema ■ Right heart failure	■ Holosystolic murmur best heard at the apex with radiation to the axilla
Aortic stenosis	■ Congenital ■ Degenerative ■ Biscuspid valve ■ Rheumatic heart disease	■ SOB ■ Chest pain ■ Syncope	■ Systolic ejection murmur, crescendo/decrescendo, radiating to the carotids ■ Low-volume pulse, slow rising (pulsus parvus et tardus)
Aortic regurgitation	■ Rheumatic heart diseases ■ Congenital bicuspid valve ■ Endocarditis ■ Second-degree aortic root dilatation (e.g., syphilis, ankylosing spondylitis)	■ SOB, orthopnea, PND	■ Early diastolic decrescendo murmur best heard at left 3rd/4th intercostal space
Tricuspid regurgitation	■ Endocarditis ■ Second-degree left heart failure ■ Pulmonary hypertension ■ Carcinoid	■ Pedal edema ■ Ascites ■ Fatigue	■ Holosystolic murmur left sternal border, ↑ by inspiration (Carvallo's sign) ■ Hepatomegaly (may be pulsatile)
Tricuspid stenosis	■ Rheumatic heart disease ■ Congenital ■ Carcinoid	■ Fatigue ■ Abdominal discomfort (Second-degree hepatomegaly) ■ Pedal edema	■ Diastolic murmur left sternal edge ■ Hepatomegaly ■ Icterus, edema

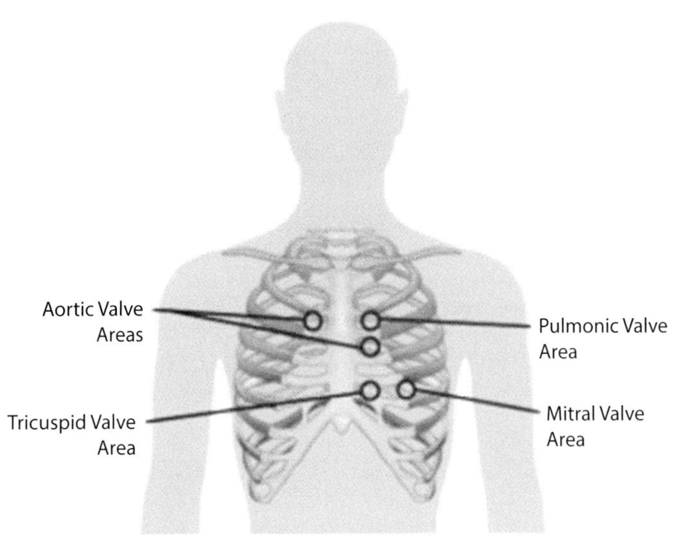

FIGURE 6-5. **Cardiac auscultation sites.** (Reproduced, with permission, from DeGowin RL. *DeGowin & DeGowin's Diagnostic Examination,* 6th ed. New York: McGraw-Hill, 1994: 359.)

- Murmur is mid-diastolic with opening snap and low-pitched rumble best heard over the left sternal border between the second and fourth interspace (see Figure 6-5).

Diagnostic Workup

- **Echocardiography** demonstrates diseased valve with increased pressure gradients across it.
- **CXR** may show straight left heart border due to enlarged left atrium and Kerley B lines from pulmonary edema.

Management

- Surgical repair or balloon valvuloplasty in symptomatic patients with severe stenosis.
- Treat for heart failure and dysrhythmias as needed.

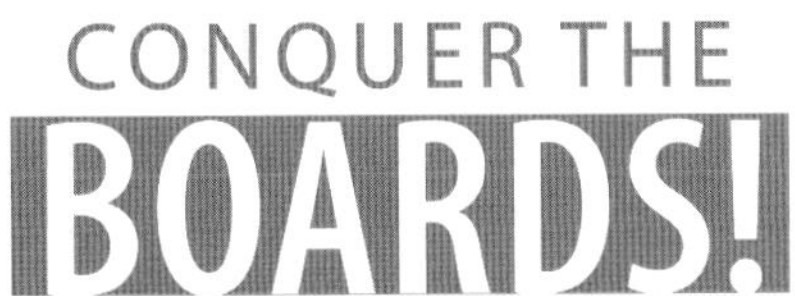

Endocarditis prophylaxis is only indicated in patients with intracardiac prosthetics, not native valvular disease.

CONQUER THE WARDS!

Patients with mitral regurgitation have a good prognosis if LV function is preserved.

MITRAL REGURGITATION

General Facts

- Mitral regurgitation can occur due to acute or chronic conditions.
- Acute causes include MI with papillary muscle rupture or infective endocarditis.
- Chronic causes include rheumatic fever, mitral prolapse that devolves to regurgitation, left ventricular dilation, or congenital abnormalities.

Clinical Features

- The extra volume in the left atrium leads to an increase in left atrial pressure, which backs up into the lungs and the right heart.
- Symptoms of CHF and right-sided failure (dyspnea on exertion, rales, cough, JVD).
- The heart tries over time to compensate for increased left atrial pressure by dilating.
- On physical examination, murmur is loud, holosystolic, and apical radiating to the axilla or back.

Diagnostic Workup

- Echocardiography demonstrating diseased/prolapsed valve.

Management

- Medical therapy for symptomatic patients has a limited role, but in patients who cannot have surgery, the treatment is similar to that for heart failure.
- Surgical therapy (valve replacement or repair) is definitive therapy if signs of LV dysfunction begin.
- Acute mitral regurgitation (from papillary muscle rupture from MI) usually results in severe CHF and requires emergent surgery.

MITRAL VALVE PROLAPSE

General Facts

- Most common valvular disorder (women are 90% of cases).
- Causes include Marfan syndrome, genetic (can be inherited as an autosomal dominant trait leading to redundant tissue in mitral valve leaflets), or idiopathic.

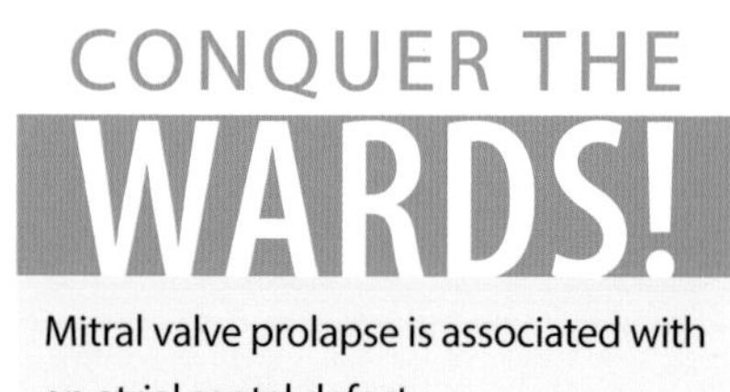

Mitral valve prolapse is associated with an atrial septal defect.

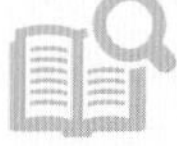

HIGH-YIELD LITERATURE

Patients with mitral regurgitation from left ventricular dilatation do better with a mitral clip: Transcatheter mitral-valve repair in patients with heart failure. *N Engl J Med.* 2018;379:2307-2318.

Clinical Features

- Often asymptomatic, but can rarely have chest pain and shortness of breath.
- On physical exam, you will find a midsystolic click followed by late systolic, high-pitched murmur (if mild regurgitation is present also), best heard at apex, wide splitting of S2.

A young woman presents with atypical chest pain and midsystolic click. *Think: Mitral valve prolapse.*

Diagnostic Workup

- Echocardiography.

Treatment

- None unless regurgitation becomes severe.

AORTIC STENOSIS

General Facts

- Degenerative calcific (calcification) disease (idiopathic, older population). Bicuspid aortic valve (most common *congenital* valve abnormality) can result in aortic stenosis around age 40.
- Mean survival for patients with aortic stenosis (AS) correlates with symptoms. Patients with angina have a 5-year prognosis, syncope 2 to 3 years, and heart failure 1 to 2 years.

CONQUER THE **BOARDS!**

Older patients will slowly decrease activity to avoid or minimize symptoms of AS. Consider a treadmill stress test to illicit symptoms to guide management.

CONQUER THE **WARDS!**

The murmur of aortic stenosis can often be heard when placing your stethoscope on the patient's clavicle.

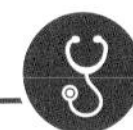

Conditions with narrow pulse pressure (small difference between systolic and diastolic blood pressure):

- Aortic stenosis
- Cardiac tamponade
- Heart failure
- Hypovolemia
- Shock/anaphylaxis

Clinical Features

- **Asymptomatic** early in course.
- Then develop **angina and syncope**, particularly during exercise. Exertion increases heart rate, which results in less filling time and decreased flow across the stenotic valve. Syncope results from decreased blood flow to the brain. **Angina** results from subendocardial ischemia as a result of LVH with decreased aortic pressure at the level of the aortic root.
- With long-standing severe AS, the left ventricle ultimately fails and CHF develops.
- On physical examination: narrow pulse pressure, paradoxical splitting of S2, carotid pulse is "parvus and tardus" (weak and slow).
- Murmur: Loud systolic ejection murmur, crescendo-decrescendo, medium pitched loudest at second right intercostal space, radiates to carotids.

Diagnostic Workup

- **Echocardiography** confirms a diseased aortic valve with increased pressure gradients and increased velocities across the narrowed valve orifice.
- **Other possible findings:**
  - Calcification of aortic valve may be seen on CXR.
  - ECG with LVH and strain pattern.

Management

- Valve replacement (surgically or percutaneous) is the only definitive treatment and is done in patients with symptoms and decreased ejection fraction. Valvuloplasty produces only temporary improvement, and the rate of restenosis is very high. It is often used in patients who need to have urgent or emergent surgery.

HIGH-YIELD LITERATURE

Aortic valve replacement can be done surgically or with a catheter based approach:
Transcatheter aortic-valve implantation for aortic stenosis in patients who cannot undergo surgery. *N Engl J Med.* 2010;363:1597-1607.

CONQUER THE **WARDS!**

Left ventricular strain on ECG is ST-segment depression with T-wave inversion in lateral leads (I, aVL, V_5, V_6).

CONQUER THE **WARDS!**

Indications for valve replacement:

- Severe AS pressure gradient
- Persistent symptoms
- Valve area <0.7 cm^2

AORTIC REGURGITATION

General Facts

- Can be caused by a dilation of the aortic root causing the valve not to close properly or a problem with the aortic valve itself.
- **Causes of aortic root dilatation:** Idiopathic, Marfan syndrome, collagen vascular disease, syphilitic aortitis.
- **Causes of aortic valve problem:** Rheumatic heart disease, endocarditis, Marfan diseases, Ehlers–Danlos syndrome, Turner syndrome, trauma.

Clinical Features

- **Murmur:**
  - High-pitched, blowing, decrescendo diastolic murmur best heard over second right interspace or third left interspace, accentuated by leaning forward.
  - **Austin Flint murmur:** Observed in severe regurgitation; low-pitched diastolic rumble due to regurgitated blood striking the anterior mitral leaflet (similar sound to mitral stenosis).
- Wide pulse pressure.

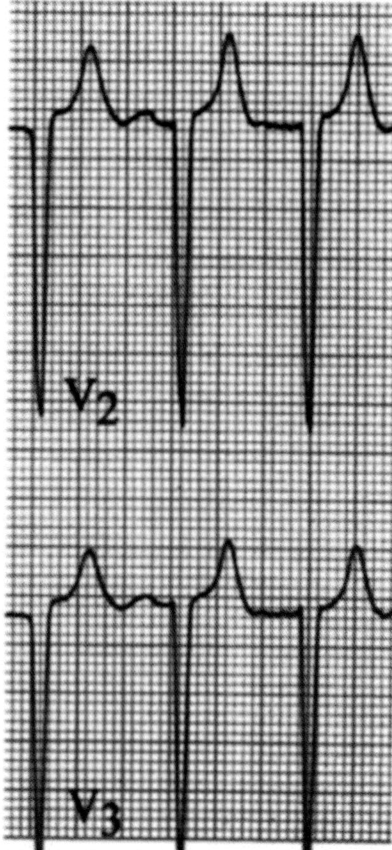

FIGURE 6-6. Left ventricular hypertrophy.

Diagnostic Workup

- **Echocardiography** confirms blood flow across closed aortic valve in diastole. As regurgitation continues, the left ventricle will dilate to accommodate increase in end diastolic volume, leading to heart failure.
- Hyperdynamic, down and laterally displaced point of maximum impulse (PMI) due to LV enlargement.
- ECG shows LVH (see Figure 6-6).

Clinical Features

- Syncope or lightheadedness.
- Angina (due to reduced diastolic coronary blood flow due to low pressure in aortic root).
- LV failure leading to dyspnea, orthopnea, and PND.
- **Other signs (eponyms are in BOLD):**
  - **Corrigan** or water-hammer pulse, "pistol shot" femoral pulses, pulsus bisferiens (dicrotic pulse with 2 palpable waves in systole).
  - **Duroziez sign:** Presence of a diastolic femoral bruit when the femoral artery is compressed enough to hear a systolic bruit.
  - **Hill sign:** Systolic pressure in the legs >20 mm Hg higher than in the arms.
  - **Quincke sign:** Alternating blushing and blanching of the fingernails when gentle pressure is applied.
  - **De Musset sign:** Bobbing of head with heartbeat.
  - **Muller sign**: Pulsating uvula due to increased stroke volume.

CONQUER THE **WARDS!**

Conditions with wide pulse pressure:

- Aortic regurgitation
- Hyperthyroidism
- Anemia
- Wet beriberi
- Stroke

CONQUER THE **BOARDS!**

Asymptomatic aortic regurgitation can be monitored until LVEF <50% or LV dilatation ≥50 mm, at which time surgery is indicated.

Management

- Aortic valve surgery is the only definitive treatment and is recommended for symptomatic patients and most asymptomatic patients.
- Medical management is only reserved for symptomatic patients who are not candidates for surgery due to other comorbidities. Medical management is similar to heart failure patients: ACE I, beta blocker, mineralocorticoid receptor antagonists, and diuretics.

TRICUSPID STENOSIS

General Facts

- Stenosis of the tricuspid valve is rare and can be caused by rheumatic heart disease, congenital causes, and systemic diseases such as carcinoid.

Clinical Features

- Right-sided heart failure (peripheral edema, JVD, hepatomegaly, ascites, jaundice).
- Murmur is diastolic, rumbling, low pitched; accentuated with inspiration. Best heard over left sternal border between fourth and fifth interspace.

Diagnostic Workup

- **Echocardiography** demonstrates diseased valve.

Management

- Surgical repair.

TRICUSPID REGURGITATION

General Facts

- Tricuspid regurgitation (TR) is a relatively common abnormality, being present in 70% of normal adults, usually in a mild form. A small percentage of patients have symptoms.
- **Etiology:**
  - **Primary TR:** The most common causes are infective endocarditis, rheumatic heart disease, and ischemic heart disease causing papillary muscle dysfunction. Other causes are trauma, carcinoid syndrome, connective tissue disorder (e.g., Marfan syndrome).
  - **Secondary TR:** Much more common than primary TR and usually caused by pulmonary hypertension leading to RV dilatation. Common causes of pulmonary hypertension leading to TR are:
    a. Left-sided heart failure
    b. Primary pulmonary disease (pulmonary embolism [PE], chronic obstructive pulmonary disease [COPD], cor pulmonale)
    c. Left-to-right shunt
    d. Pulmonic valve stenosis
    e. Hyperthyroidism

Clinical features

- Signs of right heart failure: Dyspnea, prominent JVD, hepatojugular reflux.
- Murmur: Holosystolic, blowing, medium-pitched murmur heard best along the left sternal border in the fifth interspace, accentuated with inspiration.

Diagnosis

- **Echocardiography.**
- **Other findings:**
  - **ECG** shows right ventricular hypertrophy only in severe cases. Atrial fibrillation is common.

Management

- **Medical management:** Treatment of underlying causes and diuresis for volume overload.
- **Surgical repair** is reserved for patients with severe primary TR with symptoms and is usually not done in patients with pulmonary hypertension.

CONQUER THE WARDS!

Right-sided (tricuspid or pulmonic valve) bacterial endocarditis is most frequently due to IV drug use.

CONGENITAL HEART DISEASES

ATRIAL SEPTAL DEFECT

General Facts

- An atrial septum defect (ASD) is a defect in either the ostium secundum (the central portion of the interatrial septum) or the ostium primum (the lower part). A defect in the sinus venosus can occur as well, located in the upper part of the septum.
- The defect causes shunting of oxygenated blood from the left atrium to the right, which increases pulmonary blood flow and cardiac workload.
- Pulmonary hypertension (HTN) and cardiac remodeling can occur as a consequence.

Clinical Features

- ASD leads to progressive remodeling of the pulmonary vasculature and cardiac muscle. Patients are usually asymptomatic until later-stage disease develops.
- The onset of symptoms usually starts at age 35 to 45, with dyspnea on exertion and fatigue.
- Late-stage disease can have right heart failure, arrhythmias, and paradoxical emboli.
- Eisenmenger disease is a rare late complication where the shunting can no longer be compensated for and cyanosis ensues.
- On examination, a mild systolic ejection murmur can be heard due to increased pulmonary blood flow.

CONQUER THE BOARDS!

Contrast echocardiography is colloquially called a "bubble study" due to the contrast bubbles seen during the study.

Diagnostic Workup

- The best diagnostic test is echocardiography. Contrast echocardiography can show the defect and the shunt. The contrast bubbles will travel through the defect.
- ECG may show signs of right ventricular hypertrophy, such as right axis deviation.
- Chest imaging may reveal enlarged pulmonary arteries and markings.

Management

- Most defects do not require closure, and surgical closure is recommended for severe cases of symptomatic or asymptomatic shunting.

VENTRAL SEPTAL DEFECT

General Facts

- Ventral septal defect (VSD) is a defect in the ventricular septum. It is the most common congenital cardiac malformation.
- The gradient of pressure between the left and right ventricles causes a return of flow to the right heart, leading to pulmonary hypertension.

Clinical Features

- Symptoms typically depend on the size of the defect and subsequent volume of blood flow to the right ventricle.
- Most cases are asymptomatic.
- Large defects can cause shortness of breath, dyspnea on exertion (DOE) less so than chest discomfort, and cyanosis.
- Eisenmenger syndrome, pulmonary hypertension, and heart failure can develop in late stages.
- On examination, a harsh holosystolic murmur with thrill can be heard at the fourth left intercostal space. RV lift and increased S2 can be heard.

Diagnostic Workup

- Echocardiography is the diagnostic test of choice.
- ECG may show biventricular hypertrophy.
- Chest imaging may show enlarged pulmonary artery and markings.

Management

- Most defects do not require closure if the defect is small and the patient is asymptomatic.
- Surgical closure is recommended for severe cases or patients with endocarditis.

PATENT DUCTUS ARTERIOSUS

General Facts

- Patent ductus arteriosus (PDA) is a persistence of the in utero communication between the aortic and pulmonary arteries after birth, causing a left-to-right shunt.
- Exposure to rubella in utero, high altitude, and prematurity are risk factors.

Clinical Features

- Mild cases are usually asymptomatic.
- As the shunting progresses, pulmonary HTM and cardiac remodeling occur.
- Shortness of breath and DOE can occur along with signs of heart failure.
- On examination, a loud P2 can be heard and a wide pulse pressure with bounding peripheral pulses.

Diagnostic Workup

- Echocardiography is the diagnostic test of choice. Doppler modalities may show turbulence of the blood flow where the PDA is present.
- ECG may show biventricular hypertrophy.
- Chest imaging may show enlarged pulmonary artery and markings.

Management

- Indomethacin may promote closure of the ductus.
- Surgical ligation may be needed, but may be contraindicated if severe pulmonary HTN or severe shunting is present.

COARCTATION OF THE AORTA

General Facts

- Coarctation is a narrowing that occurs in the aorta, causing significant obstruction and increasing the left ventricular afterload and cardiac workload.
- PDA usually occurs in the origin of the left subclavian artery near the ligamentum arteriosum.

Clinical Features

- PDA may cause headache, cold lower extremities due to low blood flow, and claudication with exercise.
- Upper extremities usually have high blood pressure, while lower extremities are discordant with low blood flow. This can lead to a developed upper torso and underdeveloped lower body.
- On examination, a midsystolic murmur can be heard, along with delayed femoral pulses when compared to radial pulses.

Diagnostic Workup

- Echocardiography is the gold standard by using Doppler modality and finding the abnormality and flow gradient.
- ECG may show LVH.
- Chest imaging may show "notching of the ribs."

Management

- Surgical decompression is the standard of care.
- New treatment modalities are emerging, such as minimally invasive aortoplasty procedures.

TETRALOGY OF FALLOT

General Facts

- Tetralogy of Fallot (TOF) is a complex set of abnormalities that includes VSD, right ventricular hypertrophy (RVH), and pulmonary AS with an overriding aorta.
- The complex set of cardiac anomalies leads to cyanosis.

Clinical Features

- Cyanosis is the hallmark of the condition, along with SOB and DOE.
- Episodes of hypoxia known as Tet spells can occur after crying or feeding, or when agitated. They are caused by a rapid drop in the amount of oxygen in the blood and can be relieved by squatting.
- On examination, a crescendo-decrescendo murmur can be heard in the left upper sternal border.

Diagnostic Workup

- Echocardiography is the gold standard.
- CXR may show a boot-shaped heart.

Management

- Surgery is indicated to correct the anomalies.

ARRHYTHMIAS

VENTRICULAR FIBRILLATION AND PULSELESS VENTRICULAR TACHYCARDIA

General Facts

- **Ventricular fibrillation** (see Figure 6-7) is disorganized electrical activity of the ventricular myocardium. Because the myocardium depolarizes in an irregular, disorganized fashion, regular myocardial contraction does not occur (looks like a "bag of worms").
- **Pulseless ventricular tachycardia:** Organized rapid contraction of the myocardium, with insufficient filling time and lack of forward flow resulting in loss of pulse. It may degenerate into ventricular fibrillation. Both of these conditions are medical emergencies and require immediate cardioversion and IV administration of amiodarone or lidocaine.
- Can be caused by many things, but myocardial ischemia is the most common. Long QT syndrome, torsades de pointes, Wolff-Parkinson-White (WPW) with atrial fibrillation and rapid ventricular response, and medications are other causes (Table 6-9).

CONQUER THE WARDS!

Torsade de pointes translates to "twisting of the peaks," which describes the appearance of the polymorphic VT with a rotational axis.

Clinical Features

- Ventricular fibrillation (V-fib) is not compatible with life.
- A patient with V-fib lasting more than 5 to 6 seconds will lose consciousness and suffer anoxic brain injury within minutes.

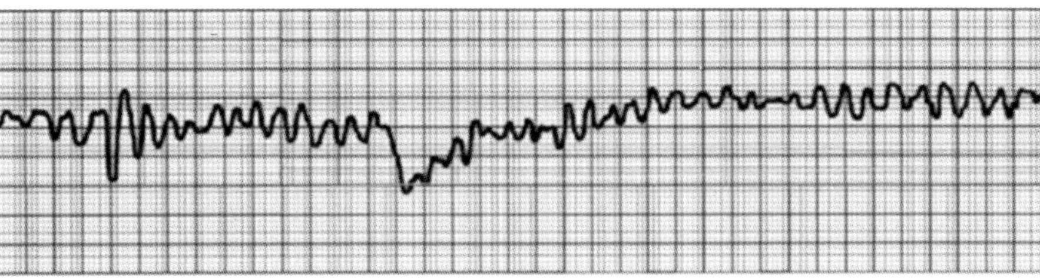

FIGURE 6-7. Ventricular fibrillation.

TABLE 6-8. Etiology of Torsade de Pointes
POINTES
Phenothiazines
Other meds (tricyclic antidepressants)
Intracranial bleed
No known cause (idiopathic)
Type I antiarrhythmics (quinidine and procainamide)
Electrolyte abnormalities (low K^+ or Mg^+)
Syndrome of long QT

Management

- V-fib patients or patients with hemodynamically unstable VT require emergent electrical cardioversion following the advanced cardiac life support (ACLS) protocol followed by IV amiodarone or lidocaine to maintain the sinus rhythm.
- In hemodynamically stable patients with VT, pharmacologic therapy can be attempted. ACLS guidelines recommend IV amiodarone, IV procainamide, or IV sotalol.
- **For prevention:**
  - ICD in patients who have underlying conditions that predispose to VT/V-fib or survivors of cardiac arrest secondary to VT/V-fib (this does not prevent the rhythm, but does treat it).
  - Electrophysiologic testing and radiofrequency ablation for accessory bypass tracts or slow VT pathways.

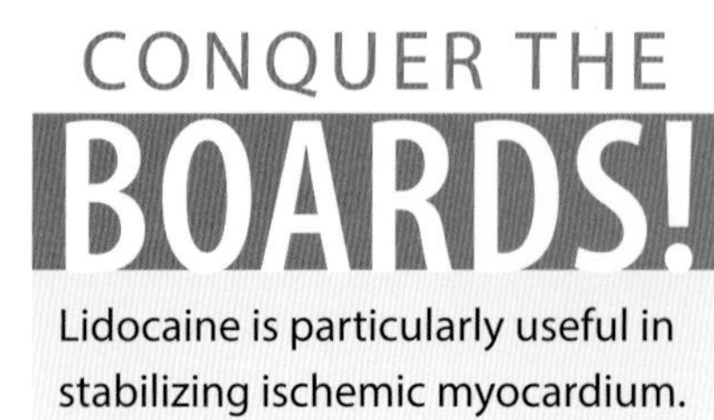

Lidocaine is particularly useful in stabilizing ischemic myocardium.

Nonsustained VT

Definition: Three or more consecutive ventricular beats at a rate of >120 beats/min and lasting less than 30 seconds.

Workup:

1. **ECG:** All patients should have an ECG, as nonsustained VT (NSVT) is often found on telemetry monitoring in the hospital.
2. **Search for underlying causes:** One episode usually does not require further investigation but the following should be considered: electrolyte imbalances, hypoxia, anemia, myocardial ischemia, and drug effect.

Management:

1. **Asymptomatic patients:** No specific treatment necessary.
2. **Symptomatic patients:** Beta blockers are first line and then amiodarone if patient remains symptomatic. Catheter ablation is only reserved for frequent, symptomatic NSVT that has failed medical treatment.

TORSADES DE POINTES

Polymorphic VT with rotating axis and prolonged QT (see Figure 6-8). Emergency – usually degenerates into ventricular fibrillation!

Management

- Magnesium IV for cardiac stabilization and then address an underlying cause. Overdrive pacing and beta blockers can also be used.
- Hemodynamically unstable patients need urgent cardioversion.

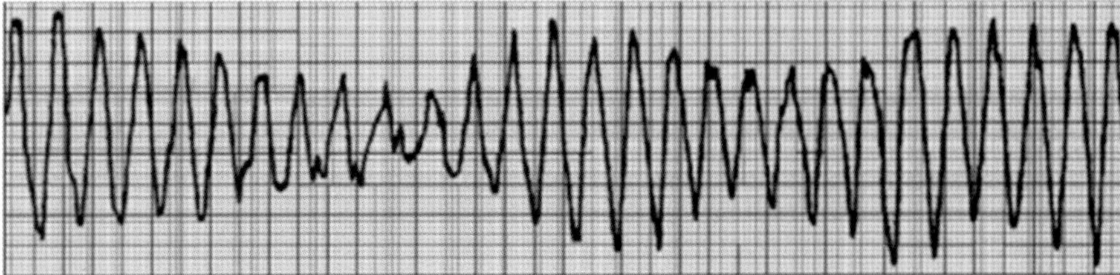

FIGURE 6-8. Torsades de pointes.

ATRIAL FIBRILLATION

General Facts

- Disorganized electrical activity of the atrial myocardium, causing ineffective atrial contractions and an irregular ventricular rhythm.
- Seen often in patients with dilated atria, related to heart failure or valvular disease.

Clinical Features

- Sensation of **palpitations** or skipped beats.
- **Lightheadedness**, fatigue comes from the fact that without the "atrial kick" that the atrial contraction provides, the cardiac output falls.
- **Thrombus** can develop in dyskinetic atrium and subsequently embolize to cause **a stroke.**
- On physical examination, pulse is irregularly irregular.

Diagnostic Workup

- **ECG:** Absent P waves. Wavy undulating baseline: R-R interval is variable (see Figure 6-9).
- **Echocardiogram**: Should be obtained on every patient in order to identify presence of clot in the left atrium and to look for underlying causes of atrial fibrillation such as valvular disease or heart failure.
- **Underlying causes:** Hypertension and coronary artery disease are the most common underlying disorders; however, other causes must also be considered (see Table 6-9).

Management

The mainstay of treatment for atrial fibrillation is rate control and anticoagulation to prevent stroke. Rhythm control can be considered, but only in symptomatic patients:

- **Rate control:** Slow rate with a calcium channel blocker like diltiazem or a beta blocker with a goal resting heart rate of less than 110 beats/min. Often just controlling the rate but not changing the rhythm can control symptoms.

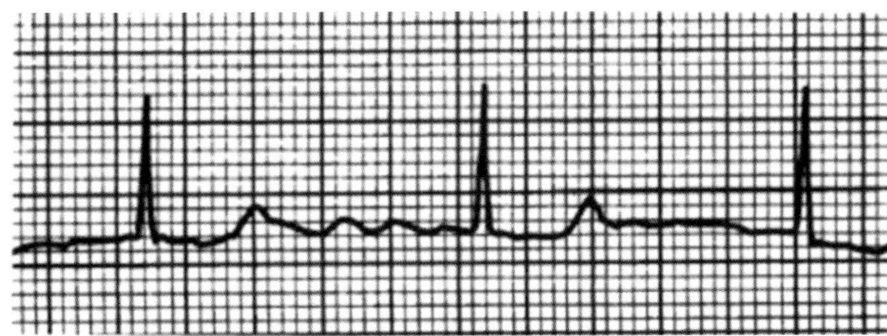

FIGURE 6-9. Atrial fibrillation.

TABLE 6-9. Etiology of Atrial Fibrillation
PIRATES
Pulmonary disease (pulmonary embolism and COPD are common)
Inflammation (pericarditis)
Rheumatic heart disease
Anemia, atrial myxoma
Thyroid disease (hyperthyroidism or hypothyroidism)
Ethanol
Sepsis

CONQUER THE WARDS!

Lightheadedness with atrial fibrillation is commonly seen in ventricles with diastolic dysfunction or aortic stenosis, conditions in which stroke volume is more preload sensitive.

CONQUER THE BOARDS!

Atrial fibrillation with rapid ventricular response in a patient with hypotension should be cardioverted.

CONQUER THE WARDS!

Very few arrhythmias result in an irregularly irregular rhythm, but among them are atrial fibrillation and multifocal atrial tachycardia.

CONQUER THE BOARDS!

The left atrial appendage is the most common location of thrombus in atrial fibrillation. It is poorly visualized on transthoracic echo, so use transesophageal echo instead.

TABLE 6-10. CHA_2DS_2-VASc Score	
Congestive HF	1
Hypertension	1
Age ≥75	2
Diabetes mellitus	1
Stroke/TIA/Thromboembolism	2
Vascular disease	1
Age 65 to 74 years	1
Sex (Female)	1

TABLE 6-11. Ischemic Risk and Anticoagulation

CHADS-VASc Total Score	Adjusted Ischemic Stroke Rate (% per year)	Anticoagulation
0	0%	No anticoagulation
1	1.30%	**Clinical judgment in conjunction with patient preference**
2	2.20%	NOAC
3	3.20%	
4	4.00%	
5	6.70%	
6	9.80%	

NOAC, new oral anticoagulants.

- **Anticoagulation:** Depending on risk factors, the incidence of stroke per year in patients changes drastically. An easy-to-use tool to assess stroke risk and in turn decide on anticoagulation is CHA_2DS_2-VASc (see Table 6-10).

All patients with a **CHA_2DS_2-VASc score** ≥**2** should be fully anticoagulated with a new oral anticoagulant such as rivaroxaban, apixaban, or dabigatran (Table 6-11). If the **CHA_2DS_2-VASc score** = **1**, it is up to patient preference, and for a score of 0 no oral anticoagulation is recommended. This is due to the fact that oral anticoagulation carries a yearly risk of intracranial bleed of around 1%.

- **Rhythm control:** In some cases the goal is to convert back to sinus rhythm. This is usually done in young patients or patients with persistent symptoms. In patients in A-fib <48 hours, synchronized cardioversion can be considered, and amiodarone and beta blockers can help maintain sinus rhythm after conversion. However, for most patients, it is difficult to tell how long they have been in A-fib. If cardioversion is being done, a TEE must be done prior to rule out clots in the heart. Radiofrequency ablation can be used for patients refractory to this, but success is variable.
- **For unstable patients with any rate or duration of rhythm:** Immediate synchronized cardioversion is indicated.

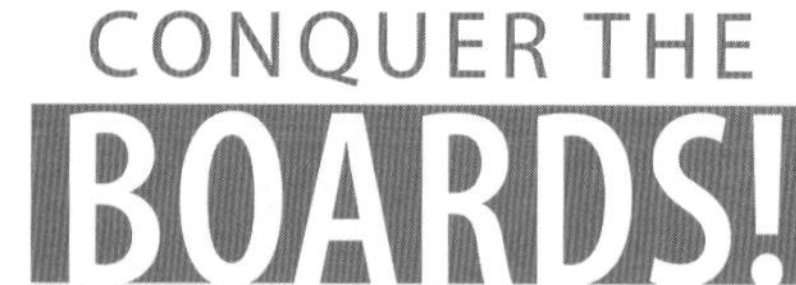

Patients cardioverted to sinus rhythm should be on anticoagulation for 4 weeks after the procedure.

HIGH-YIELD LITERATURE

Lip GYH, Nieuwlaat R, Pisters R, Lane DA, Crijns HJGM. CHA2DS2-VASc scores can predict patients at risk for stroke from atrial fibrillation:

Lip GY, et al. Refining clinical risk stratification for predicting stroke and thromboembolism in atrial fibrillation using a novel risk factor-based approach. *Chest.* 2010;137(2):263-272.

HIGH-YIELD LITERATURE

The AFFIRM writing group. Restoring sinus rhythm may not be better than rate control in atrial fibrillation: A comparison of rate control and rhythm control in patients with atrial fibrillation. *N Engl J Med.* 2002; 347: 1825-1833.

ATRIAL FLUTTER

General Facts

- Electrical activity forms a persistent circuit, usually in the right atrium, leading to a regular tachycardia.
- Seen often in patients with dilated atria related to heart failure or valvular disease, but also seen in patients with right atrial enlargement from pulmonary disease.
- Patients generally have a sensation of **palpitations** or skipped beats.

Diagnostic Workup

- **ECG:** Absent P waves. Instead, there is a "sawtooth" pattern to the baseline, most easily recognized in the inferior leads (II, III, and aVF).

Management

- Acute treatment is the same for atrial fibrillation, including anticoagulation for stroke prophylaxis and emergent cardioversion for hemodynamically unstable patients.
- Radiofrequency ablation is more effective in atrial flutter and should be considered in all patients with this condition.

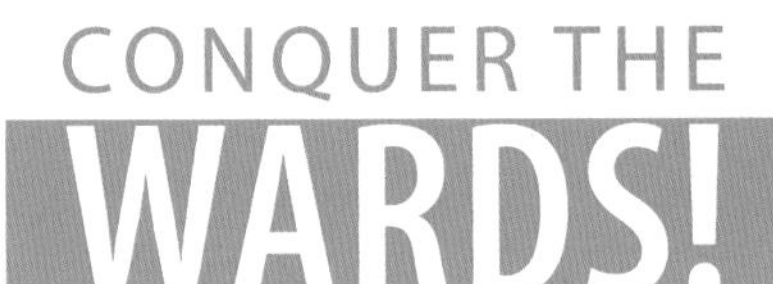

Atrial flutter often uses the cavo-tricuspid isthmus as part of the reentrant circuit. This is a good target for ablation.

WOLFF-PARKINSON-WHITE SYNDROME

General Facts

- **WPW** is a syndrome in which there is an accessory pathway that allows the electrical signal to travel from the sinus node to the ventricle, bypassing the atrioventricular (AV) node (this is called a "preexcitation syndrome"). This results in an abnormal finding on ECG (delta wave – see later) and a risk for arrhythmias.
- The accessory pathway is frequently slower than the His–Purkinje system, meaning that only a small portion of the ventricle is depolarized via the pathway before the standard conduction through the AV node and down the His–Purkinje system completes ventricular depolarization.
- **Antiarrhythmics that block the AV node** (adenosine, beta blockers, calcium channel blockers, and digoxin) **are contraindicated**—they can allow preexcitation to worsen.

CONQUER THE BOARDS!

WPW patients have a wide QRS, but not as wide as patients with a bundle branch block or ventricular depolarization.

Diagnostic Workup

- **ECG:** Shows a "delta" wave, a slurred upstroke of the QRS complex (see Figure 6-10).

CONQUER THE WARDS!

Accessory pathways are necessary to produce atrioventricular reentrant tachycardia (AVRT).

Management

- Patients with suspected WPW should have electrophysiologic testing (test that finds the abnormal electrical tract) in the electrophysiology lab and radiofrequency ablation of the bypass tract if symptomatic.
- **Unstable patients** with WPW and rapid atrial fibrillation with rapid ventricular response require emergent synchronized cardioversion.
- **Stable patients** with WPW and atrial fibrillation or wide-complex SVT are treated with procainamide, amiodarone, or sotalol.

HEART BLOCK

- **First-degree** (see Figure 6-11):
  - Prolonged PR interval (>0.20 second).
  - No treatment required.

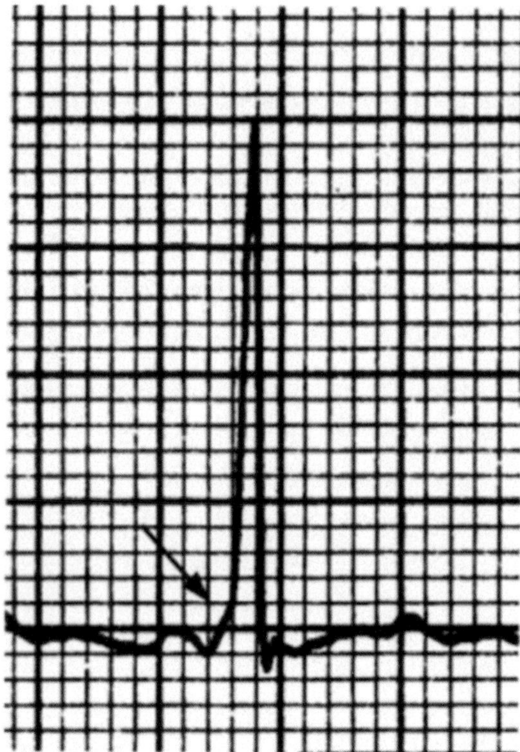

FIGURE 6-10. Wolff-Parkinson-White syndrome.

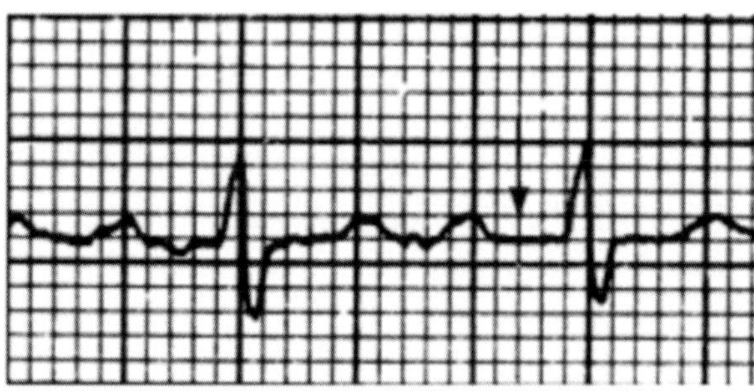

FIGURE 6-11. First-degree AV block.

CONQUER THE WARDS!

Avoid AV nodal blockers (adenosine, beta blockers, calcium channel blockers, digoxin) in patients with WPW, as it allows the atria access to the ventricle via the bypass tract. If the atria are fibrillating, this can cause the ventricle to fibrillate.

- **Second-degree** (two types – Mobitz I and II):
  - **Mobitz I (Wenckebach),** less dangerous (see Figure 6-12).
  - Progressive PR prolongation until a beat is not conducted (a P wave not followed by a QRS complex).
  - Treat with atropine or temporary pacing **only if symptoms are present**.
  - **Mobitz II,** more dangerous (see Figure 6-13).
  - Fixed prolonged PR interval followed by a nonconducted beat at a regular interval.
  - **This can degenerate into third-degree block.** Place a temporary transvenous pacemaker followed by a permanent pacemaker if rhythm persists.

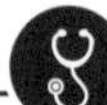

Causes of Mobitz I:

- **Inferior wall MI**
- **Digitalis toxicity**
- **Increased vagal tone**

Causes of Mobitz II:

- **Inferior wall or septal MI**
- **Conduction system disease**

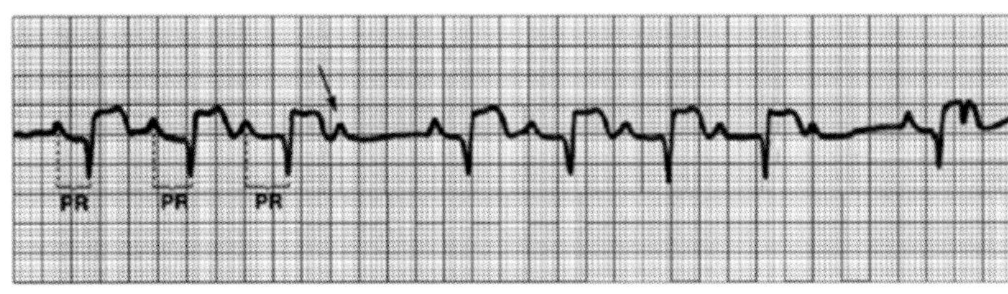

FIGURE 6-12. Wenckebach second-degree AV block (Mobitz I).

CONQUER THE WARDS!

Aging is accompanied by myocardial fibrosis. This leads to worsening conduction and heart blocks.

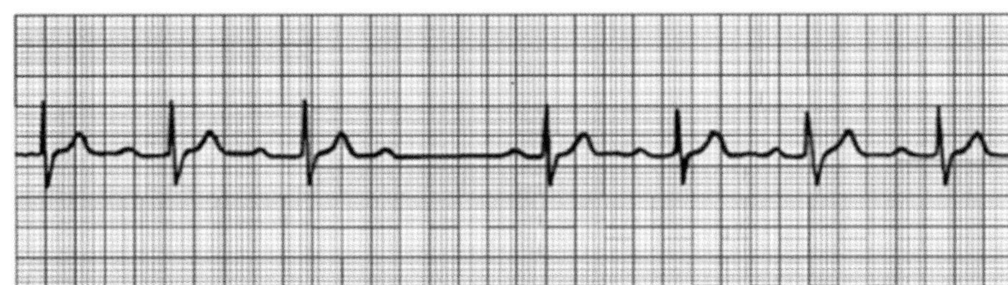

FIGURE 6-13. Mobitz II second-degree AV block.

CONQUER THE WARDS!

Third-degree AV block can arise from calcification or compression seen in calcified aortic stenosis or after aortic valve replacement.

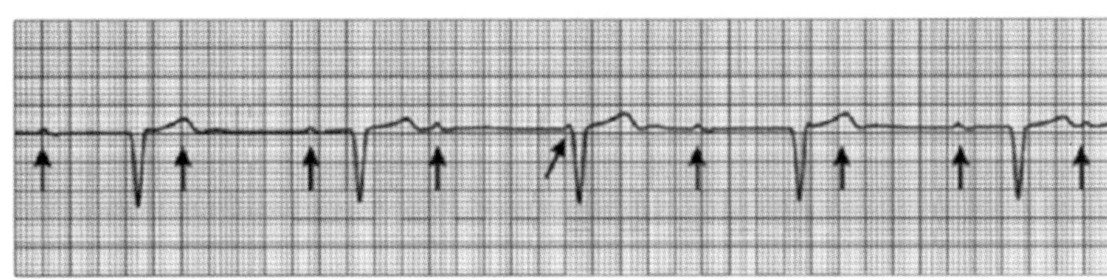

FIGURE 6-14. Complete (third-degree) AV block.

TABLE 6-12. Causes of Bradycardia
"One INCH"
If the R-R distance is at least 1 inch, consider:
Overmedication
Increased intracranial pressure
Normal variant
Carotid sinus hypersensitivity
Hypothyroidism

- **Third-degree** (complete heart block):
  - Independent atrial and ventricular activity (see Figure 6-14) (total asynchrony).
  - **Emergency:** Treat symptomatic patients with atropine and temporary pacing, followed by permanent pacemaker.
  - Always needs pacemaker, even when asymptomatic.

SINUS BRADYCARDIA

General Facts

- Defined as having a heart rate <60 with normal P waves and PR intervals.
- Causes include medications (beta blocker, calcium channel blocker, digoxin), inferior wall MI, increased intracranial pressure, normal variant (well-trained athletes can have very low resting heart rates), carotid sinus hypersensitivity, and hypothyroidism (Table 6-12).

Clinical Features

Often asymptomatic; lightheadedness and/or syncope can occur.

Management

- **Asymptomatic patients** do not require immediate treatment: Look for underlying cause. If patients can increase their heart rate with activity, then the bradycardia is not clinically significant.
- **Symptomatic patients:** Atropine +/– pacing.

HYPERTENSION

General Facts

- Hypertension accounts for more cardiovascular deaths than any other modifiable risk factor, and it is estimated that about 46% of U.S. adults have hypertension.
- There are 2 types of hypertension:

  1. **Primary** (essential hypertension, idiopathic): Essential hypertension is caused by normal cardiac output with increased peripheral vascular resistance.
  2. **Secondary HTN** (see later).

- Risk factors include diabetes, high-sodium diet, obesity, tobacco and alcohol use, family history of hypertension, and male gender.
- The classification of HTN and management goals are defined by the Joint National Committee on Prevention, Detection, Evaluation and Treatment of High Blood Pressure (JNC 8) (Table 6-13).

Diagnostic Workup

- Routine measurements of blood pressure should be used for screening; however, the diagnosis must be confirmed with one or more of the following criteria:

  1. 24-hour mean BP >125/75 mm Hg
  2. Daytime mean BP >130/80 mm Hg
  3. Nighttime mean 110/65 mm Hg

Thus, the gold standard for diagnosis of hypertension is ambulatory blood pressure monitoring. This also will help diagnose white coat hypertension if that is present.

- Next your diagnostic workup will turn to defining cardiovascular risk factors, seek secondary causes, and assess for any end-organ damage.

CONQUER THE WARDS!

Essential hypertension accounts for 90% of all cases.

CONQUER THE WARDS!

Hypertension due to pheochromocytoma is characterized by ectopic production of epinephrine and norepinephrine, causing wide swings in blood pressure.

TABLE 6-13. Blood Pressure Classifications

Stage	BP
Normal	<120 and <80 mm Hg
Elevated	120–129 and <80 mm Hg
Stage 1 hypertension	130–139 mm Hg or 80–89 mm Hg
Stage 2 hypertension	≥140 mm Hg or ≥90 mm Hg

- Always start with a thorough physical exam.
  - Blood pressure in both arms, repeated if abnormal.
  - Funduscopic examination to look for AV nicking, retinal hemorrhage, papilledema.
- **Basic labs and tests:** Your initial workup will assess for end-organ damage and may give clues to potential secondary causes of hypertension, as well as risk factors:
  - Chemistry panel should be obtained, looking at blood urea nitrogen (BUN)/creatinine, serum potassium (evidence of renal insufficiency).
  - Lipid panel to screen for hyperlipidemia.
  - **Urinalysis** to assess for microalbuminuria, hematuria, or active sediment.
  - **ECG** to assess for cardiac abnormalities such as LVH or left ventricular strain.

- **Workup for secondary causes of hypertension:** Essential hypertension is by far the most common type of hypertension, but it is still important to consider the following secondary causes when taking an initial history (Table 6-14). However, full workup for these diagnoses is not warranted

TABLE 6-14. Secondary Causes of HTN

Causes	Clinical Features	Diagnostic Approach
Renal hypertension		
Renal artery stenosis (atherosclerosis, fibromuscular dysplasia)	Abdominal bruits Femoral, carotid bruits	Renal ultrasound with dopplers
Parenchymal renal disease (CKD, PCKD, obstructive uropathy)	Ankle edema Oliguria Anasarca Hematuria	Renal ultrasound Urinalysis
Endocrine-metabolic hypertension		
Primary aldosteronism	Hypokalemia (half of patients are normokalemic)	Plasma aldosterone–renin ratio
Obstructive sleep apnea (most common secondary cause of HTN)	Fatigue Snoring Obesity Frequent nighttime a wakening	Sleep study
Uncommon endocrine causes Cushing syndrome Pheochromocytoma Hyperthyroidism Hyperparathyroidism Acromegaly	See endocrine chapter 7	See endocrine chapter 7
Drug-induced or drug-related hypertension		
Estrogen treatment ("pill hypertension") Exogenous corticosteroids, androgens Nonsteroidal antiinflammatory drugs Cocaine, amphetamine, or alcohol use Decongestants Appetite suppressants Cyclosporine, tacrolimus Some antidepressants (e.g., venlafaxine)	Careful history, looking for medication list and exposures to these medications	Drug levels if necessary

unless there are concerns based on your history and physical. Other situations where a more thorough workup for secondary causes should be obtained are:

- Refractory hypertension: Patient is on maximum doses of 3 or more antihypertensives.
- Onset of hypertension <30 years of age.
- Exacerbation of previously controlled hypertension.

Management (see figure 6-15)

- Nonpharmaceutical interventions should be recommended to all patients and can include **lifestyle modifications such as weight loss, dietary changes** (high fruits, vegetables, and low-fat dairy products, low total and saturated fats, low salt), and physical exercise.
- Therapeutic choices for hypertension will depend on the stage and patient comorbidities (see figure 6-15).
- Target BP will also depend on comorbidities and risk of cardiovascular disease.
    - Clinical CVD or 10-year Atherosclerotic Cardiovascular Disease (ASCVD) Score risk ≥10 %: a target of <130/<80 is recommended. Clinical CVDs are diabetes mellitus, chronic kidney disease, heart failure, ischemic heart disease, stroke, and peripheral artery disease.
    - Low-risk patients = No clinical CVD and 10-year ASCVD risk <10%: target blood pressure <140/<90.

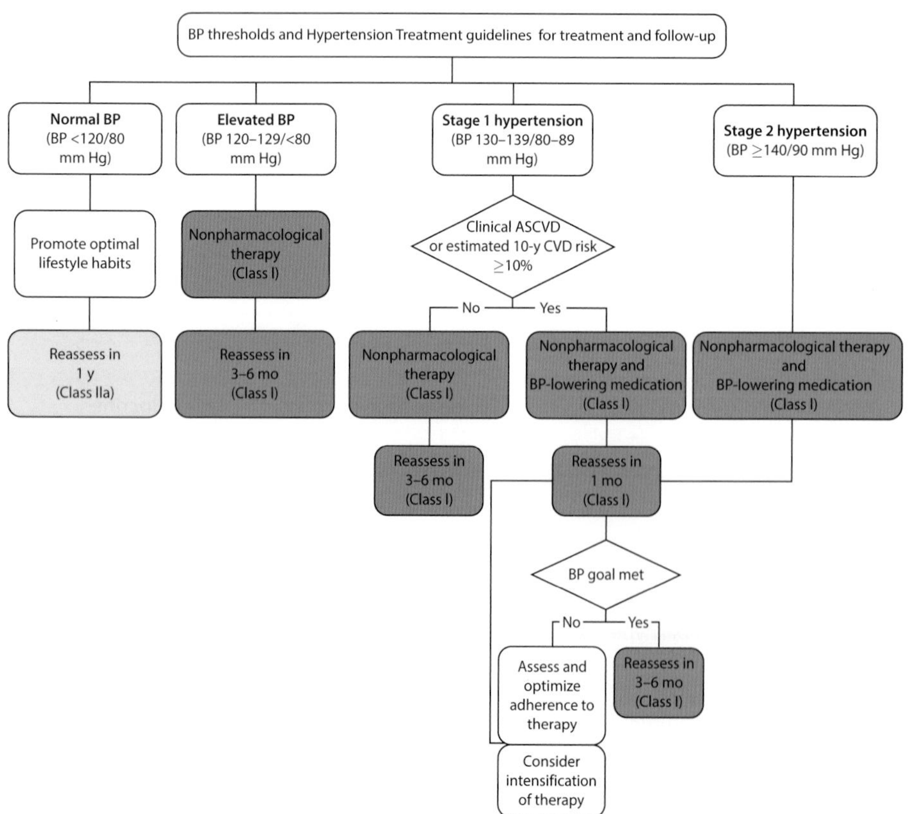

FIGURE 6-15. Hypertension Treatment Guidelines

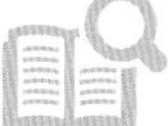

HIGH-YIELD LITERATURE

Whelton PK, Carey RM, Aronow WS, et al. 2017 ACC/AHA/AAPA/ABC/ACPM/AGS/APhA/ASH/ASPC/NMA/PCNA guideline for the prevention, detection, evaluation, and management of high blood pressure in adults: A report of the American College of Cardiology/American Heart Association Task Force on Clinical Practice Guidelines. *Hypertension.* 2018;71:e13.

Qaseem A, Wilt TJ, Rich R, et al. Pharmacologic treatment of hypertension in adults aged 60 years or older to higher versus lower blood pressure targets: A clinical practice guideline from the American College of Physicians and the American Academy of Family Physicians. *Ann Intern Med.* 2017;166:430.

- **HTN without other comorbidities:** First-line treatment is with **thiazide** diuretics, **low-dose ACE inhibitor,** or calcium channel blockers. Beta blockers are not first-line treatments in patients without other indications for them such as heart failure. Generally in stage 2 hypertension 2 agents should be started initially.
    - HTN with comorbidities will lead to more specific choices:
    - CAD: ACE inhibitor or ARB and beta blocker are first-line and then diuretics or nitrates.
    - HF: ACE inhibitor or ARB and beta blocker are first-line and then diuretics or nitrates.
    - Diabetes mellitus: ACE inhibitor or ARB, calcium channel blocker, or thiazides are all good first options.
    - Chronic kidney disease (CKD): ACE inhibitor or ARB, or diuretics are first-line.

CONQUER THE WARDS!

ACE inhibitors can be considered first-line antihypertensives in diabetics, as they are renoprotective.

CONQUER THE WARDS!

Initial drug of choice will depend heavily on underlying comorbidities. Options abound, and the specific drug of choice is controversial due to conflicting studies and heterogeneity of patients.

CONQUER THE BOARDS!

End-organ damage can be made worse by reducing pressure too rapidly in coronary and cerebral vascular beds. Intravenous agents can be rapidly titrated up or down to control BP.

HYPERTENSIVE EMERGENCY

Definition: A hypertensive emergency is characterized by severely elevated blood pressure (SBP ≥180 mm Hg and/or DBP ≥120 mm Hg) accompanied by **end-organ damage**. This is in contrast to hypertensive urgency, which is only severely elevated blood pressure.

Diagnostic Workup and Clinical Features

Presence of end-organ damage defines hypertensive emergency, and a thorough history and physical are key to diagnosing this condition. It is helpful to think about the common organs that are affected.

Neurologic: Look for signs of ischemic or hemorrhagic stroke (e.g., facial droop, unilateral limb weakness, slurred speech). There can also be signs of generalized neurologic symptoms such as delirium, agitation, stupor, seizures, and nausea and vomiting due to the increased intracranial pressure. If any of these symptoms are present, a head computed tomography (CT) should be obtained.

Cardiology: Ask patients about chest discomfort or pain, and obtain an ECG on all patients with severely high blood pressure to rule out myocardial ischemia. Dyspnea may be a sign of pulmonary edema. Also think about aortic dissection, as high blood pressure may be a result of an aortic dissection.

Renal: Obtaining BUN and creatinine are important first steps to ascertain whether there are signs of acute renal failure. Urinalysis can also be obtained.

Ophthalmology: A funduscopic exam should be performed on all patients with severely high blood pressure looking for flame hemorrhages, exudates (cotton-wool spots), or papilledema.

Pregnancy: High blood pressure may be a sign of developing eclampsia.

Management

- Reduce the mean arterial pressure by no more than 10% to 20% in the first hour and then by about 25% in the first 24 hours. The major exceptions to this rule are patients with an acute ischemic stroke, where the blood pressure should not be lower than 185/10 mm Hg, and aortic dissection, where the blood pressure must be rapidly lowered to prevent further dissection.
- Common intravenous agents used are nitroprusside drips and nitroglycerin drips because of their rapid onset of action and rapid clearance to allow for quick titration.
  - If pheochromocytoma is the cause, use phentolamine.
  - For preeclampsia-related hypertension, use magnesium or hydralazine.

AORTIC DISSECTION

General Facts

- Usually associated with a transverse tear through the intima and internal media of the aortic wall.
- Dissection can be caused by hypertension, connective tissue diseases (Marfan, Ehlers–Danlos), congenital heart disease, trauma, pregnancy, syphilis, coarctation of the aorta, and cocaine use.

Classification

- **Stanford classification:**
  - Type A: Dissection involves the ascending aorta – Requires emergent surgery.
  - Type B: Does not involve the ascending aorta – This can be medically managed.

Clinical Features

- Severe **"tearing"** chest pain, may radiate to back.
- Unequal pulses distally for descending aortic dissection.
- Aortic regurgitation murmur transmitted down right sternal border with ascending aortic dissection.
- Complications can include MI (via dissection or obstruction of coronary arteries), stroke (via dissection or obstruction of carotids), aortic regurgitation, or tamponade.

A middle-aged man comes to the emergency room (ER) with severe hypertension and a tearing pain in his back. **What do you do?** Control hypertension with labetalol and do a CT angiogram to rule out aortic dissection.

Diagnostic Features

- **CT angiography** is the diagnostic imaging modality of choice because it is easily obtained and has a high sensitivity and specificity. TEE can also diagnose aortic dissection and is used in patients who are hemodynamically unstable because it can be done at the bedside.
- **CXR:** Can be normal but often shows **widened mediastinum**, apical pleural capping, and loss of the aortic knob.

CONQUER THE **BOARDS!**

Aortic dissection in a patient with Marfan syndrome is a classic test question!.

CONQUER THE **WARDS!**

Aortic dissection due to syphilis occurs because the *Treponema* infects the vasa vasorum of the aorta.

CONQUER THE **BOARDS!**

Always get a chest film when you suspect MI—some of these patients will have aortic dissection, and thrombolysis may kill them. If there is a widened mediastinum, do not give lytics!

CONQUER THE **WARDS!**

Mean arterial pressure (MAP) is calculated as [2(dBP) + sBP] / 3.

Management

- Immediate surgical repair for type A dissection (ascending aorta).
- Medical stabilization for type B dissection (descending aorta).
- **Medical stabilization** focuses on 2 areas: heart rate control and blood pressure control. Heart rate control must be done first before blood pressure control because rapid peripheral vasodilation may result in a reflex activation of the sympathetic nervous system.
  - **Heart rate control:** Therapy for aortic dissection usually starts with a rapid-acting beta blocker such as an esmolol drip with a goal heart rate under 60 beats/min.
  - **BP control:** After the heart rate is consistently under 60 and if the systolic blood pressure remains >120 mm Hg, vasodilator agents should be used, such as nitroprusside.

BACTERIAL ENDOCARDITIS

General Facts

- Localized infection of the endocardium characterized by vegetations involving the valve leaflets or walls.
- It is best categorized by the infecting organism, which determines the course of the disease.

CONQUER THE WARDS!

Staphylococcus lugdunensis is the organism that most often causes aggressive endocarditis requiring surgical intervention.

Microbiology

- *Staphylococcus aureus,* gram-negative organisms, *Streptococcus viridans,* other oral flora, group A beta-hemolytic streptococcus, enterococci, *Staphylococcus epidermidis.*
  - **Special conditions:**
    a. **IV drug users:** *S. aureus* is the most common followed by streptococci, enterococci, and *Candida.*
    b. **Prosthetic valves** (10% to 20% of cases): *S. aureus, S. viridans,* gram-negative bacilli, fungi.
    c. **Nosocomial infections:** Indwelling venous catheters, hemodialysis.

CONQUER THE WARDS!

Streptococcus bovis endocarditis is associated with colonic neoplasms.

Clinical features

- Acute or gradual onset of fever, chills, rigors, weakness, arthralgia, anorexia, weight loss, and cutaneous lesions.
- A new cardiac murmur should always prompt further workup and in the setting of bacteremia should always prompt consideration for endocarditis.
- Metastatic infections can occur, including meningitis, septic pulmonary emboli, splenic emboli, and infarcts.
- **Other high-yield findings include:**
  - **Osler nodes:** Tender violaceous subcutaneous nodules on fingers and toes (see Figure 6-16).
  - **Splinter hemorrhages:** Fine linear hemorrhages in the middle of the nail bed (see Figure 6-17).
  - **Janeway lesions:** Multiple hemorrhagic nontender macules or nodules on the palms and soles (see Figure 6-18).
  - **Roth spots:** Retinal hemorrhages seen on fundoscopy.
  - Conjunctival hemorrhages.

CONQUER THE WARDS!

The most common organism to cause endocarditis in IV drug users is still *S. aureus.*

CONQUER THE WARDS!

S. aureus can cause perivalvular abscesses, which almost always require surgical debridement.

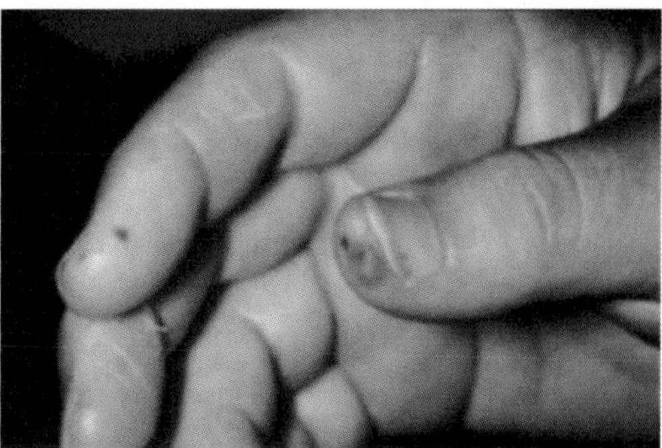

FIGURE 6-16. **Osler node.** (Photo contributor: Armed Forces Institute of Pathology, Bethesda, Maryland. Reproduced, with permission, from Knoop KJ, Stack LB, Storrow AB. *Atlas of Emergency Medicine.* 3rd ed. New York: McGraw-Hill, 2010: 375.)

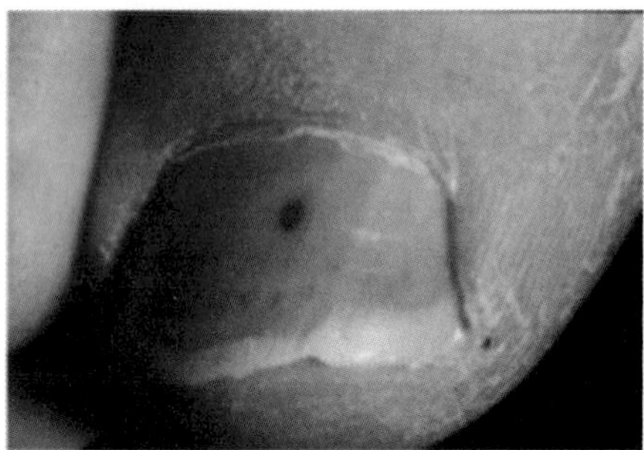

FIGURE 6-17. **Splinter hemorrhage.** (Photo contributor: Armed Forces Institute of Pathology, Bethesda, Maryland. Reproduced, with permission, from Knoop KJ, Stack LB, Storrow AB. *Atlas of Emergency Medicine.* 3rd ed. New York: McGraw-Hill, 2010: 375.)

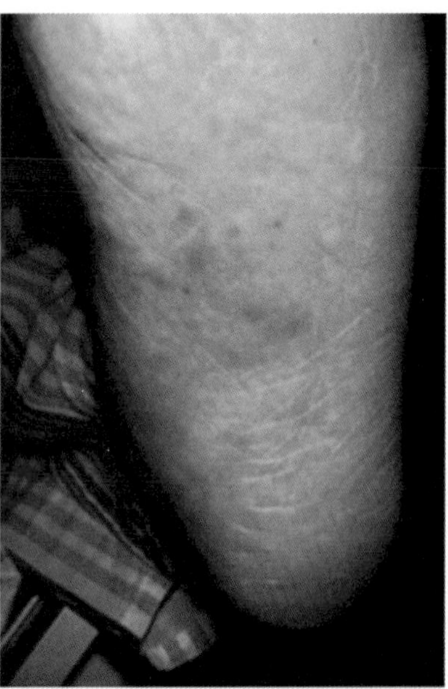

FIGURE 6-18. **Janeway lesion.** (Photo contributor: Department of Dermatology, Wilford Hall USAF Medical Center and Brooke Army Medical Center, San Antonio, Texas. Reproduced, with permission, from Knoop KJ, Stack LB, Storrow AB. *Atlas of Emergency Medicine.* 3rd ed. New York: McGraw-Hill, 2010: 374.)

Diagnostic Workup

- **Duke criteria** (patient must have 2 major, 1 major + 3 minor, or 5 minor criteria for diagnosis) (Table 6-15).

TABLE 6-15. Criteria for Rheumatoid Heart Disease

Major Criteria	Minor Criteria
■ Two positive blood cultures taken at least 12 hours apart or 3+ positive cultures taken at least 1 hour apart with typical organisms. ■ Echocardiography – vegetations are pathognomonic, but their absence does not rule out endocarditis; transesophageal echo is more sensitive.	■ Predisposing lesion on valve or IV drug use. ■ Fever >38°C. ■ Arterial emboli (Janeway lesions). ■ Osler nodes, Roth spots. ■ Positive blood cultures not meeting major criteria. ■ Echocardiogram suspicious for endocarditis but not meeting major criteria.

TABLE 6-16. Management of Native and Prosthetic Valve Endocarditis

Organism	Native Valve Endocarditis	Prosthetic Valve Endocarditis
Highly penicillin-susceptible VGS and *Streptococcus gallolyticus* (bovis)	Penicillin (PCN) OR ceftriaxone (CTX) × 4 wk OR CTX PLUS Gent × 2 wk OR Vancomycin × 4 wk	PCN OR CTX × 6 wk +/− Gentamicin (Gent) × 2 wk OR Vancomycin × 6 wk
VGS and *Streptococcus gallolyticus* (bovis) Relatively resistant to penicillin	PCN × 4 wk PLUS Gent × 2 wk OR Vancomycin × 4 wk	PCN OR CTX × 6 wk + Gent 6 wk OR Vancomycin × 6 wk
Staphylococci	Cefazolin, Nafcillin, Oxacillin, Vancomycin OR Daptomycin × 6 wk	Beta-lactam + Rifampin (RIF) × 6 wk + Gent × 2 wk OR Vancomycin + RIF × 6 wk + Gent × 2 wk
Enterococcus, PCN-S, AG-S	PCN OR Ampicillin (AMP) + Gent OR CTX × 4–6 wk	PCN OR AMP + Gent OR CTX × 4–6 wk
Enterococcus, PCN-S, AG-R	PCN OR AMP + CTX × 4–6 wk	PCN OR AMP + CTX × 4–6 wk
Enterococcus, PCN-R, AG-S	Vancomycin + Gent × 6 wk	Vancomycin + Gent × 6 wk
VRE	Linezolid OR Daptomycin × >6 wk	Linezolid OR Daptomycin × >6 wk
HACEK	CTX OR PCN OR Ciprofloxacin × 4 wk	CTX OR PCN OR Ciprofloxacin × 6 wk
Candida	Amphotericin B + 5-FC + Surgery	
Whipple	CTX × 2 wk, Doxycycline or TMP-SMX × 12 mo	CTX × 2 wk, Doxycycline or Trimethoprim sulfamethoxazole (TMP-SMX) × 12 mo
Q fever	Doxycycline plus Hydroxychloroquine >18 mo	Doxycycline plus Hydroxychloroquine >18 mo
Culture negative	Ampicillin-sulbactam + Gent × 6 wk OR Vancomycin + Gent + Ciprofloxacin × 6 wk	Ampicillin-Sulbactam + Gent × 6 wk OR Vancomycin + Gent + Ciprofloxacin × 6 wk

Management

- Management will depend on the organism and whether it is a native or prosthetic valve (Table 6-16).

TABLE 6-17. Criteria for Rheumatoid Heart Disease

Major Criteria	Major Criteria
■ Arthritis (migratory, multiple joints)	■ Fever
■ Carditis (endo-, myo-, peri-)	■ Arthralgias
■ Erythema marginatum rash	■ Elevated ESR
■ Subcutaneous nodules	■ Prolonged PR interval
■ Sydenham chorea	■ Recent streptococcal pharyngitis

RHEUMATIC FEVER

- **Rheumatic fever (RF)** is a systemic immune process that usually occurs secondary to pharyngeal streptococcal infection.
- **Rheumatic heart disease (RHD)** is the occurrence of valvular abnormalities due to immune complex deposition in valve leaflets generated by rheumatic fever.

Diagnostic Workup

- **Laboratory findings:**
  - Positive antistreptolysin-O (ASLO) antibody titers and elevated ESR.
- Diagnosis of RF requires the presence of 2 major criteria or 1 major and 2 minor criteria (Table 6-17).

Management

- **Acute:** Course of penicillin to eradicate throat carriage of group A streptococci. Aspirin for arthritis and steroids for carditis.
- **Chronic:** Monthly doses of benzathine penicillin to prevent recurrences.

> CONQUER THE WARDS!
>
> Strep throat is treated with antibiotics to reduce the incidence of rheumatic heart disease. The pharyngitis will resolve without intervention.

> CONQUER THE WARDS!
>
> HDL >60 is considered cardioprotective.

> CONQUER THE WARDS!
>
> Patients with very high triglycerides are at risk of developing pancreatitis.

DYSLIPIDEMIA

About half of all cases of CAD are associated with disorders of lipid metabolism. Formulas for calculating lipid levels:

- LDL = TC − HDL − VLDL
- VLDL = Trig / 5
- A normal total cholesterol (TC) level is <200, with borderline ranging at 200 to 240 and high at >240.
- Normal high-density lipoprotein (HDL) ranges from 30 to 100.

MAJOR LIPOPROTEINS

- **Chylomicrons:** Transport cholesterol from the gut in the bloodstream.
- **Chylomicron remnants:** Left over after lipoprotein lipase liberates free fatty acids from chylomicrons for use in tissues.
- **Very low-density lipoprotein (VLDL):** Secreted from the liver; carries cholesterol in the bloodstream.
- **Intermediate-density lipoprotein (IDL):** Metabolized from VLDL.
- **LDL:** Metabolized from IDL, it carries cholesterol in the bloodstream to tissues.
- **HDL:** Uptakes free cholesterol secreted by tissues and transports it to the liver.

Clinical Features

- **Xanthelasma:** Painless, nonpruritic, raised, yellow plaques that occur on eyelids near the inner canthi.
- **Xanthoma:** Reddish-brown papules on scalp, face, trunk, and flexor surfaces of the limbs.

Diagnostic Workup

- Serum lipid analysis is done after a 12-hour fast.
- One-time sample cholesterol levels may not represent true levels when patients are undergoing weight loss, during pregnancy, after a major surgery, or during a severe illness.
- In patients who have MI, lipoprotein levels obtained within the first 24 hours will more closely approximate true pre-MI levels than later levels, which may not return to baseline for several weeks.
- For cholesterol levels, see Table 6-18.

Management

Recent updates in cholesterol guidelines have changed how we assess patients for treatment. However, the mainstay of treatment remains lifestyle modifications and statin therapy. Statins can vary in dosage and intensity (Table 6-19).

TABLE 6-18. Cholesterol Levels Associated with Familiar Disease

	Type	Total Cholesterol Level (mg/dL)	LDL Level	VLDL	Chylomicrons
Familial hypercholesterolemia	IIa	275–500	High	Normal	Normal
Familial defective apo B100	IIa	275–500	High	Normal	Normal
Polygenic hypercholesterolemia	IIa	240–350	High	Normal	Normal
Familial hypertriglyceridemia	IV	250–750	Normal/ High	High	Normal/High
Familial lipoprotein lipase deficiency	I, (I,V)	>750	Normal/ High	Normal/ High	High
Familial apoprotein CII deficiency	I, (I,V)	>750	Normal/ High	Normal/ High	High
Familial combined hyperlipidemia	IIb	275–500	High	High	Normal/High
Dysbetalipoproteinemia	III	275–500	Normal	High	Normal/High

TABLE 6-19. Statins by Intensity and Dosage

High-Intensity Statins	Moderate-Intensity Statins
Atorvastatin 40–80 mg	Atorvastatin 10–20 mg
Rosuvastatin 20–40 mg	Rosuvastatin 5–10 mg
	Simvastatin 20–40 mg
	Pravastatin 40–80 mg
	ASCVD risk <5%, Lifestyle reduction only

TABLE 6-20. Cardiovascular Risk Factors and Recommended Interventions	
Risk Factor	Intervention
Clinical ASCVD*	High-intensity statin
LDL-C >190 mg /dL	High-intensity statin
Diabetes mellitus (age 40–75 yr)	Moderate-intensity statin
Age 40–75 yr without diabetes AND LDL-C ≥70 and <190 mg/dL	ASCVD risk ≥7.5%, Moderate-intensity statin
	ASCVD risk 5%–<7.5%, Moderate-intensity statin if it has one risk enhancer†
	ASCVD risk <5%, Lifestyle reduction only

* Clinical ASCVD includes cerebrovascular accident, transient ischemic attack, coronary artery disease, acute coronary syndrome, peripheral vascular disease, and aortic aneurysm.
† ASCVD risk enhancers include family history of premature ASVD, chronic kidney disease, metabolic syndrome, inflammatory diseases, LDL-C ≥160 mg/dL or triglycerides ≥175 mg/dL persistently after lifestyle modification.

Lifestyle Modifications: This includes:

1. Diet: Decrease saturated fat intake and eat food rich in omega-3 fatty acids such as fish. Intensive diet modifications can lower LDL by as much as 10%.
2. Exercise: Exercise increases HDL and reduces other CAD risk factors.
3. Smoking cessation.

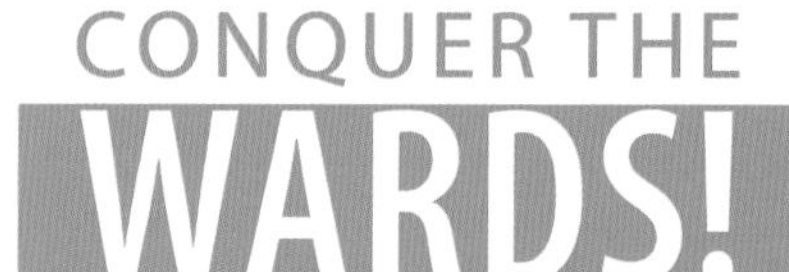

PCSK9 inhibitors can drastically reduce LDL in patients with familial hypercholesterolemia or who cannot tolerate statins.

Statin Treatment

Table 6-20 shows patients who should begin pharmacologic treatment for their hyperlipidemia along with lifestyle modifications.

- Statins can reduce LDL levels by 20% to 60% and have an impact on HDL and triglycerides (TG) as well. Statins can cause transaminitis and cause myalgias or rhabdomyolysis.
- LDL level should be rechecked 2 to 3 months after initiating treatment to gauge response.
- Ezetimibe can reduce LDL levels by 20% and is well tolerated if a patient has tolerability problems with statins. It can also be added to high-intensity statin therapy if LDL-C remains >100 mg/dL despite treatment.

Hypertriglyceridemia

- Consider therapy if triglycerides >500 mg/dL due to the increased risk of cardiovascular events and risk of pancreatitis. However, it has not been convincingly shown that lowering triglyceride levels reduces risk.
- Fibrates are usually first-line and can decrease TG by 50% and have moderate impact on LDL and HDL. Fibrates can increase the risk of myopathies with statins.
- Niacin can decrease TG by up to 40% and have a moderate impact on LDL and HDL. Niacin can cause flushing, which can be prevented with aspirin as pretreatment.

Other Regimens

- Resins can decrease LDL and HDL but increase TG. Side effects include bloating and binding in the gastrointestinal (GI) tract with other medications.
- PCSK9 inhibitors are subcutaneous injections and can have a big impact on LDL of >50%, along with moderate impact on HDL and TG.

TABLE 6-21. Common Cardiac Medications

	Medication	Main Clinical Uses	Adverse Effects
Class I: Sodium channel blockers	Lidocaine	Suppresses ventricular dysrhythmias.	Mild: drowsiness, confusion, ataxia. Severe: psychosis, seizures, AV block, respiratory depression.
	Quinidine	Suppresses ventricular dysrhythmias, atrial premature beats, A-fib.	Cinchonism: tinnitus, hearing loss, visual changes, delirium, psychosis. Also causes GI upset, promotes torsades de pointes (proarrhythmic). Potentiates many other medications.
	Procainamide	Suppresses ventricular dysrhythmias and A-fib, A-flutter, WPW.	Myocardial depression, prolonged QT and QRS, torsades de pointes, V-fib.
Class II: Beta blockers	Propranolol	SVT, thyrotoxicosis, acute MI, hypertension.	All beta blockers can cause bradycardia. Hypotension, light-headedness, fatigue, depression, and elevation of triglycerides can occur.
	Metoprolol	SVT, acute MI, hypertension.	
	Esmolol	SVT, thyrotoxicosis.	
	Labetalol	Hypertension.	
Class III: Prolongs action potentials	Amiodarone	VT, VF, A-fib, WPW.	Bradycardia, AV block, peripheral neuropathy, pulmonary fibrosis, corneal deposits, skin discoloration, hepatotoxicity. Due to high iodine content, can cause hypo- or hyperthyroidism.
	Bretylium	Ventricular dysrhythmias.	Transient hypertension, hypotension.
	Sotalol	AV reentry SVT, WPW.	Bradycardia, CHF, peripheral edema.
Class IV: Calcium channel blockers	Verapamil	Mild to moderate hypertension.	Calcium channel blockers reduce inotropy and are contraindicated in patients with heart failure, second- or third-degree heart block.
	Diltiazem	Mild to moderate hypertension.	
	Amlodipine, nifedipine	Mild to moderate hypertension.	
Other anti-arrhythmic agents	Adenosine	Supraventricular tachycardia.	Transient asystole, hypotension, flushing.
	Digoxin	Rate control of atrial tachydysrhythmia, increased inotropy for CHF.	Toxicity can occur in therapeutic range. Vomiting, anorexia, confusion, visual changes, AV block, PVCs, VT, VF. Hyperkalemia is seen with acute poisoning. Hypokalemia lowers threshold for toxicity (remember, many drugs used for CHF can cause hypokalemia). Chronic therapy can cause gynecomastia.
	Magnesium	Torsades de pointes, hypertension due to preeclampsia.	Hypotension, flushing, CNS changes, decreased reflexes, respiratory collapse.
	Epinephrine	Asystole, anaphylaxis, pressor.	May cause ischemia.
	Dobutamine	Increases inotropy.	Associated with reflex arterial vasodilatation and tachycardia.

	Medication	Main Clinical Uses	Adverse Effects
Ionotropic agents	Dobutamine	Increases myocardial contractility.	Associated with reflex arterial vasodilatation and tachycardia.
	Milrinone	Increases myocardial contractility.	Can lead to systemic hypotension
Chronotropic agents	Atropine	Asystole, symptomatic bradycardia.	Anticholinergic.
Venous/coronary dilators	Nitroglycerin	Venous and coronary artery dilator, can be used for malignant hypertension.	Hypotension, headache.
Antihypertensive agents	Nitroprusside	Malignant hypertension.	Can cause hypotension, cyanide toxicity, methemoglobinemia.
	Minoxidil	Severe hypertension.	Can cause hypotension, tachycardia, hair growth.
	Hydralazine	Moderate to severe hypertension, particularly in the setting of preeclampsia and eclampsia. Hydralazine is a direct vasodilator.	Can cause tachycardia, angina, lupus-like syndrome with a malar rash that disappears after discontinuing the drug.
	Clonidine	Central-acting agent for hypertension.	Hypotension, rebound hypertension after halting medication.
	Phentolamine	Parenteral alpha blocker used for hypertension due to pheochromocytoma, cocaine.	Hypotension, tachycardia, light-headedness.
	ACE inhibitors	Hypertension (decrease preload and afterload), nephroprotective CHF. Decrease cardiovascular events and mortality in high-risk patients >55 years old.	All ACE inhibitors are variably associated with cough and angioedema and can cause acute renal failure in patients with bilateral renal artery stenosis. Hyperkalemia.
	Angiotensin receptor blockers	Hypertension. Unclear magnitude of renal protection compared to ACE inhibitors.	Side effects similar to ACE inhibitors but less cough.
Antiplatelet agents	Aspirin	Used to prevent MI in patients with risk factors, can improve mortality from MI by about 25%.	Associated with GI bleed. Some patients can have hypersensitivity reaction to aspirin.
Antithrombotic agents	Warfarin	Long-term prevention of clots in deep vein thrombosis (DVT), A-fib, stroke, and others.	Warfarin has an initial procoagulant effect. When anticoagulating as an inpatient, use heparin coverage initially. For outpatients, start at very low doses and raise gradually.
	Heparins	Myocardial infarction, pulmonary embolism, deep venous thrombosis.	Both low-molecular-weight and unfractionated heparins can be associated with excessive bleeding.
	Tissue plasminogen activator	Myocardial infarction, pulmonary embolism, embolic CVA.	High cost. Associated with hemorrhage at various sites.

AV: atrio-ventricular; A-fib: atrial fibrillation; V-fib or VF: ventricular fibrillation; WPW: wolf parkinson white; SVT: supraventricular tachycardia; MI: myocardial infarction; VT: ventricular tachycardia; CHF: congestive heart failure; PVC: paroxysmal ventricular contractions; CVA: cerebrovascular accident.

CHAPTER 7 ENDOCRINOLOGY

OVERVIEW OF HIGH-YIELD TOPICS IN ENDOCRINOLOGY

DIABETES MELLITUS

TYPE 1 DIABETES MELLITUS

General Facts

Type 1 diabetes is characterized by absolute insulin deficiency from selective autoimmune destruction of the pancreatic beta cells, which are responsible for producing insulin.

- It accounts for <10% of all diabetes cases and mainly affects lean children, teenagers, and young adults. Usually diagnosed before age 30.
- There are strong genetic associations with linkage to the human leukocyte antigen (HLA) *DQA* and *DQB* genes. Several autoantibodies directly against the beta cells or their products are usually detectable:
  - Anti–islet cell autoantigen (anti-ICA).
  - Anti–glutamic acid decarboxylase (anti-GAD).
  - Anti-insulin antibodies.
  - Antibody to the tyrosine phosphatase IA-2.
  - Antibody to zinc 8 transporter.

Type 1B diabetes: Idiopathic, with no autoimmune markers, occurs more commonly in Asian or African ancestry.

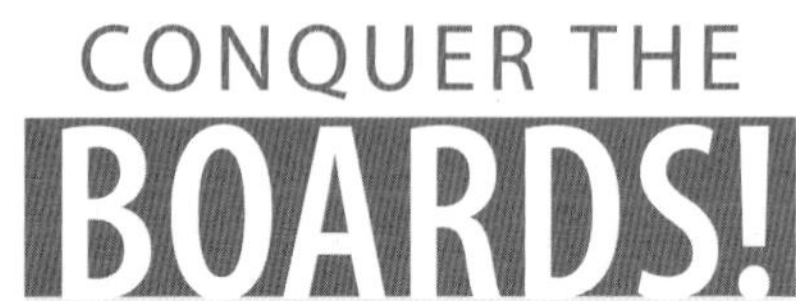

Latent autoimmune diabetes of adulthood (LADA) looks like type 1 DM in *older* patients.
Think when DKA appears in a thin adult.

A woman presents with a recurrent vaginal candidiasis that is refractory to treatment. *Think: Diabetes mellitus.* **Next step:** Get a finger stick for blood glucose.

Clinical Features

Usually presents with symptomatic hyperglycemia or diabetic ketoacidosis (DKA) (discussed later).

- Polyuria, polydipsia, weight loss, dehydration, and fatigue can occur.
- Blurred vision and recurrent infections as disease progresses.
- Dawn phenomenon: An exaggeration of the normal tendency of the plasma glucose to rise in the early morning hours before breakfast secondary to an increase in hormones, including cortisol and growth hormone (GH).

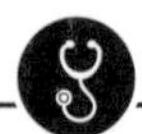

HbA_{1c} and corresponding average blood glucose levels:

HbA_{1c}	blood glucose
6:	120
7:	150
8:	180
9:	210
	(Increments of 30)

Diagnostic Workup

- Confirmed with a fasting serum glucose of >126 mg/dL on 2 occasions.
- HbA_{1c} is a measure of glucose control over the past 3 months. Most complications can be prevented if the HbA_{1c} level is kept below 7%.
- Glucosuria (causes an osmotic diuresis that leads to dehydration).

Management

- Treated solely with insulin (see Table 7-1 for types). Oral agents have no role in its management.

TABLE 7-1. Insulin Preparations and Their Pharmacokinetic Properties

Preparation	Onset	Peak (HR)	Duration (HR)
Rapid-acting			
Insulin lispro	10–15 min	1–2	3–5
Insulin aspart	10–15 min	1–2	3–5
Insulin glulisine	10–15 min	1–2	3–5
Short-acting			
Regular	30–60 min	2–4	4–8
Intermediate-acting			
Neutral protamine Hagedorn (NPH)	1–3 hr	4–10	10–18
Lente	2–4 hr	4–12	10–20
Long-acting			
Insulin detemir	2–3 hr	No peak	Up to 24 hr
Insulin glargine	2–3 hr	No peak	24 hr
Insulin degludec	2–3 hr	No peak	Up to 42 hr

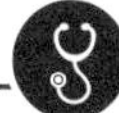

The required treatment for type 1 diabetes mellitus (DM) patients is insulin (both long and short acting), administered by subcutaneous injection. Most oral hypoglycemics have no role in management because these patients have no functioning pancreatic beta cells.

CONQUER THE **BOARDS!**

Three classes of diabetes medications promote weight loss (GLP1 agonists, SGLT2i, biguinides).

A patient presents with persistent morning hyperglycemia, despite steadily increasing his evening NPH insulin dose. He also complains of frequent nightmares. His wife brings him in because she witnessed him having a seizure in the middle of the night. *Think: Somogyi effect.* **Next step:** Check 3 AM blood glucose.

CONQUER THE **WARDS!**

Several diabetes medications have indications preventing cardiovascular events (GLP1, SGLT2i).

CONQUER THE **WARDS!**

Weight-based dosing:
Total daily dose ≈ 0.5 units/kg body weight
60 kg * 0.5 = 30 units
15 units - basal
5 units with each meal

Initiating Therapy

- Patients are usually hospitalized at the time of initial diagnosis because they often present with DKA, which is dangerous and are treated with a regular insulin drip in the intensive care unit (ICU).
- The average total daily dose of regular insulin is used as the initial dose of outpatient insulin therapy (be conservative so as not to induce hypoglycemic episodes) (Figure 7-1).
- Divide the total daily dose to give half the dose as basal (long-acting insulin) and half as bolus (rapid-acting insulin) in divided doses between 3 meals (see figure 7-1).
- Initially, the patient should monitor finger stick glucose levels 4 to 6 times a day and keep a record of the levels:
  - Choose the regimen that is easiest for the patient to follow while maintaining good blood glucose control.
- Type 1 DM patients must always take insulin to avoid ketosis, especially their long-acting insulin, even if fasting (may decrease dose).
  - **Somogyi effect:** Nighttime hypoglycemia followed by a dramatic increase in fasting glucose levels and increased plasma ketones. If the Somogyi effect is suspected, patients should check their blood glucose around 3 AM because hypoglycemia at this time confirms the diagnosis. **The morning hyperglycemia is a rebound effect**. Replacement of intermediate-acting insulin with long-acting insulin at bedtime can help this effect (try to avoid peaking of insulin effect in the middle of the night), as can a reduced long-acting insulin dose (basal).

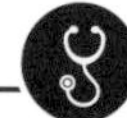

Measure finger stick glucose levels 4 times per day:

- **Morning fasting (prebreakfast)**
- **Lunch preprandial**
- **Dinner preprandial**
- **Before bed**

Postprandial can also be done 2 hours after the meal.

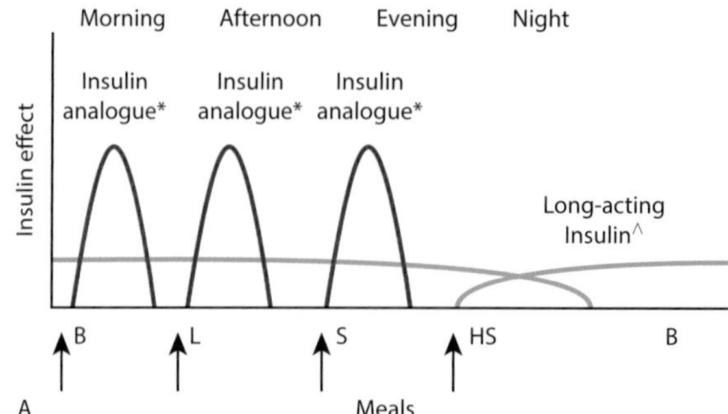

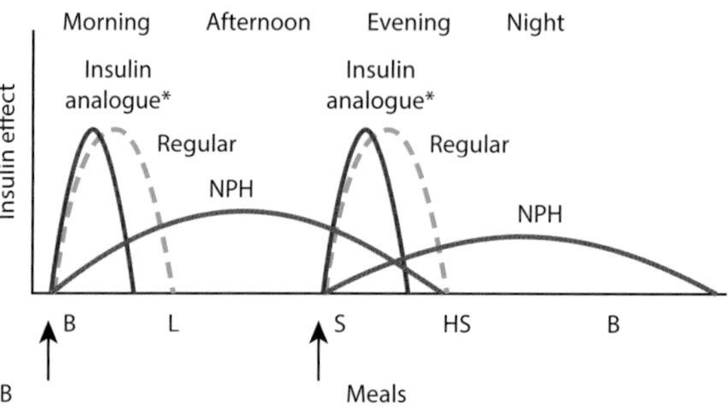

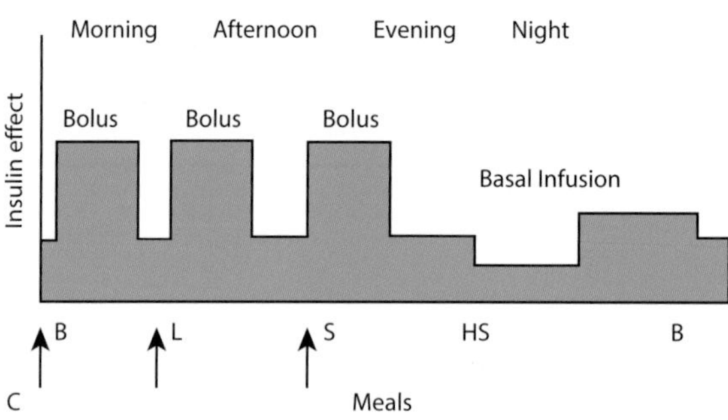

FIGURE 7-1. **Representative insulin regimens for the treatment of diabetes.** For each panel, the Y-axis shows the amount of insulin effect and the X-axis shows the time of day. B, Breakfast; HS, bedtime; L, lunch; S, supper. *Lispro, glulisine, or insulin aspart can be used. The time of insulin injection is shown with a vertical arrow. The type of insulin is noted above each insulin curve. A: Multiple-component insulin regimen consisting of long-acting insulin (Degludec, Determir, or Glargine) to provide basal insulin coverage and three shots of glulisine, lispro, or insulin aspart to provide glycemic coverage for each meal. B: Injection of 2 shots of long-acting insulin (NPH) and short-acting insulin analogue (glulisine, lispro, insulin aspart [solid red line], or regular insulin [green dashed line]). Some deliver the second dose of NPH at bedtime or also use a short-acting insulin at lunch. Only one formulation of short-acting insulin is used. C: Insulin administration by insulin infusion device is shown with the basal insulin and a bolus injection at each meal. The basal insulin rate is decreased during the evening and increased slightly prior to the patient awakening in the morning. Glulisine, lispro, or insulin aspart is used in the insulin infusion device. (Part C adapted from FR Kaufman: *Medical Management of Type 1 Diabetes*, 6th ed. Alexandria, VA: American Diabetes Association, 2012.) (From Jameson JL, Fauci AF, Kasper DL, et al, eds: *Harrison's Principles of Internal Medicine*, 20th ed. www.accessmedicine.com. Copyright © McGraw-Hill Education. All rights reserved.)

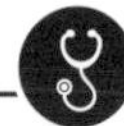

If a patient has hypoglycemic finger sticks in the morning, decrease the long-acting (basal) dose, even if the bedtime finger sticks are high.

HIGH-YIELD LITERATURE

DCCT Research Group, Nathan DM, Genuth S, Lacin J, et al. The effect of intensive treatment of diabetes on the development and progression of long-term complications in insulin-dependent diabetes mellitus. *N Engl J Med*. 1993;329(14):977-986.

Diabetes Control and Complications Trial/Epidemiology of Diabetes Interventions and Complications (DCCT/EDIC) Research Group, Nathan DM. Modern-day clinical course of type 1 diabetes mellitus after 30 years' duration: The Diabetes Control and Complications Trial/Epidemiology of Diabetes Interventions and Complications and Pittsburgh Epidemiology of Diabetes Complications Experience (1983-2005). *Arch Intern Med*. 2009;169(14):1307-1316.

TYPE 2 DIABETES MELLITUS

General Facts

- Type 2 diabetes is characterized by variable degrees of **insulin deficiency and insulin resistance**.
- It accounts for >90% of diabetes cases in the United States. Usually diagnosed after age 30, but increasingly seen in adolescents and children due to rising incidence of obesity and sedentary lifestyle.
- Concordance rate for type 2 DM in monozygotic twins is >90% (<50% in type 1).
- Commonly associated with obesity and often presents after a period of weight gain.

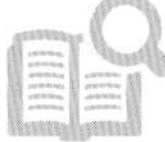

HIGH-YIELD LITERATURE

The Diabetes Prevention Program (DPP) Research Group. The Diabetes Prevention Program (DPP): Description of lifestyle intervention. *Diabetes Care*. 2002;25:2165-2171.

UK Prospective Diabetes Study (UKPDS) Group. Intensive blood glucose control with sulfonylureas or insulin compared with conventional treatment and risk of complications in patients with type 2 diabetes (UKPDS 33). *Lancet*. 1998;352:837-853.

Diabetes Prevention Program Research Group. Reduction in the incidence of type 2 diabetes with lifestyle intervention or metformin. *N Engl J Med*. 2002;346:393-403.

The Action to Control Cardiovascular Risk in Diabetes (ACCORD) Study Group. Effects of intensive glucose lowering in type 2 diabetes. *N Engl J Med*. 2008;358:2545-2559.

ADVANCE Collaborative Group. Intensive blood glucose control and vascular outcomes in patients with type 2 diabetes. *N Engl J Med*. 2008;358:2560-2572.

Etiology

- Hyperglycemia is caused by:
  - Impaired secretion of insulin.
  - Decreased cellular responsiveness to insulin.
  - Impaired inhibition of hepatic gluconeogenesis.
- The syndrome of insulin resistance (**metabolic syndrome** – see later) associated with hyperglycemia leads to obesity, hypertension, hyperlipidemia, and coronary artery disease.
- **Glucose toxicity:** Hyperglycemia itself induces impaired glucose tolerance, increased hepatic gluconeogenesis, and even impaired beta cell function.

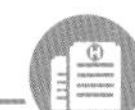

It is important for diabetics to have their feet frequently inspected to look for small cuts that may develop into ulcers and/or sources of infection. Due to neuropathy, diabetics can often have significant foot pathology and not feel anything.

Clinical Features

- Patients may be asymptomatic, or the presenting complaint may be from a complication of their diabetes, such as a soft tissue infection, blurred vision, or signs of hyperglycemia.
- Increased susceptibility to fungal infections (cell-mediated immunity is impaired by acute hyperglycemia).
- Patients with type 2 DM will suffer from DKA only in rare instances (called ketosis-prone or atypical type 2 diabetes).
- The nonketotic hyperglycemic-hyperosmolar coma (NKHC) is more common in type 2 DM, but still rare.

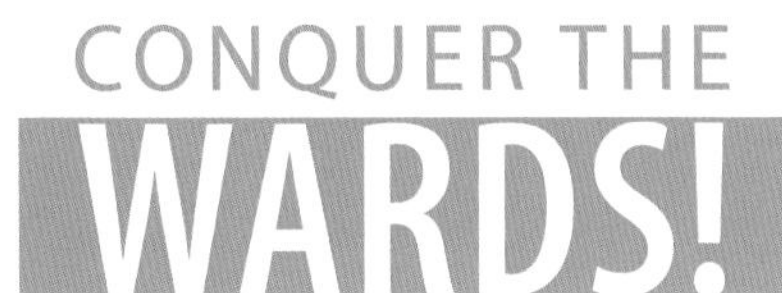

If an obese adult presents with DKA, consider ketosisprone diabetes and request antibody testing!

Diagnostic Workup

Requires any one of the following:

- Random glucose >200 mg/dL in the presence of symptoms.

- HbA_{1c} equal or above 6.5% is diagnostic and an easy point-of-care test that can be performed.
- Asymptomatic patients require a fasting glucose of >126 mg/dL on 2 separate occasions.

Use of glucose tolerance test: If patients have fasting glucose levels of >100 mg/dL and <126 mg/dL, an oral glucose tolerance test is indicated. A positive oral glucose tolerance test is a plasma glucose >200 mg/dL at 2 hours after ingesting 75 g of glucose in solution.

CONQUER THE BOARDS!

Lifestyle therapy (diet and exercise) is a critical part of the initial treatment for patients with type 2 DM.

Management

- Initial management should consist of **education, diet**, and **exercise** to achieve weight control.
- Patient education increases compliance with diet, exercise, and medication therapy. Discussions should involve when to seek medical attention, side effects of medications, proper foot care, ophthalmology visits, and symptoms of hyperglycemia and hypoglycemia.
- If glycemic control cannot be obtained with diet and exercise, oral hypoglycemic medications should be discussed and initiated. The goal of oral hypoglycemics is to control hyperglycemia, while monitoring and preventing hypoglycemia.
- Metformin is most often the initial oral agent used. The second drug choice depends on patient preferences (e.g., injection vs. oral), provider practice, and cost considerations.
- Glucose-lowering drugs: see Table 7-2.
- Patients not controlled with oral hypoglycemics or patients who develop hypoglycemia and have difficulties using oral hypoglycemics may require insulin. The transition to insulin involves extensive education and assessing options.
- In general, the goal is to provide an alternative to naturally secreted insulin in the most physiologic way. This usually involves a combination of rapid-acting insulin for postprandial hyperglycemia, along with intermediate- or long-acting insulin for glucose control between meals.
- The patient's weight, overall diet intake, and glucose measurements will help guide the selection and dosages of insulin modalities (see Type 1 Diabetes Mellitus earlier).

CONQUER THE WARDS!

Several GLP1 agonists are available as weekly injections, which patients adhere to very well!

CONQUER THE BOARDS!

Metformin and thiazolidinediones are contraindicated in patients with advanced heart failure.

ACUTE COMPLICATIONS OF DIABETES

Diabetic Ketoacidosis

Definition: Metabolic acidosis due to ketoacid accumulation secondary to severely depressed insulin levels.

General Facts

- Severe insulin deficiency causes the body to switch from metabolizing carbohydrates to metabolizing and oxidizing lipids.
- Usually precipitated by a lapse in insulin treatment, acute infection, major trauma, or stress.

CONQUER THE WARDS!

DKA is the most life-threatening acute complication of diabetes and is often the presenting syndrome of type 1 DM, but can also occur in type 2 DM, especially in people of color.

TABLE 7-2. Glucose-Lowering Drugs	
Sulfonylureas: glimepiride, glyburide, glipizide	■ HgA_{1C} change: Moderately effective, lower blood glucose by 20% and A_{1C} by 1%–2%. ■ Mechanism: Stimulates insulin secretion from the pancreas. ■ Benefits: Extensive experience; low cost; daily dosing. ■ Risks/Concerns: Hypoglycemia, especially with renal disease; weight gain; may impede ischemic preconditioning.
Meglitinides: repaglinide (Prandin), nateglinide (Starlix)	■ HgA_{1C} change: Reduce A_{1C} by 1%–2%. ■ Mechanism: Increase insulin production by the pancreas. ■ Benefits: Less hypoglycemia, targets postprandial glucose, mimics physiological insulin secretion. ■ Risks/Concerns: Short-acting glucose-lowering drugs, should be taken before each meal; slightly less effective compared to sulfonylureas.
Biguanides: metformin	■ HgA_{1C} change: Reduce A_{1C} by 1%–2%. ■ Mechanism: Decreases liver's glucose production and slightly increases muscle glucose uptake. ■ Benefits: No weight gain; no hypoglycemia when used alone (it may even lead to initial weight loss). ■ Risks/Concerns: Major side effects are gastrointestinal (GI) symptoms; most serious side effect is lactic acidosis (50% mortality). ■ Contraindications: Within 24–48 hours of injection of radiographic contrast material; renal disease with glomerular filtration rate (GFR) <60 mL/min or creatinine >1.5 (increased risk of lactic acidosis); liver disease; congestive heart failure (CHF); excessive alcohol intake. ■ *Note: Unless contraindicated, it is the first choice for an oral hypoglycemic agent.*
Thiazolidinediones: troglitazone, rosiglitazone, pioglitazone	■ HgA_{1C} change: Reduce A_{1C} by 0.5%–1.4%. ■ Mechanism: Decreases insulin resistance at the muscle and liver. ■ Benefits: No hypoglycemia; may improve high-density lipoprotein (HDL) cholesterol and triglycerides. ■ Risks/Concerns: Slow onset of action (takes 4–6 weeks to see an effect on blood glucose); weight gain (subcutaneous insulin-sensitive fat); fluid retention; major side effect is hepatotoxicity, which requires liver monitoring; expensive. ■ Contraindications: Class III and IV heart failure and liver disease. Recently, there has been a concern for increased cardiovascular disease that led to a Food and Drug Administration (FDA) warning.
Alpha-glucosidase inhibitors: acarbose, miglitol	■ HgA_{1C} change: Reduce A_{1C} by 0.5%–1.0%. ■ Mechanism: Slows the digestion of carbohydrates. ■ Benefits: No weight gain; no hypoglycemia when used alone. ■ Risks/Concerns: Major side effects are GI symptoms (transient diarrhea, nausea, and abdominal pain); caution use with irritable bowel disease (IBD), intestinal obstructions; expensive.
DPP-4 Inhibitors: sitagliptin (Januvia), linagliptin (Tradjenta), saxagliptin (Onglyza), alogliptin (Nesina)	■ HgA_{1C} change: Reduce A_{1C} by 0.5%–1.0%. ■ Mechanism: Increases insulin production and decreases the liver's production of glucose. ■ Benefits: No weight gain; less hypoglycemia. ■ Risks/Concerns: Low side-effect profile – upper respiratory infection (URI) symptoms, nausea, and diarrhea; require dose adjustment in renal insufficiency; expensive.
GLP-1 analogue: exenatide (Byetta, Bydureon), dulaglutide (Trulicity), liraglutide (Victoza), semaglutide (Ozempic)	■ HgA_{1C} change: Reduce A_{1C} about 0.8%. ■ Mechanism: Enhances insulin secretion, decreases liver's glucose output, and may suppress appetite. ■ Benefits: Weight loss; less hypoglycemia; cardiovascular benefit (some). ■ Risks/Concerns: Nausea and vomiting; hypoglycemia risk increased when combined with sulfonylurea; hypertriglyceridemia.
SGLT2 inhibitors: empagliflozin (Jardiance), canagliflozin (Invokana), dapagliflozin (Farxiga), ertugliflozin (Steglatro)	■ HgA_{1C} change: Reduce A_{1C} 0.8%–1%. ■ Mechanism: Reduce proximal tubule glucose reabsorption in the kidney, causing glucosuria. ■ Benefits: Weight loss; lowers blood pressure (BP), less hypoglycemia, cardiovascular benefit (some). ■ Risks/Concerns: Polyuria, genital mycotic infections, urinary tract infections, DKA.
Pramlintide (Symlin):	■ Synthetic analogue of the human hormone amylin that is cosecreted normally with insulin. ■ Adjunctive therapy in patients with type 1 or 2 diabetes mellitus. ■ It is used in patients who fail to achieve good glycemic control, despite intensive insulin therapy, with or without metformin and/or sulfonylureas. ■ Its use is associated with weight loss.

Pathophysiology

- Insulin deficiency causes hyperglycemia, which induces an osmotic diuresis (**severe dehydration**). Profound dehydration, sodium loss, and potassium loss occur.
- The body believes there is no glucose because the cells aren't getting any, which triggers the oxidation of free fatty acids from adipose tissue. The liver converts these free fatty acids into an alternative energy source: **ketones** (acetoacetic acid and beta-hydroxybutyric acid), which causes the metabolic ketoacidosis.
- There is respiratory compensation for this metabolic acidosis (fast breathing [i.e., Kussmaul], blowing off CO_2).
- **Other findings:**
  - Acetone is produced from spontaneous decarboxylation of acetoacetic acid. The acetone is disposed of by respiration, and its odor is present on the patient's breath (fruity odor).

Clinical Features

- **Polyuria** and **polydipsia**, nausea, vomiting, and vague abdominal pain.
- Lethargy and fatigue are later components and may progress to coma.
- Signs of dehydration are present, and patients may be hypotensive and tachycardic.
- Kussmaul respirations (rapid deep breaths) may be present, and acetone (fruity) odor on the patient's breath.

CONQUER THE WARDS!

When calculating the anion gap in DKA, use the actual Na, not the corrected Na.

CONQUER THE WARDS!

Urine ketones only tests for acetoacetic acid.

Diagnostic Workup

- DKA is characterized by the triad of:
  - Hyperglycemia: Usually between 350 and 500 mg/dL and rarely more than 800 mg/dL. Higher glucose levels are more consistent with hyperosmolar hyperglycemic states.
  - Anion gap metabolic acidosis (pH <7.30 and bicarb <18)
  - Ketones: Both in the blood and in the urine.
- If DKA is suspected, initial workup consists of the following tests:
  - **Diagnosis: These tests should always be sent:** Serum glucose, arterial blood gas, serum ketones, and urinalysis to look for ketones, complete blood count (CBC), plasma osmolality (differentiates DKA from hyperglycemic hyperosmolar syndrome [HHS]), electrocardiogram (ECG, see later) and electrolytes (basic metabolic panel, magnesium, phosphorous).
  - **Underlying cause:** Whenever someone is diagnosed with DKA, it is important to look for an underlying cause. A thorough history and physical is the first step, but common causes of DKA are:
    a. Infection: Commonly a urinary tract infection, cellulitis, pneumonia, viral URIs, viral gastroenteritis. **Always send a CBC** and consider chest radiographs.
    b. Pancreatitis: Consider getting a serum amylase and lipase if the patient has symptoms.
    c. Ischemia: DKA can be a sign of a myocardial infarction or stroke, since patients with diabetes are at high risk for cardiovascular disease. ECG and ruling out myocardial infarction should be considered.
  - **Electrolyte disturbances:**
    a. *Pseudohyponatremia* (not real hyponatremia) is due to a normal response to the osmotic shifts of severe hyperglycemia. The sodium reading in the lab value does not accurately represent what the true

sodium is. The "corrected" sodium concentration is obtained by adding 1.6 mEq of sodium for each 100 mg/dL of glucose above normal.

b. Potassium: Can be low due to glucose osmotic diuresis but is more commonly normal or high even though total body stores are low. This is because insulin usually shifts potassium from the extracellular space to the intracellular space. Because DKA is an insulin-deficient state, all the intracellular potassium moves into the bloodstream.

c. Phosphate: Is often high as well due to a similar process as potassium.

Management

- **Treatment:** There are 4 main treatments for DKA:
  - Intravenous fluids: DKA patient usually has severe volume deficits, and it is important to adequately resuscitate them.
  - Insulin: Regular insulin is used with a bolus 0.1 units/kg followed by 0.1 units/kg continuous insulin infusion. Patients are also not allowed to eat during treatment.
  - Replace potassium.
  - Correct acidosis: Fluids and insulin help correct the underlying cause of the acidosis; however, some patients whose pH drops below 6.9 need bicarbonate infusions to help correct the acidosis more quickly.
- **Close monitoring:** One of the tenets of DKA management is close monitoring. Usually, this requires the following labs be drawn:
  1. Glucose every hour to adjust the insulin drip.
  2. Arterial blood gas every 2 hours to monitor acidosis. Calculate anion gap every 2 hours.
  3. Basic metabolic panel every 2 hours to monitor potassium, creatinine, and sodium.
- **High-yield facts:**
  1. Usually 0.9% normal saline is used, but D5 should be added when the glucose is below 200 mg/dL to prevent hyperglycemia and to act as a substrate for continued removal of the acids in the blood.
  2. The insulin drip should only be stopped once the anion gap has closed and should be continued for 2 hours after initiation of subcutaneous insulin.

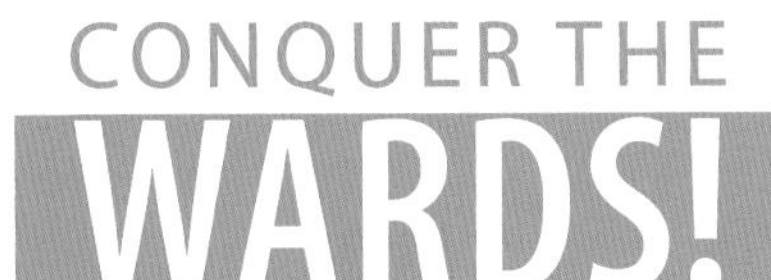

Transition to subcutaneous insulin only after anion gap has closed!

CONQUER THE BOARDS!

If initial potassium is low (<3.3 mEq/L) HOLD insulin and give potassium to avoid severe hyponatremia.

Complications

- Mortality rate is approximately 10%.
- Hypotension and coma present at admission are negative prognostic indicators.
- Major causes of death are circulatory failure, hypokalemia, and infection.

HYPERGLYCEMIC HYPEROSMOLAR SYNDROME

General Facts

- HHS is defined by a plasma osmolarity >320 mOsm/L and a plasma glucose level >600 mg/dL but a **normal bicarbonate level, normal PH**, and no significant evidence of ketosis.
- Occurs in patients with **type 2 DM**. The diagnosis is considered in any elderly patient with altered mental status and dehydration, particularly with known diabetes.
- Common causes include medication noncompliance, severe infection or sepsis, dehydration, diuretics, and glucocorticoids.

HHS most commonly occurs in patients unable to affect their own environment (e.g., nursing home residents) or in elderly residents with impaired thirst mechanism and lack of access to water.

Pathophysiology

- Patients usually have a period of symptomatic hyperglycemia before the syndrome develops.
- When fluid intake becomes insufficient, **extreme dehydration** ensues because of the hyperglycemia-induced osmotic diuresis.

Clinical Features

- Altered mental status is a key symptom with signs of profound dehydration.
- Seizures and transient neurologic deficits may occur.

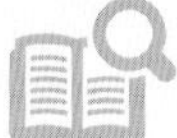

HIGH-YIELD LITERATURE

Gosmanov AR, Gosmanova EO, Dillard-Cannon E. Management of adult diabetic ketoacidosis. *Diabetes Metab Syndr Obes.* 2014;7:255-264.

Kitabchi AE, Umpierrez GE, Miles JM, Fisher JN. Hyperglycemic crises in adult patients with diabetes. *Diabetes Care.* 2009;32:1335-1343.

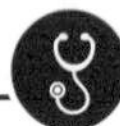

Hypoglycemia due to oral hypoglycemic agents lasts about 24 hours. Patients with sulfonylurea (and/or long-acting insulin analogues) overdose should be admitted to the hospital for at least 24 hours for monitoring and continuous glucose administration.

Diagnostic Workup and Management

- Diagnosis and management of HHS are similar to DKA with intravenous (IV) fluids, continuous insulin drop, and potassium repletion. However, it's even more important to adequately hydrate patients prior to starting an insulin drip.

HYPOGLYCEMIA

General Facts

- Common causes include **drug-induced** (most common cause, due to insulin or sulfonylureas), alcohol, adrenal insufficiency, shock, insulinomas, hypopituitarism, or severe liver or renal disease.

CONQUER THE WARDS!

Hypoglycemia is the most common cause of altered mental status in hospitalized patients.

Pathophysiology

- Glucose transport across the blood–brain barrier is regulated by adrenergic nervous system activity. The adrenergic outflow causes the typical sympathetic stimulatory symptoms of hypoglycemia, and the lack of glucose to the brain results in altered mental status.
- When there is hypoglycemia, glucagon is secreted by the pancreatic alpha cells. It increases plasma glucose levels and stimulates gluconeogenesis in the liver.

For alcoholics and people with malnutrition, always give thiamine prior to glucose to prevent Wernicke encephalopathy.

Clinical Features

- History of insulin or sulfonylurea treatment.
- Adrenergic symptoms: Diaphoresis, anxiety, tremor, feeling faint, palpitations, and hunger.
- Central nervous system (CNS) manifestations: Confusion, inappropriate behavior (sometimes mistaken for alcohol intoxication), visual problems, stupor, and coma.

CONQUER THE WARDS!

Low finger stick glucose needs to be confirmed with low plasma glucose, as it may not be accurate (e.g., shock, ischemic fingers)

Diagnostic Workup

- Abnormally low serum glucose is <55 mg/dL (may need 72-hour fasting to precipitate).

- Distinguish medication-induced vs. endogenous cause: Send C-peptide level to distinguish between endogenous (high C-peptide) and exogenous (low C-peptide) insulin because synthetic insulin has no C-peptide.
- For endogenous insulin, determine where it is coming from: Measure insulin level, anti-insulin antibodies, insulin-like growth factor 2 (IGF2), sulfonylurea panel, and beta-hydroxybutyrate, and see glucose response to glucagon.

Management

- Once hypoglycemia is confirmed or if a serum glucose level is not immediately available, IV glucose should be given. If IV access is not available, intramuscular, intranasal, or subcutaneous **glucagon** should be administered.
- Only if the patient's mental status is OK should you try giving food (PO); otherwise, they may aspirate.
- Whenever dextrose is administered for hypoglycemia and alcoholism or nutritional deficiency is suspected, administer **thiamine** prior to glucose to prevent **Wernicke encephalopathy**.
- Continue checking glucose levels, as they can drop again quickly (rebound hypoglycemia), or if from a medication, it may have a long half-life and still be on board.
- If hypoglycemia is refractory to glucose administration, consider adrenal insufficiency and give steroids.

CONQUER THE BOARDS!

Satisfy Whipple triad before more testing (e.g., blood glucose [BG] 58, healthy young woman, no symptoms = not pathologic).

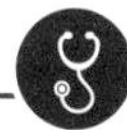

Whipple triad of hypoglycemia:

1. **Plasma glucose <60 mg/dL**
2. **Symptoms of hypoglycemia**
3. **Improvement of the symptoms with administration of glucose**

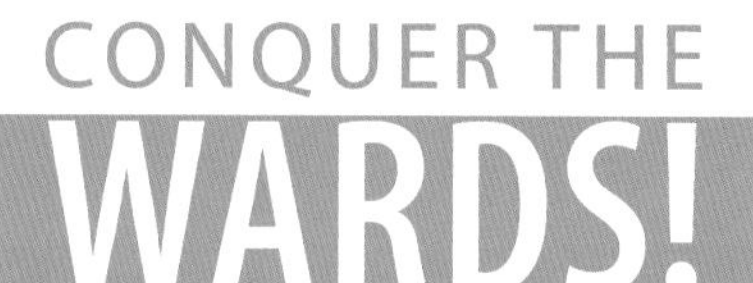

CONQUER THE WARDS!

Most often diabetes microvascular complications occur top-down: retinopathy, then nephropathy, then neuropathy.

HIGH-YIELD LITERATURE

Cryer PE, Axelrod L, Grossman AB, et al. Evaluation and management of adult hypoglycemic disorders: An Endocrine Society Clinical Practice Guideline. *J Clin Endocrinol Metab*. 2009;94(3):709-728.

CHRONIC COMPLICATIONS OF DIABETES MELLITUS

Diabetic Retinopathy

General Facts

- The highly vascular retina is commonly involved in long-standing diabetes. Diabetes is responsible for most cases of legal blindness in adults in the United States.

Progression

- **Background diabetic retinopathy:** Early changes include hard exudates, microaneurysms, and minor hemorrhages on funduscopic examination.
- **Preproliferative retinopathy:** Presence of "cotton-wool spots," which are indicative of retinal infarcts.
- **Neovascularization/proliferative retinopathy:** Abnormal vessels form on the retina that can cause damage. They are abnormal in both appearance and structure and are prone to retinal and vitreous hemorrhage.

CONQUER THE BOARDS!

Blurred vision in the setting of hyperglycemia is most often from lens changes in the eyes, not retinopathy. Don't change the glasses prescription until BG is controlled!

Diagnostic Workup

- Regular and careful screening by an ophthalmologist is necessary to detect the early changes of diabetic retinopathy.

Management

- Control blood glucose level and blood pressure.
- Controlling plasma lipids may also slow the progression of eye disease.
- Ophthalmologist can do laser ablation of abnormal vessels.

DIABETIC NEPHROPATHY

General Facts

- Diabetes is the most common cause of renal failure in the United States.
- Diabetic nephropathy begins with a period of glomerular hyperfiltration and intraglomerular hypertension. Subsequently, glomerular injury develops, with the eventual loss of filtration capacity, leading to azotemia.
- Progresses from a small amount of a small protein (microalbumin) to large amounts of a large protein.
  - Microalbuminuria (30 in 300 mg/day).
  - Macroalbuminuria (>300 mg/day).
  - Nephrotic syndrome (>3.5 g/day).

CONQUER THE WARDS!

False-positive microalbumin-to-creatinine ratios occur commonly (especially menstruating women), so repeat before starting medications.

Conquer the boards: Angiotensin-converting enzyme (ACE) inhibitors and angiotensin II receptor blockers reduce albuminuria and slow the progression of renal disease in diabetic patients with and without hypertension.

Diagnostic Workup

- Annual measurement of microalbumin-to-creatinine ratios on spot urine samples and serum creatinine concentrations to screen for diabetic kidney disease.

Management

- Aggressive blood pressure control, particularly with ACE inhibitor or angiotensin II receptor blockers.
- Control glucose level.

DIABETIC FEET

General Facts

- Diabetic patients frequently have peripheral vascular disease and peripheral neuropathy. These place the diabetic foot at extreme risk for ulceration, infection, and, ultimately, possible amputation.

Clinical Features

- Cold feet, claudication, and leg discomfort on ambulation (relieved with rest) are key symptoms.
- Numbness, burning, or tingling sensation of the hands and feet in a glove-and-stocking distribution can occur as well.

Diagnostic Workup

- Frequent, careful examination of the feet in routine physician visits.
- Detect sensory deficits in the foot (monofilament test) to screen for DM neuropathy.

Management

- Glucose control, is critical and maintaining A1c at goals.
- Use of comfortable, protective, and well-fitting shoes and plain cotton socks to protect from trauma, along with ongoing foot care by a podiatrist, is important.
- Aggressive treatment of the diabetic foot ulcer or infection with broad-spectrum antibiotics, often for longer periods. Debridement if necessary.

HIGH-YIELD LITERATURE

American Diabetes Association. Standards of medical care in diabetes – 2018. *Diabetes Care*. 2019;42(Suppl 1): S1-S156.

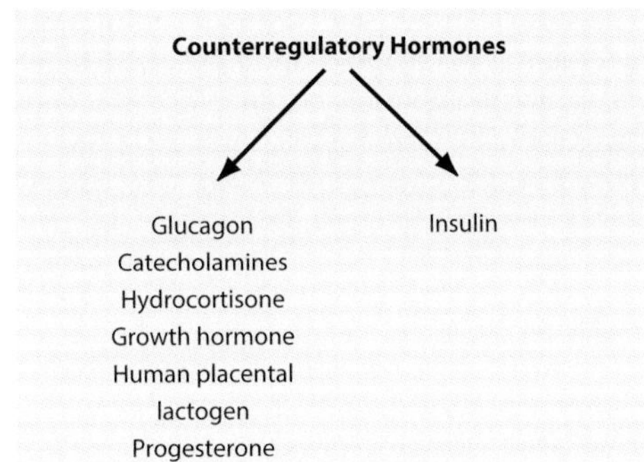

FIGURE 7-2. Glucose Regulation

Pituitary adenomas are part of multiple endocrine neoplasia (MEN) type I (pituitary, pancreas, parathyroid). See Figures 7-2 and 7-3.

DISORDERS OF THE PITUITARY GLAND

PITUITARY TUMORS

- Anterior pituitary lobe (adenohypophysis): Derivative of Rathke pouch during embryogenesis. Evagination of the roof of the developing mouth.
- Posterior pituitary lobe (neurohypophysis): Composed of hypothalamic neuronal axon terminals; storage and release site for hormones produced by these neurons.
- For specific hormones, see Table 7-3.

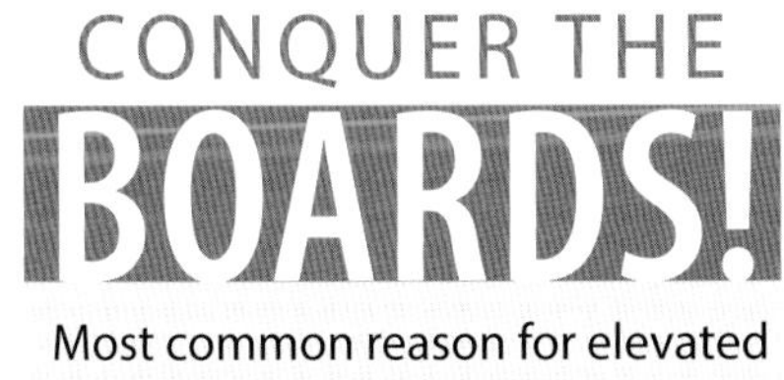

Most common reason for elevated prolactin is pregnancy!

General Facts

- Most are benign and slow growing, constituting ~10% of intracranial tumors.
- Anterior pituitary: Craniopharyngiomas, adenomas.
- Posterior pituitary: No primary tumors.
- Metastases and meningiomas are occasionally seen in the pituitary.
- Pathology/manifestations arise from:
  - Excess hormone production.
  - Compression of suprasellar structures.
  - Destruction of normal pituitary parenchyma.
  - Compression of pituitary stalk leads to increased prolactin due to loss of inhibition by dopamine.

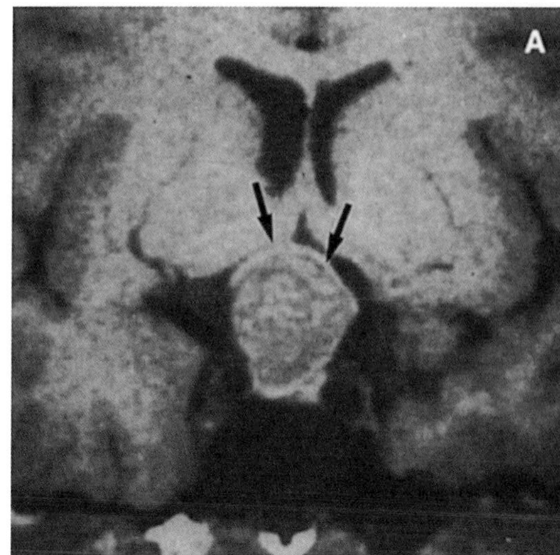

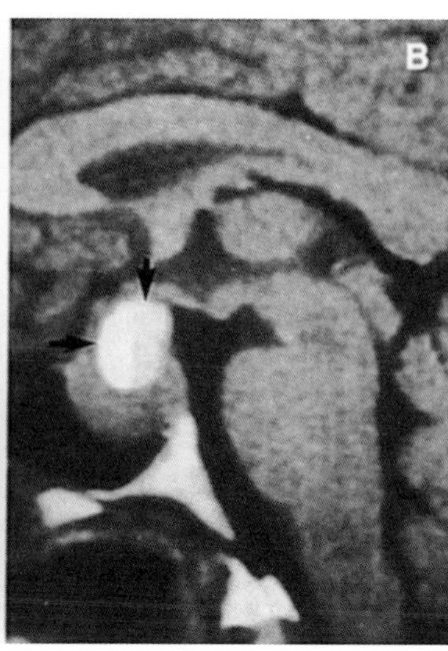

FIGURE 7-3. **Pituitary tumor. A:** The coronal magnetic resonance (MR) image shows a large nonfunctioning pituitary adenoma (arrows) with pronounced suprasellar extension and chiasmal compression. **B:** A sagittal MR image of another large pituitary adenoma shows spontaneous hemorrhage within the suprasellar portion of the adenoma (arrows). (From Hypothalamus and Pituitary Gland. In: Gardner DG, Shoback D. Greenspan's Basic & Clinical Endocrinology, 10th ed. New York, McGraw Hill, 2017, Fig. 4-16. Used with permission from David Norman, MD.)

TABLE 7-3. Pituitary Hormones and Their Functions

Anterior Lobe	Main Stimulatory Actions	Hypothalamic Stimulus
Adrenocorticotropic hormone (ACTH, corticotropin)	■ Growth and secretion of adrenal cortex to make cortisol and sex hormones	■ CRH
Growth hormone (GH, somatotropin)	■ Secretion of somatomedin C (insulin-like growth factor) ■ Body growth	■ GRH
Thyroid-stimulating hormone (TSH, thyrotropin)	■ Growth of thyroid gland ■ Production of T_3 and T_4	■ TRH
Follicle-stimulating hormone (FSH)	■ Spermatogenesis in the male ■ Ovarian follicle growth in the female	■ GnRH
Luteinizing hormone (LH)	■ Testosterone secretion in the male ■ Ovulation in the female	■ GnRH
Prolactin	■ Milk production ■ Maternal behavior	■ PRH (stimulates) ■ Dopamine (inhibits)
Melanocyte-stimulating hormone (MSH)	■ Skin pigmentation	
Posterior Lobe		**Releasing Stimulus**
Antidiuretic hormone (ADH; vasopressin, AVP)	■ Retains water, producing concentrated urine	■ Osmoreceptors ■ Thirst, pain, nausea
Oxytocin	■ Milk letdown ■ Contractions of labor	■ Touch receptors in uterus, genitalia, and breast

CRH, corticotropin-releasing hormone; *GNRH*, gonadotropin-releasing hormone; *GRH*, growth-releasing hormone; *PRH*, prolactin-releasing hormone; *TRH*, thyrotropin-releasing hormone.

PITUITARY ADENOMAS

- **Prolactinoma** is the most common pituitary tumor. Women present with galactorrhea, infertility, or oligomenorrhea. Men present with hypogonadism or infertility and usually later than women. Prolactin levels correlate with tumor size. Treat with dopamine agonists (cabergoline or bromocriptine) to reduce prolactin, resolve symptoms, and shrink tumor.
- **Nonfunctioning tumors** are the second most common pituitary tumors. Symptoms include visual changes or slightly high prolactin levels due to mass effect, which disrupts the inhibitor signal that dopamine has on prolactin-producing cells. Treat with surgery.
- Less common pituitary adenomas include **somatotrophs** (GH; see Acromegaly), **corticotrophs** (ACTH), and **thyrotrophs** (TSH).
- **Pituitary microadenomas** (<10 mm) are found in ~15% of asymptomatic women by magnetic resonance imaging (MRI); in the absence of progression (assessed by follow-up MRI), they are clinically insignificant.

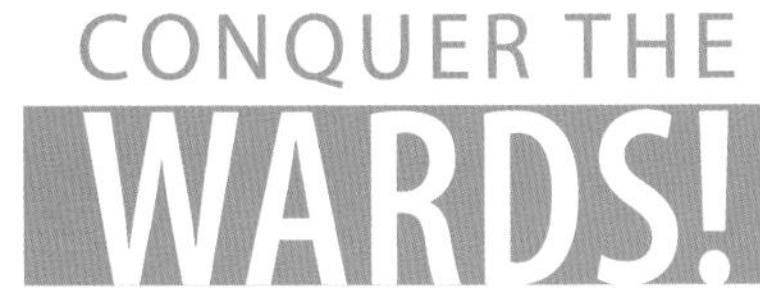

Microadenoma: <1 cm
Macroadenoma: ≥1 cm

CRANIOPHARYNGIOMAS

- Arise from embryologic remnants of Rathke pouch.
- Most common tumors of suprasellar region in children.
- Solid or cystic; usually calcified.

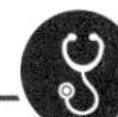

Patients rarely complain of "tunnel vision" (bitemporal hemianopsia) or a deficit when the defect is confined to the temporal visual fields. They more typically just report increased clumsiness, bumping into things, or car accidents.

Clinical Features

- Headache.
- Compression of optic chiasm:
  - Superior bitemporal quadrantanopia: Early visual defect, since compression begins on inferior surface of chiasm.
  - Bitemporal hemianopsia ("tunnel vision"): Classic finding; occurs when tumor has reached a significant size.
- Signs of increased intracranial pressure (ICP) are rare, as tumors are usually diagnosed before they reach the requisite dimensions.

Diagnostic Workup for Pituitary Adenomas and Craniopharyngiomas

- **MRI:** This is the test of choice because it is more sensitive than computed tomography (CT) scans and can detect microadenomas. Must perform with gadolinium contrast.
- **Hormone studies:** Detect excesses or deficiencies, give information about type of tumor; useful when tumor cannot be detected radiographically.
- If a patient presents with manifestations of a specific disease (such as acromegaly, Cushing disease, etc.), always start with hormonal workup prior to diagnostic imaging. That is because of the high prevalence of incidentalomas in the general population.

Management of Pituitary Adenomas and Craniopharyngiomas

- Medications: Dopamine agonists for prolactinomas (dopamine inhibits prolactin). Hormone replacement for hypopituitarism.
- Surgery: Indicated whenever there are neurologic symptoms (except prolactinoma).
- Radiotherapy: Most often surgical adjunct, but has a delayed response (minimum 3 to 6 months).

HIGH-YIELD LITERATURE

Freda PU, Beckers AM, Katznelson L, et al. Pituitary incidentaloma: An Endocrine Society Clinical Practice Guideline. *J Clin Endocrinol Metab*. 2011; 96(4): 894-904.

Huang W, Molitch ME. Evaluation and management of galactorrhea. *Am Fam Physician*. 2012;85(11):1073-1080.

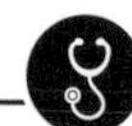

Acromegaly: The changes in a patient's appearance occur over many years and may not be apparent to the patient or his family. Old photos may suggest the diagnosis.

CONQUER THE **BOARDS!**

The most common cause of death is cardiovascular in patients with acromegaly (e.g., heart failure).

CONQUER THE **WARDS!**

Uncontrolled type 2 DM out of proportion to body habitus along with facial coarseness: Think acromegaly.

CONQUER THE **WARDS!**

Due to delay in diagnosis, most tumors are macroadenomas and may not be completely resectable.

ACROMEGALY

General Facts

- Disorder of excess GH production marked by progressive enlargement (-megaly) of peripheral (acral) body parts.
- Pituitary somatotroph (cells that make GH, or somatotropin) adenoma is by far the most common cause.
- Ectopic GH secretion; hypothalamic tumors secreting growth hormone–releasing hormone (GHRH) are rare.

Clinical Features

- **Progressive enlargement of peripheral body parts**, particularly head, hands, and feet.
- **Joint pains and hyperhidrosis** (excessive sweating) are present in most patients.
- Progressive and irreversible **organomegaly**, especially cardiomegaly. Patients may present with decompensated heart failure prior to diagnosis.
- **Impaired glucose tolerance** due to the anti-insulin actions of GH.
- **Hyperphosphatemia** due to GH's influence on tubular resorption of phosphate.
- **Gigantism** in children due to excess linear growth prior to epiphyseal closure.

Diagnostic Workup

- **Serum IGF-I levels** is the best single test for a diagnosis of acromegaly. It is made by the liver under stimulation by GH, is elevated in acromegalics, and does not fluctuate as does GH itself.
- **GH levels** are highly variable, so testing will yield inaccurate results. Always check IGF-I if acromegaly is suspected.
- **Oral glucose suppression test:** Lack of GH suppression by glucose load. This confirms the diagnosis if IGF-1 levels are equivocal.
- **MRI of pituitary** should be obtained as well.

Management

- Surgery (transsphenoidal [most often] or transfrontal adenectomy, depending on the size and location of the tumor).
- Radiation therapy can be adjunct to surgery if IGF-1 levels remain elevated after surgery. It has a delayed effect and takes months to years to work.
- Medications: Dopamine agonist (cabergoline) for mild disease. Somatostatin analogues (octreotide, lanreotide) or GH receptor blocker such as pegvisomant can also be used.

HIGH-YIELD LITERATURE

Katznelson L, Laws ER, Melmed S, et al. Acromegaly: An Endocrine Society Clinical Practice Guideline. *J Clin Endocrinol Meta*. 2014;99(11):3933-3951.

HYPOPITUITARISM

General Facts

- Hypopituitarism can be caused by a variety of conditions, such as tumors, surgical destruction, systemic or local causes, and Sheehan syndrome.
  - **Tumors** causing dysfunction either by invasion, replacement, or compression. It can affect normal pituitary parenchyma, pituitary stalk, and hypothalamic parenchyma.
  - **Surgical destruction** of pituitary or hypothalamus: Either therapeutic or as a result of an unrelated neurosurgical procedure.
  - **Sheehan syndrome:** Pituitary gland enlarges during pregnancy due to hyperplasia of lactotrophs without commensurate increase in blood supply; if hypotension occurs during childbirth, pituitary infarction can result.
  - **Systemic** (rare): Hemochromatosis, sarcoid, lymphocytic hypophysitis (more common in women in late pregnancy and postpartum).
  - **Infectious** (rare): Tuberculosis (TB), neurosyphilis.

A 29-year-old woman presents with an inability to lactate after childbirth. Delivery was complicated by blood loss and hypotension. *Think: Sheehan syndrome.* **Next step:** Check prolactin level, screen for hypopituitarism, and MRI of the brain with contrast.

Clinical Features

- **ACTH deficiency:** See Adrenal Insufficiency section.
- **GH deficiency:** Growth retardation in children. Muscle weakness, unfavorable fat distribution and lipid profiles, lower quality of life in adults.
- **Prolactin:**
  - Deficiency: Failure to lactate after childbirth.
  - Excess: Amenorrhea and galactorrhea in women, gynecomastia in men. Infertility and decreased libido in both.
- **TSH deficiency:** See Hypothyroidism section.
- **Luteinizing hormone (LH)** and **follicle-stimulating hormone (FSH) deficiency:** Amenorrhea in women; decreased libido and infertility in both.
- In slow-growing tumors, GH, FSH, and LH levels are affected early. Adrenocorticotropic hormone (ACTH), thyroid-stimulating hormone (TSH), and prolactin levels decline only with advanced disease.
- **Antidiuretic hormone (ADH) deficiency:** Known as diabetes insipidus (discussed in separate section later). Rare with pituitary adenomas.

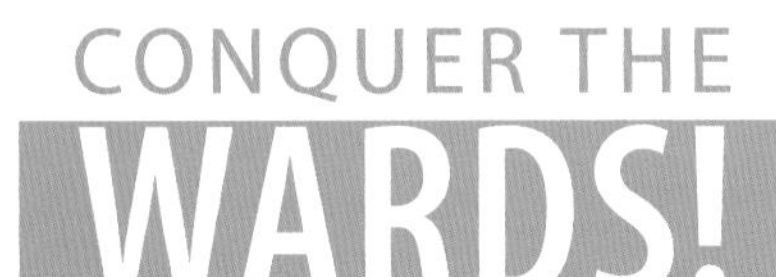

As tumors near the pituitary grow, they commonly damage normal pituitary hormones in the following order:
GH → FSH/LH → TSH/ACTH

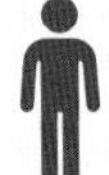

A 36-year-old woman complains of amenorrhea for 1 year, increasingly bad headaches, clumsiness, and sporadic nipple discharge; beta-hCG levels are normal. *Think: Prolactinoma.* **Next step:** Check serum prolactin level, MRI of the brain.

Diagnostic Workup

Evaluation of target organ function is usually required: Tests include imaging studies (usually an MRI), hormone levels, and response to exogenous pituitary hormones.

- **ACTH:** ACTH levels are expected to be low or normal, but not as important as cortisol measurements. Morning (8 AM) cortisol level is the most useful test for adrenal insufficiency testing.

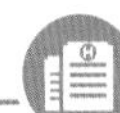

Drugs that inhibit dopamine activity also cause hyperprolactinemia: tricyclic antidepressants, prochlorperazine, haloperidol, methyldopa, metoclopramide, and cimetidine.

- **GH:** GH levels are pulsatile and unreliable on their own. Evaluation requires IFG-1 level as well. Stimulation testing is next step if results are not clear. This can be done by giving glucagon, or by inducing hypoglycemia with insulin – both trigger a rise in serum GH. GH is drawn at 30, 60, and 90 minutes post stimulus and compared to normal values.
- Prolactin levels are rarely low even with hypopituitarism (with extensive destruction). This is a clinical diagnosis along with imaging.
- TSH and thyroxine (T_4) are measured together. If the T_4 is low and the TSH is normal or low, this supports hypothyroidism.
- **LH and FSH:** In women, LH and FSH levels vary with the menstrual cycle, so the timing of the levels is important; postmenopausal women have high LH and FSH levels normally.
- **ADH** levels normally vary according to plasma osmolality. Testing is discussed in Diabetes Insipidus section.

CONQUER THE BOARDS!

Postmenopausal women should have elevated LH and FSH levels. Low or "normal" range suggests hypopituitarism.

Management

- Address underlying cause: Tumor, infection, systemic disease.
- **Hormone replacement:**
  - ACTH: glucocorticoid replacement (hydrocortisone, prednisone, dexamethasone).
  - Prolactin: No treatment for deficiency.
  - GH deficiency: GH injections daily.
  - TSH deficiency: Thyroid hormone replacement (levothyroxine).
  - FSH and LH deficiency can be treated with estrogen/progesterone replacement in women (fertility is usually not restored unless GNRH is given in a pulsatile fashion via a pump) and testosterone replacement in men.
  - ADH deficiency: Desmopressin (DDAVP) is given often twice daily.

HIGH-YIELD LITERATURE

Fleseriu M, Hashim IA, Karavitaki N, et al. Hormonal replacement in hypopituitarism in adults: An Endocrine Society Clinical Practice Guideline. *J Clin Endocrinol Metab*. 2016;101(11): 3888-3921.

Psychogenic polydipsia: Psychiatric disorder of compulsive water drinking, most common in young to middle-aged women. Presents with polyuria and dilute urine, distinguished from DI by *low* plasma osmolality.

ANTIDIURETIC HORMONE DISORDERS

DIABETES INSIPIDUS

- **Central diabetes insipidus (DI):** Inadequate pituitary release of ADH.
- **Nephrogenic DI:** Lack of renal response to ADH.

General Facts

- **Central DI:**
  - Idiopathic: Accounts for 50% of cases.
  - Posterior pituitary or hypothalamic damage (tumor, trauma, neurosurgery).
  - Systemic: Sarcoidosis, neurosyphilis, encephalitis.
- **Nephrogenic DI:**
  - Familial.
  - Chronic renal disease.
  - Sickle cell anemia (renal papillary necrosis).
  - Drugs: Lithium, demeclocycline, methoxyflurane.

CONQUER THE BOARDS!

Lithium causes several endocrinopathies: Nephrogenic DI, hypercalcemia (parathyroid hormone [PTH] mediated), hypothyroidism.

Clinical Features

- Polyuria (3 to 15 L/day).
- Thirst and polydipsia.
- Dilute urine (specific gravity <1.005).

Diagnostic Workup

- Dilute, polyuria with inappropriately high-to-normal serum osmolality (280 to 310 mOsm/kg).
- **Water deprivation test:** Must be done to diagnose DI. In this test fluids are withheld and urine osmolality measured hourly. When serum sodium is >145 mEq/L and serum osmolality is >295 mOsm/kg, this should stimulate ADH release and urine osmolality should be high (>700 mOsm/kg). If not, then exogenous ADH (desmopressin) is given:
  - Central DI: Low urine Osm → high urine Osm
  - Nephrogenic DI: Low urine Osm → low urine Osm

CONQUER THE WARDS!

The most common serum sodium level in a patient with diabetes insipidus is NORMAL!
Intact thirst keeps sodium normal by increased water intake.

Management

- **Desmopressin (DDAVP):** Analogue of ADH, useful in **central DI**.
- **Thiazide diuretics:** Paradoxically decreases urine output in patients with DI by increasing sodium and water resorption in the proximal tubule, leading to decreased water delivery to the ADH-responsive sites in the collecting ducts. They are the only therapy useful in **nephrogenic DI**.
- **Chlorpropamide:** Oral hypoglycemic with a side effect of potentiating secretion and action of endogenous ADH. Partial function must exist for this therapy to be of use.

SYNDROME OF INAPPROPRIATE ANTIDIURETIC HORMONE SECRETION

General Facts

- Idiopathic overproduction via the hypothalamic–posterior pituitary axis. Often associated with disorders of the CNS (encephalitis, stroke, head trauma) and pulmonary disease (TB, pneumonia).
- Ectopic production by malignant tumors, particularly small cell lung cancer and pancreatic carcinoma.
- Pharmacologic stimulation of the hypothalamic–pituitary axis: Carbamazepine, chlorpropamide, clofibrate, vincristine.

Clinical Features

- Attributable to hyponatremia

Diagnostic Workup

- Hyponatremia, low serum osmolality, normal volume status (euvolemic), high urinary sodium, and osmolality of urine greater than serum.
- Normal adrenal and thyroid functions.

Management

- Fluid restriction is a key intervention.
- Hypertonic saline in severe hyponatremia.
- Demeclocycline: Due to causing nephrogenic DI, reserved for cases not responding to fluid restriction.
- Direct vasopressin (V2) receptor antagonists: **The vaptans**.

HIGH-YIELD LITERATURE

Schrier RW, Gross P, Gheorghiade M, et al. Tolvaptan, a selective oral vasopressin V2-receptor antagonist, for hyponatremia. *N Engl J Med*. 2006;355:2099-2112.

Verbalis JG, Adler S, Schrier RW, Berl T, Zhao Q, Czerwiec FS. Efficacy and safety of oral tolvaptan therapy in patients with the syndrome of inappropriate antidiuretic hormone secretion. *Eur J Endocrinol*. 2011;164:725-732.

- Conivaptan only for hospitalized patients (IV only).
  - Tolvaptan oral for chronic hyponatremia (syndrome of inappropriate antidiuretic hormone secretion [SIADH] or hypervolemic [liver, cardiac failure])

CONQUER THE **WARDS!**

Hyperthyroidism is from too much thyroid hormone production, whereas **thyrotoxicosis** is the state of too much hormone.

THYROID DISORDERS

HYPERTHYROIDISM

General Facts

- Increased synthesis and secretion of free thyroid hormones resulting in hypermetabolism.
- Ten times more common in women than in men, with an annual incidence of 1 in 1000 women.
- Graves disease (most common cause, 80% of cases in the United States).
- Can also be caused by toxic multinodular goiter, toxic adenoma, iatrogenic (lithium therapy, amiodarone), inadvertent toxic ingestion, or factitious (thyrotoxicosis factitia) transient hyperthyroidism (subacute thyroiditis), or ectopic thyroid hormone secretion (struma ovarii).

CONQUER THE **BOARDS!**

Causes of large tongue (macroglossia):

- Acromegaly
- Myxedema
- Amyloidosis

Pathophysiology

- High levels of free thyroid hormones increase levels of cellular metabolism, cause a state of hypermetabolism, and amplify catecholamine signals.

Clinical Features

- Heat intolerance, sweating, palpitations (hyperthyroidism is a common cause of atrial fibrillation), weight loss, and tremor are key symptoms.
- Nervousness, anxiety, weakness, fatigue, diarrhea, and hyperdefecation can also occur.

CONQUER THE **WARDS!**

Patients may experience onycholysis (Plummer nails) from excess thyroid hormone, where the nail raises up away from the nail bed.

Diagnostic Workup

- Measure TSH, free T_4, and free T_3 (if the T_4 level is normal) (see Table 7-4).
- Radioactive iodine uptake scans can help assess location and pattern of uptake in the thyroid gland and elsewhere (Table 7-5).

Management

- Depends on underlying disorder (see later for specifics).

HIGH-YIELD LITERATURE

Ross DS, Burch HB, Cooper DS, et al. 2016 American Thyroid Association Guidelines for diagnosis and management of hyperthyroidism and other causes of thyrotoxicosis. *Thyroid*. 2016;26:1343-1421.

TABLE 7-4. Laboratory Evaluation of Patients for Thyroid Disease

Disorder	Laboratory Test Results Suggestive of Diagnosis in the Appropriate Clinical Setting
Hyperthyroidism	
Graves disease	TSH low; free T_4 high; in some cases, T_3 is elevated and free T_4 is normal; TRAbs elevated
Toxic multinodular goiter	TSH low; free T_4 and T_3 normal or high; normal or increased radioactive iodine uptake; thyroid scan with multiple areas of increased uptake surrounded by suppressed uptake in non-tumor tissue
Toxic adenoma	TSH low; free T_4 and T_3 normal or high; normal or increased radioactive iodine uptake; thyroid scan with focal increased uptake in tumor surrounded by suppressed uptake in non-tumor tissue
Subacute thyroiditis	TSH low; free T_4 and T_3 high; increased; decreased radioactive iodine uptake
T_3 Thyrotoxicosis	TSH low; free T_4 normal and T_3 high; normal radioactive iodine uptake
Hypothyroidism	
Hashimoto thyroiditis	TSH high; T_4 normal and then low, preceding a decline in T_3; anti-TPO and/or antithyroglobulin antibody positive
Ablative hypothyroidism	TSH high; free T_4 and T_3 low following procedure that ablates thyroid
Infantile hypothyroidism	TSH high; free T_4 low in a newborn or infant
Euthyroid sick syndrome	TSH normal to high; free T_4 normal; T_3 low; T_3 high; concentrations of TSH and thyroid hormones vary throughout disease course

TABLE 7-5. Thyroid disorders and Iodine Scan Results

Disease	Iodine Uptake Scan
Graves	Elevated iodine uptake and homogenous on scan
Toxic multinodular goiter	Heterogenous uptake on scan
Autonomous thyroid nodule	Single area of uptake
Thyroiditis: Subacute, radiation, silent/painless, postpartum	Low uptake on scan
Exogenous: Amiodarone, iatrogenic, factitious, iodine induced	Low uptake on scan
Other causes: Struma ovarii, trophoblastic tumor, metastatic follicular carcinoma, TSH-producing adenoma	Low uptake on scan Possible uptake outside of thyroids (in tumor or adenoma)

THYROID STORM

General Facts

- Exaggerated manifestation of hyperthyroidism with fever and CNS, cardiovascular (CV), and GI dysfunction.
- Mortality is high (20% to 50%) even with the correct treatment.
- Can be caused by infection, trauma, surgical procedures, DKA, myocardial infarction (MI), cerebrovascular accident (CVA), pulmonary embolism (PE), withdrawal of antihyperthyroid medications, iodine administration, thyroid hormone ingestion, or idiopathic causes.

Clinical Features

- Overactivated sympathetic nervous system causes most of the signs and symptoms of this syndrome, including fever >101°F, tachycardia, diarrhea, abdominal discomfort, and exhaustion.

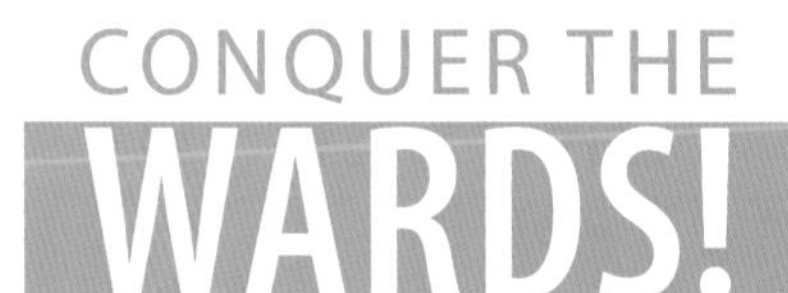

Look up the Burch and Wartofsky score for thyroid storm!
It is used to evaluate the likelihood of thyroid storm based on presentation.

- High-output congestive heart failure (CHF) and volume depletion can occur.
    - Continuum of CNS alterations (from agitation to confusion when moderate to stupor or coma with or without seizures when most severe).
- Jaundice is a late and ominous manifestation.

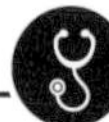

Never send any thyroid storm patient for a procedure involving iodine contrast before giving a thionamide (propylthiouracil or methimazole).

Diagnostic Workup

- This is a clinical diagnosis, and since most patients present in need of emergent stabilization, treatment is initiated empirically.
- Patients may have inadequately treated hyperthyroidism.
- May also occur in the setting of unintentional or intentional toxic ingestion of synthetic thyroid hormone in the hypothyroid patient.

CONQUER THE BOARDS!

Never give iodine (Lugol or potassium iodine) until after the thionamide has started to take effect.

Management

- **Primary stabilization is the most important first step, with focus on airway protection,** oxygenation, circulation (pulse/blood pressure [BP]) and continuous cardiac monitoring, and IV hydration.
    - **Beta blocker therapy** (e.g., propranolol) is given to block adrenergic effects and block peripheral conversion of T_4 to T_3.
    - Treat fever with acetaminophen and cooling blanket (not aspirin, which displaces T_4 from thyroid-binding protein).
- Address the thyroid hormone itself with **propylthiouracil (PTU)** or **methimazole** to block synthesis of new thyroid hormone and **iodine** to decrease release of preformed thyroid hormone.
    - **Corticosteroids** are also given to prevent peripheral conversion of T_4 to T_3 and to treat "relative" adrenal failure occurring due to a high metabolic rate.
    - Treat any possible precipitating factors that may be present (e.g., MI, infection, etc.).

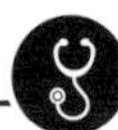

Graves disease (and Hashimoto thyroiditis) are sometimes associated with other autoimmune diseases (type 1 diabetes mellitus, vitiligo, myasthenia, pernicious anemia, collagen diseases).

GRAVES DISEASE

General Facts

- Autoimmune disease causing hyperthyroidism due to antibody that stimulates TSH receptor.
- Antibody is produced that interacts with the receptor for TSH, resulting in continuous excess secretion.
- The cause of the exophthalmos (infiltrative ophthalmopathy) in Graves disease is unknown, but is thought to be due to immunoglobulins that interact with self-antigens in the extraocular muscles and on orbital fibroblasts.

CONQUER THE WARDS!

Symptoms SPECIFIC to Graves disease: Exopthalmos, thyroid bruit, pretibial myxedema.

Clinical Features

- Diffusely enlarged thyroid, exophthalmos, pretibial myxedema, tachycardia, and palpitations are all common symptoms.
- In elderly patients the presentation is less classic. Apathy can be present without the common hyperactivity signs (apathetic hyperthyroidism). Cardiovascular features may be prominent, and hyperthyroidism may not be suspected initially.

CONQUER THE BOARDS!

Older patient presenting with new-onset atrial fibrillation and weight loss = classic apathetic Graves disease: Check TSH!

Diagnostic Workup

- Checking **TSH, T_4, and T_3 is the first step:** Low or undetectable TSH levels with elevated free thyroid hormones (some with elevated T_3 only: T_3 toxicosis).

- After hyperthyroidism is established, check **TSH receptor antibodies** or **thyroid-stimulating immunoglobulin (TSI) levels**, since Graves disease is by far the most common cause of hyperthyroidism.
- If antibodies do not establish the diagnosis, **radioactive iodine uptake on a radionuclide imaging (I-123)** should be done. In Graves disease, there will be elevated and diffuse uptake.

Management

- **Antithyroid therapy is the first-line treatment.** Surgery and ablation can be considered after the patient is euthyroid. But antithyroid therapy alone can lead to remission.
  - Usually accomplished with **methimazole (MMI)**. MMI is as effective as PTU when administered at one-tenth of the PTU dosage.
  - PTU inhibits peripheral T_4 to T_3 conversion but is more toxic (liver failure).
  - Treatment for 12 to 18 months to start, as 40% to 50% obtain remission with methimazole alone.
  - *Complications:* Granulocytopenia/agranulocytosis – If patient develops fever or sore throat, check CBC (otherwise not routine). Liver injury – Watch for jaundice, abdominal pain, and dark urine, and check liver function tests (LFTs). Rash – If minor, you can treat; in rare cases this may be Stevens–Johnson syndrome.
  - **Methimazole is contraindicated in first-trimester pregnancy – use PTU.**
- **Beta blockers**, with propranolol as the most commonly used agent, and atenolol as an alternative that can be used in once-daily dosage. Should be used only as adjunctive therapy because it does not treat the underlying problem.
- **Definitive therapy:**
  - **Radioactive iodine ablation therapy (I-131)** can produce the same effects as surgery without the surgical complications, but commonly results in hypothyroidism (may be delayed over time). Radiation thyroiditis commonly appears within 7 to 10 days after therapy and is associated with accelerated release of thyroid hormone into the blood. Rarely, this results in thyrotoxic crisis.
  - **Thyroidectomy** is still used for younger patients or when ablation therapy is unsuccessful. Delayed complications include hypoparathyroidism (can be life threatening) and hypothyroidism.

> CONQUER THE **WARDS!**
>
> PTU has fallen out of favor and is only used in rare circumstances: first-trimester pregnancy, thyroid storm (some), reaction to MMI.

> CONQUER THE **BOARDS!**
>
> When monitoring pa-tients on methimazole, TSH levels lag thyroid hormone levels to normalize.
> Dose changes are initially based on free T_4 changes and not TSH.

HYPOTHYROIDISM

General Facts

- Clinically evident hypothyroidism occurs in 2% of women and in 0.2% of men.
- The incidence increases with age, usually between 40 and 60.
- Insufficient thyroid hormone production, by far most commonly from thyroid gland failure (primary hypothyroidism).
- Overt hypothyroidism with classic symptoms and subclinical hypothyroidism with more mild symptoms.

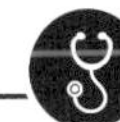

Hashimoto thyroiditis (chronic lymphocytic thyroiditis) is the most common cause of hypothyroidism in North America.

Etiology (see Table 7-7)

- **Primary hypothyroidism** (thyroid gland dysfunction) can be caused by Hashimoto thyroiditis, previous treatment for hyperthyroidism, hypothyroid

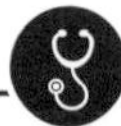

Muscle weakness and cramps occur in both hyperthyroidism and hypothyroidism. In hyperthyroidism, creatinine phosphokinase (CPK) will be normal. In hypothyroidism, it may be elevated.

CONQUER THE WARDS!

In clinical practice there is no meaningful difference between secondary and tertiary hypothyroidism. Group them together in your mind!

CONQUER THE WARDS!

Queen Anne sign (sign of Hertoghe) is the loss of outer one-third of the eyebrows.

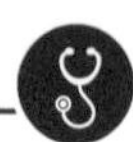

Consider evaluating thyroid function tests in any patient with hypercholesterolemia.

phase of thyroiditis (painless, subacute), radiation therapy to the neck (for other malignancy), iodine deficiency or excess, medications (lithium, amiodarone), or prolonged treatment with iodine-containing substances.

- **Secondary hypothyroidism** (pituitary dysfunction) can be caused by postpartum necrosis (Sheehan syndrome), space-occupying pituitary neoplasm, pituitary surgery or infiltrating disease (TB) causing TSH deficiency.
- **Tertiary hypothyroidism** (deficiency in thyrotropin-releasing hormone [TRH] secretion; hypothalamic dysfunction) can be caused by granulomas, neoplasm, or secondary to radiation.

Clinical Features

- **General signs:** Cold intolerance, fatigue, lethargy, weakness, and weight gain are common symptoms.
- **Musculoskeletal:** Muscle weakness, cramps, arthralgias, and cold intolerance can occur as well.
- **GI:** Constipation.
- **Skin** findings include dry, coarse, thick, and cool skin along with nonpitting edema of the skin and eyelids. Hair can turn brittle and coarse; loss of outer one-third of eyebrows.
- **Cardiac:** Distant heart sounds may be present if pericardial effusion is present. Bradycardia may occur.
- **Neurologic: Delayed relaxation phase of deep tendon reflexes** (very specific). Cerebellar ataxia can be present. Peripheral neuropathies with paresthesias and carpal tunnel syndrome are neurologic manifestations.
- **Severe hypothyroidism:** Slow speech with hoarse voice (from myxedematous changes in vocal cords) and decreased or altered mentation can occur in severe cases.

HIGH-YIELD LITERATURE

Chaker L, Bianco AC, Jonklaas J, et al. Hypothyroidism. *Lancet*. 2017;390:1550-1562.

CONQUER THE WARDS!

Weight-based replacement dosing of levothyroxine (e.g., after thyroidectomy): 1.6 mcg/kg body weight, e.g., 100 kg × 1.6 mcg/kg = 160 mcg. Choose closest available dose (150 mcg daily).

Diagnostic Workup

- See Table 7-6 for results of thyroid tests and Table 7-7 for different thyroid conditions.
- Also, **in Hashimoto thyroiditis:** May show **increased antithyroglobulin and antimicrosomal antibody titers (aka anti-TPO antibody).**

Management

- For mild disease, start therapy with low-dose **levothyroxine** and increase dose every 6 to 8 weeks, depending on the patient's response (*start low, go slow*).
- Elderly patients and patients with coronary artery disease should be started on a low dose of levothyroxine because high doses may precipitate angina pectoris.

TABLE 7-6. Laboratory Evaluation of the Thyroid

Thyroid State	T_4	FT_4	T_3	FT_3	TSH	TRH
Hypothyroidism						
First degree	↓	↓	↓	↓	↑	↑
Second degree	↓	↓	↓	↓	↓	N
Third degree	↓	↓	↓	↓	↓/N	↓
Peripheral unresponsiveness	↑/N	↑/N	↑/N	↑	↓/N	↑/N
Hyperthyroidism						
Pituitary tumor (secretes TSH)	↑	↑	↑	↑	↑	↓
Graves disease	↑	↑	↑	↑	↓	↓
T_3 thyrotoxicosis	N	N	↑	↑	↓	↓
T_4 thyrotoxicosis	↑	↑	N	N	↓	↓
Toxic nodular goiter	↑	↑	↑	↑	↓	↓

TABLE 7-7. Primary, Secondary, and Transient Thyroid Disorders

Primary	Secondary	Transient
• **Autoimmune:** Hashimoto, atrophic thyroiditis • **Iatrogenic:** Thyroidectomy, external irradiation of neck for malignancy, radioactive iodine treatment • **Drugs:** Iodine excess, lithium, antithyroid drugs, p-aminosalicylic acid, interferon α, aminoglutethimide, tyrosine kinase inhibitors • **Congenital:** Absent or ectopic thyroid, dyshormonogenesis, receptor mutations • **Iodine deficiency** • **Infiltrative diseases:** Amyloidosis, sarcoidosis, hemochromatosis, scleroderma	• **Hypopituitarism:** Tumors, pituitary surgery or irradiation, infiltrative disorders, Sheehan syndrome, trauma • **Isolated TSH deficiency** or inactivity • Hypothalamic disease: Tumors, trauma, infiltrative disorders, idiopathic	• Silent thyroiditis, including postpartum thyroiditis • Subacute thyroiditis • Withdrawal of supraphysiologic thyroxine treatment in individuals with an intact thyroid • After I-131 treatment or subtotal thyroidectomy for Graves disease

- **Monitoring therapy:**
  - In first-degree hypothyroidism, it is adequate to measure the TSH level every few months, which should fall well within the normal range.
  - In second-degree hypothyroidism, measure the free T_4 level, which should fall well within the normal range.

SUBCLINICAL HYPOTHYROIDISM

Elevated TSH level with normal thyroid hormone levels (free T_4) with absent or mild clinical symptoms.

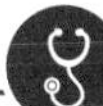

Thyroid peroxidase autoantibodies (TPO Ab) are indicative of autoimmune thyroid disease and have predictive value for progression to overt hypothyroidism or development of drug-induced thyroid dysfunction.

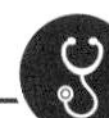

Hypothermia is often missed by tympanic thermometers. Use a rectal probe if hypothermia is suspected.

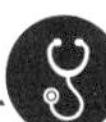

Infection is a common precipitant of myxedema coma; panculture and empiric antibiotic therapy with broad-spectrum antibiotics is recommended for all affected patients.

CONQUER THE BOARDS!

Patients with subclinical hypothyroidism are more likely to develop overt disease: positive antibodies.

CONQUER THE BOARDS!

Patient difficult to wean from ventilator with no other obvious cause: Think hypothyroidism.

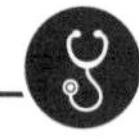

Differential diagnosis of myxedema coma:

Severe depression or primary psychosis
Drug overdose or toxic exposure
CVA
Liver failure
CO_2 narcosis
Hypoglycemia
CNS infection

CONQUER THE WARDS!

No single test can diagnose myxedema coma or thyroid storm: Think of as a spectrum of severe hypothyroidism/hyperthyroidism with altered mental status (AMS) and hypothermia/hyperthermia as most concerning.

CONQUER THE WARDS!

Get a random cortisol at presentation and then treat with steroids empirically.
Once cortisol level returns to normal can reduce/eliminate and rule out adrenal insufficiency.

Clinical Features

- There are usually 2 distinct patterns: Patients who will eventually develop first-degree hypothyroidism or clinical euthyroidism with persistent mildly elevated TSH.

Management

Thyroid replacement therapy is necessary only in the following circumstances:

- All patients with TSH >10.
- Patients with TSH >5 if:
  - Goiter or antithyroid antibody or symptoms of hypothyroidism.
- Pregnant women or women thinking of becoming pregnant.

MYXEDEMA COMA

General Facts

- A life-threatening complication of hypothyroidism with profound lethargy or coma, usually accompanied by hypothermia. Mortality is 20% to 50% even if treated early.
- Can be precipitated by sepsis, prolonged exposure to cold weather, CNS depressants (sedatives, narcotics), trauma, surgery, or medication nonadherence (especially with history of thyroidectomy).

Clinical Features

- Altered mental status, which typically starts with confusion and progresses to lethargy and then to coma.
- Hypothermia can be profound, with rectal temperatures <35°C (95°F).
- Bradycardia or circulatory collapse, peripheral edema, pericardial effusion, pleural effusion, anasarca (severe), hypoventilation, and respiratory acidosis.
- Delayed relaxation phase of deep tendon reflexes; areflexia if severe (this is an important clue).

A 75-year-old female presents with progressive obtundation and nonarousal. Core temperature is 35°C; cold, doughy skin; delayed deep tendon reflex in the relaxation phase. Urine analysis with many leukocytes and gram-negative rods. *Think: Myxedema coma.*

Diagnostic Workup

Lab tests for the patient presenting with signs and symptoms of myxedema coma (in descending order):

- TSH, free thyroxine (FT_4), cortisol level, CBC with differential, complete metabolic panel (CMP) (electrolytes, creatinine, glucose, liver function).
- Blood and urine cultures to assess for underlying precipitants.
- Urine toxicology screen to rule out reversible drug precipitants.
- Arterial blood gas (ABG) to rule out hypoxemia and CO_2 retention.
- Chest radiograph and CT of the brain.

Management

- Airway management with mechanical ventilation if necessary (ABCs, etc.).
- Pharmacologic therapy, including IV levothyroxine and glucocorticoids (until coexisting adrenal insufficiency is excluded).
- Prevent further heat loss, monitor patient in ICU, and maintain appropriate IV hydration (D5 and half normal saline).
- Rule out and treat any precipitating causes (antibiotics for suspected infection).

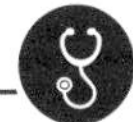

Corticosteroids are given empirically in myxedema coma before T_4 is given due to a concern that associated Addison disease exists. Giving only T_4 could precipitate an addisonian crisis.

THYROIDITIS

General Facts

- Inflammation of the thyroid.
- Can be divided into 3 common types (Hashimoto, subacute, and silent) and 2 rarer forms (suppurative and Riedes).
- **Hashimoto thyroiditis:** Autoimmune disorder that involves CD4 lymphocyte-mediated destruction of the thyroid. The lymphocytes are specific for thyroid antigens, but the precipitant is unknown. Marked by antibodies: TPO, anti-Tg antibody.
- **Subacute thyroiditis:** Possibly a postviral condition because it usually follows a viral URI. Not considered an autoimmune reaction.
- **Silent thyroiditis:** Usually occurs **postpartum** and is thought to be autoimmune mediated.
- **Suppurative thyroiditis:** Usually a bacterial infection, but fungi and parasites have also been implicated in some cases. Immunocompromised hosts, or those with retained thyroglossal duct.
- **Riedel thyroiditis:** Fibrous infiltration of the thyroid of unknown etiology; also called fibrous thyroiditis.

A patient who comes in with fever, anxiety, and a painful neck should be worked up for thyroiditis (pain!). Thyroid function tests will show decreased TSH with increased T_4 but decreased uptake on iodine scan. **Next step:** *Prescribe a nonsteroidal antiinflammatory drug (NSAID) or steroid.*

CONQUER THE WARDS!

Hashimoto disease: Even though called thyroiditis, you often don't see patients during the hyperthyroid phase. Most common cause of hypothyroidism in the United States is Hashimoto thyroiditis.

Clinical Features

- **Hashimoto:** There may be signs of hyperthyroidism or hypothyroidism depending on the stage. Usually, there is diffuse, firm enlargement of the gland, but it may be of normal size if the disease has progressed.
- **Subacute:** Tender, enlarged gland; severe neck pain; often mistaken for pharyngitis. Fever and signs of hyperthyroidism are initially present. Hypothyroidism may develop. Very high erythrocyte sedimentation rate (ESR).
- **Silent:** Similar to subacute except there is no tenderness of the gland (painless thyroiditis).
- **Suppurative:** Fever with severe neck pain. Focal tenderness of involved portion of the gland.
- **Riedel:** Slowly enlarging, rock-hard mass in the anterior neck. Tight, stiff neck. Must differentiate from thyroid cancer. Hypothyroidism may occur if advanced. Fibrosis may involve mediastinum.

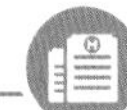

The thyroid in Hashimoto and silent thyroiditis is nontender, which distinguishes it from other forms of thyroiditis.

CONQUER THE BOARDS!

Thyrotoxic patient (weight loss, palpitations, heat intolerance, etc.) with a TENDER thyroid: Think subacute thyroiditis, not Graves disease.

A 35-year-old female with symptoms of hyperthyroidism and a recent flu presents with neck pain and an elevated ESR. *Think: Subacute thyroiditis.* **Next step:** Check thyroid function tests.

CONQUER THE WARDS!

Reidel is described as "woody" thyroid: Tremendously firm and nonobile.

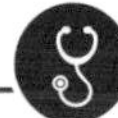

Differential diagnosis of thyroiditis:
The hyperthyroid stage of Hashimoto, subacute, or silent thyroiditis; may mimic Graves disease. Riedel must be differentiated from thyroid cancer. Subacute thyroiditis can be mistaken for oropharyngeal or tracheal infections or for suppurative thyroiditis.

Diagnostic Workup

- **History:**
  - Presentation following viral URI is suggestive of subacute thyroiditis.
  - Presentation after penetrating injury to the neck is suggestive of suppurative processes.
  - Postpartum presentation is suggestive of silent thyroiditis.
- **Laboratory examination:**
- TSH and FT_4 : Results depend on which phase of thyroiditis the patient currently is in (may be low, normal, or high).
  - White blood cell (WBC) count with differential should be obtained to look for leukocytosis and left shift (subacute and suppurative).
  - Antimicrosomal antibodies (anti-TPO) to support Hashimoto diagnosis.
  - Serum thyroglobulin levels are elevated in subacute and silent thyroiditis (test is very nonspecific).
- **Imaging studies:** Radioactive iodine uptake (RAIU) can be useful to distinguish Graves disease (increased RAIU) from subacute thyroiditis (decreased RAIU) in a thyrotoxic patient.

Management

- Control symptoms of hyperthyroidism, if present, with propranolol.
- Pain management in patients with subacute thyroiditis should be accomplished with NSAIDs. If ineffective, begin a tapering course of steroids.
- IV antibiotics and abscess drainage, if present, should be performed in suppurative thyroiditis.
- **Do not** give PTU or methimazole in thyroiditis – the mechanism is release of preformed hormone from an inflamed gland, *not* overproduction of hormone by the gland.
- Treat hypothyroidism, if symptoms develop, with levothyroxine. Reevaluate in the future, as it may be temporary phenomenon.

Prognosis

- **Hashimoto:** Most patients do not completely recover their total thyroid function.
- **Subacute:** Hypothyroidism persists in 10%.
- **Silent:** Hypothyroidism persists in 6%.
- **Suppurative:** Full recovery is common.
- **Riedel thyroiditis:** Hypothyroidism occurs when the entire gland undergoes fibrosis.

THYROID NODULE

General Facts

- Common (1% of men and 5% of women).
- Incidence increases after age 45.
- Increased cancer risk: History of neck irradiation, family history of thyroid cancer.

Clinical Features

- Mostly asymptomatic.

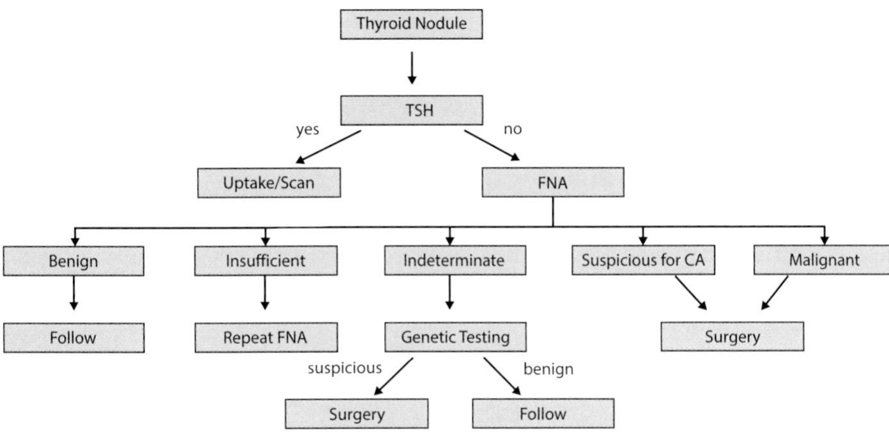

FIGURE 7-4. **Initial approach to the thyroid nodule.**

- Compressive symptoms: Dysphagia, shortness of breath (stridor), hoarseness.
- Physical exam: Likelihood of malignancy increases with nodule >2 cm, regional lymphadenopathy, fixation to tissues, age <40, male sex, family history of thyroid cancer, history of head and neck irradiation.
- Pemberton sign: Large goiter compressing the superior vena cava and causing facial plethora.

Diagnostic Workup

- **Thyroid ultrasound** is performed to evaluate the size and number of thyroid nodules. Ultrasound features are also useful for diagnosis: hypoechoic, microcalcification, irregular borders, extrathyroidal extension, solid, taller than wide all raise malignancy risk. See Figure 7-4.
- **TSH** is the next step prior to fine needle aspiration (FNA) or thyroid uptake scan. If TSH is low, then thyroid uptake scan. If TSH is not low, then FNA to assess for malignancy.
- **FNA** is the best way to assess for malignancy risk.
- **Thyroid uptake and scan (RAIU)**, using I-123 preferably, classifies nodules as hyperfunctioning (hot nodules, highly unlikely to be malignant) or hypofunctioning (cold nodules, more likely to be malignant).
- FNA result interpretation: Uses Bethesda Classification System:
  - Benign: Follow with ultrasound imaging.
  - Malignant/suspicious for malignancy: Surgery.
  - Nondiagnostic (not enough sample): Send for repeat FNA.
  - Indeterminate nodules: Carry 10% to 30% risk depending on category.
    - Genetic testing: Changes likelihood of malignancy for deciding on surgery.

CONQUER THE WARDS!

Incidental thyroid nodules are exceedingly common. Often found after imaging completed for another reason (e.g., CT chest for shortness of breath).

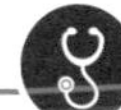

Measurement of serum thyroglobulin is useful for following thyroid cancers in response to treatment, but a serum thyroglobulin level is not useful in distinguishing benign from malignant nodules.

THYROID CANCER

General Facts

- Incidence ~9/100,000, with 2:1 female predominance.
- Risk increases with age and plateaus after age 50; worse prognosis if <20 years old or >65 years old.
- Risk factors include history of childhood head or neck irradiation, large nodule (>4 cm), enlarging neck mass, and family history.

CONQUER THE BOARDS!

Patient with medullary thyroid cancer concern on FNA needs to be evaluated for pheochromocytoma: MEN II syndromes.

Causes of hypercalcemia:

PTH mediated (PTH high or inappropriately normal):

- **Primary hyperparathyroidism**
- **Tertiary hyperparathyroidism**
- **Lithium use**
- **Familial hypocalciuric hypercalcemia (FHH)**

Non-PTH mediated (PTH low)

- **Bone metastases**
- **Sarcoidosis**
- **Hyperthyroidism**
- **Thiazide diuretics**
- **Immobilization**
- **Excess supplement intake (calcitriol, calcium supplement)**
- **Paget disease (only if patient is immobilized)**

Classification

Two types – follicular (epithelial) and parafollicular:

- **Epithelial** (3 histologic types):
  - Papillary: Most common, has best prognosis.
  - Follicular: Early metastasis.
  - Anaplastic: Rare, worst prognosis.
- **Parafollicular** (also called medullary thyroid cancer):
  - Calcitonin is increased from parafollicular C-cells.
  - Seen in MEN IIa and IIb.

Management

- Thyroidectomy.
- Radioiodine ablation of residual cancer and micrometastasis.
- Oral T_4 suppressive therapy after surgery to suppress TSH that is thought to promote thyroid growth.
- Careful monitoring of TSH and thyroglobulin levels (a rise indicates recurrence of the cancer).

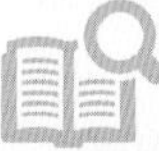

HIGH-YIELD LITERATURE

Haugen BR, Alexander EK, Bible KC, et al. American Thyroid Association Management Guidelines for Adult Patients with Thyroid Nodules and Differentiated Thyroid Cancer: The American Thyroid Association Guidelines Task Force on Thyroid Nodules and Differentiated Thyroid Cancer. *Thyroid*. 2016;26(1):1-133.

Gharib H, Papini E, Valcavi R, et al. American Association of Clinical Endocrinologists, American College of Endocrinology, and Associazione Medici Endocrinologi Medical Guidelines for Clinical Practice for the Diagnosis and Management of Thyroid Nodules – 2016 Update. *Endocrine Practice*. 2016; 22(Suppl 1):1-60.

PARATHYROID DISORDERS

HYPERPARATHYROIDISM

- **Primary:** Hypersecretion of PTH by the parathyroid glands (*the rest of this section refers to first degree only*).
- **Secondary:** Glandular hyperplasia and elevated PTH in an appropriate response to hypocalcemia (due to renal failure, GI disturbances, etc.).
- **Tertiary:** Continued elevation of PTH after the disturbance causing second-degree hyperparathyroidism has been corrected.

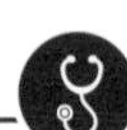

Before you send a patient with first-degree hyperparathyroidism to surgery, make sure you are not dealing with FHH. Urine calcium is usually <50 mg/24 hr. It is autosomal dominant with 100% penetrance and is benign. No treatment, only reassurance, of patient and family members.

General Facts

- Most common in middle-aged and elderly women.
- PTH secretion is stimulated by decreased serum levels of Ca^{2+} and inhibited by high levels, except in adenomas and carcinomas, in which feedback inhibition is lost.

Etiology

- Parathyroid adenoma: 85%, 1 gland involved.
- Parathyroid hyperplasia: 14%, all 4 glands involved.
- Parathyroid carcinoma: 1%, 1 gland involved.
- Associated with MEN I and IIa.
- Neck irradiation increases risk.

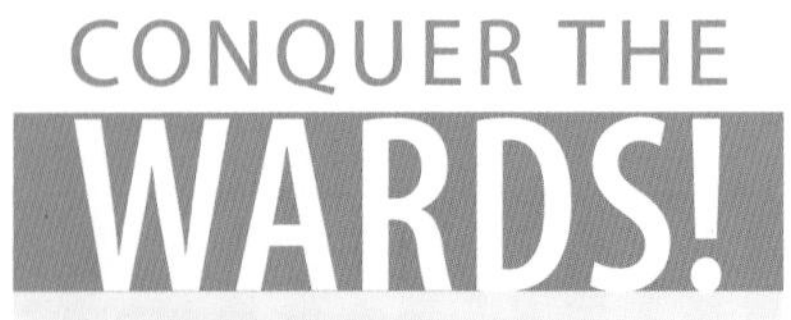

Remember symptoms of hypercalcemia: **Bones** (fractures), **Stones** (kidney), **Groans** (constipation, abdominal pain), **Psychiatric overtones** (confusion, AMS)!

Clinical Features

- Many patients are asymptomatic, and the disease gets discovered during routine blood work.
- Symptoms range from mild to severe.
- Generally, with **serum calcium** levels above 13.5 mg/dL, patients experience fatigue, polyuria, weakness, nausea, vomiting, abdominal pain, and changes in mental status from confusion to lethargy to obtundation and coma.
- Milder elevations in calcium can result in mild neurocognitive impairment.

Diagnostic Workup

- Elevated serum Ca^{2+}, low serum phosphate.
- High serum PTH (or inappropriately normal).

Management

- Assess for surgical indications: All symptomatic patients (mainly fractures, kidney stones), calcium elevation – greater than 1 mg/dL above upper limit lab normal, age <50, estimated GFR [EGFR] <60 mL/min, osteoporosis (T score <–2.5) or elevated urinary calcium (>400 mg/day).
- **Surgery:**
  - Adenoma: Remove with intraoperative PTH monitoring.
  - Hyperplasia: Either 3.5 glands removed or 4 glands removed with the half a gland reimplanted in the forearm or strap muscle in neck.
- **Emergency measures:**
  - Hydration with normal saline (salt leads to increased urinary calcium excretion), followed by loop diuresis (for volume control only).
  - Calcitonin acts rapidly but loses its efficacy after several days.
  - Bisphosphonates to block bone resorption (IV pamidronate, IV zoledronic acid).

HYPOPARATHYROIDISM

General Facts

- Condition characterized by PTH deficiency with equal incidence in men and women.
  - Can be idiopathic, due to DiGeorge syndrome (congenital aplasia or hypoplasia of thymus caused by missing gene on chromosome 22), postsurgical (i.e., thyroidectomy), infiltrative carcinoma, irradiation, or hypomagnesemia (magnesium is necessary for parathyroid gland to secrete PTH).

CONQUER THE BOARDS!

Next step after elevated calcium is to measure PTH level.
High or high normal = PTH mediated (short differential)
Low = all others.

CONQUER THE WARDS!

Surgical success for parathyroidectomy:
Greater than 50% drop in PTH after adenoma resected (intraoperative monitoring).

CONQUER THE WARDS!

Elevated calcium?
Ask for albumin (or ionized calcium). Corrected calcium = Serum Ca + 0.8 mg/dL * (4.0 g/dL – patient's albumin).

CONQUER THE BOARDS!

Severe hypercalcemia is treated with large-volume normal saline, calcitonin, and IV bisphosphonates.
Dialysis is also an option if this treatment is contraindicated or not working!

HIGH-YIELD LITERATURE

Bilezikian JP, Brandi ML, Eastell R, et al. Guidelines for the management of asymptomatic primary hyperparathyroidism: Summary statement from the Fourth International Workshop. *J Clin Endocrinol Metab*. 2014;99:3561-3569.

Insogna KL. Primary hyperparathyroidism. *N Engl J Med*. 2018;379(11):1050-1059.

CONQUER THE WARDS!

Chvostek sign: Tap anterior to ear = facial twitch (CN VII irritation)
Trousseau sign: Inflate arm BP cuff to a level above systolic pressure = carpopedal spasm.

Vitamin D acts on the intestines to increase absorption of calcium and phosphate. It is formed in the skin via sunlight as a previtamin and is converted to an inactive intermediate form (25-OH vitamin D) in the liver before being converted to its active form 1,25-$(OH)_2$ vitamin D (calcitriol) in the kidney.

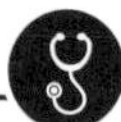

Pseudohypoparathyroidism presents the same as hypoparathyroidism, except that the pathophysiology in pseudohypoparathyroidism is tissue resistance to PTH, so that PTH is high (distinguishing feature). Pseudohypoparathyroidism is associated with Albright hereditary osteodystrophy (round facies, short stature, short fourth metacarpal bone, and subcutaneous calcification).

CONQUER THE BOARDS!

Young person presenting with abdominal pain, vomiting, and hyperkalemia = think Addison disease.
Next test random cortisol or ACTH stimulation.

A 30-year-old woman presents with perioral paresthesias and a long QT interval on ECG. She recently had surgery for a thyroid goiter. *Think: Hypoparathyroidism* (due to neck surgery with probable accidental resection of the parathyroids). **Next step:** Check serum calcium, PTH, and vitamin D levels.

Clinical Features

- Seizures, perioral paresthesia, fasciculations, tetany, and muscle weakness.
- CNS irritability, confusion, and seizures can occur in severe cases.
- Chvostek and Trousseau signs.

Diagnostic Workup

- Low serum calcium and high serum phosphorus.
- Normal or low PTH with normal 25-OH vitamin D and low 1,25-$(OH)_2$ vitamin D.
- QT prolongation on ECG in severe cases.

Management

- Treat severe, life-threatening hypocalcemia with IV calcium.
- Maintenance therapy with calcitriol and oral calcium supplementation.

ADRENAL DISORDERS

ADRENAL INSUFFICIENCY

General Facts

- More common in women (2:1) in its autoimmune form.
- **Primary insufficiency (Addison disease):** Inability of the gland to produce hormones. It is caused by autoimmune causes (80%); TB (15%) most commonly. Other causes are neoplasms, sarcoid, amyloid, disseminated fungal infections, hemochromatosis, AIDS, adrenal hemorrhage due to trauma, anticoagulants, or coagulopathies and Waterhouse-Friederichsen syndrome (fulminant septicemia).
- **Secondary insufficiency** can occur after suppression of hypothalamic–pituitary–adrenal axis by exogenous steroids (most common), Sheehan syndrome (postpartum pituitary necrosis), pituitary tumor, surgery, or autoimmune destruction of pituitary.
- **Tertiary insufficiency** is due to hypothalamic failure. Not clinically different from secondary.

Clinical Features

Primary Adrenal Insufficiency

The primary deficiencies caused by adrenal insufficiency that lead to symptoms are lack of cortisol and low mineralocorticoid production.

1. Lack of cortisol

   General symptoms: Fatigue (>80%), weight loss (66% to 76%), muscle and joint pain (40%)

   GI symptoms: Nausea, vomiting, and abdominal pain occur in about 50% of patients

   Specific symptoms:

   - **Hyperpigmentation** of mucosa, areolae, hand creases, knees, elbows, and knuckles (first degree only). Caused by pituitary overproduction of prohormone proopiomelanocortin as the body tries to increase cortisol production. It is cleaved into ACTH and MSH, which are increased in melanin synthesis.
   - **Hypoglycemia**.

2. Low aldosterone: Due to adrenal failure causing renal sodium loss, which leads to dehydration and hyponatremia:
   - **Orthostatic hypotension.**
   - **Hyperkalemia**.
   - **Salt craving.**

Secondary Adrenal Insufficiency

Patients with secondary adrenal insufficiency generally do not have hyperpigmentation or the symptoms of low aldosterone. They do have the general symptoms listed earlier, and **hypoglycemia** is more common. Generally their presentations are more chronic and less acute.

Addisonian or adrenal crisis is an acute complication of adrenal insufficiency characterized by shock, dehydration, confusion, vomiting, hyponatremia, hyperkalemia, and hypoglycemia. It is precipitated by sepsis, hemorrhage, trauma, and other stressors.

Primary adrenal insufficiency results in increased levels of ACTH. Melanocyte-stimulating hormone (MSH) and ACTH are cleaved from the same propeptide, so elevated ACTH results in increased skin pigmentation.

CONQUER THE **WARDS!**

Patients with secondary adrenal insufficiency generally do not have hyperpigmentation or the symptoms of low aldosterone. They do have the general symptoms listed earlier, and hypoglycemia is more common. Generally their presentations are more chronic and less acute.

An 18-year-old man with hemophilia A who was recently mugged (receiving multiple blows to the back and abdomen) is now complaining of dizziness, abdominal pain, dark patches on his elbows and knees, and uncontrollable cravings for pizza and French fries. *Think: First-degree adrenal insufficiency.* **Next step:** ACTH stimulation test.

Diagnostic Workup

- **Morning cortisol** is usually the first step. Morning cortisol is not sensitive or specific for adrenal insufficiency, but it can strongly suggest it. A level less than 3 μg/dL is highly suggestive for adrenal insufficiency and a level >18 μg/dL makes adrenal insufficiency unlikely.
- **ACTH stimulation test.** This should be done in all patients where adrenal insufficiency is being considered.
  - Give dose of ACTH and measure serum cortisol levels at 0, 30, and 60 minutes. A peak level <18 to 20 μg/dL confirms adrenal insufficiency.
  - **ACTH level:** Measuring the plasma ACTH at time 0 of an ACTH stimulation test will tell you whether it is primary adrenal insufficiency (high ACTH) or secondary adrenal insufficiency (low or normal ACTH).
  - **Other lab values:** Hyperkalemia, hyponatremia, extracellular fluid (ECF) volume contraction, and metabolic acidosis due to aldosterone deficiency (first degree only) can also be seen.

Secondary adrenal insufficiency can be distinguished from Addison disease by:

- Absence of hyperpigmentation
- Normal aldosterone secretion
- Other signs of hypopituitarism, such as hypothyroidism and hypogonadism, suggest presence of pituitary lesion or tumor

CONQUER THE WARDS!

Emergent treatment is required for patients in adrenal crisis! IV normal saline and IV steroids (hydrocortisone) can be lifesaving.

Management

- Glucocorticoid replacement (e.g., hydrocortisone) for all patients, usually with a morning and afternoon dose to mimic the normal diurnal cycle.
- Instruct patients to increase their glucocorticoid dose in times of stress and infection.
- Patients with Addison disease should also receive mineralocorticoid replacement therapy (e.g., fludrocortisone).

CUSHING SYNDROME AND CUSHING DISEASE

General Facts

- **Cushing syndrome:** Symptoms caused by excess cortisol production.

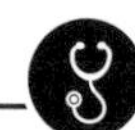

The most common source of glucocorticoid excess is exogenous corticosteroid therapy.

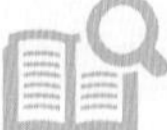

HIGH-YIELD LITERATURE

Bornstein SR, Allolio B, Arit W, et al. Diagnosis and treatment of primary adrenal insufficiency: An Endocrine Society Clinical Practice Guideline. *J Clin Endocrinol Metab.* 2016;101:364-389.

Charmandari E, Nicolaides NC, Chrousos GP. Adrenal insufficiency. *Lancet.* 2014;383(9935):2152-2167.

- **Cushing disease:** Cushing syndrome caused by excess ACTH secretion by pituitary.
- More common in females.
  - Can be caused by exogenous corticosteroid therapy, pituitary tumors (Cushing disease), adrenal adenomas or ectopic ACTH production (such as small cell lung carcinoma, pheochromocytoma, medullary thyroid carcinoma, and carcinoids).

CONQUER THE WARDS!

Exogenous steroids are not just oral! Ask about topical, intraarticular, intranasal, inhaled, and even over-the-counter (OTC) supplements.
Drug–drug interactions can also happen (e.g., HIV meds and intranasal steroids).

Clinical Features

- Hypertension.
- Central obesity (apple-shaped habitus, moon facies, thin extremities) and hyperglycemia.
- Posterior cervical fat pad enlargement (buffalo hump), facial plethora, and hair loss.
- Fragile, easily bruised skin; abdominal purplish striae (wide).
- Proximal muscle weakness.
- Hirsutism.

Small cell lung carcinoma is frequently associated with ectopic ACTH production.

Diagnostic Workup

The diagnosis of Cushing is challenging. The first step is always a thorough history to rule out exogenous uses of steroids. Following is an explanation of the variety of tests that are used.

- **Late-night salivary cortisol:**
  - Midnight collection of saliva (can be done by patient at home) on 2 separate nights.
  - Cortisol should be low in the late evening; if elevated supports Cushing syndrome.

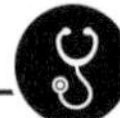

Patients with ectopic ACTH production often do not have all the mentioned symptoms; they usually have only hypertension and muscle weakness due to hypokalemia.

- **24-hour urine free cortisol:**
  - Should be completed twice and be 2 to 3 times higher than upper limit of normal to be considered positive.
  - Cortisol should be low in the late evening; if elevated supports Cushing syndrome.
- **Low-dose dexamethasone suppression test:**
  - Dexamethasone 1 mg is given at midnight; plasma cortisol measured at 8 AM.
  - If <1.8 μg/100 mL, excludes Cushing as a diagnosis.
- **ACTH:**
  - Low (<10) = adrenal source.
  - High/normal or high = pituitary or ectopic source.
  - **Corticotropin-releasing hormone (CRH) stimulation test:** CRH is given IV, and ACTH and cortisol levels are drawn.

A 42-year-old woman on long-term steroids for asthma has excess adipose tissue in her neck and upper trunk, a wide "moon face," and very fine hair. *Think: Cushing syndrome* (due to exogenous steroids).

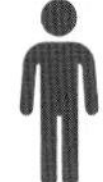

A 44-year-old woman has hypertension, muscle cramps, and excessive thirst. *Think: Hyperaldosteronism.*

Management

- **Pituitary adenomas:**
  - Transsphenoidal surgery:
    a. Success marked by postoperative cortisol insufficiency, which usually requires steroid replacement.
  - Pituitary irradiation can be considered for failed surgery.
- **Medical therapy:**
  - Target pituitary: Cabergoline, pasireotide.
  - Target adrenal: Ketoconazole, metyrapone, mitotane, etomidate.
  - Target cortisol receptor: Mifepristone.
  - Bilateral adrenalectomy if all else fails.
- **Adrenal adenoma:** Unilateral resection, followed by 3 to 12 months of glucocorticoid replacement (normal adrenal needs time to recover from suppression).
- **Bilateral adrenal hyperplasia:** Bilateral resection with lifelong replacement of glucocorticoids and mineralocorticoids.
- **Ectopic ACTH production:**
  - Remove source of neoplasm if possible.
  - Bilateral adrenalectomy if unsuccessful.

CONQUER THE **BOARDS!**

Ectopic ACTH syndrome is associated with severe cortisol excess that can occur quickly (may not have time to develop classic Cushing features, e.g., thin, smoker with severe hypokalemia and hyperglycemia).

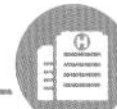

Screening tests for Cushing syndrome in suspected patients include the midnight salivary cortisol, 24-hour urine free cortisol test, and the low-dose (1 mg) dexamethasone-suppression test.

CONQUER THE **WARDS!**

Each test for Cushing syndrome has limitations: Late-night saliva (night shift workers), urine cortisol (renal impairment), dexamethasone suppression (medications: e.g., oral contraceptive pills [OCPs], antiseizure).

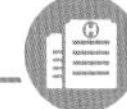

The most sensitive screening test for primary aldosteronism is the plasma aldosterone–plasma renin activity ratio.

Secondary causes of hypertension:

Renovascular hypertension
Primary aldosteronism
Pheochromocytoma
Cushing syndrome
Renal disease
Acromegaly

PRIMARY HYPERALDOSTERONISM

General Facts

- Primary hyperaldosteronism, also called Conn syndrome.
- One to two percent of all patients with hypertension.
- Most frequent in ages 30 to 60.
- Adrenal tumor more common in women.
- Can be due to a unilateral aldosterone-producing adenoma (most common cause) or bilateral hyperplasia of zona glomerulosa (idiopathic).

CONQUER THE BOARDS!

Resistant hypertension (3 or more medications) and hypokalemia (spontaneous or diuretic-induced): Think primary aldosteronism = measure morning aldosterone and renin levels.

A young man is evaluated with persistent hypertension. He was diagnosed at a routine examination. His blood pressure has remained high despite diet, weight loss, and compliance with therapy, which includes 4 BP medications. *Think: Secondary hypertension.*

Clinical Features

- Usually asymptomatic.
- Hypertension.
- May see signs of hypokalemia (muscle cramps, palpitations).

Multiple endocrine neoplasia type I: (3 Ps)

Pituitary tumors

Pancreatic islet tumors

Hyperparathyroidism due to **P**arathyroid hyperplasia

Diagnostic Workup

- **Screening:**
  - **Measure plasma aldosterone to plasma renin activity ratio**; a ratio >20 suggests hyperaldosteronism. Aldosterone levels also usually are >10 to 15 ng/mL.
- **Confirmation:**
  - Saline suppression or oral salt loading doesn't lower aldosterone as expected in patients with primary hyperaldosteronism.
- **Localization:**
  - CT scan may show adrenal nodule.
  - Adrenal vein sampling (AVS) often needed to confirm laterality before surgery.
- **Other findings:**
  - Hypokalemia and metabolic alkalosis.
  - Aldosterone escape: After initial edema and weight gain, patients usually diurese and shed the edema.

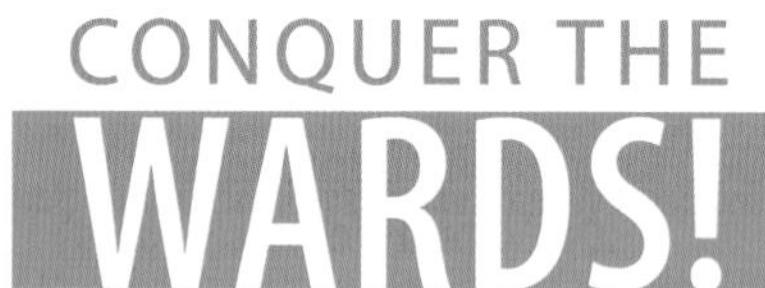

Renin (mostly) and aldosterone levels are influenced by antihypertensive medications. Be sure to check what medications the patient is on when interpreting testing!

Management

- Adrenalectomy for unilateral tumor.
- Medical management for hyperplasia or bilateral tumors:
  - Spironolactone or eplerenone (aldosterone receptor blocker).
  - Low-sodium diet.
  - Maintenance of ideal body weight, regular exercise, smoking cessation.

PHEOCHROMOCYTOMA

General Facts

- Tumor of the adrenal medulla resulting in catecholamine excess.
- Equal incidence in men and women. Tumors in women are 3 times as likely to be malignant.

Etiology

- Sporadic.
- MEN types IIa and IIb.
  - MEN IIa: Pheochromocytoma, medullary thyroid cancer, and parathyroid hyperplasia.
  - MEN IIb: Pheochromocytoma, medullary thyroid cancer, and mucosal neuromas.
- Neurofibromatosis.
- Succinyl dehydrogenase (SDH) mutations.
- Von Hippel–Lindau disease: Pheochromocytoma, retinal angiomas, CNS hemangioblastomas, renal cell carcinoma, pancreatic pseudocysts, ependymal cystadenoma.

CONQUER THE WARDS!

5 Hs
Headache
Hot (diaphoretic)
Hyperhidrosis
Hypertension
Heart (palpitations)

CONQUER THE WARDS!

Rule of 10s:
10% are extra-adrenal.
10% are bilateral.
10% are malignant.
10% are familial.

HIGH-YIELD LITERATURE

Lenders JWM, Duh Q, Eisenhofer G, Gimenez-Roqueplo AP, Grebe SKG, Murad MH. Pheochromocytoma and paraganglioma: An Endocrine Society Clinical Practice Guideline. *J Clin Endocrinol Metab*. 2014;99:1915-1942.

Clinical Features

- Patients experience "paroxysmal attacks" of high blood pressure.
- Physical exam usually normal outside of an attack.
- Symptoms of catecholamine (sympathetic) excess will predominate during an attack.
- Tremor, anxiety, and weight loss.

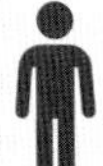

A 38-year-old woman on labetalol presents with poorly controlled hypertension, frequent headaches, and palpitations. *Think: Pheochromocytoma.* **Next step:** Stop labetalol and check urine metanephrines/catecholamines and serum metanephrines.

The classic symptoms of pheochromocytoma consist of hypertension with the triad of headaches, palpitations, and diaphoresis.

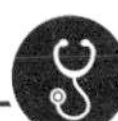

Patients with pheochromocytoma may carry an incorrect diagnosis of anxiety disorder.

Urinary excretion of metanephrine, normetanephrine, and catecholamines may be used to confirm the presence of excess catecholamine production.

Diagnostic Workup

- **24-hour urine catecholamines and metanephrines:** Often the first-line test when you suspect pheochromocytoma. Can be repeated during an episode if initially negative.
- **Plasma fractionated free metanephrines:** If you have a high suspicion for pheochromocytoma.

CONQUER THE WARDS!

Paragangliomas can occur anywhere along the sympathetic chain: Look from base of the neck to the pelvis!

- Once you have these tests confirming pheochromocytoma then CT or MRI to look for an adrenal mass. If these tests are negative with clinical impression and biochemical tests being positive, consider a **MIBG scan**. MIBG is a compound that resembles metanephrine and is taken up by pheochromocytoma and paraganglioma tissues.

Treatment

- Alpha-adrenergic blockade (may also add beta blocker), BP control, and volume expansion.
- Surgical resection.

BONE DISORDERS

OSTEOMALACIA

General Facts

- Disease of impaired bone mineralization.
- Termed *rickets* in the pediatric population.

Etiology

- Decreased Ca^{2+} absorption.
- Dietary calcium deficiency: Rare, avoidance of dairy products.
- GI disorders: Malabsorption syndromes, gastrectomy, dumping syndrome.
- Vitamin D deficiency.
- Hepatobiliary and pancreatic disease: Loss of bile acids or pancreatic lipase reduces absorption of fat-soluble vitamins.
- Extremely low-fat diets.
- Renal osteodystrophy: Decreased renal hydroxylation of vitamin D.
- Decreased serum PO_4.
- Renal tubular acidosis, Fanconi syndrome, hypophosphatasia.
- Tumor-induced osteomalacia (TIO): Often small mesenchymal tumors producing fibroblast growth factor 23 (FGF 23).

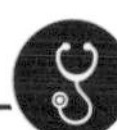

Prior to surgery for tumor resection, the patient must be properly alpha blocked with phenoxybenzamine or other alpha blockers to prevent an intraoperative hypertensive crisis. Also, prior to starting beta blocker therapy, alpha blockers must be on board to prevent unopposed alpha receptor stimulation.

Clinical Features

- Bone pain and weakness.
- Difficulty walking: Broad-based waddling gait with short strides.
- Thoracic kyphosis.

Diagnostic Workup

- **Radiographs:**
  - Show diffuse, nonspecific osteopenia.
  - Vertebrae may be biconcave from compression by intervertebral disks.
  - Pseudofractures (radiolucent lines perpendicular to bone cortex).
- **Labs:**
  - Ca^{2+} and PO_4 low to normal.
  - High alkaline phosphatase.
  - PTH may be elevated in response to low Ca^{2+}.
  - FGF 23 for suspected TIO.

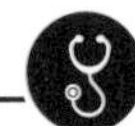

Abnormalities of vitamin D synthesis and metabolism are common in osteomalacia.

Management

- Address underlying disorder.
- Calcium, vitamin D supplements.

Oncogenic osteomalacia can be cured with removal of the tumor.

OSTEOPOROSIS

General Facts

- Systemic disorder resulting in a reduction of bone mass that leads to increased risk of fracture; early diagnosis and treatment are important.
- **Risk factors for osteoporosis** include female gender, old age, postmenopause, tobacco use, sedentary lifestyle, and family history of osteoporosis.
- The **Fracture Risk Assessment Tool (FRAX)** can be used to assess the 10-year probability of hip fracture and major osteoporotic fracture. FRAX considers the age, family history of the patient, bone mineral density, smoking history, and steroid use to quantify this risk.

CONQUER THE BOARDS!

Fragility fractures (fractures with fall from standing height) constitute a diagnosis of osteoporosis regard-less of bone mineral density (BMD) scoring.

Clinical Findings

- Osteoporosis has no clinical manifestations until a fracture occurs.
- Common fractures seen in osteoporosis:
  - **Vertebral body fracture** (compression fracture) is the most common fracture in osteoporosis and is usually diagnosed incidentally on a chest radiograph. But can cause pain and loss of height.
  - **Hip fractures.**
  - **Colles fracture:** Distal radius fracture.

CONQUER THE WARDS!

FRAX score calculators can be found online.

Diagnostic Workup

- **Osteoporosis** is diagnosed by the presence of one of the following:
  - Fragility fracture at spine, wrist, humerus, rib, or pelvis. A fragility fracture is defined as those occurring spontaneously or from minor trauma, such as a fall from a standing height. For example, a vertebral compression fracture alone diagnoses osteoporosis.
    OR
  - T score ≤ -2.5 standard deviations (SD) at any site on a dual-energy x-ray absorptiometry (DEXA) scan (not a bone scan).
    OR
  - Clear elevated risk of fracture as calculated by the FRAX. The 10-year probability of a major fracture is ≥20% or the 10-year probability of hip fracture is ≥3%.
- **Screening:** Since early diagnosis and treatment are key to preventing fractures, consider the indications for a screening DEXA scan:
  - Women age ≥65 years old.
  - Postmenopausal women age <65 years who have at least one risk factor for osteoporosis other than menopause.
  - Postmenopausal women who present with fractures or radiographic findings consistent with osteoporosis.
  - Corticosteroid therapy for >3 months.
  - Primary hyperparathyroidism.

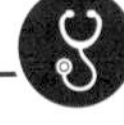

Bone Mineral Density Scoring

T score ≥ -1 = normal bone mass

T score -2.5 to -1 = osteopenia

T score ≤ -2.5 = osteoporosis

T score ≤ -2.5 + fragility fracture = Severe osteoporosis

CONQUER THE WARDS!

Rare complications of long-term bisphosphonate therapies: Osteonecrosis of jaw and atypical femoral fractures. Benefits far outweigh the risk!

- **Differential diagnosis:** It is also important to consider other diagnoses that can cause bone fractures and reduced bone mineral density:
  - Malignancy: Multiple myeloma, lymphoma, leukemia, and metastatic carcinoma
  - Hyperparathyroidism
  - Osteomalacia
  - Paget disease of bone

Management

- **Lifestyle measures:** The following should be adopted in all postmenopausal women. This includes exercise, smoking cessation, and avoidance of heavy alcohol use. Patients should receive in their diet and supplementation 1200 mg of elemental calcium daily and 800 international units of vitamin D daily.
- **Pharmacologic treatment:**
  - Oral bisphosphonates are the treatment of choice. They should be started in all patients diagnosed with osteoporosis and in patients with osteopenia (T scores between −1.0 and −2.5) and high risk for fracture via the FRAX score. Bisphosphonates (alendronate or zoledronic acid most commonly) prevent resorption and decrease incidence of fractures when used in conjunction with vitamin D and calcium supplementation.
  - Denosumab: A monoclonal antibody against RANK ligand (similar effect to bisphosphonates) and is used only in patients who cannot tolerate bisphosphonates or have impaired renal function.
  - Parathyroid analogue (e.g., teriparatide) can be considered in men or postmenopausal women with severe osteoporosis or who have failed bisphosphonates.

Bisphosphonates and teriparatide (PTH analogue) are the agents that decrease nonvertebral fractures in osteoporosis.

HIGH-YIELD LITERATURE

Cosman F, de Beur SJ, LeBoff MS, Lewiecki EM, Tanner B, Randall S. Clinician's guide to prevention and treatment of osteoporosis. *Osteoporos Int*. 2014;25:2359-2381.

Qaseem A, Forciea MA, McLean RM, et al. Treatment of low bone density or osteoporosis to prevent fractures in men and women: A clinical practice guideline update from the American College of Physicians. *Ann Intern Med*. 2017;166:818-839.

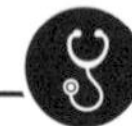

When alkaline phosphatase is elevated, send gamma-glutamyl transpeptidase (GGT) to determine if hepatic or bone (elevated in liver but not bone).

PAGET DISEASE OF BONE

General Facts

- Chronic disease of adult bone in which localized areas of bone become hyperactive and the normal bone matrix is replaced by radiographically dense but weak and enlarged bone.
- Cause is unknown, but it is suspected that a viral infection plays a role.
  - Rare for age >40 years, 3:2 male predominance.
  - Hyperactive bone turnover causes increased bone formation.
  - Pelvis, femur, skull, tibiae, and vertebrae all affected.
  - Enlarged multinucleated osteoclasts.

Paget disease is associated with elevated serum alkaline phosphatase levels and typical radiographic abnormalities; most patients are asymptomatic.

Clinical Features

- Most patients are asymptomatic, and Paget is incidentally found on radiographs with areas of hyperlucency surrounded by a hyperdense border or routine labs find an elevated alkaline phosphatase.
- Symptomatic patients:
  - **Skull:** Increasing hat size.
  - **Long bones:** Swelling or lengthening of a long bone, causing gait disturbance.
  - **Spine:** Dull aching pain, usually in the back; may radiate to the buttocks or lower extremities.
  - **Vestibular bones:** Rarely hearing loss due to involvement of the ossicles or auditory canal impinging on cranial nerve VIII.
  - **Complications** include pathologic fractures, urinary stones, and rarely a "high-output" cardiac failure due to high vascularity of lesions.

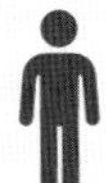

A patient is found to have an elevated alkaline phosphatase during a routine blood test. No other abnormalities were found. Further workup revealed this was bone specific. *Think: Paget disease.*

CONQUER THE BOARDS!

Headache and hearing loss: Think Paget disease – order alkaline phosphatase (bone specific) and bone scan if positive.

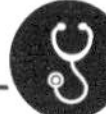

The primary indication for treatment in Paget disease is the presence of symptoms and lytic involvement of vertebrae, skull, weight-bearing bones, or areas adjacent to major joints.

Management

- Most patients require no treatment. However, patients with symptoms usually require treatment or patients with extremely high alkaline phosphatase.
- Indications for therapy are excessive pain, neural compression, profound alteration in posture or gait, high-output heart failure, hypercalcemia, and hypercalciuria, with or without renal calculi.
- **Bisphosphonates** containing nitrogen (e.g., alendronate, risedronate, or IV zoledronic acid) are first-line treatment. They help decrease bone reabsorption and are usually well tolerated.
- Calcitonin may be instituted as well in cases with cardiac failure or neurologic deficits. Calcitonin also has an analgesic effect.

The therapy of choice for uncomplicated Paget disease is a nitrogen-containing bisphosphonate.

HIGH-YIELD LITERATURE

Singer FR, Bone HG, Hosking DJ, et al. Paget's disease of bone: An Endocrine Society Clinical Practice Guideline. *J Clin Endocrinol Metab*. 2014;99(12):4408-4422.

CHAPTER 8 HEMATOLOGY/ ONCOLOGY

OVERVIEW OF HIGH-YIELD TOPICS IN HEMATOLOGY/ ONCOLOGY

BENIGN RED CELL DISORDERS

IRON-DEFICIENCY ANEMIA

General Facts

- Iron-deficiency anemia (IDA) occurs due to decreased iron stores resulting in decreased hemoglobin synthesis.
- The most common causes of IDA are blood loss, menorrhagia in premenopausal women, gastrointestinal blood loss, hookworm infection in tropical areas, malnutrition/malabsorption (e.g., bariatric surgery, *Helicobacter pylori* gastritis, celiac sprue), and pregnancy.

Clinical Features

- The most common signs and symptoms of IDA are fatigue, exertional dyspnea, and decreased exercise tolerance.

CONQUER THE WARDS!

IDA is the most common cause of anemia worldwide.

CONQUER THE BOARDS!

A young man or postmenopausal woman with IDA needs aggressive workup with colonoscopy and endoscopy to evaluate for colon cancer.

CONQUER THE WARDS!

Differential for low MCV includes thalassemia, anemia of chronic diseases, and sideroblastic anemia.

CONQUER THE BOARDS!

Both ferritin and transferrin saturation are decreased in IDA; however, ferritin is increased in anemia of chronic diseases

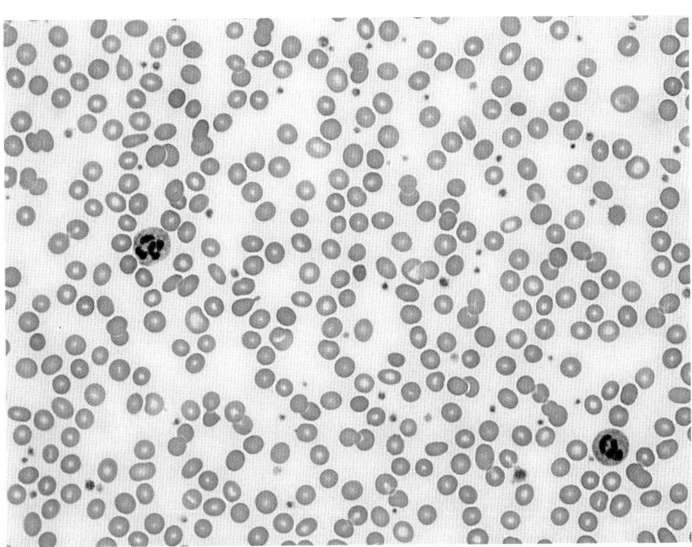

FIGURE 8-1. **Iron-deficiency anemia.** (Source: https://images.app.goo.gl/4aWst8iZk4e5WGy39.)

- Koilonychias (spoon nails), pica (ingestion of clay or ice), glossitis (red, beefy, glossy, swollen tongue without papillae), and cheilosis (crusting of angle of the mouth) are other symptoms to look for.

Diagnostic Workup

- The diagnosis of IDA is made based on lab values, as listed:
  - Microcytosis, that is, low mean corpuscular volume (MCV) less than 80 (Figure 8-1).
  - High red cell distribution width (RDW) more than 15%.
  - Low iron.
  - Low ferritin (<30 ng/mL indicates iron deficiency).
  - High total iron-binding capacity (TIBC).
  - High transferrin.
  - Low transferrin saturation (TSAT), less than 16%.

Management

- IDA is treated by first identifying the cause.
- Supplementation with oral ferrous sulfate can be used to correct the iron deficiency and to build iron stores. Oral iron can be hard to tolerate with gastrointestinal side effects like dyspepsia, nausea, etc. being the main cause of lack of compliance. Using stool softener along with oral iron can help improve symptoms of constipation.
- Consider intravenous (IV) iron formulations if patient is not able to tolerate oral iron.
- Hypersensitivity reactions and even anaphylactic shock have been reported with IV iron formulations, so slow administration and very careful patient selection and monitoring are recommended.

CONQUER THE BOARDS!

Causes of folate-deficiency anemia—
Pregnant MAN
Pregnancy and lactation
Malabsorption (celiac and Crohn disease)
Alcoholism
Nutritional (toast and tea elderly diet)

CONQUER THE WARDS!

Management with IV iron formulations can be dangerous! Make sure the patient is in a setting where nursing can monitor closely for reactions.

CONQUER THE WARDS!

HIV patients on highly active antiretroviral therapy (HAART) can have macrocytic anemia due to azathioprine (AZT).

HIGH-YIELD LITERATURE

Evaluation of unexplained or refractory IDA:
Hershko C, Camaschella C. How I treat unexplained refractory iron deficiency anemia. *Blood*. 2014;123:326-333.

MACROCYTIC ANEMIA

- Macrocytic anemia can be thought of as megaloblastic or non-megaloblastic.
- Causes of megaloblastic macrocytic anemia include folate deficiency and vitamin B_{12} deficiency.
- Causes of non-megaloblastic macrocytic anemia include liver dysfunction, hypothyroidism, drugs, and bone marrow disorders.

CONQUER THE BOARDS!

Causes of macrocytosis—
FEeD THeM
Folate and vitamin B_{12} deficiency
Ethanol and liver disease
Drugs (AZT, methotrexate)
Thyroid (hypothyroidism)
Hemolysis (reticulocytosis)
Myelodysplastic syndrome

FOLATE DEFICIENCY

General Facts

- Macrocytic anemia due to folate pathway abnormalities.
- Most common causes of folate deficiency include pregnancy, malabsorption (Crohn disease and celiac sprue), alcoholism, and malnutrition. Green vegetables are an excellent source of folate; overcooking or lack of adequate intake can lead to anemia.

Clinical features

- Suspect folate deficiency in a patient who consumes "tea and toast" diet and/or has alcohol abuse and presents with macrocytic anemia, diarrhea, glossitis, and cheilosis.

CONQUER THE BOARDS!

Folate deficiency can be differentiated from vitamin B_{12} deficiency by the lack of neurologic abnormalities.

Diagnostic Workup

- Diagnosis of folate deficiency is made based on:
  - High MCV.
  - Hypersegmented neutrophils seen on peripheral smear.
  - High homocysteine levels.
  - Low red blood cells (RBCs).
  - Low serum folate levels.

Management

- Folate deficiency is treated with oral folate supplementation.

CONQUER THE BOARDS!

Folic acid is absorbed in the upper third of the small intestine, so conditions like short gut syndrome will lead to folate deficiency.

B_{12} DEFICIENCY

General Facts

- A macrocytic anemia due to B_{12} deficiency.
- Most common causes of vitamin B_{12} deficiency include pernicious anemia (lack of intrinsic factor), lack dietary B_{12} intake (vegan diet or no-dairy diets), fish tapeworm (*Diphyllobothrium latum*), or malabsorption (celiac, Crohn disease, bacterial overgrowth, and ileal resection).
- A hallmark of vitamin B_{12} deficiency is neurologic symptoms that present after the anemia. The neurologic symptoms may include dementia or "megaloblastic madness":
  - Subacute combined degeneration of the dorsal (sensory) and lateral (upper motor neuron) spinal cord columns from myelin deficiency.
  - Symmetrical, affecting the legs and beginning with paresthesias and ataxia (loss of vibration and position sense) and progressing to weakness, spasticity, clonus, and hyperreflexia (upper motor neuron symptoms).

CONQUER THE WARDS!

Average age of diagnosis of pernicious anemia is 60 or older in adults.

Diagnostic Workup

- Diagnosis of vitamin B_{12} deficiency is made based on a complete blood cell count (CBC), looking for high MCV and hypersegmented neutrophils.
- Also look for high homocysteine levels, high methylmalonate in urine, and low serum B_{12} levels.

Management

- Vitamin B_{12} deficiency is treated with intramuscular (IM) vitamin B_{12} injections.

PERNICIOUS ANEMIA

General Facts

- Pernicious anemia is caused by an inability to absorb vitamin B_{12}.
- The parietal cell in the stomach produces hydrochloric acid (HCl) and intrinsic factor (IF). Vitamin B_{12} needs hydrogen ions from HCl to bind to IF, which carries vitamin B_{12} to the terminal ileum, where it is absorbed.
- In pernicious anemia, autoantibodies are made against the IF and/or the parietal cells, thus impairing the absorption of vitamin B_{12}. As the parietal cells get destroyed, chronic gastritis and eventually gastric cancer can ensue.

Clinical Features

- Same as B_{12} deficiency; insidious onset.
- Associated with chronic gastritis, vitiligo, and gastric cancer.
- Pernicious anemia can be associated with other autoimmune processes like vitiligo.

Diagnostic Workup

- Anti-IF antibody is the diagnosis of choice (IF-Ab).
- Anti–parietal cell antibody is less sensitive.
- Schilling test (now obsolete): First give IM radioactive vitamin B_{12}. Then give oral radioactive iodide. If there is no pernicious anemia, B_{12} will be absorbed and will "spill" in a 24-hour urine specimen (>10%) as tissue receptors are already saturated.

Management

Give IM B_{12} shots for life. Newer studies show oral B_{12} in high doses (300 to 1000 μg/day) is also equally effective.

GLUCOSE-6-PHOSPHATE DEHYDROGENASE (G6PD) DEFICIENCY

General Facts

- G6PD deficiency is an X-linked disease that results from a deficiency of glutathione in the RBCs. This deficiency is more common in those with Mediterranean (Italians, Greeks, Arabs) and African ancestry.
- G6PD is an enzyme needed to make nicotinamide adenine dinucleotide phosphate (NADPH), which is needed to make glutathione. It helps protect RBCs from the oxidative stress of free radicals.
- Infections, diabetic ketoacidosis, and medications such as sulfa drugs (trimethoprim-sulfamethoxazole, primaquine), quinolones, and fava beans cause hemoglobin (Hb) to precipitate within cells and cause hemolysis.
- Cells with precipitated Hb have **Heinz bodies**, which are removed by the spleen, resulting in **bite cells**.

Clinical Features

- Acute hemolysis causing anemia, with sudden onset of jaundice (high indirect bilirubin).
- Dark urine (hemoglobinuria) and abdominal and back pain can occur.
- Acute tubular necrosis can occur due to hemoglobinuria.

CONQUER THE BOARDS!

Causes of normocytic normochromic (normal size, normal shape) anemia include:

- Bone marrow problems (aplastic bone marrow, leukemia, myelodysplastic syndromes, etc.)
- Destruction (hemolytic anemias)
- Early nutritional anemias (iron, B_{12}, folate)

CONQUER THE BOARDS!

Causes of vitamin B_{12} deficiency—**VITAMIN B**

Vegan diet
Ileal resection
Tapeworm
Autoimmune (pernicious anemia)
Megaloblastic anemia
Inflammation of terminal ileum
Nitrous oxide
Bacterial overgrowth

CONQUER THE BOARDS!

ABCs of G6PD deficiency: **ABCDEFG**

Antimalarials
Bactrim/bite cells
Ciprofloxacin
DKA
InfEction
Fava beans (can be Fatal without transfusion)
G6PD deficiency

A 31-year-old Italian male with back pain, dark urine, jaundice, and anemia after 2 days of ciprofloxacin. *Think: G6PD deficiency.* **Next step:** Check peripheral smear, looking for "bite cells"; transfuse if severe anemia; and check renal function.

CONQUER THE BOARDS!

Check the G6PD assay 3 weeks after an acute episode because in acute situations younger RBCs that still have the G6PD enzyme reveal a falsely high level. The G6PD deficiency causes a decreased half-life of enzyme, so older RBCs without G6PD die.

CONQUER THE WARDS!

Pure red cell aplasia (anemia only) can be seen in sickle cell patients after parvovirus B19 infection (erythema infectiosum).

Diagnostic Workup

- Evidence of intravascular hemolysis, such as increased indirect bilirubin elevated and decreased haptoglobin and hemoglobinuria.
- Smear will show reticulocytes, **bite cells**, and **Heinz bodies**.
- Negative Coombs tests (nonautoimmune).
- G6PD assay.

APLASTIC ANEMIA

General Facts

- Marrow failure resulting in **pancytopenia** from stem cell defect, which is usually from immune-mediated injury (idiopathic or after exposure to radiation, drugs, infections, or certain chemicals).
- Common causative viral infections include viral hepatitis and **parvovirus B19**.
- Drugs include **chloramphenicol**, benzene, and dichlorodiphenyltrichloroethane (DDT).

Clinical Features

- Anemia: Weakness, fatigue, and pallor.
- Thrombocytopenia and ymptoms such as of mucosal bleeding and spontaneous bleeding.
- Neutropenia can lead to fevers and infections with typical organisms.

Diagnostic Workup

- Low reticulocyte count and normal MCV.
- Bone marrow biopsy will show hypocellular marrow with lots of white fat cells.

Management

- Immunosuppression (anti–thymocyte globulin [ATG], cyclosporine, and steroids).
- Young patients: Bone marrow transplant if immunosuppression fails.

ANEMIA OF CHRONIC DISEASE

General Facts

- Anemia caused by chronic diseases (infectious, malignant, and rheumatologic).
- Impairment in iron mobilization is the likely etiology, from chronic inflammation, cytokines, and an acute-phase reactant called hepcidin.

- These patients have features similar to IDA despite adequate iron stores on lab evaluation.
  - Chronic infections (tuberculosis, fungal diseases, etc.), malignancies, and rheumatologic diseases (systemic lupus erythematosus [SLE], rheumatoid arthritis) are common causes.

Diagnostic Workup

- Normocytic to microcytic anemia and normal erythropoietin.
- Increased ferritin (acute-phase reactant), decreased **TIBC and transferrin** (unlike IDA), and decreased serum iron.

Management

- Treat the underlying cause.

HEMOGLOBINOPATHIES

Normal electrophoresis pattern in adult:

- Hemoglobin A (96%): α2/β2 (normal hemoglobin).
- Hemoglobin F (3%): α_2/γ_2 (fetal hemoglobin, normal until 6 months of age).
- Hemoglobin A2 (1%): $\alpha_2\delta_2$.
- There are 2 alpha genes and 1 beta gene on each chromosome, making a total of 4 alpha genes and 2 beta genes.

ALPHA-THALASSEMIA

General Facts

- Genetic defect causing gene deletions of α chains.
  - αα/– thalassemia trait is most common in Asians (hydrops fetalis may result if heterozygotes mate and their offspring lack any alpha genes).
  - α-/α- thalassemia trait is most common in Africans.
- Ineffective production of α globin chains causes overproduction of β chains that results in unstable soluble tetramers, which can precipitate within the cell. Because of this instability, α-thalassemia can cause chronic hemolysis. Severity depends on how many of the 4 foci get deleted or mutated.

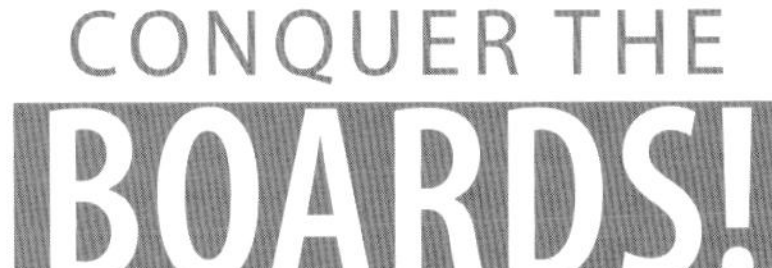

Yersinia enterocolitica is a significant cause of morbidity in patients with thalassemia and other iron overload syndromes (cirrhosis and hereditary hemochromatosis).

Clinical Features

- 1/4 foci involved = silent thalassemia: Asymptomatic.
- 2/4 foci involved = thalassemia trait: Mild anemia (very low MCV).
- 3/4 foci involved = hemoglobin H (HbH) disease: A significant amount of HbH, consisting of β_4 tetramers in circulation, resulting in moderate to severe microcytic, hypochromic, or hemolytic anemia with marked splenomegaly.
- 4/4 foci involved = hemoglobin Bart syndrome, hydrops fetalis (**Bart drops a (α) fetus**): Incompatible with life. Fetal death.

- HbH has an extremely high oxygen affinity, and failure to release oxygen in peripheral tissues results in severe congestive heart failure (CHF) and anasarca, termed *hydrops fetalis*.

Diagnostic Workup

- Blood smear: Microcytic anemia, hypochromia, target cells, Heinz bodies.
- HbH precipitates on staining with brilliant **cresyl blue**.

BETA-THALASSEMIA

General Facts

- Genetic defects, including deletions, abnormalities of transcription and translation, and instability of messenger RNA (mRNA) in β-globin hemoglobin.
  - Ineffective production of β-globin chains causes α globin chains to accumulate in the cell.
  - The accumulation of α chains forms insoluble aggregates that damage cell membranes.
  - A partial compensatory increase of the δ and γ chains yields elevated levels of HbA_2 ($\alpha_2\ \delta_2$) or HbF ($\alpha_2\ \gamma_2$).

Clinical Features

- β-Thalassemia major (Cooley anemia): Associated with jaundice, hepatosplenomegaly, and jaundice.
- β-Thalassemia minor: Mild or no anemia.

Diagnostic Workup

- Elevated HbF and HbA_2 measurements on hemoglobin electrophoresis.

Management

- β-Thalassemia major: Aggressive transfusions, splenectomy to enhance survival of RBCs, bone marrow transplant.
- β-Thalassemia minor: No treatment indicated.

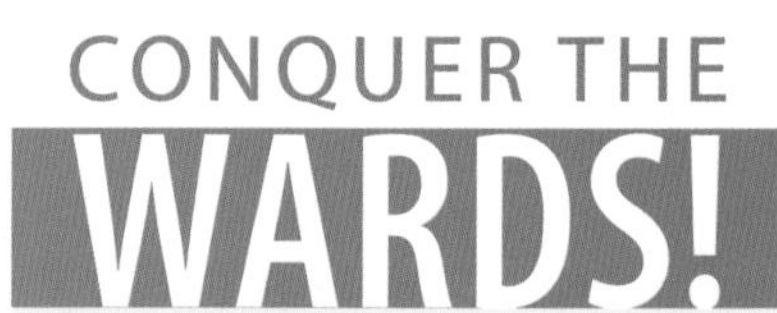

Sickle cell patients should always be on folate! Chronic hemolysis causes folate loss and deficiency, B19 infection (erythema infectiosum).

SICKLE CELL ANEMIA

General Facts

- Autosomal recessive genetic disease characterized by the presence of hemoglobin S in RBCs.
- Hemoglobin S is formed by substitution of valine for glutamic acid in the sixth position of the β-hemoglobin chain.
- This change causes Hb S to polymerize in hypoxic conditions, distorting the red cell into the classic crescent or sickle shape. The decreased deformability can cause hemolysis and vascular occlusion, causing crisis (Figure 8-2).
- Sickle cell trait: Heterozygous for sickle gene.
- Sickle cell disease: Homozygous for sickle gene.
- Populations at risk include populations from the Mediterranean, Middle East, Africa and India.

Clinical Features

- Acute vasoocclusive pain crisis (VOC) typically manifests as acute-onset generalized pain in the back, extremities, chest and abdomen, and joints.
- VOC is caused by vascular sludging and thrombosis, which can lead to organ failure secondary to infarction, dehydration, fever, and leukocytosis.
- Acute chest syndrome: Hypoxia, chest pain, shortness of breath, infiltrates caused by occlusion of pulmonary vasculature by sickled cells and/or infection. It is the most common cause of death in sickle patients and is an emergency requiring exchange transfusion with normal red cells. Treat with exchange transfusion.
- Priapism can occur acutely or chronically. This is a medical emergency, as permanent damage can occur. Genitourinary evaluation is needed.
- Chronic disease manifestations include aseptic necrosis of the femoral head, pigmented gallstones (increased bilirubin), hematuria, renal papillary necrosis, pulmonary hypertension, high-output cardiac failure, and secondary hemochromatosis.
- Increased susceptibility to infections occurs due to functional asplenism (due to repeated infarction). This carries a higher risk of sepsis with encapsulated organisms (*Streptococcus pneumoniae*, *Salmonella* osteomyelitis, and *Haemophilus influenzae*).
- Ischemic retinopathy and cerebrovascular accidents (CVAs) occur at a younger age than the general population.

Diagnostic Workup

- Hemoglobin electrophoresis will show Hb S.
- Blood smear: Howell–Jolly bodies (cytoplasmic remnants of nuclear chromatin that are normally removed by the spleen), sickled cells.
- Blood tests show anemia and evidence of hemolysis: Increased reticulocyte count, increased indirect bilirubin, and leukocytosis.

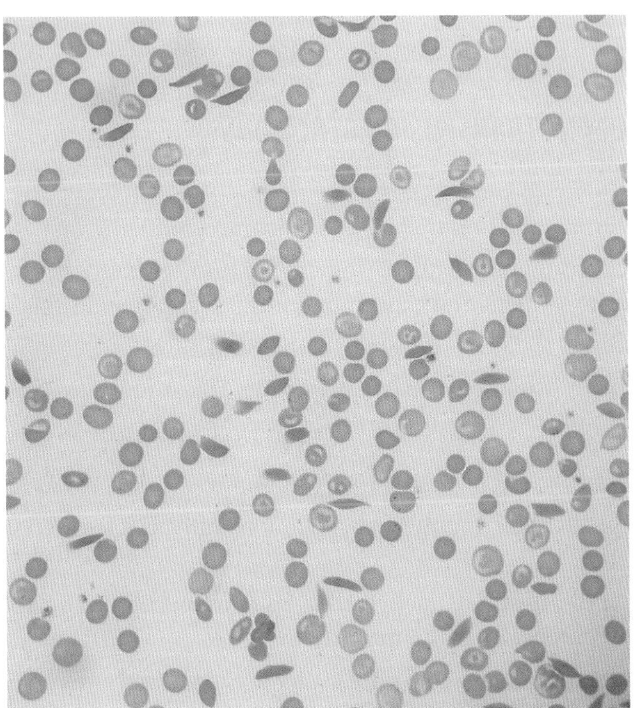

FIGURE 8-2. Sickle anemia. (Source: https://images.app.goo.gl/SYVgBueeyL9hhZ616.)

CONQUER THE **BOARDS!**

Indications for exchange transfusion in sickle cell disease:
Stroke/TIA
Acute chest syndrome
Priapism
Third-term pregnancy
Intractable vasoocclusive crisis

CONQUER THE **WARDS!**

Signs of SCA:
SICKLE
Splenomegaly/Sludging
Infection
Cholelithiasis/acute Chest syndrome
Kidney (hematuria, papillary necrosis)
Liver congestion/Leg ulcers
Eye changes

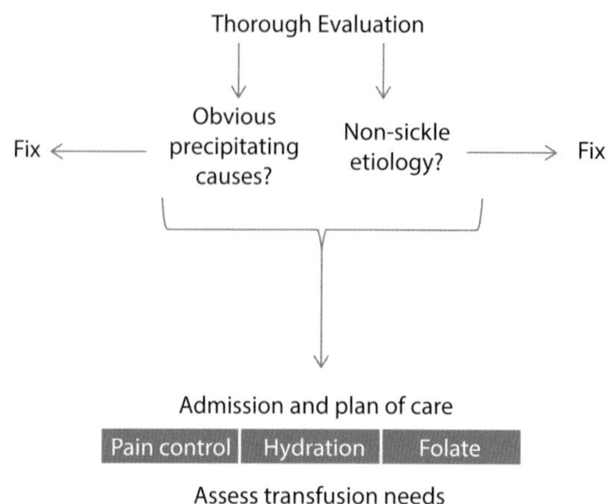

FIGURE 8-3. Approach to Sickle Cell Crisis

Management

- **Acute crisis:** Analgesia and hydration (and antibiotics if signs of infection) (Figure 8-3).
- **Acute chest syndrome:** Respiratory support, exchange transfusion, and empiric antibiotics for pneumonia.
- **Long-term treatment:**
  - **Hydroxyurea** acts by increasing the amount of fetal hemoglobin; may increase frequency of crisis.
  - *H. influenzae* and pneumococcal **vaccines** for prophylaxis.
  - Frequent follow-up.

HEMOLYTIC ANEMIAS

Hemolysis can be caused by multiple different conditions. The clinical features can help you identify them (Table 8-1).

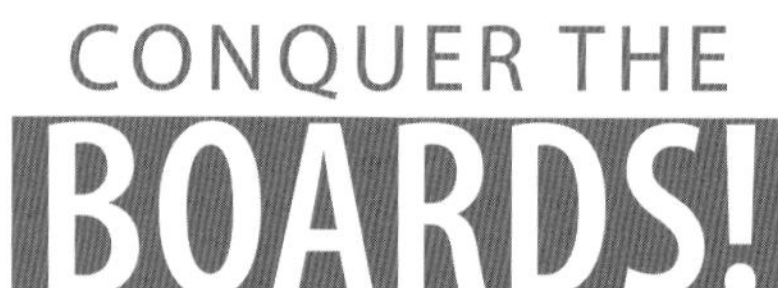

General anesthesia is a frequent setting for blood transfusion. In this setting, immediate hemolytic transfusion reaction should be suspected with:

- Severe hypotension
- Coagulopathic oozing
- Hemoglobinuria/pink urine
- Fevers

TRANSFUSION REACTIONS

ACUTE HEMOLYTIC TRANSFUSION REACTIONS

General facts

- Life-threatening reaction due to ABO incompatibility.
- These reactions involve naturally occurring host IgM anti-A, and anti-B, which fix complement and cause rapid intravascular hemolysis.
- Direct Coombs test is positive (antibodies on RBCs).
- **Usually due to human error** (improper identification or mislabeling of blood).

Clinical Features

- Begins soon after starting the transfusion, **usually as a sudden clinical deterioration**.
- Fever +/– chills, **dyspnea**, tachycardia, **back pain**, chest pain, abdominal pain, and hypotension are common symptoms.
- Sequelae includes acute renal failure (acute tubular necrosis [ATN]), shock, disseminated intravascular coagulation (DIC), and death (40%).

TABLE 8-1. Clinical Features of Hemolytic Anemias

Hemolytic Anemia	Feature
Immune-mediated hemolytic anemia	■ Presence of autoantibodies to one's RBCs, resulting in hemolysis. ■ Reticulocytosis (bone marrow pushes out immature RBCs). ■ Increased indirect bilirubin (by-product of lysed cells [globin]). ■ Increased lactic dehydrogenase (LDH; by-product of lysed cells) and haptoglobin (binds free hemoglobin released from lysed cells). ■ Direct Coombs test (presence of antibody on RBC surface). ■ Splenomegaly (site of clearance).
Warm hemolytic anemia	■ Most common form of immune-mediated hemolytic anemia. ■ **IgG** antibodies to different RBC antigens (e.g., Rh). ■ Do not usually fix complement (IgG). ■ Active at body temperature. ■ **Treat with steroids.** Transfuse if severe anemia. Splenectomy for steroid resistant. ■ Seen with chronic lymphocytic leukemia (CLL), leukemias, SLE, and other autoimmune diseases, and drugs (penicillin, sulfas, and antimalarials). ■ Sixty percent of cases are idiopathic.
Cold hemolytic anemia	■ **Immunoglobulin M (IgM)** antibodies. ■ Active at cool temperatures (dissociate at 30°C) such as in distal body parts (blue fingers and toes). ■ **Fixes complement** (IgM). ■ Presence of a high titer of cold agglutinins. ■ Seen acutely with ***Mycoplasma*** and **infectious mononucleosis** (resolve spontaneously) and chronically with **lymphomas** and **Waldenström macroglobulinemia**. ■ Degree of hemolysis is variable. ■ **Treatment includes keeping warm**; corticosteroids don't work well.
Paroxysmal cold hemoglobinuria	■ Also called cold hemolysis (hemoglobinuria after exposure to cold). ■ **IgG** antibodies against P group antigen (Donath–Landsteiner antibodies). ■ Active at cool temperatures, dissociate at 30°C to cause hemolysis. ■ **Fix complement**. ■ Clinically characterized by **acute intermittent massive hemolysis** and hemoglobinuria following exposure to cold.

IgG, immunoglobulin G; *LDH*, lactate dehydrogenase; *RBC*, red blood cell; *SLE*, systemic lupus erythematosus.

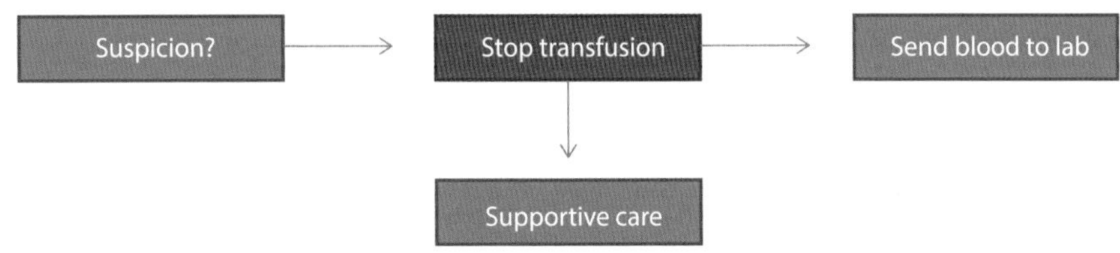

FIGURE 8-4. Immediate management of transfusion reactions.

Management

- Discontinue transfusion immediately (Figure 8-4)!
- Hemodynamic support, supportive care, and IV fluids.
- Recheck compatibility of blood with blood bank by sending blood back to lab.

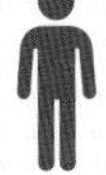

A young woman in the hospital was transfused 2 units of red cells after severe bleeding in childbirth. Several hours later, she developed acute shortness of breath, fever, and hypoxia. **Next step:** Chest x-ray. X-ray findings demonstrate diffuse bilateral infiltrates. What is the likely diagnosis? Transfusion-related acute lung injury (TRALI).

CONQUER THE **WARDS!**

Bystander hemolysis happens due to hemolysis of antigen-negative RBCs being destroyed by delayed hemolytic transfusion reactions.

DELAYED HEMOLYTIC TRANSFUSION REACTIONS

General Facts

- **Mild** and occurs days to weeks after transfusion.
- Patient received a transfusion in the past and is now having immune response after being re-exposed to the antigen. Due to **anamnestic antibody response to a minor antigen** (Rh or Kidd, **not ABO**).
- Pretransfusion antibody level low; screening and crossmatch tests usually negative.
- Signs of mild hemolysis: Has high lactate dehydrogenase (LDH), high total bilirubin, low haptoglobin.

Clinical Features

- **Common symptoms include fever, anemia, or asymptomatic**. Rarely, there are serious manifestations that look more like acute transfusion reactions.

Management

- Milder than acute reactions, and usually no treatment or just supportive care is required.

FEBRILE NONHEMOLYTIC TRANSFUSION REACTIONS

General Facts

- These are common reactions that last only a few hours.
- Due to host immune response against transfused leukocytes/platelets or cytokines from donor leukocytes.

Clinical Features

- Chills followed by fever within a few hours of transfusion; typically mild.

Management

- Discontinue transfusion (can occur after) to rule out acute hemolysis (see Acute Hemolytic Transfusion Reactions section).
- Can give Tylenol and Benadryl as prophylaxis, although studies have shown no benefit.
- Not routinely recommended; however, the use of leukocyte-reduced blood products may reduce the incidence of febrile nonhemolytic transfusion reactions.

Allergic Reactions to Plasma

- Rare. Usually occurs in patients with congenital IgA deficiency; have anaphylactic reactions to the IgA in donor blood. Anti-IgA antibodies present.
- Can get hives, bronchospasm, anaphylaxis.
- Treatment: Maintain airway and give epinephrine.

Transfusion-Related Acute Lung Injury

- Sudden severe respiratory distress similar to adult respiratory distress syndrome (ARDS).
- Occurs within 6 hours of transfusion.

CONQUER THE **BOARDS!**

Learn how to differentiate between ITP, aplastic anemia, and MDS:

- ITP has normal RBCs, normal WBCs, only low platelets with giant (young) platelets on the peripheral smear. Usually don't give platelets – treat with steroids or IVIG.
- Aplastic anemia has low RBCs, low WBCs, and low platelets (all cell lines low). No dysmorphic cells on smear.
- Myelodysplastic syndrome (MDS) can have any one or all lineages low. The smear can show dysplastic neutrophils (hypolobulated), and RBCs with ringed sideroblasts.

- Incidence ~1 in 5000 transfusions (all types of blood products).
- Caused by donor Ab against recipient granulocytes, agglutination of granulocytes and complement activation in the pulmonary vascular bed, capillary endothelial damage, and eventual fluid leak into the alveoli.
- Symptoms include chills/fever, chest pain, hypotension, cyanosis, dyspnea, and crackles/rales.
- **Chest x-ray (CXR)** shows diffuse pulmonary edema (diffuse congestion).
- Resolves within 48 to 96 hours without residual effects (interim ventilatory support often required).
- Treatment is supportive.

COAGULATION

IDIOPATHIC THROMBOCYTOPENIA PURPURA

General Facts

- Immune-mediated thrombocytopenia of unknown etiology.
- Antibodies against a platelet surface antigen are developed, and the antibody–antigen complexes effectively decrease platelet count by being removed from circulation.

Clinical Features

- Petechiae and purpura over the trunk and limbs can occur spontaneously and with minimal trauma.
- Mucosal bleeding can occur as well.

Diagnostic Workup

- CBC will show low platelet counts.
- It is a diagnosis of exclusion; thus, absence of other factors to explain thrombocytopenia is also key.
- Antiplatelet antibodies are **not useful** for the diagnosis of idiopathic thrombocytopenic purpura (ITP).

Management

- Corticosteroids acutely to improve platelet count.
- Intravenous immunoglobulin (IVIG) for severe cases.
- **Platelet transfusion** if significant bleeding present.
- A splenectomy can be performed electively to reduce recurrence.

THROMBOTIC THROMBOCYTOPENIA PURPURA

- **ADAMTS13** is the protease that normally cleaves these multimers, but is deficient in this condition.
- **This is a medical emergency with mortality approaching 90% if untreated.**

CONQUER THE BOARDS!

Causes of thrombocytopenia, think **PLATELETS:**
Platelet disorders: TTP, ITP, DIC
Leukemia
Anemia
Trauma
Enlarged spleen
Liver disease
EtOH (alcohol)
Toxins (benzene, heparins, aspirin, chemotherapy agents, etc.)
Sepsis
And RBCs with ringed

CONQUER THE BOARDS!

Classic pentad for TTP—
RAT FaN
Renal dysfunction
Anemia (hemolytic)
Thrombocytopenia
Fever
Neurologic dysfunction

- Usually caused by an immune process that clears ADAMTS13 after an infection, but some cases are genetic.
- Infection (especially HIV and *Escherichia coli* O157:H7), malignancy, drugs (antiplatelet agents, chemotherapy agents, contraceptives), autoimmune disorders, and pregnancy can cause thrombotic thrombocytopenia purpura (TTP).

CONQUER THE **WARDS!**

Thrombocytopenia presents as oozing from mucosal sites (gums) and petechiae. Petechiae = Platelet Problem. Factor deficiencies (e.g., hemophilia) present with large bleeds (typically hemarthrosis).

Clinical Features

- **Classic pentad** – not all have to be present: Fever, altered mental status (waxing and waning), renal dysfunction (hematuria, oliguria), thrombocytopenia (mild to severe), and microangiopathic hemolytic anemia.

Diagnostic Workup

- A CBC will reveal thrombocytopenia and microangiopathic hemolytic anemia.
- **Schistocytes on peripheral smear**, decreased haptoglobin, elevated LDH, and elevated total bilirubin (see Figure 8-5).
- Renal failure can occur due to microangiopathy.
- Fever and altered mental status can also occur.

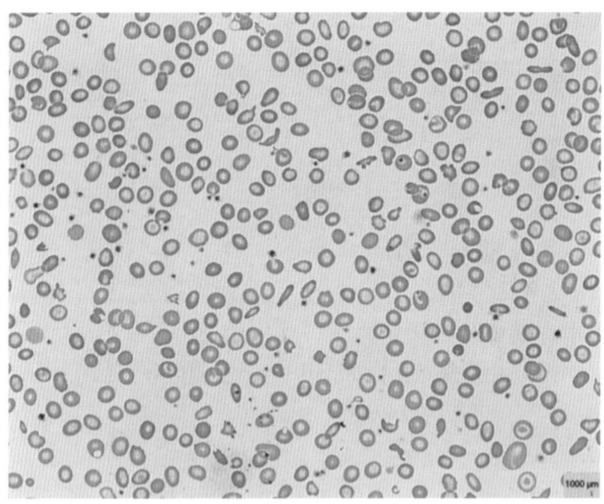

FIGURE 8-5. Schistocytes on peripheral smear. (Source: https://images.app.goo.gl/CKUSJJjJ-1EDMZbrJ9.)

CONQUER THE **BOARDS!**

E. coli O157:H7 is the causative organism in a bloody diarrhea syndrome that has been associated with the subsequent development of HUS. HUS differs from TTP in severity and lack of neurologic symptoms.

Management

- **Plasma exchange** (plasmapheresis) is the **mainstay** of treatment.
- **Do not transfuse platelets! It will continue to feed the TTP and will not halt the end-organ damage.**
- Fresh frozen plasma may help (contains missing ADAMTS13).

DISSEMINATED INTRAVASCULAR COAGULATION

General Facts

- Acquired coagulation defect that results in consumption of coagulation factors, including **fibrinogen**, causing bleeding and thrombosis.
- Usually secondary to exposure of blood to procoagulants such as tissue factor (fetus, bacteria) and cancer procoagulant, resulting in depletion of clotting factors and microangiopathic hemolytic anemia.
- Can be acute and life threatening or can be chronic, as seen with malignancies.
- Can be caused by a variety of inciting events, including obstetric problems (retained dead fetus, abruptio placentae, second-trimester abortion, amniotic fluid embolism, preeclampsia), sepsis (particularly with gram-negatives, *Rickettsia*, hemolytic uremic syndrome [HUS], malaria), local tissue damage (snake bites, burns, frostbite), extensive trauma, and chronic illness such as malignancy or liver disease.

Clinical Features

- Diffuse, systemic bleeding (not from a single site).
- Usually have some other severe underlying condition also (e.g., sepsis).

Diagnostic Workup

- Decreased fibrinogen, thrombocytopenia along with elevated prothrombin time (PT), activate partial thromboplastin time (aPTT), and thrombin time (TT).
- Presence of fibrin split products (elevated D-dimers) and evidence of microangiopathic hemolysis (schistocytes) on peripheral smear.

Management

- Treat underlying cause.
- Platelets, fresh frozen plasma (FFP), and cryoprecipitate to control bleeding can support until underlying cause is under control.

CONQUER THE BOARDS!

SPELL Etiology of DIC—
How do you "SPELL" DIC?
Sepsis/Surgery/Snake bite
Pregnancy
Extensive trauma
Liver disease/Leukemia
Local tissue damage

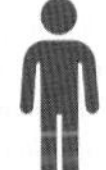

A 50-year-old woman who is in the intensive care unit (ICU) for sepsis has purpura and gingival bleeding on day 2 of her hospital stay and blood coming from her urinary catheter. PT and PTT are increased and fibrinogen is decreased. *Think: DIC.* **Next step:** Transfuse FFP and cryoprecipitate.

VON WILLEBRAND DISEASE

General Facts

- Genetic disease, most commonly autosomal dominant, characterized by **lack or functional defect** of von Willebrand factor (vWF).
  - Three types of disease:
    a. **Type 1** (by far the most common, and will likely be the one on the exam): Decrease in amount (quantitative defect), autosomal dominant inheritance.
    b. **Type 2: Qualitative defect** of vWF (several subtypes but all with functional defect).
    c. **Type 3:** Severe decrease (**essentially absent**) in vWF.

CONQUER THE **WARDS!**

Unlike in vWD, bleeding time in hemophilia A is unaffected because no abnormality with platelets is present. More importantly, hemophilia typically has bleeding into a joint (hemarthrosis), and vWF is usually mucosal bleeding or post–surgical procedure bleeding.

Clinical Features

- Mostly asymptomatic.
- Often have history of very heavy menstruation or bleeding with dental procedures and then might have an episode of severe bleeding during a major surgery.

Diagnostic Workup

- Test 3 parameters: the amount of vWF (vWF antigen); the function of vWF (ristocetin aggregation test, also called ristocetin cofactor assay); and size (multimers). **PTT can also be elevated because vWF carries factor 8**.
- **Type 1:** vWF antigen decreases; ristocetin aggregation test shows a decrease in proportion to the decrease in antigen. Multimers normal in size.
- **Type 2:** vWF antigen normal or decreased; ristocetin test is low – out of proportion to any decrease in the vWF antigen; multimers usually small (these are abnormal proteins).
- **Type 3:** Both vWF antigen and ristocetin test **very low**.

Management

- Mild bleeding or minor surgery: DDAVP (desmopressin) increases vWF levels by releasing it from endothelium.
- Serious bleeding or major surgery: vWF and factor 8 concentrates.

A young man presents with bleeding profusely after having his tooth pulled. Labs demonstrate normal platelets and normal PT but a prolonged aPTT. What is the likely diagnosis? *von Willebrand disease.* First-line treatment? *Desmopressin.*

CONQUER THE **BOARDS!**

von Willebrand disease is the most common bleeding disorder.

HEMOPHILIA

General Facts

Sex-linked recessive disease (only males are affected) causing a deficiency of factor VIII or IX. Hemophilia A is factor VIII deficiency, and hemophilia B is factor IX deficiency (Christmas disease). They are both X-linked recessive.

Clinical Features

- Dependent on amount of active factor (usually measured as a percentage of normal):
  - **5% to 25% factor VIII or IX activity (mild):** Abnormal bleeding when subjected to surgery or dental procedures; excessive bleeding following **circumcision** of newborns is a clue.
  - **1% to 5%** (moderate) **and** <1% (severe) factor VIII or IX activity: Deep tissue bleeding (muscles), **typically** intraarticular hemorrhages **or** hemarthrosis (**usually knees**).

Diagnostic Workup

- Prolonged aPTT, normal bleeding time.
- Clinical picture, family history, and the factor VIII and IX coagulant activity level.

Management

- Recombinant factor VIII or IX.
- DDAVP (desmopressin) for patients with mild hemophilia A but not hemophilia B.

HEMATOLOGIC MALIGNANCIES

Hematologic malignancies include any cancer of blood cells. In the context of malignancies, the term clone or clonal refers to a process in which the abnormal cells or process has **arisen from a single precursor**. This is the basic concept of cancer. When there is an abnormal growth of a specific cell, it is important to determine if they are clonal (cancer or precancer) or **polyclonal** (from multiple parent cells and usually a **reaction** to another process). For example, if the lymphocytes in a patient with a lymphocytosis are clonal, then the patient has leukemia; if they are polyclonal, these cells are likely reacting to an infection.

> CONQUER THE BOARDS!
>
> Most common leukemia in adults = AML
> Most common leukemia in children = ALL

ACUTE LEUKEMIAS

- Acute leukemia is a disease in which patients present with a relatively sudden acute illness, which can be manifested by bleeding or extreme weakness or infection. This is in contrast to chronic leukemias, in which the patients can be asymptomatic for months or years and are often picked up on routine blood tests. Any leukemia is a cancer of the blood.
- **Two basic types: lymphocytic and myeloid.** Each has subsets within: acute lymphocytic leukemia (ALL) and acute myelocytic leukemia (AML), discussed in detail later.

Pathophysiology

- The clonal progenitor cells (*lympho**blast*** or *myelo**blast***) proliferate, eventually taking over the bone marrow and inhibiting the growth of normal cells.
- Clinical manifestations occur because of the loss of normal bone marrow elements and by infiltration of the body's tissues by malignant cells.

> A 22-year-old woman recently received her first dose of chemotherapy for acute lymphocytic leukemia (or could be lymphoma). She has extreme fatigue and a fever. Labs reveal a high LDH with low calcium and high phosphate. What is the likely diagnosis? Tumor lysis syndrome. **Next step:** Aggressive hydration and then allopurinol. What are you worried about? Renal failure. Also arrhythmias from low calcium and high potassium.

Clinical Features

- **Acutely ill!**
- Anemia: Weakness, fatigue, pallor, cardiopulmonary compromise.
- Neutropenia: Infections, fever.
- Thrombocytopenia: Petechiae, purpura, hemorrhages.
- Marrow infiltration: Bone pain.

Diagnostic Workup

- **Initial finding:** Numerous **blasts** found on the peripheral smear (large, immature cells with large nuclei, unclumped chromatin).
- **Bone marrow biopsy** showing >20% infiltration with blasts (usually almost entirely made of blasts).

> CONQUER THE BOARDS!
>
> In a patient with APL, it is prudent to start ATRA as soon as the diagnosis is suspect.
>
> A white count more than 10 indicates high-risk APL.
>
> APL has high risk of DIC, so close monitoring of coagulation profile, including fibrinogen, and replacement with factors or cryoprecipitate is very important.

A patient presents to the emergency room (ER) feeling extremely weak. CBC shows Hgb 7.2 g, platelets of 9, and white blood cells (WBCs) of 49,000. **Next step:** Check coagulation factors, correct coagulopathy emergently (platelets and blood products), then perform bone marrow biopsy.

- **Other tests** (used for leukemias and lymphomas):
  - **Flow cytometry:** Evaluates which proteins are expressed on the cell surface; expression of different proteins is associated with different stages of development (i.e., blasts), and specific constellations of proteins are associated with different lymphomas.
  - **Fluorescent in situ hybridization (FISH):** A sensitive method to look for specific cytogenetic lesions associated with different leukemias and lymphomas.

Management

Please see Table 8-4 for a complete list of the various chemotherapies available for selected malignancies.

- Three steps of chemotherapy:
  - *Induction:* High doses of chemotherapy are used to induce remission.
  - *Consolidation:* Chemotherapy is then administered to eradicate residual, undetectable malignant cells.
  - *Maintenance:* Ongoing chemotherapy to keep the number of malignant cells low.
- Complete remission is the goal in cancer patients. This is achieved if normal marrow elements are being produced and less than 5% residual blasts are present in the bone marrow.

CONQUER THE BOARDS!

At presentation of acute leukemias the following need to be closely monitored:

- Risk of neutropenic fevers
- Tumor lysis syndrome
- Coagulopathy
- Hyperleukocytosis

ACUTE MYELOCYTIC LEUKEMIA

General Facts

- More common in **adults**.
- Association with history of benzene exposure.
- Eight subtypes: M0 to M7:
  - M0 to M3 have granulocytic differentiation.
  - M4 and M5 are monocytic precursors.
  - M6 has predominance of erythroblasts.
  - M7 is mainly megakaryocytic.

Clinical Features

- Fatigue, hemorrhage, or bruising (30%).
- Infection of lung, skin (25%).
- Splenomegaly is rare (25%) compared to other types of leukemia.

CONQUER THE BOARDS!

Tumor lysis syndrome is seen in leukemias (especially after initiation of chemotherapy) and other aggressive hematologic malignancies. Rapid cell breakdown, high uric acid, hyperkalemia, hyperphosphatemia, hypocalcemia, acute renal failure, and high LDH. Treated with fluids, correcting electrolyte imbalance, and allopurinol.

Diagnostic Workup

Specific characteristics:

- M3—Acute promyelocytic leukemia: Associated with DIC, Auer rods, t(15;17); in which there is a defect in the vitamin A receptor, treatment is different than others: all-trans retinoic acid (ATRA – vitamin A) + chemotherapy. Prognosis is better than other AMLs (90% response rate). There is an increased risk of differentiation syndrome in patients with M3 acute leukemia.
- **AML** related to **prior exposure to chemotherapy or radiation therapy** (for a previous cancer) has a poor prognosis. Likewise, AML that evolves from **underlying myelodysplasia (myelodysplastic syndrome [MDS])** (often seen in elderly) has a **poor prognosis.**
- M5: Associated with gingival hyperplasia due to deposition of the malignant cells.

- M4, M5: Central nervous system (CNS) and skin manifestations.
- t(8;21) seen in M2 and t(15;17) seen in M3 have better prognosis.

Management

- **Induction:** Cytarabine + an anthracycline (daunorubicin)—50% to 80% receive remission.
- **Consolidation:** Same chemotherapy as induction.
- **Maintenance:** Clinical trials determining best drugs.
- Stem cell transplantation is also potentially curative, usually for relapsing or high-risk patients.
- M3 treated with ATRA in addition to chemotherapy.

CONQUER THE BOARDS!

Signs of LEUKEMIA
Light skin (pallor)
Energy (low)
Underweight
Kidney failure
Excess heat (fever)
Mottled skin (hemorrhages)
Infections
Anemia

ACUTE LYMPHOCYTIC LEUKEMIA

General Facts

- Primarily a disease of children, but accounts for 20% of adult leukemias.
- Generally, prognosis is inversely related to age. Younger patients (kids to young adults) have good prognosis, but older patients have a poor prognosis.
- Three subtypes:
  - **L1** occurs in 80% of ALL cases in **children**.
  - **L2** occurs in most **adult cases**.
  - **L3** cell is leukemic manifestation of Burkitt lymphoma t(8;14) involving *c-myk* gene.

CONQUER THE BOARDS!

M3 = Acute promyelocytic anemia or APL: DIC (main cause of death), t(15;17) treated with ATRA, better prognosis.
M5 = gingival hyperplasia.

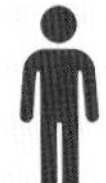

A 27-year-old woman presents to your office with night sweats, weakness, and weight loss. Laboratory work reveals anemia, thrombocytopenia, and a WBC of 47,000. Peripheral smear demonstrates blasts with intracytoplasmic rods. How do you confirm the diagnosis? *Bone marrow aspiration and biopsy*. What is the likely diagnosis? *Acute promyelocytic leukemia (M3)*. What translocation would you find on cytogenetic studies? *t(15;17)*.

Clinical Features

- Acute onset, with malaise, fever, lethargy, weight loss, bone pain, infection, and hemorrhage.
- **Lymphadenopathy**, can have mediastinal mass as well as CNS and testicular involvement.
- Splenomegaly and hepatomegaly can be seen as well.

CONQUER THE BOARDS!

ATRA affects the maturation of immature cells in M3 and reduces the life-threatening DIC that can worsen with chemotherapy.

Diagnostic Workup

- Blasts in peripheral blood is a hallmark of the disease.
- Blasts taking over bone marrow can be seen on bone marrow biopsy; other cells decrease.
- 25% to 30%: Philadelphia chromosome (chromosome 22) arising from t(9;22) – poorer prognosis.

Management

- **Various regimens – you don't have to know details of chemotherapy types.**

- General concept is that there is an induction, consolidation, and maintenance, as with AML (AML maintenance is only in specific patients).
- ALL treatment goes on for about 2 years, as opposed to AML treatment, which is shorter.
- The other difference is that ALL patients typically require CNS prophylaxis/treatment (intrathecal chemotherapy, usually given through lumbar puncture).
- **Induction:** Four or five drugs such as vincristine, prednisone, daunorubicin, L-asparaginase, and cyclophosphamide are used.
- **Consolidation:** Cell-cycle, phase-specific antimetabolites.
- **Maintenance:** Low-dose chemotherapy is standard.
- Specific case: Patients with Philadelphia chromosome often need to go straight to bone marrow transplantation because their prognosis is so poor.

CONQUER THE **BOARDS!**

CML is a Philadelphia chromosome–positive myeloproliferative neoplasm that often presents with high myeloid counts, especially high basophil count. Enlarged spleen is another characteristic unique to CML.

Philadelphia chromosome t(9;22) represents a poor prognosis in ALL. In the setting of a myeloid disorder, it is diagnostic for CML, which has a good prognosis.

CHRONIC LEUKEMIAS

Chronic leukemias—chronic myelogenous (or myelocytic leukemia and chronic lymphocytic leukemia)—differ from acute leukemias in that these patients are often **asymptomatic for years** before having clinical problems. Though ultimately life threatening, they are rarely an emergency on presentation. **Patients generally look clinically well—not acutely ill.**

CHRONIC MYELOCYTIC LEUKEMIA

- A clonal proliferation (cancer) of cells in the myeloid lineage.
- One of several myeloproliferative disorders (others are polycythemia vera, essential thrombocythemia, and general myeloproliferative disease).
- It has 25% risk per year of transforming to acute leukemia (blastic transformation).

Pathophysiology

- Philadelphia chromosome t(9;22) causes fusion of Bcr and Abl, forming a protein (a tyrosine kinase) that constantly sends cell proliferation signals.
- Phases:
  - **Chronic phase** (most common presentation): High peripheral white counts (can be several hundred thousand **myeloid cells of varying stages of maturation—most not blasts**), large spleen (can cause early satiety and abdominal fullness). **These patients are often asymptomatic!** (You will likely be tested on the chronic phase, so focus on this!)
  - **Accelerated phase:** More than 15% blasts in peripheral blood. RBCs and platelets begin to decrease. Symptoms of bone pain and weakness start.
  - **Blastic phase:** Looks like an **acute leukemia** with many blasts (>20% in the peripheral blood and marrow). Sick patient—severe **fatigue and weakness!**

A 60-year-old male presenting with fever, **petechiae, bleeding gums,** and fatigue for 2 weeks is found to have a hemoglobin of 6, platelets of 30,000, and WBC of 80,000 composed of 80% blasts with Auer rods. *Think: APL.* **Next step:** Stabilize patient, treat infection, and give blood products as needed, then bone marrow biopsy (check cytogenetics for targeting therapy because t(15;17) will benefit from ATRA).

Diagnostic Workup

- Examining the peripheral blood smear shows leukocytosis with **immature myeloid cells of varying stages of maturation** (some totally mature neutrophils too). This is in contrast with any acute leukemia in which there are monotonous immature cells (blasts).
- Bone marrow biopsy and cytogenetics showing Philadelphia chromosome t(9;22) are diagnostic.
- Leukocyte alkaline phosphatase is *low* in CML cells (*high* in infectious causes of leukocytosis).

Management

- **Imatinib** (Gleevec) and other next-generation tyrosine kinase inhibitors inhibit Philadelphia chromosome and induce indefinite remission (a revolutionary breakthrough!). It is the treatment of choice. Side effects include bone marrow suppression and cardiac toxicity.
- **Allogenic bone marrow transplant** may still have a role for younger or refractory patients.

CONQUER THE **BOARDS!**

Ninety percent of patients with CML have the Philadelphia chromosome t(9;22).

CHRONIC LYMPHOCYTIC LEUKEMIA

General Facts

- Most common type of leukemia in the Western world and is **often asymptomatic**.
- Malignant clonal disorder of **mature B lymphocytes** (rarely T cells) that **can but does not always** progress to cause lymphadenopathy, splenomegaly, and bone marrow failure.
- Generally a chronic disorder that can last for years.
- Identical to small lymphocytic lymphoma (SLL)—which is the term when the disease is confined only to lymph nodes.
- Some patients have immune dysfunction that leads to infection or autoimmune processes.
- **Richter transformation** is typically highly refractory to treatment.

Clinical Features

- Many are asymptomatic, and a routine CBC shows a lymphocytosis (see Table 8-2).
- Lymphadenopathy, splenomegaly, and cytopenias in later stages.
- At later stages of disease, patient may have classic "B" symptoms of fever, night sweats, and weight loss.
- Can have infections, **hemolytic anemia (classic complication)**, or ITP from a dysfunctional immune system.

CONQUER THE **BOARDS!**

Richter transformation is a rare transformation to an aggressive large cell lymphoma.
Patients with CLL can have autoimmune hemolytic anemia, ITP, and a high risk of infections due to cytopenias.

A 32-year-old male presents to his doctor with fullness after only eating a small portion of food. Otherwise, he feels fine. His CBC is normal except for a WBC count of 120,000. Peripheral smear shows myeloid cells in varying stages of maturation. Likely diagnosis? *CML*. What would you likely find? *t(9;22) on cytogenetics*. What would you treat with? *Imatinib*.

Diagnostic Workup

- Often suspected or found incidentally on routine CBC (increased lymphocytes, >5000 needed to make diagnosis but often >100,000). Diagnosis is made with flow cytometry of peripheral blood demonstrating CLL clone.
- Peripheral smear will reveal **numerous mature-appearing lymphocytes** (small cells with dense nuclei and scant cytoplasm).
- Lymph node biopsy can also be used for diagnosis.

Stage/Survival

TABLE 8-2. Survival by RAI Stage

RAI Stage	Survival
0 Lymphocytosis only	>10 yr
I Adenopathy	6–7 yr
II Splenomegaly	6–7 yr
III Hb <10	2–3 yr
IV Thrombocytopenia	2–3 yr

Management

- **Observation only for early asymptomatic patients in early stages.**
- There is no cure, but many therapies and combinations are effective, including fludarabine (purine analog), rituximab (antibody to CD20), and chlorambucil (alkylating agent).
- Autoimmune hemolytic anemia can be treated with steroids.
- Frequent infections with hypogammaglobulinemia can be treated with IVIG.

A 72-year-old man presents for a normal checkup. He feels great, and the exam is entirely normal except for some palpable small axillary lymph nodes. Laboratory revealed a normal CBC except a WBC of 80,000 made up of primarily lymphocytes. What is your most likely recommendation? *Observation.*

A 75-year-old man has had chronic lymphocytic leukemia (CLL) for 8 years and has never required treatment. Over the past 2 weeks he has had dramatic weakness, night sweats, and rapidly enlarging nodes, and he has lost 10 pounds. What do you suspect? *Richter transformation.*

Why is a lymphocyte count of 200,000 an emergency in a patient with acute leukemia but not so in a patient with CLL? CLL cells are small and nonsticky mature cells that have little risk of hyperviscosity. Acute leukemic cells are large, sticky blasts that can cause sludging in the CNS or pulmonary vasculature.

MYELOPROLIFERATIVE DISORDERS

General Facts

- Myeloproliferative diseases are a group of disorders originating from clones of different granulocyte cell lines: neutrophils (CML), RBC (polycythemia vera), or platelets (essential thrombocytosis).

- General myeloproliferative disease (neutrophils, RBCs, and platelets all elevated) and primary myelofibrosis are other types of myeloproliferative diseases.
- In any of these disorders, there may be a mixed picture, with more than just the primary cells being elevated (e.g., patients with polycythemia vera may have elevated neutrophils as well as RBCs).
- Patients with any of these disorders are at risk for progression to AML or myelofibrosis (ultimately resulting from the cytokine secretion of myeloid cells). CML is discussed in the Chronic Leukemias section.

CLL patients can commonly have either de novo hemolytic anemia or treatment-associated hemolytic anemia after receiving a purine analog (fludarabine).

POLYCYTHEMIA VERA

A myeloproliferative disease that results in increased RBCs.

Etiology

- **Primary polycythemia vera (PV):** A primary bone marrow cause (low erythropoietin). This is a clonal process.
- **Secondary PV** (other causes that result in increased erythropoietin); nonclonal.
- Hypoxia (high altitudes, lung disease).
- Smoking (due to carboxyhemoglobin).
- Paraneoplastic (usually renal cell carcinoma and hepatoma aberrantly producing erythropoietin).

Epidemiology

- Males are more commonly affected.
- More common in people >60.

Clinical Features

- Ruddy complexion, along with pruritus after shower.
- Abdominal fullness (from splenomegaly).
- Can lead to thrombosis (deep venous thrombosis [DVT], stroke, myocardial infarction [MI]), bleeding and transformation to AML or to myelofibrosis.

Diagnostic Workup

- Hemoglobin usually >16.5 g/dL (females) and >18.5 g/dL (males) and low erythropoietin in primary causes (must rule out secondary causes).
- Ninety percent of patients with PV have a JAK2 mutation.

Management

- Serial phlebotomy to keep hematocrit (Hct) down and aspirin.
- Add hydroxyurea in elderly or history of thrombosis.

CONQUER THE **BOARDS!**

Secondary causes of erythrocytosis include obstructive sleep apnea and chronic obstructive pulmonary disease (COPD).

JAK2 (V617F) mutation is a driver mutation in about 90% PV and about 40% to 50% ET.

CONQUER THE **BOARDS!**

Patients with ET and platelet count more than 100,000 are at high risk for acquired von Willebrand disease.

CONQUER THE **BOARDS!**

Ruxolitinib, a JAK2 inhibitor, is used for symptoms of splenomegaly and itching.

ESSENTIAL THROMBOCYTOSIS

- Elevation of platelets—the most benign of the myeloproliferative diseases.
- Often, patients are **asymptomatic**. They are at **risk for thrombosis or bleeding.**
- One must rule out secondary causes of thrombocytosis to make the diagnosis. Examples of secondary causes: iron deficiency (classically

associated with high platelets) and reactive (platelets can go up in response to any inflammatory process).

- **Treat with aspirin + either hydroxyurea or anagrelide** (used to suppress platelet production).

PRIMARY MYELOFIBROSIS

- Also called agnogenic myeloid metaplasia.
- Can occur either de novo or as a progressive manifestation of other myeloproliferative diseases.
- Other causes of bone marrow fibrosis are M7 AML and hairy cell leukemia, among other conditions.
- Often presents with weakness from severe anemia and symptoms from splenomegaly or hepatomegaly (both caused by extramedullary hematopoiesis).
- Peripheral smear shows teardrop cells and immature cells (cells forced out of the marrow).
- Treatment is steroids or thalidomide—and neither work well.

MYELODYSPLASTIC SYNDROME

- A clonal myeloid disorder (not usually classified as a myeloproliferative disorder) in which abnormal myeloid precursors give rise to dysplastic and ineffective myeloid cells.
- Can manifest in multiple ways and levels of severity.
- Patients can have a single cell line affected (i.e., **anemia**) or be pancytopenic.
- It is typically a disease of the **elderly**, but can also result from prior chemotherapy ("treatment-induced MDS").
- Peripheral smear often shows nucleated RBCs (pushed out from bone marrow) or **dysmorphic neutrophils**.
- There are various treatments with moderate efficacy, though no cure.
- Hypomethylating agents (decitabine or 5-azacitadine) are recent advancements, but often transfusion support is the only treatment used.
- Complications include infection, transformation to AML, or myelofibrosis.

LYMPHOMAS AND MULTIPLE MYELOMA

HODGKIN LYMPHOMA

Pathophysiology

- Follicular B cells undergo a transformation to malignant cells.
- The malignant cell in Hodgkin lymphoma is called the **Reed–Sternberg cell.**
- Often, biopsies reveal few Reed–Sternberg cells surrounded by numerous immune and inflammatory cells.
- Two major types of Hodgkin lymphoma exist:
  - **Classical,** composed of the subtypes nodular sclerosing (most common), mixed cellularity, lymphocyte depleted, and lymphocyte rich. Reed–Sternberg cells have very little similarity to their normal B-cell counterpart in this group.
  - **Nonclassical** has only one subgroup, which is the lymphocyte predominant.

Epidemiology

- Bimodal distribution having peaks in thirties and seventies.
- Some cases have an association with Epstein–Barr virus (EBV).

Clinical Features

- Typically presents with cervical lymph node enlargement or a mediastinal mass.
- "B" symptoms: Fever, night sweats, weight loss without trying.
- Pruritus is another classic symptom of Hodgkin lymphoma.

Diagnostic Workup

- Lymph node biopsy (excisional) demonstrating the presence of Reed–Sternberg cells.
- Staging:
  - **Stage I:** One lymph node enlarged.
  - **Stage II:** More than one node on same side of the diaphragm.
  - **Stage III:** Nodes on both sides of the diaphragm.
  - **Stage IV:** Extranodal involvement (e.g., bone marrow).
  - If there are "B" symptoms, add a "B" to any stage (i.e., one node + "B" symptoms = stage IB).

Management

- Usually a good prognosis, particularly in young patients.
- Numerous regimens exist but currently ABVD (**A**driamycin, **B**leomycin, **V**inblastine, and **D**acarbazine) is the treatment of choice.
- Occasionally, radiation has a role in bulky lymph nodes or when there is only one site of disease.

Non-Hodgkin Lymphoma

Non-Hodgkin lymphoma can arise from B or T lymphocytes, but B-cell lymphomas are far more common. They can be divided into **aggressive or indolent types**:

- **Aggressive or high-grade lymphomas** (e.g., large B-cell lymphoma, Burkitt lymphoma, lymphoblastic lymphoma) are often symptomatic with "B" symptoms. Untreated survival is short, but many cases are highly curable with treatment.
- **Indolent or low-grade lymphomas** (e.g., follicular lymphoma, marginal zone lymphoma) are often asymptomatic and slow growing, but with time can cause symptoms and clinical deterioration. Untreated patients can survive for years, but even with treatment, these diseases are usually not curable. Typically treated only if symptomatic.

Clinical Features

These symptoms can occur in any lymphoma, even in advanced stages of indolent lymphomas:

- "B" symptoms (fatigue, fever, night sweats, weight loss, infections).
- Lymphadenopathy.
- Cytopenias from bone marrow involvement.

Diagnostic Workup

- Lymph node biopsy: This is critical to evaluate the tissue architecture.
- Flow cytometry: This evaluates which proteins are expressed on the cell surface; specific constellations of proteins are associated with different lymphomas (this method is also important in any leukemia diagnosis).
- **FISH** is a sensitive method to look for specific cytogenetic lesions associated with different leukemias and lymphomas.
- Unlike Hodgkin disease, histology of the nodes is a major predictor of prognosis.

Management

- Add rituximab to chemotherapy for all B-cell lymphomas.
- Do not treat asymptomatic indolent lymphomas.

Specific Types

- **Follicular lymphoma:**
  - Typically a low-grade lymphoma seen in the middle aged or elderly.
- Commonly asymptomatic, painless, diffuse, long-standing lymphadenopathy in a middle-aged individual.
- Bone marrow involvement and disseminated disease are present in the majority of patients.
- Classic cytogenetic lesion is t(14;18) involving BCL-2 (antiapoptosis protein).
- Divided into low, intermediate, and high grades; high-grade behaves like an aggressive lymphoma.
- **Treat only if symptomatic**. Among many acceptable treatments/combinations are alkylating agents (cyclophosphamide), monoclonal antibodies (rituximab), and corticosteroids.
- **Diffuse large cell lymphoma:**
  - Most common intermediate/high-grade lymphoma.
  - May present in a variety of extranodal sites, particularly the gastrointestinal tract and the head and neck.
  - **Often curable.** Treat with chemotherapy—R-CHOP (**R**ituximab, **C**yclophosphamide, Doxorubicin [**H**ydroxydaunomycin], Vincristine [**O**ncovin], **P**rednisone).
- **Lymphoblastic lymphoma:**
  - Very high-grade lymphoma often seen in children; behaves like an acute leukemia.
  - Derived from thymic T cells and often presents with large mediastinal mass.
  - Often seen in children.
  - Associated with testicular, CNS, and marrow involvement.
- **Adult T-cell leukemia/lymphoma:**
  - Associated with HLTV-1 virus, seen in patients from Japan and the Caribbean.
  - Often presents with hypercalcemia.
  - Although high grade, not typically curable.
- **Burkitt lymphoma:**
  - High-grade lymphoma more common in children than adults.
  - Endemic type (African) associated with EBV and jaw lesions.

- Nonendemic type: Diffuse lymphadenopathy.
- Classic cytogenetic lesion is t(8;14) involving the *c-myc* gene.
- Bone marrow can have a "starry sky" appearance (from macrophages eating away the necrotic cells and leaving spaces between cells).
- Treatment includes high-dose cyclophosphamide, methotrexate, and cytarabine and intensive CNS prophylaxis.

- **Mantle cell lymphoma:**
  - Has both high- and low-grade features.
  - Can be very aggressive (high-grade feature) but usually relapses after treatment (low-grade feature).

MULTIPLE MYELOMA

General Facts

- Plasma cells normally produce antibodies to fight infections. Multiple myeloma is the clonal proliferation of plasma cells usually characterized by the **presence of monoclonal immunoglobulin** or **immunoglobulin fragments (light chains)** in the serum and urine.
- Other manifestations include bone destruction **(lytic lesions)** and **hypercalcemia**.
- Patients also can get renal failure, usually from protein damage.
- Typically elderly; twice as common in African Americans than whites.

Clinical Features

Patients can present with a pathologic fracture (where a lytic lesion was), hypercalcemia, renal failure, weakness, infection, hyperviscosity from high protein, and anemia from bone marrow failure.

Diagnostic Workup

- **Serum and urine electrophoresis (SPEP/UPEP):** These will detect the presence of a monoclonal protein in the serum or urine. Light chains (without the rest of the immunoglobulin) are referred to as **Bence Jones proteins.**
- **Immunofixation** is another method to detect monoclonal proteins.
- **Bone marrow biopsy** shows elevated plasma cells (normal is <5%).
- Other possible findings:
  - Peripheral blood smear: **Rouleaux formation, anemia.**
  - Radiography: **Lytic lesions** on x-ray (needs whole-body skeletal survey or x-rays, not bone scan).
  - **Elevated total protein** on chemistry.

Management

- There is no cure.
- Multiple effective therapies exist, including older chemotherapies (melphalan) and newer (bortezomib and lenalidomide). Steroids are effective.
- Autologous bone marrow transplant (use the person's own stem cells) is also used.
- Bisphosphonates may delay or prevent lytic lesions and decrease hypercalcemia.

CONQUER THE **BOARDS!**

Clover leaf cells are seen in HTLV-associated leukemia/lymphoma.

CNS and testes can represent sanctuary sites in lymphomas.

Bone and CNS metastasis signify high-risk disease.

CONQUER THE **WARDS!**

Patients with BRCA1 mutations tend to have triple negative breast cancer and higher risk of ovarian cancer.

Patients with BRCA2 mutations tend to have hormone receptor–positive cancer and higher risk of pancreatic, prostate, gastric cancer, and melanoma.

Men with BRACA2 mutations start prostate cancer screening at age 40.

Adverse effects of chemotherapy agents:

Cisplatin: Nephrotoxicity

Bleomycin and **Meth**otrexate: Pulmonary fibrosis (**bleo**mycin blasts the lungs with **METH**ane)

Vin**cristine** = neurotoxic, palsies (**Kristine** lost her **nerves**)

Doxo**rubi**cin = cardiotoxic (**Rubi** lost his heart.)

Tamoxifen = uterine cancer (selective estrogen antagonist at breast is an agonist at uterus causing uterine hyperplasia/cancer)

Asparaginase = pancreatitis

CYclophosphamide = hemorrhagic **CY**stitis

A 60-year-old man with punched-out lytic lesions in the skull and mild anemia. *Think: Multiple myeloma.* **Next step:** Check SPEP and UPEP.

A 68-year-old man presents with low back pain, hypercalcemia, anemia, and azotemia. *Think: Multiple myeloma* (common triad of back pain, anemia, and renal insufficiency).

CONQUER THE **BOARDS!**

Mutations in the *CDH1* gene are associated with gastric cancer and lobular breast cancer. Prophylactic gastrectomy is recommended in carriers.

CONQUER THE **BOARDS!**

In patients with DCIS lumpectomy +/– radiation, decreased risk of invasive breast cancer in ipsilateral breast.

Systemic therapy (with tamoxifen or aromatase inhibitors) decreases risk of invasive breast cancer in ipsilateral and contralateral breast.

SOLID TUMOR MALIGNANCIES

BREAST CANCER

Epidemiology

Breast cancer is the second most common cause of **cancer death** in women in the United States (most common is lung cancer, as in men). One in eight women will develop breast cancer in their lifetime. Breast cancer is rare in men and accounts for 1% of all breast cancer.

Mutations in the p53 (tumor suppressor gene associated with Li Fraumeni syndrome), *BRCA1, BRCA2, erbB2* (HER-2/neu), and *PTEN* (Cowden syndrome) genes account for about 10% of breast cancer cases.

Risk Factors

- Age, prior breast cancer, family history, previous benign biopsy, increased estrogen exposure.
- **Causes of estrogen exposure:** Early menarche, late menopause, nulliparity/late pregnancy, no breastfeeding.
- Oral contraceptives **do not** increase risk, but hormone replacement therapy **does** increase risk.
- *BRCA1* and *BRCA2* have increased risk of breast (50% to 85%) and ovarian cancer (50%). Prophylactic bilateral mastectomy and oophorectomy should be considered.
- Ductal carcinoma in situ (DCIS) and lobular carcinoma in situ (LCIS).

Screening

- **Breast exams:**
  - Annually by physician (starting at age 20).
  - Monthly self-exam (best time is 3 to 5 days after onset of menses) does not decrease mortality.
- **Mammograms:**
  - Not done if <35 years because of a dense breast.
  - 40 to 49 years: Every 1 to 2 years is controversial but recommended by most.
  - 50+: Annually until age 70, then only if life expectancy is >10 years.
- **Evaluation of breast masses:**
  - Cancer is usually, although not always, painless.
  - Sonography—differentiate cystic from solid masses.
  - Fine-needle aspiration (FNA).
  - **Excisional/open biopsy**—definitive diagnosis.
  - **Diffusely inflamed and indurated breast (peau d'orange**—looks like the skin of an orange): Signifies inflammatory breast cancer in which the cancer has infiltrated the dermal lymphatics. Typically very aggressive with poor prognosis.

Prognosis

Prognosis depends on staging, tumor grade, and hormone receptor status (estrogen/progesterone positive is better).

Management

- For **nonmetastatic disease:** Surgical resection.
  - Breast conservation (lumpectomy) is usually possible, but mastectomy is required for very large tumors (>7 cm) and other specific situations (for example, multifocal breast cancer or small breasts, etc.)
  - If lumpectomy only, adding radiation reduces the risk of local recurrence (but not mortality).
  - Adjuvant systemic (chemotherapy) treatment is needed if tumor >2 cm or there are axillary lymph nodes.
  - Special cases:
    a. In estrogen/progestin receptor–positive patients, tamoxifen (an estrogen/progesterone receptor blocker) is used in premenopausal women and an aromatase inhibitor should be used for postmenopausal women.
    b. Trastuzumab (Herceptin) and pertuzumab is used for HER-2/neu-positive patients.
    c. Chemotherapy typically used includes Adriamycin, cyclophosphamide, and taxanes, or a combination of 2 of the 3.
- For **metastatic disease:** Chemotherapy, hormonal therapy, and/or trastuzumab can be used, depending on receptor status.

CONQUER THE **BOARDS!**

The overall survival of patients who underwent breast conservation (i.e., lumpectomy followed by radiation) vs. those who underwent mastectomy for breast cancer was not inferior at 20 years of follow-up.

CONQUER THE **WARDS!**

Krukenberg tumors: Metastasis to ovaries. Suspected in bilateral ovarian tumors. Evaluate for gastric, appendiceal, gastrointestinal primaries.

CONQUER THE **BOARDS!**

Avoid radiation in patients with Li–Fraumeni syndrome.

HIGH-YIELD LITERATURE

Length of therapy for adjuvant hormonal therapy:

Gray RG, Rea D, Handley K, et al. aTTom: Long-term effects of continuing adjuvant tamoxifen to 10 years versus stopping at 5 years in 6,953 women with early breast cancer. *J Clin Oncol*. 2013;31(Suppl 18):5.

Davies C, Pan H, Godwin J, et al. Long-term effects of continuing adjuvant tamoxifen to 10 years versus stopping at 5 years after diagnosis of oestrogen receptor-positive breast cancer: ATLAS, a randomised trial. *Lancet*. 2013;381(9869): 805-816.

> CONQUER THE **WARDS!**
>
> Prognostic factors are those that indicate natural history of the tumor—for example, histologic grade of the tumor, Ki-67, etc. Predictive factors are those that indicate response to a treatment—for example, hormone receptor–positive breast cancer responds to hormonal therapy.

OVARIAN CANCER

Epidemiology

- Ovarian cancer is the fourth most common cause of death from cancer among women of all ages in the United States.
- Most patients present in advanced stages.

Clinical Features

Abdominal bloating, early satiety, **enlarging pants size,** ascites (all nonspecific symptoms).

Risk Factors

- Increased **risk**: Older age at first pregnancy/nulliparous; family history/ BRCA1 and BRCA2.
- Decreased **risk** (by prolonging periods of anovulation): Childbearing and breastfeeding, oral contraceptives, tubal sterilization.

Figo Staging

- **Stage I:** Ovary only.
- **Stage II:** Ovary + pelvic extension.
- **Stage III:** Ovary + peritoneal carcinomatosis with ascites (70% of patients)—but confined to abdominal cavity.
- **Stage IV:** Metastasis outside of abdominal cavity.

Screening

Not recommended.

Prognosis

Forty percent 5-year survival depending on stage and presentation.

Management

- Surgery alone for stages IA and IB.
- Surgery (debulking) followed by chemotherapy (paclitaxel + platinum agent) for more advanced stages (**surgical debulking is done even when there are metastases**).

CERVICAL CANCER

Cervical cancer is a consequence of sexually transmitted infection of human papillomavirus (HPV) types 16 and 18 and other high-risk HPV (31, 33, 45, 52, 58) accounting for 70%.

Risk Factors

- HPV, human immunodeficiency virus (HIV), smoking.
- Early age at first intercourse.
- Large number of sexual partners.

Clinical Features

- Foul-smelling vaginal discharge.
- **Postcoital** and irregular vaginal bleeding.
- Pelvic pain.
- Dyspareunia.

Screening

- Yearly Papanicolaou (Pap) smear test starting at age 21 in virgins or age at first sexual intercourse until age 65. Perform every 2 to 3 years if 3 consecutive negative Pap smears.
- Counsel patients about protective effect of barrier contraceptives.

Figo Staging

- **Stage I:** Confined to cervix.
- **Stage II:** Cervix + uterus but not to pelvic wall or lower third of vagina.
- **Stage III:** Invades pelvic wall or lower third of vagina.
- **Stage IV:** Invades other organs in pelvis (bladder) or distant metastases.

Management

- Colposcopic-directed cervical or cone biopsy for carcinoma in situ (stage 0).
- Radical hysterectomy for disease invading the cervix (**stage I**). Fertility preservation, if desired, may be possible in limited disease.
- Radiation therapy (usually with *cis*-platinum chemotherapy) for disease that invades beyond the cervix (**stages II to IV**) but without distant metastasis.
- Recurrent or distant metastasis: Radiation for palliation and/or chemotherapy.

Prognosis

Depends on nodal status and stage:

- **Stages I and II:** 5-year survival is 80%.
- **Stage III:** 5-year survival is 40%.

CONQUER THE BOARDS!

Gleason score of 6 is low, and these tumors are considered well differentiated and slow growing.

Gleason score of 8 to 0 is high, and these tumors are considered poorly differentiated and aggressive.

Gleason score of 7 is moderate, and these tumors are considered moderately differentiated.

PROSTATE CANCER

General Facts

- Prostate cancer is an adenocarcinoma that is the most common cancer in men and the third most common cause of cancer death in men in the United States.
- Incidence increases with age, with most in men older than 50 years.
- There is a higher incidence in African Americans.

Clinical Features

- Usually asymptomatic, diagnosed by elevated prostate-specific antigen (PSA).
- Dysuria and urinary hesitancy (more common with benign prostatic hyperplasia [BPH] than prostate cancer) or hematuria.
- New-onset erectile dysfunction.
- Back pain—when presenting with bone metastasis to spine.

Screening

- Screening (PSA) begins at age 50 until age 75 (or when life expectancy <10 years); start at age 40 for African American men or those with *BRCA1* or family history.
- Yearly digital rectal exam to look for nodules.
- Yearly PSA (controversial).
- For PSA >4.1, transrectal ultrasonography (TRUS) with biopsy of suspicious areas.

Staging and Management

- In addition to staging, factors that define high risk are high PSA score and high Gleason score.
- Generally, treatment is surgery or radiation for local disease.
- Prostate cancer typically grows in response to testosterone, so blocking testosterone is an important part of treatment in advanced stages.
- Those with high risk (as defined by a high Gleason score or high PSA) but local disease may benefit from adjuvant hormonal deprivation ("hormonal therapy").
- Metastatic disease can be treated with hormonal therapy alone.
- Commonly used hormonal therapies are antiandrogen agents (e.g., flutamide), gonadotropin-releasing hormone (GnRH) agonists (paradoxically, this can initially increase testosterone production), and orchiectomy.
- **T1 (nonpalpable) and T2 (palpable) disease:**
  - Prostatectomy or radiotherapy.
  - Consider both or adding antiandrogen therapy if pathologically high Gleason score or high PSA.
- **T3 disease (extracapsular extension):**
  - Radical prostatectomy or radiation.
  - Consider hormonal therapy.
- **Metastasis:**
  - Hormonal therapy.
  - Consider chemotherapy if refractory to hormonal therapy.

CONQUER THE BOARDS!

Seminomas do not secrete AFP and have a good prognosis with over 90% cure rate.

Nonseminomas are AFP-producing tumors. If AFP is elevated, it is automatically considered nonseminoma.

AFP can be increased in liver cancer, viral hepatitis, and liver disease.

Prognosis

Ten-year survival rates are 75% when the cancer is confined to the prostate, 55% for those with regional extension, and 15% for those with distant metastases.

TESTICULAR CANCER

General Facts

- A common cancer in men age 20 to 40 and is seen more frequently in whites.
- Though other types exist, 95% are germ cell tumors.

Classification

- Germ cell tumors are divided into **seminomas (50%)** and **nonseminomas (50%)**.
- Nonseminomas have the following subtypes: choriocarcinoma (secretes human chorionic gonadotropin [hCG]; hence causes gynecomastia); endodermal sinus tumor (yolk sac tumor; secretes alpha-fetoprotein [AFP]); embryonal carcinoma (secretes hCG and AFP); teratoma (cell types from more than one layer—ecto-, meso-, or endoderm).

Clinical Features

- Painless testicular mass or persistent swelling is cancer unless proven otherwise.
- Metastases may present as back pain (retroperitoneal), para-aortic/supraclavicular nodes, or dyspnea (lung metastases).

Diagnostic Workup

- **Do not perform scrotal biopsy** (risk of seeding retroperitoneum by disruption of fascial planes).
- **Orchiectomy from inguinal approach.** Ultrasound should be done prior to surgery to rule out infections or benign conditions such as varicoceles.
- Tumor markers: **LDH for seminoma** (if hCG or AFP is elevated, it is automatically considered a nonseminoma regardless of LDH), **hCG for choriocarcinoma**, and **AFP for yolk sac tumor**.

Management

- Cure rates are high, even in advanced stages, due to the chemosensitivity of nonseminomas and the radiation sensitivity of seminomas.
- **Nonseminoma:** Orchiectomy, retroperitoneal lymph node dissection (RPLND), and chemotherapy for lymph node involvement or metastasis. Patients without lymph node involvement or metastases have a 95% cure rate.
- **Seminoma:** Orchiectomy and retroperitoneal radiation have 98% cure rate for nonmetastasized seminomas; chemotherapy for metastases.

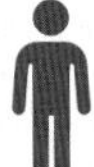

A 23-year-old man presents with gynecomastia and substernal pain, and physical exam reveals painless testicular mass. *Think: Malignancy.* **Next step**: CXR. Finding? *Mediastinal mass = germ cell tumor. Young men with mediastinal mass. Think: Lymphoma or germ cell tumor.*

RENAL CELL CANCER

Presentation

- Triad of flank mass, hematuria, and abdominal pain. Diagnosed with abdominal CT scan.
- Paraneoplastic syndromes: Hypercalcemia, polycythemia.
- **Renal vein thrombosis** and **IVC thrombus** are classic findings (see Table 8-3).

Management

- Early stages (within kidney): Radical nephrectomy.
- Advanced stages (metastasis or invading the capsule): Interleukin-2 (IL-2) may increase remission in 10% of patients who can tolerate it; vascular endothelial growth factor (VEGF) inhibitors (sunitinib or sorafenib).

CONQUER THE **WARDS!**

Predictors of shorter survival in renal cell carcinoma: LDH more than 1.5 times upper limit of normal, hemoglobin less than lower limit of normal, corrected calcium more than 10, poor performance status, interval less than 1 year from original diagnosis to start of systemic therapy and more than equal to 2 sites of organ metastasis.

BLADDER CANCER

General Facts

Usually, cell type is transitional cell carcinoma. Rarely can be "small cell" (neuroendocrine tumor).

Risk Factors

Smoking and occupational (dye) exposure.

TABLE 8-3. Paraneoplastic and Distant Effects of Tumors		
Effect	**Molecule**	**Associated Neoplasm**
Cushing syndrome	ACTH or ACTH-like peptide.	Small cell lung carcinoma.
SIADH	ADH or ANP.	Small cell lung carcinoma and intracranial neoplasms.
Hypercalcemia	PTH-related peptide, TGF-α, TNF-α, IL-2.	Squamous cell lung carcinoma, renal carcinoma, breast carcinoma, multiple myeloma, and bone metastasis (lysed bone).
Polycythemia	Erythropoietin.	Renal cell carcinoma (hypernephroma).
Lambert–Eaton syndrome	Antibodies against presynaptic Ca^{2+} channels at NMJ.	Thymoma, bronchogenic carcinoma.
Gout	Hyperuricemia due to excess nucleic acid turnover (i.e., cytotoxic therapy).	

ACTH, adrenocorticotropic hormone; *ADH*, antidiuretic hormone; *ANP*, atrial natriuretic peptide; *IL-2*, interleukin-2; *NMJ*, neuromuscular junction; *PTH*, parathyroid hormone; *TGF*, transforming growth factor; *TNF-α*, tumor necrosis factor-α.

CONQUER THE BOARDS!

If there is no bladder muscle seen in TURBT specimen, then need to repeat procedure because you need to evaluate the bladder muscle for invasion by the cancer, since in that case the treatment will be cystectomy.

CONQUER THE BOARDS!

Hepatocellular carcinoma paraneoplastic syndrome: Hypoglycemia, hypercalcemia, elevated hemoglobin and RBCs, and hypercholesterolemia.

Presentation

Painless hematuria.

Diagnostic Workup

CT urogram and cystoscopy. Urine for cytology (10% yield).

Management

- Localized (not invading bladder muscle): Transurethral resection of bladder tumor (TURBT) + intravesical chemotherapy or bacillus Calmette–Guerin (BCG).

  Localized (invading bladder muscle): neoadjuvant chemotherapy followed by cystectomy
- Advanced: Chemotherapy.

GASTRIC CANCER

General Facts

- More than 90% of gastric cancers are adenocarcinomas.
- *H. pylori* is an important risk factor in the United States. Other risk factors include achlorhydria and tobacco use.

Clinical Features

- The most common symptom is dysphagia.
- A lymph node in the left supraclavicular region (Virchow node) is classically associated with gastric cancers. A periumbilical node (Sister Mary Joseph node) can occur as well.

Diagnostic Workup

- Endoscopy can be performed along with biopsy of the lesion; this will be sent for pathologic and histologic examination.
- Endoscopic ultrasound-guided biopsy of surrounding lymph nodes can be used to assess staging.

Management

- For local disease, options include surgery and chemotherapy.
- For metastatic disease, chemotherapy can help reduce progression.

HEPATOCELLULAR CANCER

Epidemiology

- More common in Asia.
- Seen in patients with cirrhosis, especially hepatitis B and hemochromatosis.

Screening

- Liver ultrasound +/– **AFP (tumor marker)** every 6 months in patients with cirrhosis or chronic hepatitis B.
- Magnetic resonance imaging (MRI) for more definitive diagnosis.

Management

- Depends on the degree of cirrhosis and the size of the tumor.
- For local disease, options include surgery, radiofrequency ablation, and chemoembolization.
- For metastatic disease, VEGF inhibitors (sunitinib or sorafenib) can be given.

CONQUER THE **BOARDS!**

Hepatocellular carcinoma can be diagnosed via triple-phase CT scan showing arterial hyperenhancement and venous phase washout.

PANCREATIC CANCER

General Facts

- Pancreatic cancer is the fourth most common cause of cancer-related deaths in the United States.
- Tobacco use, obesity, inactivity, and diabetes are common risk factors.
- Risk increases with age, with most cases between the age of 60 and 80.
- Adenocarcinoma is the most common type. Other types are associated with better prognosis, such as neuroendocrine pancreatic tumors.

CONQUER THE **WARDS!**

Stauffer syndrome: Cytokine-mediated paraneoplastic syndrome leading to abnormal liver function. Treatment is to remove the primary tumor in the kidney.

Clinical Features

- The most common symptom is painless jaundice due to obstruction of surrounding structures.
- Anorexia, weight loss, and abdominal pain can occur as well.

Diagnostic Workup

- Abdominal imaging via computed tomography (CT) or MRI can help characterize the tumor location, followed by interventional radiology (IR) or endoscopy-based biopsy and pathology.
- CA-19-9 may be elevated, but is not reliable, with false positives and false negatives.

Management

- For local disease, pancreaticoduodenectomy (Whipple procedure) can be curative.
- For advanced disease, a combination of chemotherapy and surgical interventions may be used.

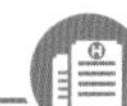

Lots of Bad Stuff Kills Glia
(Origin of brain metastases: Lung, Breast, Skin, Kidney, GI)

MISCELLANEOUS METASTATIC DISEASE

- **Liver metastasis:**
  - Liver and lung are the most common sites for metastatic disease.
  - Primary tumors that metastasize to the liver: **Colon** > **Stomach** > **Pancreas** (all three GI from portal circulation) > **Breast** > **Lung**.
- **Bone metastasis:**
  - Breast and prostate are the most common.
  - Kidney, thyroid, testes, lung, prostate, breast.

TABLE 8-4. Common Classes of Chemotherapies

Specific Drugs (Examples)	Indications	Specific Toxicity
Drug Class: Alkylating agents	**Mechanism:** Formation of DNA cross-links and hence inhibition of DNA function and synthesis.	**General Toxicities:** Myelosuppression, mucosal toxicity/mucosal ulceration, diarrhea, nausea and vomiting.
Cyclophosphamide/ Ifosfamide	HL, NHL, ALL/CLL, multiple myeloma, breast/lung/ovary/ testicular cancer.	Hemorrhagic cystitis.
Melphalan	Multiple myeloma, ovarian cancer.	Myelosuppression, hypersensitivity.
Chlorambucil	CLL, HL/NHL.	Myelosuppression, bone marrow failure.
Bendamustine	CLL, NHL.	Pancytopenia, hyperbilirubinemia.
Temozolomide	Brain cancer, malignant melanoma.	Myelosuppression, elevated LFTs.
Procarbazine	HL, NHL.	Myelosuppression, reproductive dysfunction, hemolysis (in G6PD deficiency).
Dacarbazine	HL, malignant melanoma.	Myelosuppression, metallic taste, rash.
Drug Class: Platinum compounds	**Mechanism:** Form intrastrand and interstrand DNA cross-links; bind to nuclear and cytoplasmic proteins.	
Cisplatin	NSCLC, breast cancer, bladder cancer, head and neck cancer, ovarian cancer.	Nephrotoxicity, peripheral neuropathy, myelosuppression, ototoxicity.
Carboplatin	NSCLC, breast cancer, bladder cancer, head and neck cancer, ovarian cancer.	Myelosuppression.
Oxaliplatin	Colorectal cancer, pancreatic cancer.	Myelosuppression, peripheral neuropathy.

ALL, acute lymphoblastic leukemia; *CLL*, chronic lymphoblastic leukemia; *HL*, Hodgkin lymphoma; *LFT*, liver function test; *NHL*, non-Hodgkin lymphoma; *NSCLC*, non–small cell lung cancer.

- Lung = **L**ytic.
- Breast = **B**oth lytic and blastic.
- Prostate = blastic.

- **Brain metastasis:**
  - Fifty percent of brain tumors are metastatic lesions.
  - Primary tumors metastasizing to the brain: **L**ung, **B**reast, **S**kin (melanoma), **K**idney (renal cell carcinoma), **G**I.

ONCOLOGIC EMERGENCIES

HYPERCALCEMIA

- The most common metabolic emergency of malignancy.
- Symptoms and signs include confusion, nausea, fatigue, decreased PO intake, polyuria, depression, psychosis/confusion, nephrolithiasis (**BONES, STONES, GROANS, and PSYCHIATRIC OVERTONES**).
- Can progress to severe confusion and coma.
- Electrocardiogram (ECG) may show QT interval shortening.
- Usual cancers: Multiple myeloma, breast cancer, squamous cell (lung cancer, head and neck), renal cell cancer, lymphomas.
- Either from bone metastases, parathyroid hormone (PTH)–related peptide, or 1-25 vitamin D (lymphomas).
- **Treatment:** Aggressive rehydration with normal saline, **furosemide if patient is fluid overloaded**, bisphosphonates (takes 2 to 3 days). **Calcitonin (takes 2 to 4 hours to work) as a temporizing measure has limited role due to tachyphylaxis.**

> **CONQUER THE BOARDS!**
>
> Patients with neutropenia should receive antibiotics with gram-negative, especially *Pseudomonas*, coverage.

FEBRILE NEUTROPENIA

Fever in the setting of clinically significant neutropenia (absolute neutrophil count <500).

Diagnostic Workup

- Careful history and detailed physical examination, looking for skin findings, oral abnormalities, central venous catheters, and any other symptoms.
- Chest imaging, starting with a chest x-ray and pursuing a CT of the chest if patient remains febrile.
- Blood and urine cultures.
- Beta-D-glucan and galactomannan are markers of possible fungal infection that can increase suspicion for invasive *Aspergillosis.*

Management

- Antibiotics should be started empirically and immediately; febrile neutropenia is a medical emergency (see Figure 8-6).
- Add vancomycin if hypotension, history of methicillin-resistant *Staphylococcus aureus* (MRSA), soft tissue infection, or a **central venous access** concerning for infection.
- If vancomycin is not added initially, then add it at day 3 if the patient continues to have fever and neutropenia. Add antifungals (voriconazole) on day 5 if no improvement.

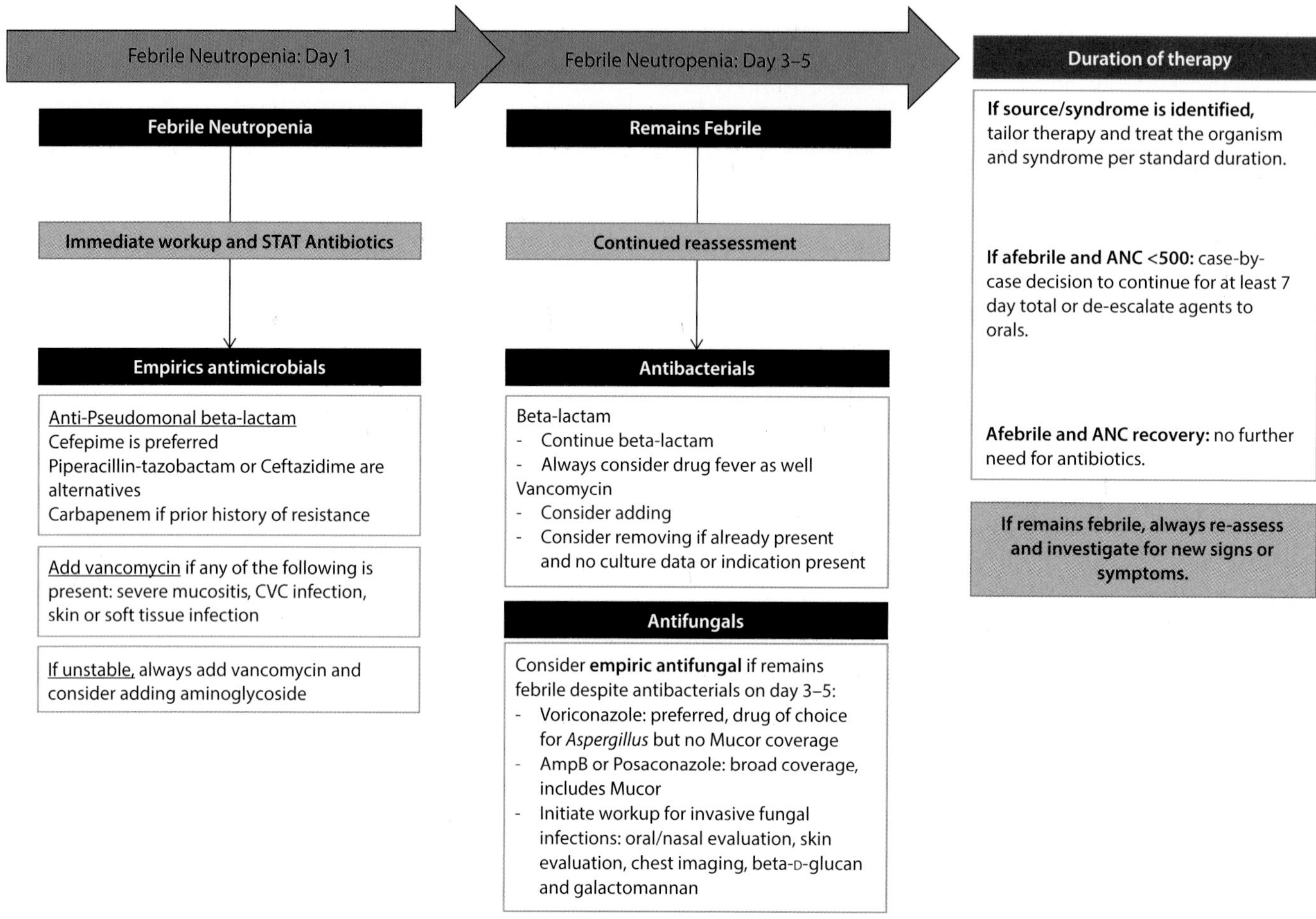

FIGURE 8-6. Management of febrile neutropenia.

TUMOR LYSIS SYNDROME

- Cell breakdown causes release of intracellular ions (potassium and phosphorus) and DNA breakdown causing **hyperuricemia**.
- Seen in leukemias, lymphomas, and after chemotherapy in bulky tumors.
- Uric acid can cause acute renal failure and gout.
- Electrolyte disturbances: Hyperkalemia, hyperphosphatemia, and hypocalcemia (from binding to phosphorus). **High LDH**.
- Treat with IV fluids, allopurinol.
- Severe cases require urine alkalinization and IV therapy with rasburicase (an enzyme that degrades uric acid).

SUPERIOR VENA CAVA SYNDROME

- Caused by obstruction of the superior vena cava (SVC) by external compression, tumor invasion, or thrombus formation in the SVC lumen.
- Symptoms include dyspnea, facial edema and plethora, cough, neck and arm edema.
- Diagnosis can be done via CT of the chest or chest x-ray.
  - Treatment includes chemotherapy, **radiation**, stenting, and in select cases, steroids.

SPINAL CORD COMPRESSION

- Compression of spinal cord secondary to vertebral collapse or extension of tumor from vertebra.
- Most commonly affects the thoracic spine.
- Back pain in cancer patient with neurologic symptoms = cord compression.
- Back pain, loss of bowel or bladder function, muscle weakness, and saddle anesthesia are the hallmark of the disease.
- A thorough examination may yield the diagnosis, with MRI of the spine with gadolinium to confirm.
- Management involves **high-dose steroids + radiation therapy** or surgical decompression.

CONQUER THE BOARDS!

The first sign of cord compression is pain. Hence, having a high index of suspicion in cancer patients with new-onset or worsening back pain is key for timely diagnosis of cord compression.

CHAPTER 9 INFECTIOUS DISEASES

OVERVIEW OF HIGH-YIELD TOPICS IN INFECTIOUS DISEASES

CONQUER THE WARDS!

Viral pneumonias are more common than perceived. A study showed they could be >30% of all pneumonias! .

PNEUMONIA

General Facts

- There are different ways to categorize pneumonia: type of germ (bacterial, viral, atypical, and fungal), how it is acquired (ventilator associated and aspiration), and location where it was acquired (community acquired and hospital acquired).
  - Location where it was acquired is most commonly used because it dictates what empiric antibiotics should be started. We will address ventilator-associated and aspiration pneumonia at the end of this section.
- **Community-acquired pneumonia (CAP):** Pneumonia diagnosed in patients within 48 hours of hospital admission who do not meet criteria for hospital-acquired pneumonia. CAP can be caused by bacterial, viral, atypical, or fungal organisms. See Table 9-1.
- **Hospital-acquired pneumonia (HAP):** Pneumonia developing at least 48 hours after hospital admission. The concept here is that for HAP, we must be worried about multidrug-resistant (MDR) bacteria, especially methicillin-resistant *Staphylococcus aureus* (MRSA), *Pseudomonas,* and MDR gram-negative bacteria. (See Table 9-1.)

TABLE 9-1. Pathogens Associated with Community- and Hospital-Acquired Pneumonia

Organisms (in order of prevalence)	CAP	Hospital Acquired[2]
Bacterial (**bold are atypical**)[1]	■ Streptococcus pneumonia (most common bacterial cause) ■ ***Mycoplasma pneumoniae*** (mostly in outpatients) ■ *Staphylococcus aureus* (especially post-influenzae, increasing prevalence) ■ *Haemophilus influenzae* (especially COPD) ■ ***Legionella pneumophila*** ■ *Klebsiella* and gram-negative rods (especially in aspiration and alcoholics)	■ *S. aureus* (28%) ■ *Pseudomonas* (22%) ■ *Klebsiella* species (10%) ■ *Escherichia coli* (7%) ■ Acinetobacter species (7%) ■ Enterobacter species (6%)
Viruses	■ Rhinovirus ■ Influenza viruses ■ Respiratory syncytial virus ■ Parainfluenza virus ■ Human metapneumovirus ■ Coronavirus ■ Adenovirus	

HIGH-YIELD LITERATURE

Impact of vaccination and the changing epidemiology of CAP:

Musher DM, Abers MS, Bartlett JG. Evolving understanding of the causes of pneumonia in adults, with special attention to the role of Pneumococcus. *Clin Infect Dis*. 2017;65:1736.

Microbiology

Risk Factors for Drug Resistance

Health care–associated pneumonias (HCAPs) depend on risk factors for MDR organisms because it will change what antibiotics you will treat with. If any of the following are present, then MDR organisms should be covered with your antibiotics:

- Antibiotic therapy within 90 days of infection.
- Current hospitalization of >2 days.
- High frequency of antibiotic resistance in the specific hospital unit.
- Immunosuppressive disease or therapy.
- Presence of HCAP risk factors for MDR, including home infusion therapy, residing in a nursing home or extended care facility, home wound care, chronic dialysis (within 30 days), or family member with MDR.

Clinical Features

- Fevers, chills, and/or rigors (80% of patients, but this can be absent in older patients).
- Increased respiratory rate greater than 24 (45% to 70% of patients).
- Cough with sputum production.
- Shortness of breath can occur at rest or with activity.
- Pleuritic chest pain at rest or with coughing.
- Mental status change in the elderly or with severe systemic infection from pneumonia.
- On examination, dullness to percussion, egophony, crackles, and decreased breath sounds can be found.

Diagnostic Workup

- **Chest x-ray (CXR)** is the most common test used to diagnose pneumonia.
- Computed tomography (CT) imaging is more sensitive but more expensive, so CXR is generally done first.
- **Serologic testing**, such as urine *Legionella* antigen, urine *Streptococcus pneumoniae* antigen, and influenza swab should be sent as well.
- **Blood cultures** are important to ensure no secondary bacteremia has occurred, but are often negative.
- **Sputum Gram stain and culture** are recommended. The utility, however, is controversial. A good sample will contain <10 epithelial cells per low-power field (the fewer the better). More than 25 leukocytes per low-power field represents a lower respiratory tract isolate.
- A **viral respiratory panel** can be obtained if you suspect a viral antigen. If positive, it can help avoid antibiotics.
- **Procalcitonin** is a new test that may not be available at all hospitals. Its utility is still under debate, but it may come up on rounds.

CONQUER THE BOARDS!

Legionella and intracellular organisms can cause temperature–pulse dissociation: normal pulse when febrile.

CONQUER THE BOARDS!

Legionella typically happens in summer, when water towers are active.

CONQUER THE WARDS!

An infiltrate alone is not enough. In order to diagnose pneumonia, your patient should have some of the clinical and physical exam findings noted, as well as an infiltrate on CXR.

HIGH-YIELD LITERATURE

Procalcitonin and pneumonia:

Self WH, Balk RA, Grijalva CG, et al. Procalcitonin as a marker of etiology in adults hospitalized with community-acquired pneumonia. *Clin Infect Dis.* 2017;65:183.

Management

Management of pneumonia will depend on epidemiologic risk factors (community vs. hospital acquired) and severity.

Assessing Severity

- Several scoring systems exist to predict prognosis and help physicians decide if patients should be treated as an outpatient or inpatient.
- The two most widely used scores are the **Pneumonia Severity Index/** Pneumonia Patient Outcomes Research Team (PSI/PORT) score and **CURB-65**.
- CURB-65 is simpler and has shown to be more sensitive and more specific in predicting mortality in pneumonia (Table 9-2).
- The most important tool you have is your clinical judgment.

CONQUER THE **BOARDS!**

Elderly inpatients, immunocompromised, or pregnant females are at higher risk of severe influenza, and treatment is recommended.

Selection of Empiric Antimicrobial Therapy

- Table 9-3 lists the typical starting medications and doses for empiric coverage of the two types of pneumonia.
- It is also important to de-escalate therapy after starting empiric antibiotics to follow up on your blood and sputum cultures.

TABLE 9-2. Pneumonia Severity Assessment

CURB-65	Points
Confusion	1
Blood urea nitrogen >19 mg/dL	1
Respiratory rate >30 breaths per minute	1
Systolic blood pressure <90 mm Hg or Diastolic blood pressure <60 mm Hg	1
Total points:	

HIGH-YIELD LITERATURE

Pneumonia prediction scores:

Shah BA, Ahmed W, Dhobi GN, et al. Validity of Pneumonia Severity Index and CURB-65 Severity Scoring Systems in community acquired pneumonia in an *Indian* setting. Indian *J Chest Dis Allied Sci.* 2010;52(1):9-17.

Table 9-3. Antimicrobial Therapy for Pneumonia

	CAP (**bold are typical**)[1]	Hospital Acquired[2]
Empiric antibiotics	**Inpatient:** Second- or third-generation cephalosporin (e.g., ceftriaxone 1 g daily) + Macrolide (e.g., azithromycin 500 mg daily) Alternative: Fluoroquinolone (e.g., levofloxacin 750 mg daily) **Outpatient**: Macrolide alone Alternative: Fluoroquinolone	**MRSA coverage:** (Vancomycin 1 g IV twice a day) + ***Pseudomonas* coverage:** Piperacillin–tazobactam 4.5 g IV q6h, cefepime 2 g IV q8h, levofloxacin 750 mg IV daily, meropenem 1 g IV q8h

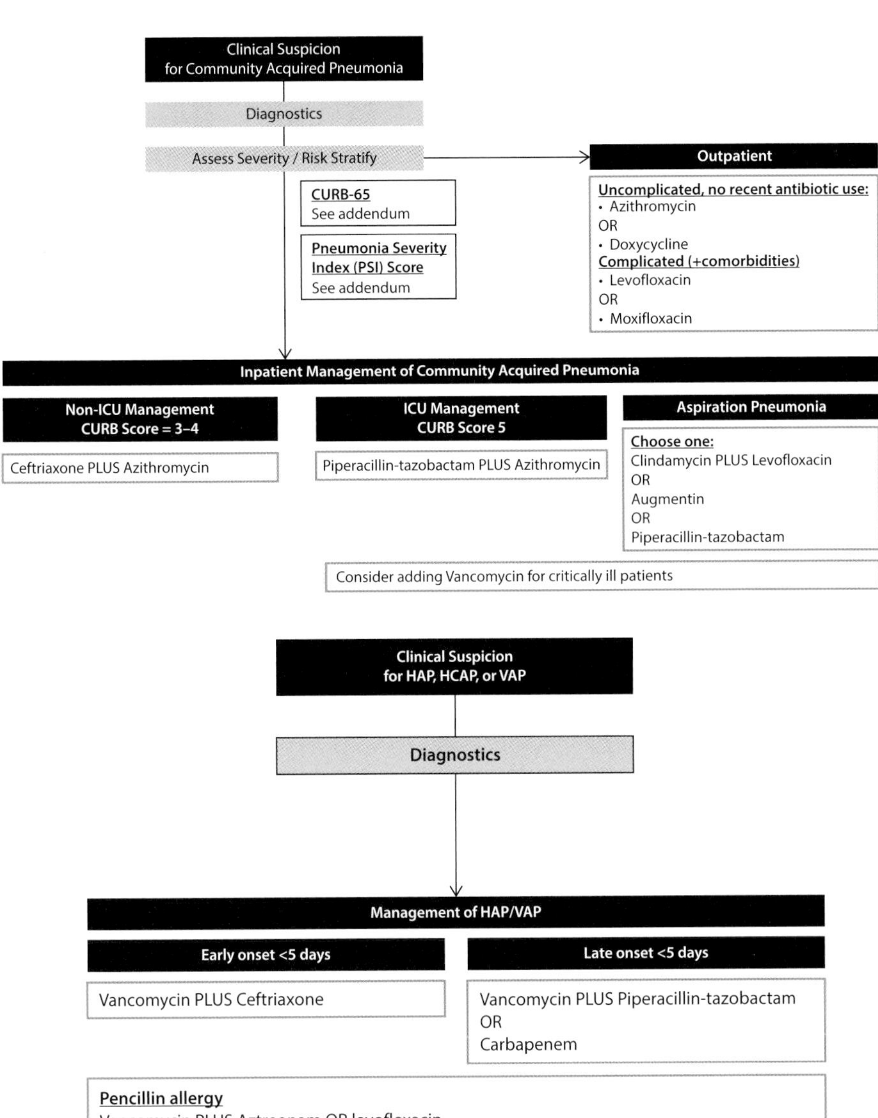

HIGH-YIELD LITERATURE

The IDSA Guidelines are the gold standard:

Mandell LA, Wunderink RG, Anzueto A, et al. Infectious Diseases Society of America/American Thoracic Society consensus guidelines on the management of community-acquired pneumonia in adults. *Clin Infect Dis*. 2007;44(Suppl 2):S27.

Kalil AC, Metersky ML, Klompas M, et al. Executive summary: Management of adults with hospital-acquired and ventilator-associated pneumonia: 2016 Clinical Practice Guidelines by the Infectious Diseases Society of America and the American Thoracic Society. *Clin Infect Dis*. 2016;63:575.

- In HAP, if your blood cultures are negative for 48 hours, consider de-escalating your antibiotic coverage to a CAP regimen.
- Duration of treatment is also an important concept. Recent guidelines and evidence support **5 days of treatment** if there is clinical improvement.

ASPIRATION PNEUMONIA

- This is a common diagnosis on the inpatient service, whether it's an admission from home or nursing home or with a patient who has respiratory distress in the hospital.
- Most aspiration pneumonias are chronic anaerobic infections with prolonged symptoms such as weight loss, foul-smelling sputum, and halitosis.
- Acute aspiration pneumonitis, a condition where patients become acutely tachypneic with increased oxygen requirements and acute infiltrates on CXR, can be confused with an aspiration pneumonia. The current guidelines are not to treat with antibiotics, but rather to support the patient with oxygen and monitor. Patients typically improve within 24 to 48 hours.
- True aspiration pneumonias can progress to chronic anaerobic necrotizing pneumonias with cavitary disease and lung abscess if untreated.
- The treatment usually involves a beta-lactam/beta-lactamase inhibitor such as amoxicillin clavulanate or clindamycin. Intravenous option includes ampicillin-sulbactam, piperacillin-tazobactam, or parenteral clindamycin.

VENTILATOR-ASSOCIATED PNEUMONIA

- This happens when patients are intubated, but treatment is the same as with HAP.

TUBERCULOSIS

General Facts

- Tuberculosis (TB) is a leading cause of death worldwide. In the United States, the incidence of TB decreased every year until 1984, when there was a resurgence during the HIV epidemic.
- Transmission occurs by inhalation of droplet nuclei produced by the cough or sneeze of a patient with pulmonary TB disease. Particles may remain suspended in the air for several hours.
- **High-prevalence groups** include HIV+ individuals, intravenous (IV) drug users, immunocompromised hosts, prisoners, homeless individuals, and persons in close contact with patients with known TB.
- TB can be classified as active TB or latent TB infection (LTBI). Active TB can be primary progressive (caused at the initial acquisition of TB prior to becoming LTBI) or reactivation (LTBI that becomes active). Most cases represent reactivation (90%).
- The risk of reactivation is 5% within the first 2 years and 5% in the lifetime after 2 years.

Sites of TB disease:

- **Lungs (85% of all cases)**
- **Central nervous system (TB meningitis)**
- **Lymphatics**
- **Genitourinary system**
- **Bones (Pott disease)**
- **Disseminated TB (miliary)**

Clinical Features

- The hallmark of active TB is chronic constitutional symptoms along with organ-specific symptoms. Latent TB, by definition, will not have active disease, and thus it is an asymptomatic phase.
- As a chronic infection, constitutional symptoms such as weight loss, anorexia, fatigue, night sweats, and fevers are common.
- **Pulmonary** symptoms such as chronic cough, hemoptysis, shortness of breath, or dyspnea on exertion can be present.

- **Radiographic** findings typical of **active TB** include upper lobe infiltrates and cavitary lung disease. Imaging can be atypical, with small nodular densities in hematogenous military TB.
- **Extrapulmonary** disease will have constitutional symptoms and end-organ manifestations that will depend on the affected organ system.

Diagnosis

- **LTBI** is diagnosed via a positive interferon gamma release assay (IGRA) or purified protein derivative (PPD) in an asymptomatic individual. The Bacillus Calmette–Guérin (BCG) vaccine can give a false-positive PPD, but this childhood vaccine is unlikely to do so in adults. Thus, a positive PPD in an adult with prior BCG immunization should not be considered a false positive (Table 9-4).
- **Active TB** is diagnosed by obtaining acid-fast bacilli (AFB) on microscopy from a clinical sample (sputum, bronchoalveolar lavage [BAL], other tissue or fluid) (Figure 9-1).
  - Three sputum samples are recommended, and the patient should be placed on airborne precautions to prevent transmission to health care workers.
  - A positive AFB from sputum should prompt a TB polymerase chain reaction (PCR) to differentiate between TB and non-TB *Mycobacteria* (NTM). Airborne precautions are not needed for NTM. A positive sputum for AFB in a patient with high suspicion for TB or a positive TB PCR is a measure of **infectivity**, the ability to infect other people.
  - A negative sputum AFB rules out infectivity but does not fully rule out TB. Cultures can take 6 weeks to grow and may yield positive results. In this scenario, the patient will have active TB but low infectivity.
  - Biopsy, AFB, culture, and *Mycobacterium* tuberculosis (MTB) PCR of all other tissues and body fluids can be performed, but the diagnosis of extrapulmonary TB is difficult due to the low sensitivity of available testing. Thus, clinical suspicion is important in making further management decisions.
  - Adenosine deaminase from pleural fluid >70 is suggestive of TB. A pleural biopsy and TB PCR can be done as well.
- Central nervous system (CNS) TB can manifest with lymphocytic pleocytosis, basal CNS abnormalities on magnetic resonance imaging (MRI), or cystic lesions known as tuberculomas.
- Renal TB can present with sterile pyuria. This occurs when leukocytes are seen on urine microscopy but Gram stain and cultures are negative (this stains bacteria but not *Mycobacteria*).

TABLE 9-4. Interpretation of PPD Skin Test

Measured Induration		
≥15 mm	≥10 mm	≥5 mm
All patients are considered infected	Considered infected if: ■ IV drug user ■ Foreign born ■ Medically underserved ■ Nursing home resident ■ Prisoner ■ Child under age 4 ■ Health care worker (you) ■ Other medical problems	Considered infected if: ■ HIV ■ Close contact ■ Abnormal CXR ■ Immunocompromised

CXR, chest x-ray; *HIV*, human immunodeficiency virus; *IV*, intravenous.

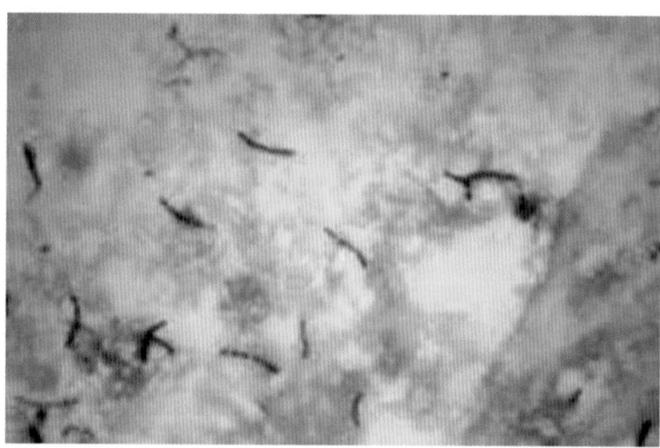

FIGURE 9-1. Acid-fast bacilli on smear. (Source: CDC, https://www.cdc.gov/tb/webcourses/tb101/page3294.html.)

Treatment

- **Latent TB:**
  - Rifampin daily for 4 months.
  - Isoniazid (INH) daily for 9 months (may be given twice weekly if directly observed therapy [DOT] is used).
  - Close contacts of active TB patients with positive PPD should be retested in 10 weeks.
  - Pregnant women should wait until after delivery for treatment unless high risk (e.g., HIV).
- **Active TB:**
  - Standard regimen for pulmonary TB: 2 months of INH, rifampin, pyrazinamide, and ethambutol followed by 4 months of INH/rifampin.
  - Pregnant with TB: 2 months of INH, rifampin, and ethambutol followed by INH and rifampin (no ethambutol) for 7 more months.
  - Meningeal, skeletal, and sometimes lymph node TB are treated with a longer duration of antituberculous antibiotics.
- People are considered no longer infectious when they are undergoing appropriate therapy, improving clinically, and have had 3 consecutive sputum smears on different days positive for TB.

Toxicity of Tuberculosis Medication

- **INH:**
  - Peripheral neuropathy (can be prevented with administration of pyridoxine).
  - Seizures in overdose: These can be very difficult to break with standard measures—remember to give pyridoxine!
  - Hepatitis (check liver function tests each month in select patients; routine testing not necessary).
- **Rifampin:**
  - Induces hepatic microsomal enzymes; also hepatotoxic.
  - Is excreted as a **red-orange compound in urine,** stool, sweat, and tears; will discolor contact lenses.
- **Ethambutol:** Optic neuritis and impaired color vision are related to cumulative dose.

A patient is brought in by ambulance in status epilepticus. The patient's family member says he has no medical history except TB. *Think*: *INH toxicity*. **Next step**: Treat with pyridoxine.

SKIN AND SOFT TISSUE INFECTIONS

General Facts

- Skin and soft tissue infections (SSTIs) are common clinical infections that are characterized by location and depth of infection.
  - **Impetigo, ecthyma, and erysipelas** are superficial or only to the dermis.
  - **Cellulitis** involves subcutaneous tissues.
  - **Necrotizing fasciitis** is an infection down to the fascia and muscles.
- Most SSTIs are caused by **streptococci and/or *Staphylococcus aureus***, with some notable exceptions such as necrotizing SSTIs, which can also include anaerobes or gram-negative pathogens.

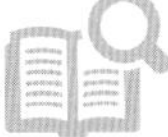

HIGH-YIELD LITERATURE

Stevens DL, Bisno, AL, Chambers HF, et al. Practice guidelines for the diagnosis and management of skin and soft tissue infections: 2014 update by the IDSA. *Clin Infect Dis*. 2014;59(2): e10–e52.

IMPETIGO AND ECTHYMA

- **Impetigo** is a superficial crusting and at times bullous infection of the skin. **Ecthyma** is localized progression into the dermis. Both infections **are more common in children**.
- **Group A streptococcus** is the primary pathogen historically, but *S. aureus* is actually now the most common cause, usually **methicillin-sensitive *S. aureus* (MSSA)**.

Clinical Features

- Impetigo starts as vesicular lesions that later develop a **golden, stuck-on-appearing crust**. There is also a less common bullous form.
- Ecthyma, as mentioned, is a deeper infection that results in ulcers with surrounding erythema.

Management

- For limited disease topical antibiotics are first line. If extensive disease, systemic therapy is used with dicloxacillin and cephalexin to cover S. aureus and streptococcus.

CELLULITIS AND ERYSIPELAS

General Facts

- **Cellulitis** is an acute spreading infection of the skin that extends to involve the subcutaneous tissues.
- **Erysipelas** is a more superficial infection (no subcutaneous tissue involvement) with group A streptococcus (Figure 9-2).
- **Group A streptococcus, other β-hemolytic streptococci, and *S. aureus*** are the most common causes.

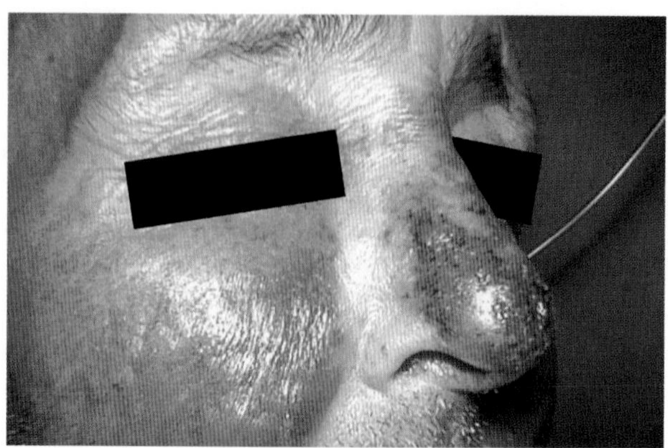

FIGURE 9-2. Erysipelas. (Source: CDC, https://phil.cdc.gov/details.aspx?pid=2874.)

Clinical Features

- **Cellulitis:** There are two types of cellulitis based on their clinical presentation, and it changes the choice of antibiotics as well as further management:
  - **Nonpurulent cellulitis** usually presents with fevers, erythema, edema, and tenderness and is usually caused by streptococcus.
  - **Purulent cellulitis** presents with nonpurulent cellulitis symptoms but has fluctuance or purulent drainage. Abscesses, folliculitis, and carbuncle (confluence of folliculitis) are common. The causative agent is often *S. aureus.*
- **Erysipelas**, as mentioned, is more superficial and is characterized by **very sharp demarcations** between the infected skin and the surrounding, uninvolved tissue. The involved tissue is **raised above the surrounding tissue** and can spread rapidly via lymphatics (lymphangitis).

Management

- **Nonpurulent cellulitis** and **erysipelas** can be managed with antibiotics alone. Oral beta-lactams can be used in mild cases, whereas IV beta-lactams with vancomycin may be needed for severe cases (Figure 9-3).

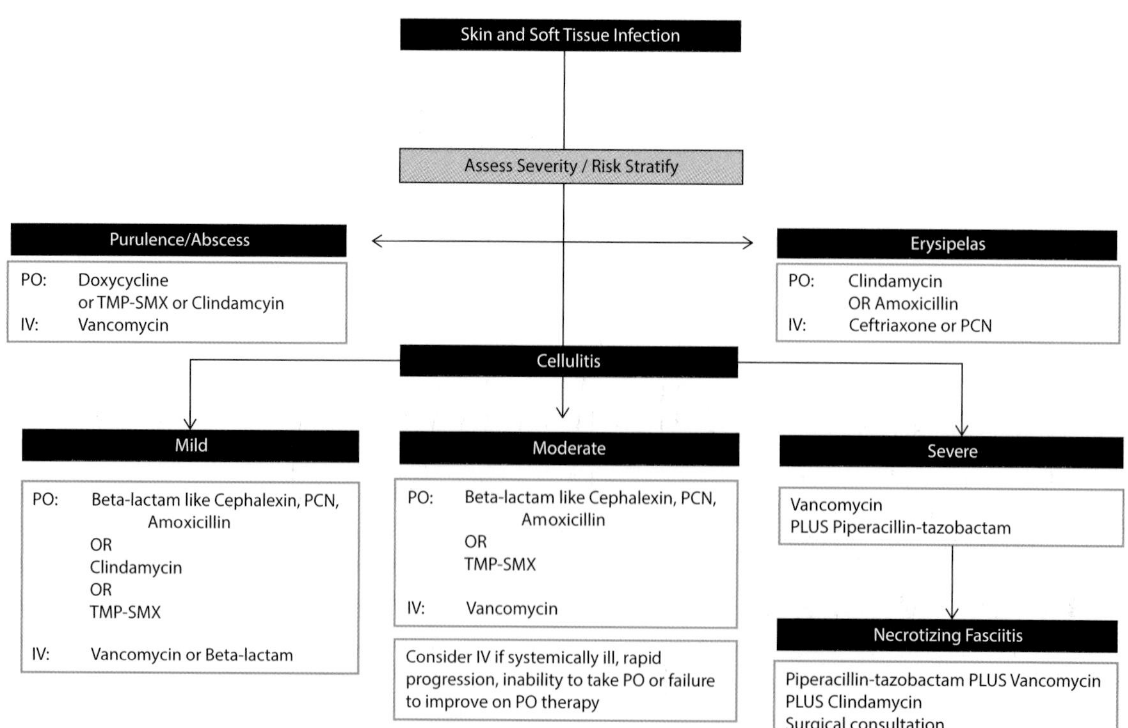

FIGURE 9-3. Management of soft tissue infections.

- **Purulent cellulitis** must undergo drainage of any drainable foci of infection (abscess, furuncle, etc.). Adjunctive antibiotics after drainage may improve outcomes.

CONQUER THE BOARDS!

Clinical scenario: An older man with cirrhosis goes swimming at the beach and then presents with fever, hypotension, and a bullous rash on his leg. What is the pathogen?

Answer:

Vibrio vulnificus. Vibrio can cause severe, necrotizing infections in patients with liver dysfunction.

NECROTIZING FASCIITIS

General Facts

- **Necrotizing fasciitis** is a life-threatening emergency characterized by deep, invasive SSTI, including involvement of the fascia, typically accompanied by marked systemic toxicity.

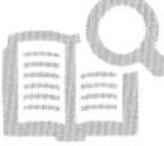

HIGH-YIELD LITERATURE

Talan DA, Mower WR, Krishnadasan A, et al. Trimethoprim-sulfamethoxazole versus placebo for uncomplicated skin abscess. *N Engl J Med*. 2016;374(9):823-832.

Stevens DL, Bisno AL, Chambers HF, et al. Practice guidelines for the diagnosis and management of skin and soft tissue infections: 2014 update by the Infectious Diseases Society of America. *Clin Infect Dis*. 2014;59(2):e10-52.

- Two types of necrotizing fasciitis are described.
  - **Type I** is a **polymicrobial infection with anaerobic bacteria** (*Bacteroides,* etc.) and aerobic gram-positives (streptococci other than group A) or gram negatives (*Klebsiella* spp., *Escherichia coli,* etc.).
  - **Type II** is usually monomicrobial, with **group A streptococcus** as the main pathogen.

Clinical Features

- **Rapid progression:** Initially patients have typical cellulitis findings, which can rapidly progress to more severe pain.
- **Pain out of proportion to palpation:** Extreme pain on palpation that is out of proportion to the skin findings. Sometimes the skin does not look red at all, and sometimes there is overt skin necrosis (bullae formation, ecchymosis) with skin crepitus.
- **Systemic toxicity:** Hypotension, tachycardia, rigors, and high fevers despite antibiotic treatment.

Diagnostic Workup

- You must have a high index of suspicion, as some of the clinical and lab signs are subtle and no different from a typical cellulitis.
- **Labs:** Show evidence of organ dysfunction and signs of systemic infection, such as a high white blood cell (WBC) count, a high C reactive protein (CRP), a high erythrocyte sedimentation rate, or a high lactate. But none of these is diagnostic.
- The LRINEC Score is an evidence-based score that can be used to calculate the probability of necrotizing fasciitis. The levels of CRP, WBC, Hgb, Na, Cr, and glucose are used to measure the severity.

- Among the patients with necrotizing fasciitis, 75% to 80% had a score ≥8, while only 7% to 10% had a score less than 6.
- **Imaging:** X-ray or CT scan is warranted if necrotizing fasciitis is suspected. Both can show gas formation in tissues or inflammation of the fascia.

Management

- **Surgery: Urgent surgical debridement of the affected tissues**. If necrotizing fasciitis is suspected, a surgical consult should be obtained urgently even before imaging (Figure 9-4).
- **Antibiotic**s should be immediately started, and empiric coverage consists of:
  - Vancomycin (anti-MRSA activity) plus piperacillin–tazobactam (a broad-spectrum beta-lactam with anaerobe coverage).
  - Clindamycin or linezolid can be added for antitoxin effects against toxin-elaborating strains of streptococci and staphylococci.

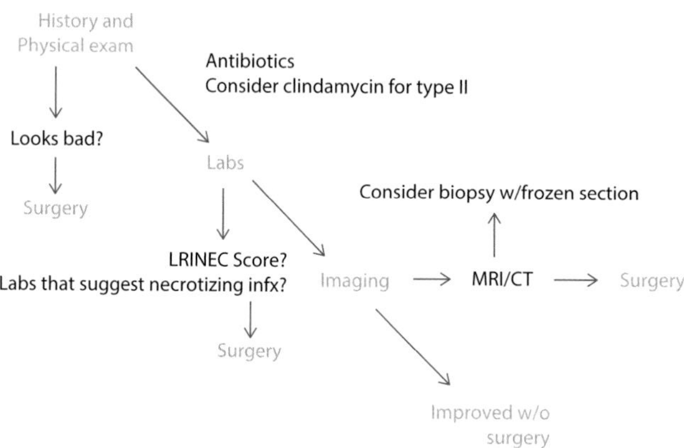

FIGURE 9-4. Workup of necrotizing fasciitis.

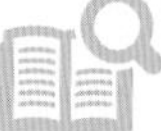

HIGH-YIELD LITERATURE

Stevens DL, Bryant AE. Necrotizing soft-tissue infections. *N Engl J Med.* 2017;377(23):2253.

Stevens DL, Bisno AL, Chambers HF, et al. Practice guidelines for the diagnosis and management of skin and soft tissue infections: 2014 update by the Infectious Diseases Society of America. *Clin Infect Dis.* 2014;59(2):e10-52

CONQUER THE WARDS!

Another medical device strongly associated with staphylococcal toxic shock syndrome is nasal packing material used for epistaxis.

TOXIC SHOCK SYNDROMES

General Facts

- **Toxic shock syndromes** (TSS) consist of an SSTI accompanied by systemic organ dysfunction, including hypotension secondary to bacterial toxin production.
- A patient with necrotizing fasciitis can also have TSS; they are simply clinical syndromes that can overlap.
- **Streptococcal TSS** secondary to group A streptococcus and its exotoxin. It most commonly begins as pharyngitis or an SSTI.
- **Staphylococcal TSS** secondary to an *S. aureus* toxin called TSST-1, historically associated with highly absorbent tampons, but also seen with packing of nose or other sites.

Clinical Features

- **Organ dysfunction + shock** (hypotension that does not respond to IV fluids) are the key hallmark.
- **Desquamating rash:** Patients with staphylococcal TSS also have a desquamating rash (also be aware that there is a toxin-mediated staphylococcal scalded skin syndrome, which causes a diffuse desquamating rash in NEONATES primarily).
- **Streptococcal TSS** typically has necrotizing skin infection as well (remember these syndromes can overlap).

Diagnostic Workup

- Diagnosis is confirmed with positive cultures from a sterile site with either group A streptococcus or *S. aureus.*

Management

- Supportive care is paramount for a patient in shock, in addition to any needed surgical debridement.
- Antibiotic therapy consists of:
  - Streptococcal TSS: Penicillin and clindamycin (for inhibition of the ribosome and reduction in toxin production).
  - Staphylococcal TSS: Vancomycin and clindamycin to ensure coverage of MRSA.

GENITOURINARY INFECTIONS

URINARY TRACT INFECTIONS

General Facts

- A **urinary tract infection (UTI)** is a general term encompassing infection anywhere from the urethral meatus to the kidneys. They are among the most common reasons patients receive antibiotics in any setting.
- The **presence of symptoms** is the most important factor in determining the need to treat.
- **An uncomplicated UTI** is one that occurs in healthy, nonpregnant females; all others are generally **complicated UTIs.**
- UTIs can be defined anatomically. For example, **cystitis** is an infection of the bladder, and **pyelonephritis** is an infection involving the renal parenchyma.
- Catheter-associated UTI (CAUTI) is a UTI in a patient with an indwelling urinary catheter.
- More common in women than men by a ratio of 30:1 from age 1 through 50; beyond age 50, the ratio is 2:1.
- Up to 60% of women have symptomatic UTIs during their lifespan, and 10% of women have UTIs each year. It is the most common infection in the elderly and in pregnancy.
- **Risk factors for UTI:** Uncircumcised men, benign prostatic hyperplasia (BPH), phimosis, recent sexual intercourse, pregnancy, postmenopausal state, use of spermicide, immunocompromised state, diabetes, catheterization, and genitourinary (GU) tract abnormalities.

Microbiology

- ***E. coli*** is the most common pathogen, accounting for 80% to 85% of community-acquired UTIs and 50% of nosocomial ones.

CONQUER THE **WARDS!**

Any male patient presenting with a UTI (especially if it is recurrent) should be investigated for evidence of **prostatitis and/or urinary obstruction**. If prostatitis is present, the patient typically has **severe pain with prostate palpation on DRE and requires prolonged antibiotic therapy (4 weeks)**.

CONQUER THE **BOARDS!**

If the urine **pH is alkaline** (>7.5), the patient likely has a urease-producing pathogen such as ***Proteus*** and she should be evaluated for **infected kidney** stones.

CONQUER THE
BOARDS!

Bugs that cause UTI:
SEEKS PP
S. saprophyticus
E. coli
Enterobacter
Klebsiella
Serratia
Proteus
Pseudomonas (especially with GU instrumentation)

- *Klebsiella* (and other enteric gram-negative bacteria), *Proteus, Pseudomonas,* and enterococci account for most of the remainder of cases.
- *Pseudomonas* is particularly important in CAUTI, infections associated with urologic procedures, and hospital-acquired infections.
- *Staphylococcus saprophyticus* can cause UTIs and even pyelonephritis in otherwise healthy young women.
- Group B streptococcus accounts for only ~1% of cases but is a clinically important pathogen in the pregnant patient at term—**always test third-trimester pregnant patients for this.**

Clinical Features

- Common complaints of UTI are dysuria, increased frequency, urgency, nocturia, suprapubic pain, cloudy, malodorous urine, or bloody urine.
- **Pyelonephritis** is a type of complicated UTI and is a clinical diagnosis characterized by fever, rigors, and especially flank pain and costovertebral angle tenderness. Treatment is similar to complicated UTI.

Diagnostic Workup

- **Initial workup** for a UTI always starts with a urinalysis and urine culture, and both clinical symptoms and urinalysis must be interpreted.
- **Urinalysis** is a rapid and cost-effective test that is fairly sensitive and specific for UTI. A urinalysis has three components: gross evaluation, urine dipstick, and microscopic examination. Following is what you will find in a UTI.
  - **Gross evaluation:** Turbid or normal.
  - **Urine dipstick:** The presence of leukocyte esterase and nitrites usually indicates a UTI.
    a. **Leukocyte esterase** correlates to pyuria—or leukocytes in the urine.
    b. **Nitrites** (made by certain common UTI bugs, e.g., Enterobacteriaceae).
- **Urinalysis** involves spinning down and directly visualizing the urine cells and sediment.
  - **WBCs:** The presence of WBCs (pyuria) (>5 WBCs is elevated) indicates infection.
  - **Red blood cells (RBCs):** Indicates hematuria, which is often seen in cystitis.
  - **Bacteria:** This can be seen in UTI, but can also be seen in colonized patients with no symptoms.

CONQUER THE
WARDS!

The three situations in which asymptomatic bacteriuria should be treated are (1) pregnancy, (2) prior to invasive urologic procedures, or (3) first 6 months post–kidney transplant. For testing purposes, treatment of pregnant patients is very important!

- **Urine culture** is the definitive test. A positive result is defined as >10,000 colony-forming units (CFUs) per milliliter with a single organism in symptomatic patients and >100,000 CFU/mL in an asymptomatic patient. Urine cultures should always be obtained for complicated UTIs due to the high rate of bacterial resistance.
- **Imaging** is not indicated for uncomplicated UTI and generally not indicated in complicated UTI. Imaging is necessary in the following situations and would usually be a renal ultrasound or CT scan with no contrast:
  - **Severely ill (hypotensive, altered mental status, and/or tachycardia).**
  - Persistent symptoms after 48 to 72 hours of appropriate antimicrobial therapy.
  - Suspected complication such as renal abscess or obstructive renal disease.

Management

- **Uncomplicated UTIs:** Treat with a short course (3 to 5 days) of oral antibiotics on an outpatient basis (Figure 9-5).
  - Nitrofurantoin and sulfamethoxazole–trimethoprim are first-line empiric agents.

- **Complicated UTIs:** As mentioned earlier, any UTI that is not in a healthy, nonpregnant female or has extended beyond the bladder is considered a complicated UTI.
  - **Empiric antibiotics** should be started based on previous microbiology data or risk factors for MDR bacteria.
  - **Complicated UTIs** can be treated for a total of 5 to 7 days, but may depend on symptomatic improvement.
  - CAUTI typically can receive 7 days of treatment with oral antibiotics if they are stable.
- **Asymptomatic bacteriuria:** Sometimes urine cultures are sent for another workup or preoperatively. Unless the patient has clinical symptoms of UTI, there is no need to treat with antibiotics.
- Consider hospitalization and IV antibiotics for high-risk patients: elderly, immunocompromised, those with indwelling catheters, sepsis, and patients who are unable to tolerate oral intake.

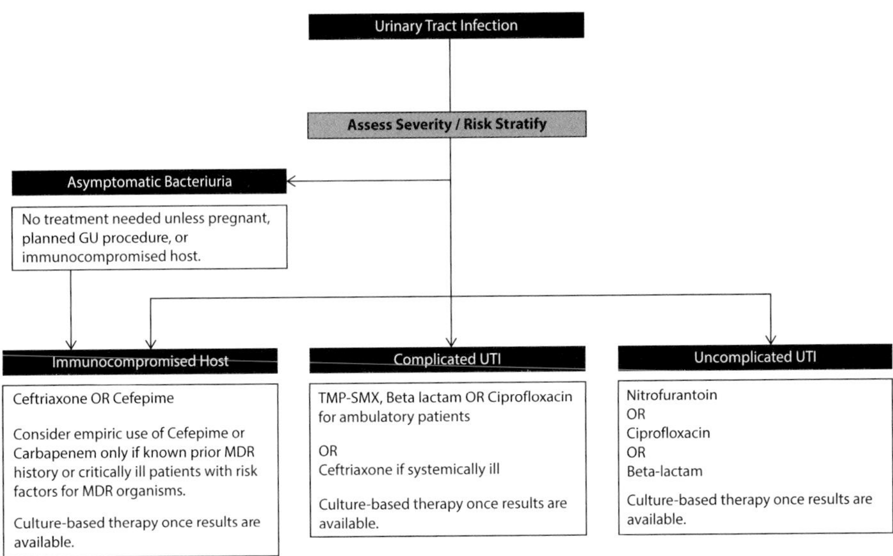

FIGURE 9-5. Management of UTI.

HIGH-YIELD LITERATURE

Levison ME, Kaye D. Treatment of complicated urinary tract infections with an emphasis on drug-resistant gram-negative uropathogens. *Curr Infect Dis Rep*. 2013;15(2):109-115.

Hoepelman AI, Meiland R, Geerlings SE. Pathogenesis and management of bacterial urinary tract infections in adult patients with diabetes mellitus. *Int J Antimicrob Agents*. 2003;22(Suppl 2):35-43.

HIGH-YIELD LITERATURE

Hooton TM, Bradley SF, Cardenas DD, et al. Diagnosis, prevention, and treatment of catheter-associated urinary tract infection in adults: 2009 International Clinical Practice Guidelines from the Infectious Diseases Society of America. *Clin Infect Dis*. 2010;50(5):625–663.

Gupta K, Hooton TM, Naber KG, et al. Practice guidelines for the treatment of acute uncomplicated cystitis and pyelonephritis in women: A 2010 update by the Infectious Diseases Society of America and the European Society for Microbiology and Infectious *Diseases. Clin Infect Dis*. 2011;52(5):e103–e120.

VAGINITIS

General Facts

- The normal flora of the vagina creates an acidic environment (pH 3.5 to 4.5) in large part through the colonization of lactobacilli to protect the vagina from pathogenic organisms.
- When this environment is disturbed, infections become possible.
- Greater than 90% of cases are caused by the following:
  - Bacterial vaginosis: Shift of bacterial flora away from *Lactobacillus.*
  - Trichomoniasis.
  - *Candida* vulvovaginitis.

CONQUER THE BOARDS!

Any patient presenting with **recurrent** *Trichomonas* should be asked if her sexual partners have been treated as well. **Without treatment of a patient's partners, reinfection can occur.**

Clinical Features

- Typically, patients will have a combination of symptoms that include vaginal pruritis, burning sensation, abnormal odor, pain, and dyspareunia.
- Specific pathogens can have additional signs and symptoms.
  - *Trichomonas* can have a fishy odor with an inflamed "strawberry" cervix.
  - *Candida* can have a cottage cheese–appearing discharge.

CONQUER THE BOARDS!

The "whiff" test: Application of KOH to the wet mount will enhance the odor of both ***Gardnerella*** and ***Trichomonas.***

Diagnostic Workup

- **Vaginal pH**: Single most important test that drives the diagnostic process. A pH test stick is applied to the vaginal sidewall.
  - **pH 4 to 4.5** – suggestive of ***Candida* vulvovaginitis.**
  - **pH >4.5** – suggestive of **bacterial vaginosis.**
  - **pH 5 to 6** – suggestive of **trichomoniasis.**
- **Microscopy** is the next test done:
  - **Wet mount**: 1 to 2 drops of 0.9% normal saline are added to a slide with vaginal discharge and examined under a microscope:
    a. **Clue cells** (epithelial cells coated with bacteria) and/or **motile trichomonads** = *Trichomonas.*
    b. **Hyphae** or **pseudohyphae** = *Candida.*
  - **Potassium hydroxide (KOH) wet mount**: This is the addition of 10% KOH to the wet mount to help confirm what is seen:
    a. **Candida –** KOH destroys cellular elements, which is helpful in identifying hyphae and budding yeast of *Candida.*
    b. **Bacterial vaginosis** – KOH enhances the odor of *Trichomonas* with a fishy (amine) odor – "whiff test."

Management

- **Metronidazole** is the treatment of choice for bacterial vaginosis and *Trichomonas.*
- Treat sexual partners as well in *Trichomonas* (sexually transmitted).
- **Azole antifungals or nystatin** for *Candida* infection.

CONQUER THE WARDS!

Warn patients against having any alcohol while on metronidazole. It can **cause a disulfiram-like reaction** (**nausea and emesis**) when ingested with alcohol.

EPIDURAL ABSCESS

General Facts

- Infection of the spine involving a vertebral body (vertebral osteomyelitis) and subsequently developing an adjacent abscess in the epidural space.
- Spinal abscesses are most commonly found in the immunosuppressed, IV drug users, and the elderly.

- An abscess can form anywhere along the spinal cord, and as it expands, it compresses against the spinal cord and occludes the vasculature.
- ***S. aureus***, gram-negative bacilli (**think *Pseudomonas* in the setting of intravenous drug use [IVDU]**), and *Mycobacterium tuberculosis* (if risk factors present) are most common causes.

Clinical Features

- Presents with a triad of pain, fever, and progressive weakness of legs (focal neuromuscular weakness).

Diagnostic Workup

- MRI can localize the lesion.
- Lumbar puncture (LP) is not required unless meningitis is suspected.
- Emergent neurosurgical evaluation is needed.

Management

- Neurosurgical management may include drainage and stabilization of the vertebra.
- Antibiotics is the definitive treatment and must be initiated early.

CONQUER THE **WARDS!**

Any patient presenting with back pain and a "red flag" symptom/risk factor should get imaging (MRI typically). Red flags include **fever, history of cancer, and new neurologic symptoms (incontinence, weakness, lack of sensation, etc.).**

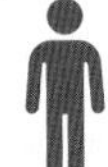

An IV drug user presents with fever of 1 week's duration and new-onset lower extremity weakness. *Think: Epidural abscess. Next step*: Order emergent MRI of spine, start empiric broad-spectrum antibiotics if positive.

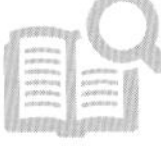

HIGH-YIELD LITERATURE

Berbari EF, Kanj SS, Kowalski TJ, et al. 2015 Infectious Diseases Society of America (IDSA) clinical practice guidelines for the diagnosis and treatment of native vertebral osteomyelitis in adults. *Clin Infect Dis*. 2015;61(6):e26-46.

HUMAN IMMUNODEFICIENCY VIRUS AND ACQUIRED IMMUNODEFICIENCY SYNDROME

General Facts

- **AIDS** is defined as an HIV-infected individual with a CD4 <200 or an AIDS-defining condition regardless of CD4 count. Major AIDS-defining conditions are:
  - Candidiasis.
  - Cervical cancer.
  - Cryptococcal disease.
  - Cytomegalovirus (CMV) retinitis.
  - Kaposi sarcoma.
  - Progressive multifocal leukoencephalopathy (*Pneumocystis jiroveci* pneumonia [PJP]).
  - CNS toxoplasmosis.

CONQUER THE **BOARDS!**

CD4 count prophylaxis thresholds:
<200: PJP prophylaxis – sulfamethoxazole–trimethoprim
<100: Toxoplasmosis – sulfamethoxazole–trimethoprim
<50: *Mycobacterium avium* complex (MAC)—azithromycin

CONQUER THE WARDS!

Patients at high risk for HIV acquisition:

- Men who have sex with men (MSM) with high-risk behavior (condomless sex, etc.)
- Heterosexual patients with high-risk behavior
- Serodiscordant couples
- IV drug users

All are candidates for pre-exposure prophylaxis (**PrEP**) with tenofovir–emtricitabine to prevent acquiring HIV.

CONQUER THE BOARDS!

Unlike PrEP, patients with a potential exposure to HIV (occupational or nonoccupational) should be on **postexposure prophylaxis** (PEP) which consists of a **full 3-drug regimen**.

First line is tenofovir–emtricitabine with dolutegravir.

CONQUER THE BOARDS!

In a patient presenting with **acute retroviral** syndrome, there is **window period of about 4 weeks** (patient has true HIV infection but the screening test is negative) even for the fourth-generation HIV Ab/Ag screening test.

The test of choice for diagnosing acute retroviral syndrome is an **HIV viral load (PCR)**.

- In the United States growing access to effective, safe antiviral medications has shifted the management of HIV from one of dealing with primarily acute AIDS complications to chronic disease management.
- **HIV transmission** is through sexual contact and via body fluids. Transmission via contaminated injection drug syringes is on the rise.

Clinical Features

Acute HIV Infection

- Some patients are asymptomatic.
- **Acute retroviral syndrome** describes a constellation of symptoms that is associated with acute symptomatic HIV infection. The symptoms are nonspecific and similar to a viral syndrome, so many are not diagnosed.
  Time course: 3 to 6 weeks after primary infection, and symptoms last about 1 week.
  Symptoms: The most common findings are fever (75% of patients), fatigue (68%), myalgia (49%), and headache (45%). Other common findings are:
  - Lymphadenopathy (39%): Typically nontender and in the axillary, cervical, or occipital nodes.
  - Pharyngitis (40%): Painful ulcerations are distinctive for HIV infection.
  - Maculopapular rash (48%).

  Nausea and diarrhea are common because the gastrointestinal (GI) tract is a primary target during acute HIV infection.

Chronic HIV infection

- Clinical latency subsequently occurs after an acute HIV infection, but continued decline of CD4 T cells occurs due to viral cytotoxicity, and CD4 counts fall approximately 50 cells/μL/year.

TABLE 9-5. Diseases Associated with CD4 Thresholds in AIDS and Prophylaxis for These Conditions

CD4 Counts			
350	**200**	**100**	**50**
■ Pneumococcal pneumonia	■ Kaposi sarcoma	■ Toxoplasmosis	■ MAC
	■ Tuberculosis	■ Disseminated *Candida*	■ Cytomegalovirus
	■ Oral thrush	■ Cryptococcosis	■ PML
	■ Oral hairy leukoplakia		
	■ PJP		
	■ Lymphoma		
Prophylaxis	**200**	**100**	**50**
	PJP: Primary prophylaxis with TMP-SMX, dapsone, atovaquone, or inhaled pentamidine	Toxoplasmosis: Primary prophylaxis with Bactrim or dapsone plus pyrimethamine plus leucovorin	MAC: Primary prophylaxis with azithromycin or clarithromycin

MAC, *Mycobacterium avium* complex; PJP, *Pneumocystis jiroveci* pneumonia; PML, progressive multifocal leukoencephalopathy (JC virus).

- AIDS (CD4 <200) ensues, usually within 6 to 10 years.
- As CD4 counts drop, patients become highly susceptible to opportunistic diseases (see Table 9-5). For more details on treatment, see the section Opportunistic Infections.

Management of HIV

Goal: The goal of HIV treatment is virologic suppression and restoration of immune function. This leads to reduction in transmission and improved morbidity and mortality.

Treatment:

- Any patient diagnosed with HIV should be started on therapy **as soon as feasible, regardless of CD4 count.**
- **HIV genotype testing** should be ordered to make sure no resistance is present and to modify the regimen if it is.
- Patients should be started on **3 drugs from at least 2 different drug classes.**

  First-line regimens include 2 nucleoside reverse transcriptase inhibitors (NRTIs) (tenofovir/emtricitabine or abacavir/lamivudine) and an integrase inhibitor (dolutegravir, etc.).
- The major drug classes for HIV therapy are reverse transcriptase inhibitors (nucleoside analogs and nonnucleoside), protease inhibitors, fusion inhibitors, and integrase inhibitors.
- **Nucleoside analog reverse transcriptase inhibitors (NRTIs):** Act as DNA chain terminator. These medications are the backbone of most HIV regimens. Important NRTIs to be familiar with are zidovudine (AZT), abacavir, emtricitabine, lamivudine, and tenofovir.
  - **Tenofovir** is the most commonly used NRTI. Main side effects are nephrotoxicity and bone toxicity (osteoporosis).
  - **Zidovudine (AZT):** First drug approved for HIV treatment. Main side effects include headache, malaise, nausea, fatigue (often subside with extended therapy), macrocytic anemia secondary to low erythropoietin (can be managed with recombinant erythropoietin injections), and proximal myopathy.
  - **Abacavir:** NRTI that is safe in renal disease. Main side effect is life-threatening hypersensitivity reaction in patients who are HLAB5701 positive. Must check HLAB5701 on EVERY patient prior to starting.
  - **Lamivudine and emtricitabine** are used in combination with the earlier-mentioned NRTIs. No major side effects to be aware of.
- **Nonnucleoside reverse transcriptase inhibitors (NNRTIs):** Bind to reverse transcriptase outside the active site and cause conformational changes that decrease enzyme activity. The most important NNRTIs include efavirenz, etravirine, and rilpivirine.
  - **Efavirenz**: No longer first line due to neurotoxicity. It may cause vivid dreams and increases the risk of suicide in patients with psychiatric comorbidities.
  - **Rilpivirine**: Well tolerated. Contraindicated in patients with HIV viremia above 100,000 copies.
  - **Etravirine**: Main side effect is a self-limited rash and possible sulfa cross-reactivity.
- **Protease inhibitors (PIs)** are potent antiretrovirals that inhibit the activity of HIV protease. They are less toxic than the reverse transcriptase inhibitors

CONQUER THE **BOARDS!**

Tenofovir can cause **Fanconi syndrome** (proximal tubular toxicity) manifested by AKI, electrolyte abnormalities, and **glucosuria without hyperglycemia**.

CONQUER THE **BOARDS!**

There are a substantial number of ARVs and many combination tablets. **Focusing on specific side effects and understanding the basic classes/mechanisms are the most important aspects.**

but have CYP450-related drug interactions. Important PIs to be familiar with include atazanavir, ritonavir, and darunavir.

- **Atazanavir**: Should be used with a pharmacologic boosting agent such as ritonavir. Main side effects are nephrolithiasis and asymptomatic indirect hyperbilirubinemia.
- **Ritonavir**: Mainly used in low doses to boost other protease inhibitors. LOTS of drug interactions.
- **Darunavir**: Main side effects are a rash and possible sulfa cross-reactivity.

- **Integrase inhibitor:** Now are first-line drugs in combination with 2 NRTIs, since they have a favorable side-effect profile. They prevent the insertion of the viral genome into host DNA. Important integrase inhibitors to be familiar with include raltegravir, elvitegravir, and dolutegravir.
  - Raltegravir: Longest clinical experience and has the fewest drug–drug interactions in its class.
  - Elvitegravir: Must be given with a boosting agent such as cobicistat.
  - Dolutegravir: High barrier to resistance and so often used before genotype testing. Major side effect is increased neuropsychiatric effects and possible neural tube defects in utero.
- **Fusion inhibitors:** Very rarely used agents in the modern era. They are mainly used in combination therapy regimens for patients with drug-resistant virus. **Maraviroc** prevents HIV binding and entry into cells by binding CCR5, and **enfuvirtide** prevents HIV virion fusion with cells by binding gp41.

CONQUER THE BOARDS!

The average AIDS patient with PJP has **symptoms for 2 to 3 weeks** before presenting for care. It is a more subacute pneumonia than typical bacterial pathogens like *S. pneumoniae*.

Special Situations

- **After needle stick:** The **occupational transmission rates after** skin puncture from blood-contaminated sharp object from person with documented HIV infection is 0.3%. **Postexposure prophylaxis** and wound cleansing after exposure decrease rate of HIV seroconversion by 79% (to 0.06% for HIV).
- **Pregnancy: HIV**-positive mothers transmit HIV to infants intrapartum, perinatally, or via breast milk. Transmission rate from untreated mother to newborn is approximately 25% perinatally, and 7% to 22% via breastmilk. This can be mitigated with antiretroviral therapy or peripartum antiretrovirals.

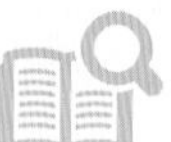

HIGH-YIELD LITERATURE

Adult and adolescent ARV guidelines:

U.S. Department of Health and Human Services. AIDSInfo. Clinical Guidelines. Accessed from https://aidsinfo.nih.gov/guidelines.

OPPORTUNISTIC INFECTIONS

Although the following diseases are often seen in patients with AIDS, they can be seen in any patient who is immunocompromised.

PNEUMOCYSTIS JIROVECI PNEUMONIA

General Facts

- Formerly known as *Pneumocystis carinii, PJP* is the most common initial AIDS-defining illness in the United States. It is seen largely in patients who are not aware of their HIV status or are not receiving/adhering to treatment.

Clinical Features

- Symptoms are gradual in onset over days to weeks.
- Most commonly fever, dry cough, and progressive dyspnea along with weight loss.
- Decreased oxygen saturation is often present at rest.

Diagnostic Workup

- **Imaging:** CXR usually shows bilateral interstitial infiltrate, but some patients can actually have a normal CXR. However, chest CT is ALWAYS abnormal in PJP.
- **Direct fluorescence antibody (DFA):** Pneumocystis cannot be cultured, so it must be seen directly using immunofluorescent staining of sputum. Initially start with **sputum induction** (where a respiratory therapist administers nebulized hypertonic saline, which liquefies airway secretions and induces expectoration of deep respiratory secretions). However, if this is not diagnostic, then **bronchoscopy** should be done for **BAL**, which is the best way to obtain samples but is more invasive.
- **Other labs:** Lactate dehydrogenase (LDH) can be sent and is often elevated, but it is a nonspecific test. 1-3-Beta-D-glucan can be elevated in PJP, as it is a component of the PJP cell wall; however, many institutions do not have this test.

A 34-year-old patient with uncontrolled HIV presents with 2 weeks of weight loss, dry cough, dyspnea, **hypoxemia**, and vague bilateral infiltrates on chest x-ray. *Think: PJP.* **Next step:** Provide supplemental oxygen and start TMP-SMZ.

Management

- **TMP-SMZ is the drug of choice** and should be empirically started if PJP is suspected in a patient with a low CD4 (Figure 9-6).
- **Glucocorticoids** should be started in any AIDS patient with severe PJP defined as **PaO_2 <70 mm Hg or Alveolar–arterial (A-a) oxygen gradient*** **>35 mm Hg.** It should be started no later than 36 to 72 hours after starting TMP-SMZ. Steroids decrease mortality by approximately 50%.
- Patients get worse before they get better and will not improve until the end of the first week of treatment.
    - May give pentamidine for patients intolerant of TMP-SMZ.
- **Prophylaxis in patients with CD4 <200 or previous PJP:** Give TMP-SMZ or dapsone in sulfa-allergic patients or aerosolized pentamidine for those unable to take systemic prophylaxis.

TOXOPLASMOSIS

General Facts

- Most common cause of secondary CNS infection in AIDS.
- Seroprevalence in the United States is 15%.
- Toxoplasmic encephalitis occurs in one-third of all seropositive AIDS patients without prophylaxis.

*Many online calculators are available but require you to know FiO_2 patient is breathing, arterial blood CO_2, and arterial PaO_2, and high gradients result from impaired diffusion in the lung.

CONQUER THE **WARDS!**

Toxoplasmosis in an AIDS patient is **nearly always a reactivation disease**, so if a patient has a negative toxoplasma IgG test, it essentially rules out the diagnosis.

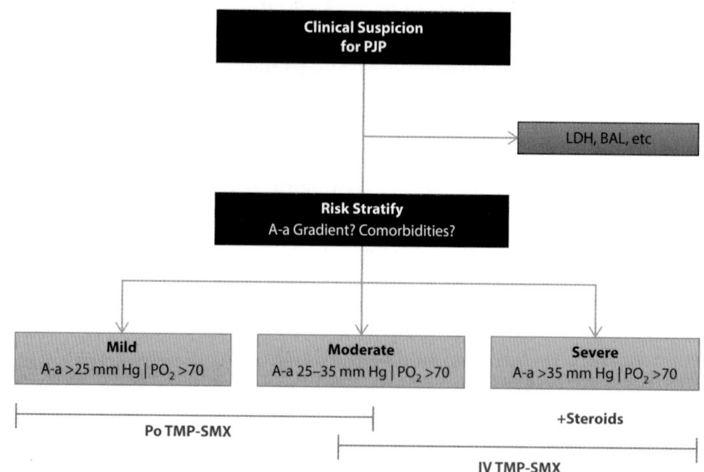

FIGURE 9-6. Management of PJP.

Clinical Features

- Common manifestations include fever, headache, and focal neurologic deficits (90%).
- Seizure, hemiparesis, and aphasia also occur.

Diagnostic Workup

- MRI or head CT with contrast shows **multiple ring-enhancing lesions** (Figures 9-7 and 9-8).
- IgG antibodies to *Toxoplasma*.
- It is usually a clinical diagnosis, comparing the likelihood of toxoplasmosis with other causes of ring-enhancing lesions in HIV patients, chief among them lymphoma.

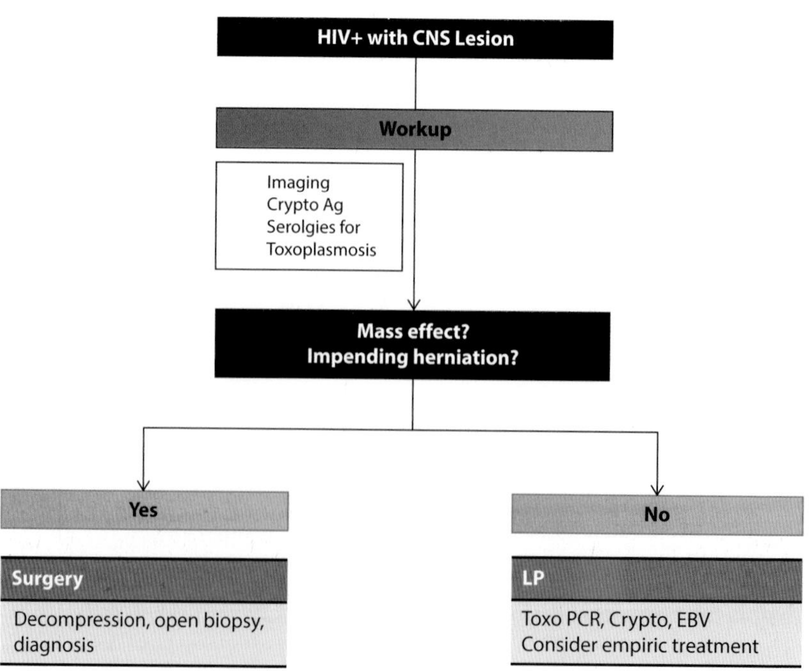

FIGURE 9-7. Management of brain lesions.

Management

- **Pyrimethamine** and **sulfadiazine** is the drug regimen of choice. Watch for leukopenia as the major side effect (treat leukopenia with folinic acid).
- Lifelong treatment for toxoplasmosis is necessary, due to relapse rate of 50% within 6 months.
- TMP-SMZ given for PJP prophylaxis is also effective as prophylaxis against toxoplasmic encephalitis. Patients with CD4 count <100 should receive prophylaxis against *Toxoplasma.*

PROTOZOAL DIARRHEA IN AIDS

General Facts

- Diarrhea caused by opportunistic pathogens, including cryptosporidia, microsporidia, *Cyclospora*, and *Isospora belli.*

Clinical Features

- All can present with protracted, watery diarrhea, usually in patients with CD4 <10.

Management

- All HIV patients with diarrhea should have stool cultures done for the noted pathogens and *Clostridium difficile.*

  Cryptosporidia and **microsporidia** are treated with paromomycin or erythromycin.
- ***Isospora:*** TMP-SMZ.
- Main treatment is to reconstitute the immune system with antiretrovirals (ARVs).

A 32-year-old HIV-positive patient with a low CD4 count presents with 3 months of watery diarrhea. *Think: Cryptosporidiosis.* **Next step:** Check stool for ova and parasites (O&P). Effective antiretroviral treatment is best therapy + nitazoxanide or paromomycin.

MYCOBACTERIUM AVIUM COMPLEX

General Facts

- Disseminated *Mycobacterium avium* is a marker of advanced immune suppression; it typically occurs when CD4 count is <50.
- Median survival after *Mycobacterium avium* complex (MAC) diagnosis is 6 to 8 months (without treatment).

Clinical Features

- Fever, cough, weight loss, and night sweats are the most common symptoms.
- Lymphadenopathy, abdominal pain, and diarrhea can also occur.

A 29-year-old HIV-positive patient presents with CD4 count of 100, unexplained fever, and elevated alkaline phosphatase. *Think: MAC.*

Diagnostic Workup

- **Induced sputum:** Initially will show long, slender, AFB on stain and confirmed with culture of sputum.
- **CXR**: 25% have bilateral lower lobe interstitial infiltrate.
- Alkaline phosphatase level is sometimes elevated.

Management

- Clarithromycin or azithromycin and ethambutol.
- Prophylaxis: Azithromycin or clarithromycin when CD4 drops below 50.

TUBERCULOSIS AND HIV

- Estimated to be the cause of death in 13% of AIDS patients worldwide.
- HIV increases risk of developing active TB by 15 to 30 times.
- HIV disease progresses more rapidly in patients with active TB.

An AIDS patient being treated for TB has clinical worsening of his TB following initiation of antiretroviral therapy. *Think: Immune reconstitution inflammatory syndrome (IRIS).* **Next step:** Supportive care and/or corticosteroids.

CANDIDIASIS

General Facts

- *Candida* infections are the most common fungal infections in HIV-negative patients, and virtually all HIV patients experience some form of *Candida* infection during their illness.
- Candidiasis is often the first sign of immunosuppression and the first AIDS-defining illness in HIV patients.
- Thrush is the most common *Candida* infection, with white, cheesy exudates on the posterior oropharynx.
- *Candida* infections of the lungs, esophagus, trachea, and bronchi, along with **esophagitis,** can happen in advanced AIDS.

Management

- Oral and vaginal *Candida*: Oral fluconazole; topical nystatin or clotrimazole troches are also effective.
- Severe cases, including esophageal candidiasis, must be treated with systemic therapy (oral itraconazole or oral/IV fluconazole).

CONQUER THE WARDS!

Think of three main causes of infectious esophagitis in an AIDS patient:

- **HSV**
- **CMV**
- ***Candida***

Diagnosis typically made by **EGD with biopsy.**

CRYPTOCOCCAL MENINGITIS

General Facts

- *Cryptococcus neoformans* is the leading cause of **meningitis** in AIDS patients.
- Highest risk when CD4 count is <50.

Clinical Features

- **Subacute meningoencephalitis, with fever,** nausea, and vomiting (40%); altered mental status; headache; and meningeal signs.
- Symptoms of elevated intracranial pressure, such as vision changes, vomiting, and headache, can also occur.

CONQUER THE BOARDS!

A critical component of managing cryptococcal meningitis is **lowering the intracranial pressure (if elevated opening pressure on LP)**, either via serial lumbar puncture or lumbar drain placement.

Diagnostic Workup

- **Imaging:** This is often done first, given the altered mental status, but a variety of findings on CT or MRI can be seen and are not diagnostic. Findings can range from normal to mass lesions such as cryptococcomas, hydrocephalus, or ring-enhancing or cystic lesions.
- **LP:** Must be done to diagnose cryptococcal antigen in cerebrospinal fluid (CSF) or serum is usually diagnostic.
- India ink stain of CSF shows organism, but this test is now rarely done.

Management

- Amphotericin B for 6 weeks in combination with flucytosine for CSF disease.
- Because 50% of patients relapse after therapy is stopped, fluconazole should be given for at least 1 year, but may need to be continued indefinitely until CD4 recovers.

ASPERGILLUS FUMIGATUS

- *Aspergillus* infections are a major issue for patients with neutropenia related to hematologic malignancy, chemotherapy, or stem cell transplant (less so in AIDS). In immunocompetent patients with chronic lung disease, *Aspergillus* can cause fungus ball (aspergilloma) in preexisting lung cavities or chronic pulmonary infection.
- Mold with acute-angle branching and septated hyphae.
- Acquired through inhalation of spores in soil and decay.
- Immunocompetent individuals can get an allergic hypersensitivity reaction; not invasive (wheezing); treat with steroids.
- Invasive aspergillosis is seen in immunocompromised patients and can present as rapidly progressive, necrotizing pulmonary infiltrates and tracheobronchitis. Can cause life-threatening hemoptysis.
- Lung biopsy is needed for definitive diagnosis.
- Extrapulmonary sites: Sinusitis, CNS, skin, and osteomyelitis.
- Voriconazole is the drug of choice for *Aspergillus* (shown to be superior to amphotericin; see later).

CONQUER THE

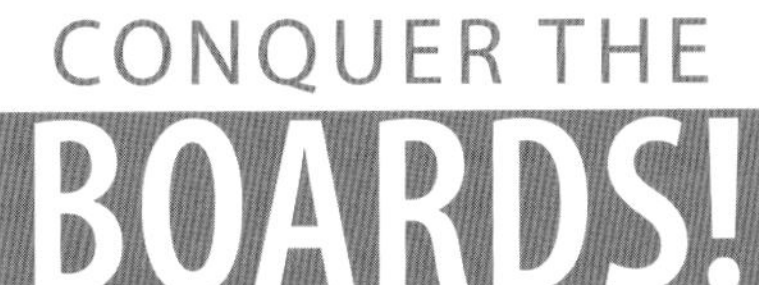

Allergic bronchopulmonary aspergillosis (ABPA): A hypersensitivity reaction in immunocompetent people, causing severe obstructive lung disease, wheezing, and bronchiectasis. Treat with steroids. Not an infection!

HIGH-YIELD LITERATURE

Herbrecht R, Denning DW, Patterson TF, et al. Voriconazole versus amphotericin B for primary therapy of invasive aspergillosis. *N Engl J Med.* 2002;347:408.

CYTOMEGALOVIRUS

General Facts

- Ninety-five percent of HIV-positive patients are CMV IgG positive, and clinical syndromes most often represent reactivation of latent infection (see Figure 9-8).

Clinical Features

- **CMV retinitis** is a dreaded HIV complication; presents with painless, progressive vision loss; may complain of "floaters."
- CMV can also cause many other end-organ infections (pneumonia, hepatitis, colitis).

CONQUER THE BOARDS!

The main toxicity of ganciclovir is **bone marrow suppression.** Patients need close monitoring for cytopenias.

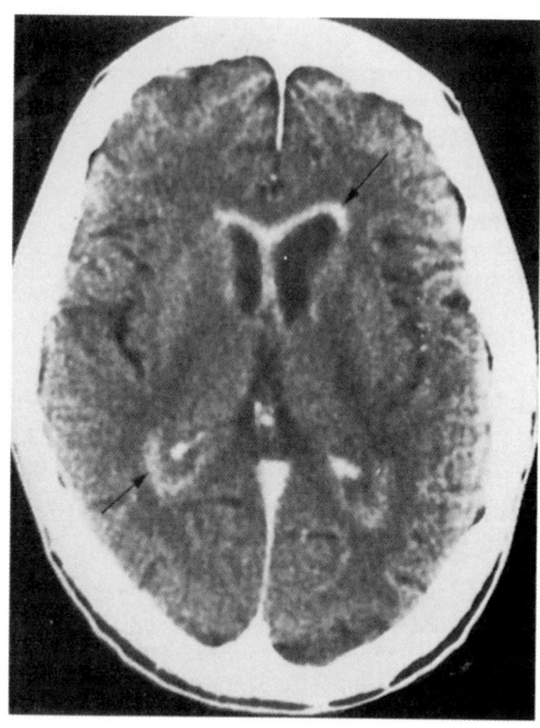

FIGURE 9-8. Cytomegalovirus infection in an AIDS patient. Note diffuse periventricular enhancement. (Reproduced, with permission, from Lee SH, Rao K, Zimmerman RA [eds]. *Cranial MRI and CT.* New York: McGraw-Hill, 1999.)

Diagnostic Workup

- Fundoscopy shows **perivascular hemorrhage and exudates** in CMV retinitis.
- Systemic CMV reactivation can be diagnosed via blood CMV PCR.

Management

- **Ganciclovir** (ocular injections can be used for eye disease) is the drug of choice for serious CMV infections. Resistant viruses can be treated with foscarnet.
- CMV Ab–negative patients should receive blood products from CMV-negative donors if at all possible.

HERPES SIMPLEX VIRUS

- Herpes simplex virus (HSV) in HIV manifests as recurrent orolabial, genital, and perianal lesions.
- Can cause herpetic esophagitis (beefy red and painful esophagus).
- Can cause recurrent **herpetic whitlow** (painful nodular lesions usually found on fingers).
- Treat with acyclovir, famciclovir, or valacyclovir.

An HIV-positive patient presents with a painful, poorly healing, perirectal lesion. The patient has gotten acyclovir for HSV multiple times but now is not responding. *Think: Acyclovir-resistant HSV.* Treat with foscarnet.

VARICELLA-ZOSTER VIRUS AND HIV

- **Shingles:** The reactivation of chickenpox (or varicella-zoster) can happen in any person but is very common in AIDS patients.
  - Reactivation of latent infection.
  - Usually an early complication of HIV.
  - Painful, vesicular skin eruptions.
  - Can have extensive involvement of several dermatomes, but also may just follow one dermatome, which would classically be seen wrapping around the flank but not crossing the midline.
  - Treatment with acyclovir or famcyclovir may shorten the disease course.
- **Primary varicella-zoster virus (VZV) infection** (chickenpox) may be *lethal* in the HIV patient. Treat aggressively with acyclovir and hyperimmune globulin.
- **Acute retinal necrosis syndrome:**
  - From VZV in the eye/orbital area (trigeminal nerve varicella-zoster or orolabial HSV).
  - Presents with pain, keratitis, and iritis.
  - Fundus exam shows widespread, pale gray peripheral lesions.
  - Often complicated by retinal detachment.

HEPATITIS

- Patients with HIV likely have risk factors for viral hepatitis (hepatitis B virus [HBV] and hepatitis C virus [HCV]) and they should be screened.
- Patients with HBV and HIV have less severe inflammatory liver disease because of immunosuppression.

KAPOSI SARCOMA

General Facts

- Incidence has been decreasing since first recognized as an HIV-associated neoplasm.
- Mostly in homosexual men.
- Associated with **human herpes virus type 8 (HHV-8)**.

Clinical Features

- Multiple **vascular nodules appearing** in the skin, mucous membranes, and viscera.
- Appearance is purplish macular or papular nodule on skin or discoloration of the oral mucosa.
- Lesions often occur in sun-exposed areas.
- Pulmonary involvement can occur; presents as shortness of breath.
- May be seen with a normal CD4 count.

Diagnostic Workup

- Biopsy of suspicious lesion.

Management

- Always treat with ARVs.

CONQUER THE WARDS!

Herpes zoster (shingles) can cause **pain PRIOR to the development of the rash**. Keep zoster on the differential diagnosis for any patient with pain in a dermatomal distribution.

CONQUER THE BOARDS!

A patient with ZVZ in the CN V1 is at risk of herpes zoster ophthalmicus with eye involvement and **needs an ophthalmologic exam.** If the patient has a **vesicle on the tip of the nose, they are at very high risk** (nasocilliary nerve supplies that area and leads to the eye) and is called "Hutchinson sign."

CONQUER THE WARDS!

Some antiretrovirals treat both HIV and HBV:

- **Tenofovir**
- **Lamivudine**
- **Emtricitabine**

CONQUER THE WARDS!

An AIDS patient with vascular-appearing skin lesions should be evaluated for **Kaposi sarcoma vs. bacillary angiomatosis (caused by *Bartonella henselae*).**

- Can use topical all-trans retinoic or local radiation. Occasionally can use systemic chemotherapy.

LYMPHOMAS

General Facts

- Six percent of patients develop lymphoma at some point during their disease.
- Incidence is increased 120-fold in HIV compared with general population.
- **Three main types occur in HIV:** Diffuse large B-cell lymphoma (70%), Burkitt lymphoma (20%), or primary CNS lymphoma (rare, strongly associated with **Epstein-Barr virus** [EBV])

Clinical Features

- Dependent on the site of the tumor.
- Persistent unexplained fever, focal seizures if in CNS, and rapidly growing mass lesion in the oral mucosa.
- Eighty percent have extranodal disease.

Management

- ARV + systemic chemotherapy.

> CONQUER THE **BOARDS!**
>
> Important AIDS-associated malignancies:
> - **Cervical cancer (HPV)**
> - **Kaposi sarcoma (HHV-8)**
> - **CNS lymphoma (EBV)**
> - **Non-Hodgkin lymphoma**

BIOTERRORISM AGENTS

General Facts

- Inhalational agents are expected to be the most common form used in bioterrorism due to ease of inoculation.
- Suspected or confirmed cases should be reported to local or state departments of health.
- Antibiotics for treating patients infected in connection with a bioterrorist event are included in the national pharmaceutical stockpile maintained by the Centers for Disease Control and Prevention (CDC), as are ventilators and other emergency equipment.
- This information is compiled from the **CDC** website, where the latest surveillance information is available: http://www.cdc.gov.

HIGH-YIELD LITERATURE

CDC bioterrorism resources:

CDC. Emergency preparedness and response. Available at https://emergency.cdc.gov/bioterrorism/index.asp.

ANTHRAX

General Facts

- Incubation is usually <1 week.
- Transmission can be via contact with skin, inhalation of aerosolized spores, or consumption of undercooked meats. There is no person-to-person transmission of anthrax.

Clinical Features

- **Initial phase** consists of nonspecific symptoms such as low-grade fever, nonproductive cough, malaise, fatigue, myalgias, profound sweats, and chest discomfort.

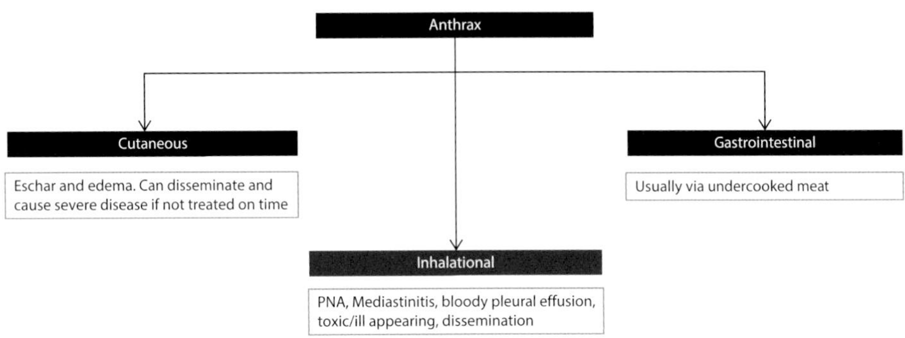

FIGURE 9-9. Clinical presentations of anthrax.

- **Physical exam** may reveal rhonchi; otherwise, normal.
- **One to five days after initial symptoms**: High fever and severe respiratory distress (dyspnea, stridor, cyanosis) occur. Shock and death occur within 24 to 36 hours. An interim period of a few days of wellness can occur between the 2 stages, or they may occur in rapid succession (Figure 9-9).
- Hemorrhagic meningitis can also be seen.

Diagnostic Workup

- Gram-positive bacilli on peripheral blood smear or CSF can be found.
- **CXR** demonstrates **widened mediastinum with clear lung fields.**
- Nasal swab for PCR available for **epidemiologic surveillance**; not approved to make individual patient decisions.

Management

- Initiate antimicrobial therapy immediately upon suspicion of inhalational anthrax (or sepsis/meningitis) with 3-drug therapy: first line is ciprofloxacin or doxycycline. Always add drugs that have CNS penetration and that can help with toxin production (Figure 9-10).

1. Main Therapy
Ciprofloxacin
OR Doxycycline

2. CNS Penetration
Carbapenem

3. Toxin Production
Linezolid
OR Clindamycin

4. Adjunctive Therapy
mAb
Steroids
Drainage of Effusions

FIGURE 9-10. Clinical presentations of anthrax.

- Exposed individuals should receive prophylaxis with ciprofloxacin or doxycycline for 60 days and anthrax immunization.
- Vaccine available for military personnel and lab workers who handle the organism directly.

CONQUER THE BOARDS!

A patient with exposure to aerosolized anthrax needs to be decontaminated with soap and water. After that they **do NOT require isolation (no person-to-person transmission).**

CONQUER THE BOARDS!

In the absence of a bioterrorism attack *Y. pestis* is spread by rodents (who carry fleas harboring the bacteria) such as **prairie dogs and rats**. Most cases in the United States occur in the **southwestern states.**

PNEUMONIC PLAGUE

General Facts

- There are three types of plague: pneumonic, bubonic, and septicemic.
- The most common form is bubonic (lymphadenitis, groin most common site), which is not transmitted person to person (only transmissible if there is pulmonary involvement).
- Caused by ***Yersinia pestis***. Indications that plague had been artificially disseminated would be the occurrence of cases in locations not known to have enzootic infection, in persons without known risk factors, and in the absence of prior rodent deaths.
- Transmission is via inhalation of respiratory droplets (CAN be transmitted person to person—need droplet isolation), with an incubation period of 2 to 4 days.

Clinical Features

- Fever, headache, weakness, and rapidly developing pneumonia with shortness of breath, chest pain, cough, and sometimes bloody or watery sputum.
- Pneumonia progresses for 2 to 4 days and causes respiratory failure and shock.

Diagnostic Workup

- Gram stain of sputum or blood may reveal gram-negative bacilli or coccobacilli.
- Wright, Giemsa, and Wayson stain will often show **bipolar staining**.
- Antigen detection, immunoglobulin M (IgM) enzyme immunoassay, immunostaining, and PCR.

Management

- Start an aminoglycoside (streptomycin or gentamicin) within 24 hours of appearance of symptoms.
- Other effective agents include tetracycline, doxycycline, and chloramphenicol.
- Isolation of patients using respiratory droplet precautions, but then are no longer contagious after 48 hours of antibiotic treatment.

A laboratory confirmation of *Y. pestis* is made on autopsy of a healthy 40-year-old living in a big city. There was no history of handling an animal carcass or any travel to an endemic area. *Think: This could be a sentinel event for a bioterrorist attack. Be on the lookout for cases of severe acute respiratory illness in others very shortly.*

- Postexposure prophylaxis for people who have had direct, close contact with infected patients (7-day course of **doxycycline or levofloxacin**).
- A plague vaccine is not currently available for use in the United States.

CONQUER THE BOARDS!

Smallpox is one of the few conditions that requires **airborne isolation** (need N95 mask) along with **tuberculosis, VZV, measles, and SARS**.

SMALLPOX

General Facts

- A viral condition caused by variola. Humans are the only natural hosts of variola.

- Spreads primarily through **respiratory viral shedding** (inhaled). Face-to-face contact is required.
- Can be spread through direct contact with infected bodily fluids or contaminated objects, with an incubation period of 7 to 17 days

Clinical Features

- **A prodrome of 2 to 4 days** with high fever, malaise, head and body aches, and sometimes vomiting. Patients are acutely ill, in contrast to varicella infection.
- **The rash is typical**, with small red spots on the tongue and in the mouth that become sores that break open and spread large amounts of the virus into the mouth and throat; person becomes most contagious at that time. Subsequently, the rash appears on the skin, starting on the face and spreading to the arms and legs **(centrifugal)** and then to the palms and soles. The bumps become raised, filled with fluid, and then pustules. They subsequently scab and form scars (Table 9-6).

CONQUER THE BOARDS!

The rash of smallpox consists of lesions that are all at the **same stage of development**. In contrast, the lesions of varicella are at all different stages.

Table 9-6. Differentiating Features Between Chickenpox, Monkeypox, and Smallpox

Chickenpox	Monkeypox	Smallpox
Lesions in all stages	Lesions in all stages	Lesions in same stage
	Exposure to prairie dogs	Terrorism
+/– palms/soles	– palms/soles	+ palms/soles

Diagnostic Workup

- PCR or enzyme-linked immunosorbent assay (ELISA) of throat swab, or culture of fluid from pustules or CSF.

Management

- Patients are quarantined for 17 days or until scabs fall off.
- Treatment consists of fluid replacement and antibiotics for any second-degree bacterial infections.

Prevention

- Smallpox vaccine contains live *vaccinia* virus, a weaker relative of the *variola* virus that causes smallpox. Some military and first responders are vaccinated.

TULAREMIA

General Facts

- Bacterial zoonosis caused by *Francisella tularensis* (small nonmotile, aerobic, non-spore-forming, gram-negative coccobacillus), found in water, moist soil, hay, straw, and decaying animal carcasses, mostly in southcentral and western United States in summer.
- Humans infected through bite of an exposed tick, fly, or mosquito or by direct contact with infectious animal (often carcasses) or environment (soil, water, food).
- No person-to-person transmission (no need for patient isolation).
- Rodents are reservoir (on testing, often **exposure to rabbits** is mentioned or implied).
- Incubation is usually 3 to 5 days, but can be as long as 14 days.

Clinical Features

- Sudden onset of high fever, chills, diarrhea, headache, myalgia, and cough.
- If inhaled, hemorrhagic inflammation, pneumonia, and pneumonitis.
- Airborne *F. tularensis* can also cause ocular involvement, ulcers in broken skin, and oropharyngeal disease.

Diagnostic Workup

- Gram stain, DFA, or immunohistochemical stains of respiratory secretions and blood.
- Confirmation of disease is via rising titers of *F. tularensis* serologies.

Management

- **Streptomycin** is drug of choice.
- Gentamicin, tetracyclines, and chloramphenicol are also effective.

TICK-BORNE DISEASES

LYME DISEASE

General Facts

- A tick-borne illness caused by *Borrelia burgdorferi,* a microaerophilic spirochete transmitted by *Ixodes scapularis* tick (deer tick) found in the **northeastern United States and Wisconsin**, in wooded areas.

Clinical Features

- **Erythema chronicum migrans** is the pathognomonic skin rash that starts at the bite and progresses until there is central clearing.
- **Initial stage:** Fevers, headaches, arthralgias, and myalgias.
- **Second stage** (weeks to months): Recurring rash, myocarditis with **first-, second-, or third-degree heart block**; meningitis; cranial nerve palsy; peripheral neuropathy.
- **Third stage:** Migratory or **oligoarthritis**.

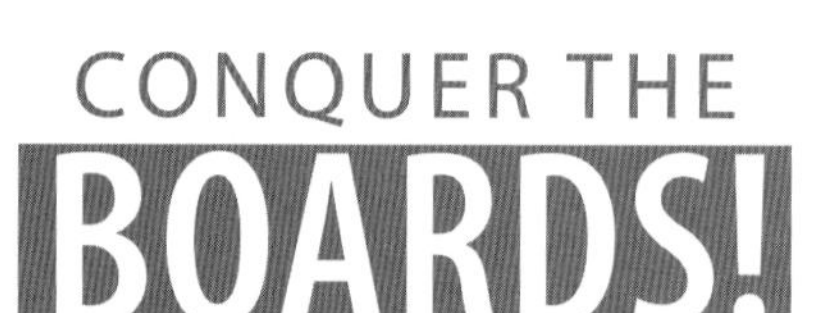

If a the patient has tick exposure on a test, **doxycycline is the treatment!**

Diagnostic Workup

- ELISA followed by Western blot. **If clinical suspicion is high, treat the patient before serologies come back.**
- Treat with **doxycycline** or amoxicillin if there is no cardiac or central neurologic involvement.
- Treat with penicillin or cephalosporin (IV ceftriaxone) if there is any cardiac or neurologic involvement.

A 42-year-old woman who recently camped in the woods of Vermont presents to the emergency room with one-sided facial droop. *Think: Lyme disease (often presents with Bell palsy).* **Next step:** Check Lyme serologies and electrocardiogram (ECG) to rule out cardiac involvement.

EHRLICHIOSIS

General Facts

Two types: Human monocytic ehrlichiosis (HME) and human granulocytic ehrlichiosis (HGE). *Ehrlichia chaffeensis* is the intracellular bacterium that causes HME, and *Ehrlichia phagocytophila* is the intracellular bacterium that causes HGE.

- HME is caused by the bite of the *Lone star* tick, while HGE is caused by the bite of the *Ixodes* tick.

Clinical Features

- Nonspecific flulike symptoms, high fever, headache, malaise, **leukopenia,** and **thrombocytopenia** are most common presentations.

Diagnostic Workup

- A thorough history, including geographic exposures, can help with the diagnosis. HME in southern United States and HGE in northern United States.
- A peripheral smear may show the presence of morulae in monocytes for HME and in granulocytes for HGE.
- Serum PCR can detect the organism.

Management

- Tetracycline or doxycycline.

ROCKY MOUNTAIN SPOTTED FEVER

General Facts

- *A tick-borne illness caused by Rickettsia rickettsii,* gram-negative coccobacillus, found in the **southeastern United States**. It is transmitted by the bite of the wood tick *Dermacentor andersoni* or the dog tick *Dermacentor variabilis.*

Clinical Features

- Patients initially present with fever, nausea, severe headache, vomiting, and history of recent tick bite.
- After 3 to 4 days of symptoms, rash starts as a nonpruritic, maculopapular rash on the distal extremities, starting on the wrists and ankles and then **involving the palms and soles**, then progresses centrally to the trunk and face.
- Can be fatal if not treated aggressively.
- Disseminated intravascular coagulation (DIC) and pneumonia are serious complications of infection.

Diagnostic Workup

- Usually a clinical diagnosis.
- Diagnosis can be confirmed via indirect immunofluorescence assay or latex agglutination.

Management

- Tetracyclines (doxycycline) are the drug of choice.

CONQUER THE **WARDS!**

A patient from the Appalachian Mountain region with symptoms suggestive of RMSF (usually including rash on the palms/soles) should be **treated immediately with doxycycline** (do NOT wait for confirmatory testing).

BABESIOSIS

General Facts

- A tick-borne infection of RBCs caused by *Babesia microti,* an intra-RBC parasite (like malaria) transmitted by the *Ixodes* tick in the northeast and midwest United States.

Clinical Features

- Fever, chills, myalgias, and **hemolytic anemia.**
- Watch for coinfection with other tick-borne illnesses!

CONQUER THE **BOARDS!**

For your coinfections, remember the phrase "Ana gives lime juice to her babies:

- Anaplasmosis
- Lyme disease
- Babesiosis

All three can be present in the same patient via coinfection!

CONQUER THE **BOARDS!**

If a patient from the NE United States with tick exposure and a febrile illness **does not improve** with empiric treatment for Lyme disease (such as doxycycline), think of **Babesiosis (coinfections can occur as they are carried by the same *Ixodes* tick)**

Diagnostic Workup

- Thick and thin smears of whole blood reveal ring-shaped trophozoites and the characteristic cross-shaped tetrad of merozoites known as the ***Maltese cross*** within RBCs.

Management

- Management is based on severity and degree of parasitemia.
- The drug of choice is a combination of quinine and clindamycin.

MALARIA

General Facts

- An infection caused by the ***Plasmodium*** parasite with the ***Anopheles*** mosquito as vector.
- Three hundred million to five hundred million malaria cases, with 3 million deaths, occur annually worldwide.
- Multiple *Plasmodium* species exist with varying geographic distribution. ***Plasmodium falciparum*** causes the most deaths, endemic in Africa. ***Plasmodium vivax*** is endemic in India and Central America. ***Plasmodium ovale*** and *P. vivax* can cause persistent infection in the liver and recur. ***Plasmodium malariae*** causes milder disease.

Clinical Features

- The organisms grow in the liver, then spread to the blood to reproduce in RBCs.
- When the RBC is full, it bursts, releasing the organism and exposing it to the host immune system; RBCs burst at the same time, causing the characteristic intermittent fever.
- ***P. falciparum* causes more severe disease** because it infects erythrocytes of all ages. It can cause a microvascular blockade that leads to local anoxia affecting the brain (delirium, seizures), kidneys, lungs (pulmonary edema, acute respiratory distress syndrome [ARDS]), intestines (nausea, vomiting, diarrhea, abdominal pain), liver, and blood.
- Symptoms of fever and chills occur about 1 to 4 weeks after infection.
- Other symptoms include headache, increased sweating, back pain, myalgias, diarrhea, nausea, vomiting, and cough.
- Anemia, thrombocytopenia, and elevated liver enzymes may be present.

Diagnostic Workup

- Thick and thin blood smears **show parasites in RBCs.**

Management

- Chloroquine for *P. falciparum* acquired in chloroquine-sensitive regions.
- **Artemisinin-based combination regimen** (artemether–lumefantrine, for example) when there is chloroquine resistance or resistance is not known.
- Combination IV therapy (quinidine or artesunate [not available readily in the United States; must call the CDC] + tetracycline or clindamycin) for critically ill patients.
- Contact the CDC.

Prevention

- Prophylactic chloroquine or mefloquine for travelers to endemic areas.
- Check CDC recommendations.
- Use DEET-containing insect repellent and avoid mosquitos.

Antimicrobial Classes and Spectrum

Figures 9-11 and 9-12 illustrate the spectrum of antimicrobial coverage. Table 9-7 has details on common antibiotic classes.

Gram Negative
Gram Positive
Anaerobes
Pen G, Pen VK
Amino penicillins: Amoxicillin, Ampicillin
Synthetics: Nafcillin etc
Extended-spectrum: Piperacillin-tazobactam
1st Gen Cephalosporins
2nd Gen Cephalosporins
3rd Gen Cephalosporins (Ceftriaxone)
4th Gen Cephalosporins (Cefepime)
5th Gen Cephalosporins (Ceftaroline)
Carbapenems
Aztreonam
Vancomycin

FIGURE 9-11. Spectrum of beta-lactams and vancomycin.

Gram Negative
Gram Positive
Anaerobes
Aminoglycosides
Linezolid
Clindamycin
Metronidazole
Moxifloxacin
Ciprofloxacin
Levofloxacin
Tetracyclines
Macrolides

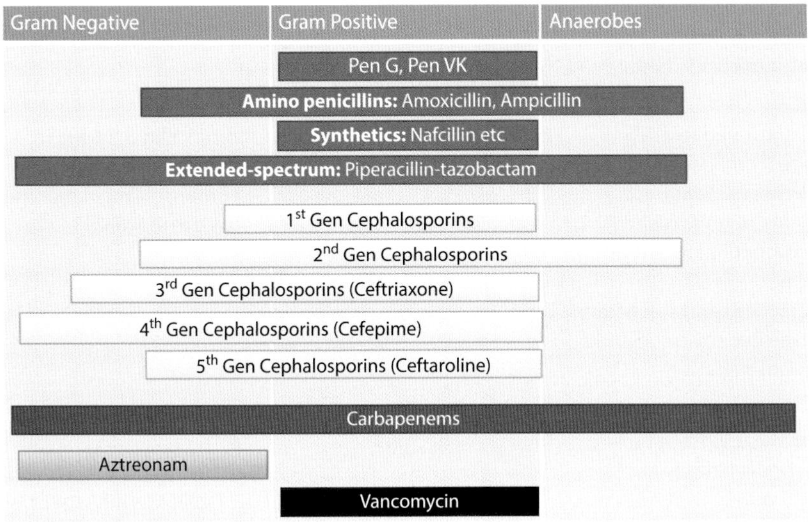

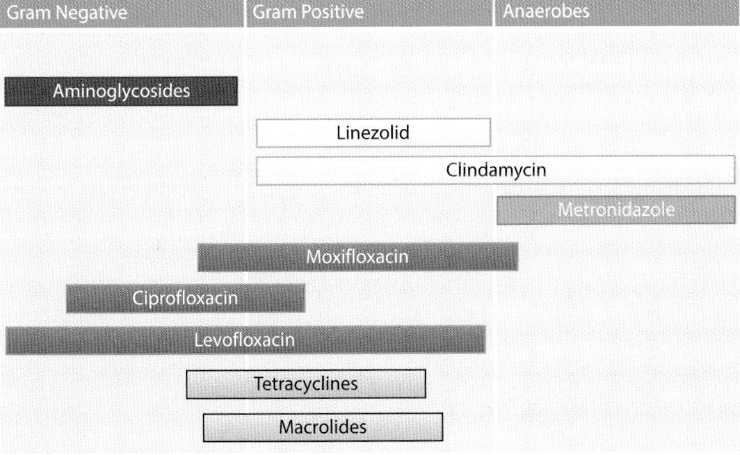

FIGURE 9-12. Spectrum of activity for select antimicrobials.

CONQUER THE BOARDS!

Mefloquine is the prophylaxis drug of choice for **pregnant patients** traveling to endemic areas.

TABLE 9-7. Common Antibiotic Classes			
Antimicrobial	**Antimicrobial Spectrum**	**Side Effects**	**Common Clinical Use**
Class: Beta-lactams Inhibition of bacterial cell wall synthesis by inhibiting enzyme transpeptidases by binding to penicillin-binding proteins.			
Penicillins			
Penicillins (natural): ■ PCN VK ■ PCN G ■ PCN benzathine	■ **Gram**-positive organisms: *Listeria*, *Streptococcus* species, *Bacillus anthracis*. ■ ***Treponema pallidum* (syphilis)**, meningococci, dental infections.	Anaphylaxis, rash, pruritus, diarrhea.	**Syphilis.**
Aminopenicillins: ■ Amoxicillin (PO) and (amoxicillin + clavulanic acid) ■ Ampicillin (IV) and (ampicillin + sulbactam)	■ Added gram-negative coverage *(H. influenzae, E. coli,* **Proteus**, *Salmonella)* and *Enterococcus faecalis* when compared to natural penicillins. ■ Clavulanic acid and sulbactam add anaerobic coverage and some gram-negative.	GI side effects.	Ampicillin is added in patients >60 or immunocompromised in meningitis to cover *Listeria.*
Antistaphylococcal: ■ Oxacillin (IV) ■ Dicloxacillin (PO) ■ Nafcillin (IV)	Added activity against beta-lactamase/penicillinase producing *S. aureus* (but does not cover MRSA).	Interstitial nephritis.	■ Oxacillin and nafcillin are first line for non-MRSA cellulitis if IV agent is required. ■ Dicloxacillin (or cephalexin) is first-line oral agent for nonpurulent cellulitis.
Antipseudomonal: ■ Piperacillin (piperacillin/tazobactam) ■ Ticarcillin (ticarcillin/clavulanic acid)	Covers *Pseudomonas aeruginosa* and anaerobes (when in combination with beta-lactamase inhibitor like tazobactam and clavulanic acid).		Commonly used in hospital for broad pneumonia or gut coverage, including *Pseudomonas* and anaerobes. Also good for resistant bugs in UTIs.
Cephalosporins	Gram-negative coverage ↑ with increasing generations.		About 5% cross-reactivity with penicillin (less with higher generations).
First generation: ■ Cefazolin (IV) ■ Cephalexin, cefadroxil (PO)	MSSA and *Streptococcus,* plus some gram-negative (e.g., *E. coli*).	■ Rash, hypersensitivity reaction. ■ GI upset.	Cephalexin is first-line oral agent for simple cellulitis. Cefazolin is first line for MSSA bacteremia.
Second generation: ■ Cefuroxime, cefoxitin, cefotetan (IV) ■ Cefaclor, cefprozil, cefuroxime axetil (PO)	■ *E. coli, Klebsiella, Proteus, Haemophilus influenzae, Moraxella catarrhalis* ■ Cefotetan and cefoxitin cover some anaerobes also.		

(Continued)

TABLE 9-7. Common Antibiotic Classes (*Continued*)			
Antimicrobial	Antimicrobial Spectrum	Side Effects	Common Clinical Use
Third generation: ■ Cefotaxime, ceftriaxone, ceftazidime (IV) ■ Ceftibuten, cefpodoxime, cefotaxime, cefdinir (PO)	■ Second-generation coverage plus: Enterobacteriaceae, *Serratia, Neisseria gonorrhoeae.* ■ Used for pneumonias and gonorrhea.		**Ceftriaxone:** (1) combined with azithromycin = first line for community-acquired pneumonia; (2) empiric treatment for meningitis (covers *Streptococcus pneumoniae* + *Neisseria*); (3) pyelonephritis.
Fourth generation: Cefepime	■ Ceftazidime and cefepime have activity against *Pseudomonas aeruginosa.* ■ Cefepime has MSSA and streptococcal coverage.		Cefepime is first line in neutropenic fever (with or without vancomycin) due to *Pseudomonas* coverage.
Carbapenems		Cross-reactivity in penicillin allergic patients <5%.	
■ **D**oripenem ■ **I**mipenem ■ **M**eropenem ■ **E**rtapenem	■ **Very** broad coverage: gram positive (but not MRSA), gram negative, and anaerobes (but ertapenem does not cover *Acinetobacter, Pseudomonas aeruginosa*). ■ Cilastatin is given with imipenem, as it prevents its hydrolysis in the renal tubules, and maintains the drug for longer.	Lowers seizure threshold.	■ Imipenem is used for very broad coverage for hospital infections/neutropenic fevers/immunocompromised patients. ■ Ertapenem very good for gut coverage.
Monobactam			
■ Aztreonam	■ Covers only aerobic gram- negative. ■ Effective in chromosomal produced beta-lactamases, but not ESBL gram negative.		■ Safe in penicillin-allergic patients. ■ Vancomycin + aztreonam is a common in-hospital regimen for gram-positive and gram-negative coverage in penicillin-allergic patients.
Class: Fluoroquinolones Inhibit bacterial DNA synthesis by inhibiting DNA gyrase/ topoisomerase IV.			Gram-positive coverage ↑ with increasing generations (whereas cephalosporin generations ↑ gram-negative coverage).
First generation: Nalidixic acid **Second generation:** ■ Ofloxacin ■ Ciprofloxacin	■ *E. coli, Salmonella, Shigella, Enterobacter, Campylobacter,* and *Neisseria.* ■ Intracellular organisms such as *Chlamydia, Mycoplasma, Legionella, Brucella.*	■ Tendonitis/tendon rupture (black box warning). ■ QTc prolongation. ■ May damage growing cartilage and cause an arthropathy; not used in children.	■ Ciprofloxacin's excellent gram-negative coverage good for UTIs, gut infections, infectious diarrhea. ■ Moxifloxacin/levofloxacin good for pneumonias (gram positive and gram negative and atypicals).
		■ No longer first line for uncomplicated infections (such as UTI) due to side-effect profile and concerns about growing resistance.	

(*Continued*)

TABLE 9-7. Common Antibiotic Classes (*Continued*)			
Antimicrobial	Antimicrobial Spectrum	Side Effects	Common Clinical Use
Third generation (respiratory): ■ Levofloxacin ■ Trovafloxacin **Fourth generation (respiratory):** ■ Moxifloxacin ■ Gemifloxacin	A respiratory quinolone covers the bugs listed earlier, plus more gram-positive coverage, including penicillin-resistant *S. pneumoniae* and *S. aureus.*		
Class: Aminoglycosides Prevents bacterial protein synthesis by binding to the 30S ribosomal subunit.			
■ **T**obramycin ■ **A**mikacin ■ **G**entamicin	■ Aerobic gram-negative bacteria. ■ Synergistic activity with beta-lactams, especially for endocarditis caused by streptococci, staphylococci, and enterococci.	■ Nephrotoxicity, ototoxicity. ■ Avoid in patients with myasthenia gravis (causes neuromuscular blockade). ■ Poor agents as monotherapy in serious infections.	■ Often combined with cefepime for double coverage against *Pseudomonas* in neutropenic patients. ■ Combined with beta-lactam for synergy in endocarditis.
Class: Macrolides Inhibits bacterial protein synthesis by binding reversibly to 50S ribosomal subunits.		Erythromycin and clarithromycin inhibit CYP3A4 enzymes.	
■ Erythromycin ■ Clarithromycin ■ Azithromycin	■ **Erythromycin:** Some gram positive (including pneumococci, group *A streptococci*) and some gram negative and treponemes, mycoplasmas, *Chlamydia,* and rickettsiae. ■ **Clarithromycin:** More potent against streptococci + atypicals + *Helicobacter pylori.* ■ **Azithromycin:** Good for atypical bugs (especially atypical pneumonias), plus some gram positive, some gram negative, and chlamydia and gonorrhea.	■ **Erythromycin:** GI upset, cholestatic hepatitis. ■ **Azithromycin:** GI upset (less common than erythromycin), LFT abnormalities. ■ **Clarithromycin:** Metallic taste.	■ Azithromycin is front line in uncomplicated community acquired pneumonias. ■ For more severe community acquired pneumonias, combined with ceftriaxone. ■ Macrolides are also mainstays of therapy for nontuberculous *Mycobacteria.*
Class: Tetracyclines Blocks protein synthesis by binding to 30S ribosomes. ■ Minocycline ■ Doxycycline ■ Tetracycline ■ Demeclocycline	■ More active against gram-positive than gram negative. ■ Some microorganisms, such as *Rickettsia* and *Chlamydia.* ■ Some atypical *Mycobacteria.*	■ Photosensitivity. ■ Gray/yellow discoloration of teeth. ■ Pseudotumor cerebri.	■ Can be used for community-acquired MRSA skin and soft tissue infections. ■ Treatment for chlamydia and gonorrhea and *Rickettsia* (Rocky Mountain spotted fever) as well as other tick borne illness (Lyme, *Ehrlichia*, etc.).
Miscellaneous			
■ Vancomycin (a glycopeptide) inhibits bacterial cell wall synthesis by inhibiting elongation of peptidoglycan and cross-linking.	■ Covers only gram positive including MSSA (second line), MRSA, but not some enterococci (VRE). ■ Used orally for treatment of *Clostridium difficile.*	■ **Red man syndrome:** Histamine-related reaction; avoid by giving slowly. ■ Nephrotoxicity.	MRSA.

(*Continued*)

TABLE 9-7. Common Antibiotic Classes (*Continued*)

Antimicrobial	Antimicrobial Spectrum	Side Effects	Common Clinical Use
■ Polymyxin B penetrates into and disrupts phospholipids in cell membranes.	Good for gram-negative aerobic bacilli except *Proteus, Serratia,* and *Providencia* species.	■ Nephrotoxicity, neurotoxicity. ■ Neuromuscular blockade. ■ Paresthesias around the lips, tongue, and extremities; peripheral neuropathy.	■ Reserved as a last-line agents for multidrug-resistant gram-negative bacteria (MDR *Pseudomonas*, carbapenem-resistant Enterobacteriaceae, *Acinetobacter*).
■ Linezolid inhibits bacterial protein synthesis by binding to 23S ribosomal RNA of the 50S subunit.	■ Bacteriostatic against *Staphylococcus* and *Enterococcus* species. ■ Bactericidal against *Streptococcus* species.	■ Myelosuppression. ■ Linezolid is an MAOI and therefore can cause serotonin syndrome when used with SSRIs or TCAs.	■ Used primarily for VRE and MRSA infections.
■ Daptomycin binds to bacterial membranes resulting in depolarization, loss of membrane potential, and cell death.	Gram-positive coverage: *Staphylococcus, Streptococcus,* and *Enterococcus.*	■ Myopathy and rhabdomyolysis. ■ Produces false elevations in PT/INR. ■ Not for lung infections, as it is denatured by pulmonary surfactant.	Covers MRSA and VRE.

ESBL, extended-spectrum beta-lactamase; *INR,* international normalized ratio; *LFT*, liver function test; *MAOI*, monoamine oxidase inhibitor; *MRSA*, methicillin-resistant *Staphylococcus aureus; MSSA*, methicillin-sensitive *S. aureus; PT*, prothrombin time; *SSRI*, selective serotonin reuptake inhibitor; *TCA*, tricyclic antidepressant; *UTI*, urinary tract infection; *VRE*, vancomycin-resistant *Enterococcus.*

CHAPTER 10 PULMONOLOGY

OVERVIEW OF HIGH-YIELD TOPICS IN PULMONOLOGY

PULMONARY FUNCTION TESTS

- **Spirometry:** Measures the rate at which the lung volume *changes* during forced breathing.
- **Forced vital capacity (FVC):** Patient inhales maximally, then exhales as rapidly and completely as possible for >6 sec. The exhalation and subsequent inhalation are recorded as a flow volume curve.
- **FEV_1:** The volume of air exhaled in the first second of the FVC maneuver.
- FEV_1, FVC, and the ratio between them (FEV_1/FVC) are important parameters to determine the nature of lung disease and severity (see Table 10-1). The values obtained in a patient are compared with the expected normal values for that age, sex, height, and ethnic background.
- Normal FEV_1 ≥80% of predicted.
- Normal FVC ≥80% of predicted.
- Normal FEV_1/FVC ratio ≥0.7.
- **Obstructive lung disease:** FEV_1 is disproportionately reduced compared to FVC; therefore, FEV_1/FVC ratio is low. FEV_1/FVC ratio of <70% is a key parameter to diagnose obstruction. Seen with airway diseases like chronic bronchitis, emphysema, and asthma.
- **Restrictive lung disease:** Seen with interstitial lung diseases, neuromuscular diseases (amyotrophic lateral sclerosis [ALS], myasthenia gravis, Guillain–Barré), chest wall disorders (obesity, kyphoscoliosis). Both FEV_1 and FVC are low, but their ratio is usually normal or elevated.
- **Lung volume measurements:** Lung volumes such as total lung capacity (TLC), functional residual capacity (FRC), and residual volume (RV) can be measured by using body plethysmography or helium dilution techniques. This is used to confirm restrictive lung disease.
- **Diffusion capacity of carbon monoxide (DL_{CO}):** Using trace amounts of CO in the inhaled gas mixture, diffusion of alveolar air across pulmonary capillaries can be assessed. DL_{CO} helps identify diseases where gas exchanged is limited, such as interstitial lung disease and emphysema.

OBSTRUCTIVE PULMONARY DISEASES

CHRONIC OBSTRUCTIVE PULMONARY DISEASE

General Facts

Chronic bronchitis and emphysema are forms of chronic obstructive pulmonary disease (COPD). COPD is defined by a chronic obstruction to expiratory airflow, largely irreversible, as evidenced by a decrease in FEV_1. The term *COPD* is preferred to describe both chronic bronchitis and emphysema, as many patients have elements of each disease.

TABLE 10-1. Pulmonary Function Tests

Normal Spirometry	Obstructive Lung Disease	Restrictive Lung Disease
■ FVC normal ■ FEV_1 normal ■ FEV_1/FVC >0.7	■ FVC normal or ↓ ■ FEV_1 ↓ ■ FEV_1/FVC <0.7 ■ Lung volume normal or ↑	■ FVC ↓ ■ FEV_1 normal or ↓ ■ FEV_1/FVC >0.7 ■ Lung volume *always* ↓

- **Chronic bronchitis:** Defined as a chronic productive cough on most days for ≥3 months in each of 2 successive years; may or may not be accompanied by chronic expiratory airflow obstruction.
- **Emphysema:** Permanent enlargement of the air space distal to the terminal bronchioles due to destruction of alveolar septa. A pathologic entity whose clinical correlate is chronic expiratory airflow obstruction with evidence of hyperinflation. Centrilobular emphysema affects the respiratory bronchioles and surrounding alveoli, while panlobular or panacinar emphysema occurs in patients with alpha-1-antitrypsin deficiency.
- COPD has a higher prevalence in men, with smoking and alpha-1-antitrypsin deficiency as risk factors.

CONQUER THE **WARDS!**

Patients with severe emphysema will lose weight for a variety of reasons, including energy lost due to work of breathing.

Clinical Features

- Clinical presentation usually involves slowly progressive shortness of breath (SOB) on exertion.
- On physical examination, a barrel chest, decreased air entry with prolonged expiration, and wheezes can be found.

Diagnostic Workup

- The diagnostic approach to COPD is to perform pulmonary function tests (PFTs) to both diagnose and quantify the degree of disease. An obstructive pattern (low FEV_1, low FEV_1/FVC) will be seen on PFTs that is not reversible with bronchodilator therapy.
- The Global Initiative for Chronic Obstructive Lung Disease (GOLD) is the most widely used staging system, which also helps guide treatment and gives information on prognosis. There are two GOLD staging systems. The first uses FEV_1, which is important in diagnosis and estimating prognosis (see Table 10-2).

The second staging system considers symptoms and exacerbations and helps guide treatment.

- **Other testing:**
  - **Chest imaging** can be performed, with x-rays showing hyperinflated lungs and low and flattened diaphragm, and computed tomography (CT) showing more radiographic details, including loss of alveolar walls and extent of disease in emphysema. Imaging can help assess for other underlying causes.
  - **Arterial blood gas (ABG)** may show decreased O_2 and increased CO_2, and may be useful to help assess the need for supplemental O_2 or positive-pressure ventilation.
  - **Electrocardiogram (ECG)** may show right-sided strain pattern.

CONQUER THE **BOARDS!**

Pink puffers (emphysema):
- Barrel-shaped chest
- Thin and emaciated
- High Pco_2, normal to low PO_2

Blue bloaters (chronic bronchitis):
- Right heart failure
- Polycythemia
- High Pco_2, low PO_2

TABLE 10-2. COPD – GOLD Criteria

Stage	FEV_1	Mortality in 3 Years
0: At risk	-	–
1: Mild	FEV_1 ≥80% predicted	?
2: Moderate	50% ≤FEV_1 <80% predicted	11%
3: Severe	30% ≤FEV_1 <50% predicted	15%
4: Very severe	FEV_1 <30% predicted or FEV_1 <50% predicted plus chronic respiratory failure	24%

Management

- The management of COPD will depend on the GOLD stage of the disease. Addressing modifiable risk factors is also a key part of management. See Table 10-3.
- **Smoking cessation** is the only intervention proven to slow down the loss of pulmonary function.
- **Oxygen can improve** COPD symptoms, exercise tolerance, and **mortality**. Oxygen should be given to patients with a resting Pao_2 of <55 mm Hg or Pao_2 of 55 to 59 or oxygen saturation <88%. **A walking oxygen test** (patient walks for 6 minutes while continuously monitoring their oxygen saturation) should also be done, as patients whose oxygen saturation drops below 88% qualify for oxygen.
- **Vaccinations:** Infection is a common cause of COPD exacerbations. Influenza and pneumococcal vaccines should be given yearly.
- Beta-agonists and anticholinergics improve FEV_1 modestly, improve symptoms, and reduce exacerbations.
- Inhaled corticosteroids (e.g., fluticasone, budesonide) are helpful in patients with severe COPD (FEV_1 <50% predicted) and frequent infective exacerbations.

TABLE 10-3. COPD Management

Stage	Symptoms	Exacerbations in Past Year	First-Line Treatment	Symptoms Persist
All Groups	–	–	Smoking cessation PNA and influenza vaccines	–
A	Mild or infrequent symptoms (breathlessness with strenuous exercise) or CAT* <10	0–1 without hospitalization	Short-acting inhaler PRN (SABA or SAMA)	Try alternative class (e.g., if on a SABA and switch to SAMA)
B	Moderate to severe symptoms (must walk slower due to breathlessness) or CAT ≥10	0–1 without hospitalization	Short-acting inhaler PRN Plus Long-acting bronchodilator (LABA or LAMA)	LAMA + LABA
C	Mild or infrequent symptoms (breathlessness with strenuous exercise) or CAT <10	≥2 with hospitalization	Short-acting inhaler PRN Plus Long-acting bronchodilator (LABA or LAMA)	LAMA + LABA Or LABA + ICS
D	Moderate to severe symptoms (must walk slower due to breathlessness) or CAT ≥10	≥2 with hospitalization	Short-acting inhaler PRN Plus 2 long-acting bronchodilators (LABA and LAMA)	Add ICS

ICS, inhaled corticoid steroid; *LABA*, long-acting beta-agonist; *LAMA*, long-acting muscarinic antagonist; *SABA*, short-acting beta-agonist; *SAMA*, short-acting muscarinic antagonist.
* COPD Assessment Test, which asks 8 questions about cough, phlegm, chest tightness, exercise tolerance, home activities, ability to leave the house, sleeping, and energy on a 5-point scale (catestonline.org).

HIGH-YIELD LITERATURE

Rabe KF, Watz H. Chronic obstructive pulmonary disease. *Lancet*. 2017;389(10082):1931-1940.

ACUTE EXACERBATIONS OF COPD

General Facts

- Acute exacerbations of COPD (AECOPD) are defined as a sudden worsening of COPD symptoms, including SOB, and increased quantity and color of phlegm.
- Infectious or environmental factors may trigger AECOPD.

Clinical Features

- Patients typically have an acute worsening of symptoms, with increased sputum production or cough.
- SOB, hypoxia, or hypercapnia can occur.
- Patients with severe hypercapnia can develop altered mentation.
- On examination, wheezing may be present on lung fields.

Diagnostic Workup

- **Chest imaging** is important in order to assess any underlying infiltrate or pneumonia that may be the cause of the overall decompensation.
- **ABG** to assess CO_2 levels and pH. Patients who have an increased Pco_2 on ABG and a low pH may require bilevel positive-pressure ventilation to help remove the Pco_2.
- **Procalcitonin** is a novel test that can help differentiate between bacterial infections and viral infections. It can be useful in helping you determine the need for antibiotic therapy in lower respiratory tract infections. There are conflicting studies on the use of procalcitonin in AECOPD, but it may be helpful in cases with low clinical suspicion.

Management

- The first step is to triage the level of care that your patient needs. Many exacerbations can be successfully treated at home, but some patients may need care in the intensive care unit (ICU). This decision is based on the severity of their SOB, oxygen saturation, and ABG findings.
- Immediate short-acting bronchodilators must be started at either close intervals or continuously. Initially this may be done with nebulizers but can be converted to inhalers if their symptoms improve. In the hospital, however, all patients should receive bronchodilator nebulizers.
- Corticosteroids for 5 to 7 days have been shown be decrease treatment failure, decrease hospital length of stay, and increase FEV_1 in acute exacerbations of COPD and are the mainstay of therapy for AECOPD. Oral steroids have been shown to be as efficacious as intravenous (IV) steroids, but IV can be used in severe cases or if patients cannot tolerate oral medications.
- Antibiotics for acute infective exacerbations of COPD reduce the duration of symptoms by 20% and decrease hospital admissions by 50%. It appears that this is independent of the choice of antibiotic. Most centers favor the use of azithromycin (Figure 10-1).

HIGH-YIELD LITERATURE

Bremmer DN, DiSilvio BE, Hammer C, et al. Impact of procalcitonin guidance on management of adults hospitalized with chronic obstructive pulmonary disease exacerbations. *J Gen Intern Med.* 2018;33(5):692-697.

Daubin C, Valette X, Thiollière F, et al. Procalcitonin algorithm to guide initial antibiotic therapy in acute exacerbations of COPD admitted to the ICU: A randomized multicenter study. *Intensive Care Med.* 2018;44(4):428-437.

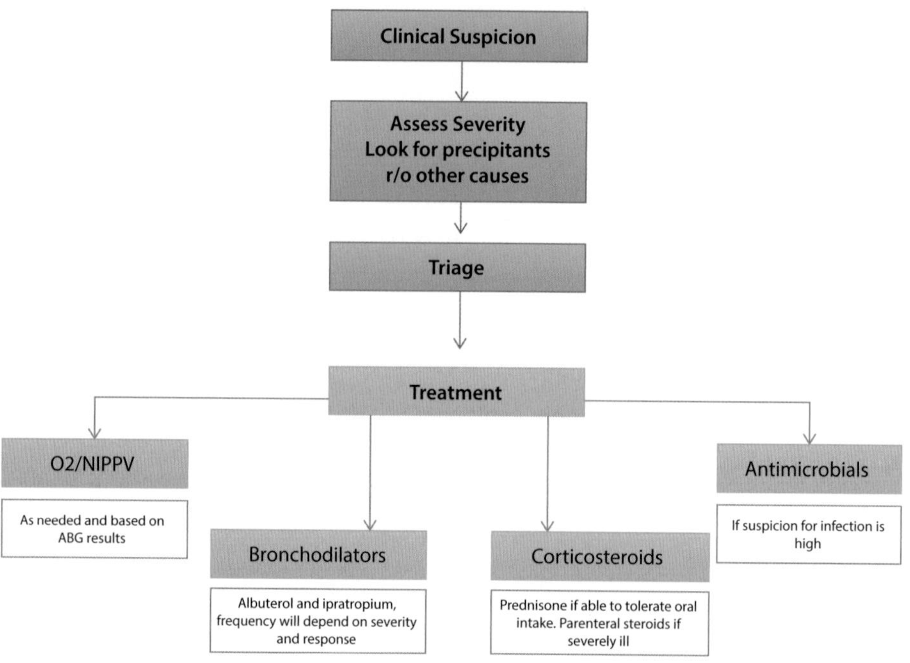

FIGURE 10-1. Management of COPD exacerbations.

> **CONQUER THE WARDS!**
>
> NSAIDs can precipitate an asthma attack. Watch for this in a patient with a history of asthma who takes ibuprofen for a headache.

ASTHMA

General Facts

- A chronic condition characterized by the following triad:
  - Airway inflammation.
  - Airway hyperresponsiveness leading to bronchoconstriction.
  - Reversible airflow obstruction (as opposed to COPD).
- Exposure to various allergens from pets, dust, and pollen can cause inflammation and airway hyperreactivity.
- Once airway hyperreactivity is established, an asthma attack may be induced by nonspecific triggers like exercise, cold air, or strong smells.

> **CONQUER THE WARDS!**
>
> Remember that not all that wheezes is asthma! COPD, heart failure, obstruction, and lung cancer can all cause wheezing.

Clinical Features

The hallmark of airflow obstruction associated with asthma is its variability from day to day, at different times of the day, and from season to season. Predominant symptoms include:

- Chest tightness, wheezing, and SOB.
- Cough is usually dry (especially at night).
- In **cough-variant asthma**, cough is the patient's only symptom and diagnosis is made by response to asthma-specific treatment.
- On physical exam, during an attack:
  - Wheezing on exhalation.
  - Increased expiratory phase.
  - In severe attacks, you will see **accessory muscle use, decreased breath sounds (no wheezing)**, and inability to complete a full sentence.

> **CONQUER THE WARDS!**
>
> If an asthmatic in respiratory distress has a normal pH and normal P_{CO_2}, beware of impending
> : intubate (he is tiring out).

Diagnosis

- **PFTs** are required for diagnosis and will show an obstructive pattern that is reversible with bronchodilators.
- **Bronchoprovocation testing** with methacholine and exercise in dry air can be used in patients with normal PFTs in whom asthma is suspected.

- **Peak flow:** After asthma has been diagnosed, measuring peak flow is a good way to monitor asthma response to treatment both in exacerbations and for chronic management.

Management

- A stepwise approach in asthma treatment is used, depending on the severity of disease (Table 10-4). The severity of the disease is based on the following symptoms:
  - Asthma symptoms per week.
  - Nighttime awakenings per month.
  - Use of rescue bronchodilator per week.
  - Interference with normal activity.
- **Rule of 2s:** If any of these symptoms is greater than 2, the asthma severity is in the persistent range and requires chronic inhaler therapy.
- **Allergen removal:** Common environmental triggers should be addressed, including smoking, dust, pets, carpets, cockroaches, and seasonal allergens.

Following are descriptions of the medications used in treatment:

- **Short-acting β_2 agonists (SABAs)** are rapid-onset medications that can provide quick relief. They include albuterol and terbutaline. SABAs can be delivered via metered-dose inhaler (MDI) or nebulizer to help promote bronchodilation. Nebulizers are preferred for inpatient management of exacerbations.
- **Ipratropium bromide** is a rapid-onset medication delivered by nebulizer or MDI that can help dry up bronchial secretions. The effects of beta-agonists and ipratropium bromide are additive, and this combination is usually used on an inpatient basis.
- **Inhaled corticosteroids (ICS):** Consistent use has been shown to reduce the frequency of symptoms, improve quality of life, and decrease exacerbations.

TABLE 10-4. Classification and Management of Asthma

		Persistent			
	Mild Intermittent (Step 1)	Mild (Step 2)	Moderate (Step 3)	Severe (Step 4)	Severe (Step 5)
Clinical history					
Asthma symptoms/wk	**≤2/wk**	**>2 days/wk**	**Daily**	**Throughout the day**	
Nighttime awakenings/month	**≤2/month**	**>2x/month**	**>1x/week**	**Daily**	
Rescue inhaler use/wk	**≤2 days/wk**	**>2 days/wk**	**Daily**	**Several times a day**	
Interference with normal activity	**None**	**Mild limitation**	**Some limitation**	**Severe limitation**	
Treatment (all levels have SABA PRN)	SABA PRN	Low-dose ICS	Low-dose ICS + LABA	Medium-dose or high-dose ICS + LABA	High-dose ICS + LABA + oral steroids or omalizumab

ICA, inhaled corticosteroids; *LABA*, long-acting beta-agonist; *PRN*, as needed; *SABA*, short-acting beta-agonist.

- **Long-acting β_2 agonists (LABAs)** such as salmeterol or formoterol are helpful to improve symptoms and reduce exacerbations when used in combination with ICS.
- **Oral steroids** (take 6 hours to work): Reduce inflammation and are generally used in asthma exacerbations. Oral and IV forms are equivalent in efficacy. Treatment in acute exacerbations is usually as long as symptoms are present, and these drugs usually do not need to be tapered.
- **Omalizumab:** Anti-IgE agent that can be used in severe persistent asthma with positive allergen skin tests and is given subcutaneously every 2 to 4 weeks.
- **Alternative agents:**
  1. **Leukotriene receptor antagonists (LTRAs)** such as montelukast are an alternative medication for chronic management of asthma and can be used instead of low-dose ICS in mild persistent asthma, instead of LABA in moderate persistent asthma, and added to LABA and ICS in severe persistent asthma.
  2. **Mast-cell modulators** such as cromolyn can help with exercise-induced bronchospasm and are typically used in younger patients.
  3. **Methylxanthines** such as theophylline are no longer regularly used for asthma due to the narrow therapeutic window and the frequency of adverse effects, including nausea, vomiting, headache, and in severe toxicity, seizures, and arrhythmias.

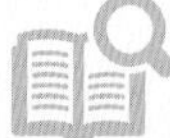

HIGH-YIELD LITERATURE

Lazarus SC. Clinical practice. Emergency treatment of asthma. *N Engl J Med.* 2010;363(8):755-764.

CONQUER THE BOARDS!

Most common organisms to colonize the bronchiectatic lung:
- Haemophilus influenzae
- Staphylococcus aureus
- Pseudomonas aeruginosa

BRONCHIECTASIS

General Facts

- A chronic condition characterized by pathologic dilatation of the medium-sized airways. Usually caused by an abnormal inflammatory response to an initial infectious or toxic insult. The resulting airway damage allows bacterial colonization, buildup of secretions, and continued bronchial inflammation and destruction.
- **Localized bronchiectasis is** usually the result of previous pneumonia or atypical infections such as nontuberculous mycobacterial disease or COPD.
- If **severe or bilateral,** cystic fibrosis, immotile cilia syndromes (Kartagener syndrome), or immunodeficiencies that lead to chronic pulmonary infections should be considered (common variable immune deficiency [CVID], hypogammaglobulinemia)

Clinical Features

- Chronic cough, often with large amount of expectoration.
- Hemoptysis is often the major or only presenting symptom.
- Wheezing and failure to thrive.

Diagnostic Workup

- **High-resolution CT scan** will detect bronchial dilatation and destruction in 60% to 100% of cases.

Management

- Chest physiotherapy and postural drainage: Patients are placed in different positions to use gravity to help drain mucus, and a therapist will clap or vibrate the patient's chest to help further dislodge mucus. There are also vests that vibrate the chest.
- Antibiotics as needed, based on culture data.
- Bronchodilators and mucolytics to help with expectoration and SOB.

OBSTRUCTIVE SLEEP APNEA–HYPOPNEA SYNDROME

General Facts

Brief periods of breathing cessation (apnea) or marked reduction in tidal volume (hypopnea) occurring during sleep due to occlusion of upper airways.

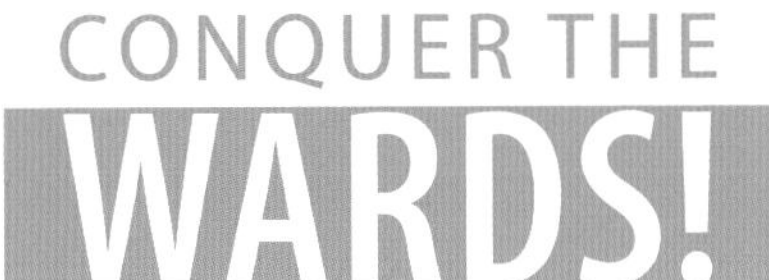

Think of OSAHS if your patient is obese and reports feeling tired throughout the day.

Clinical Features

- Snoring, persistent daytime sleepiness, and morning headache are the most common symptoms.
- Obesity and hypertension may be present secondary to obstructive sleep apnea–hypopnea syndrome (OSAHS).
- Large neck circumference and high Mallampati scores are clues as well.

Diagnostic Workup

- Diagnosis is made with polysomnography (sleep study).
- Obstructive sleep apnea (OSA) is defined by ≥5 episodes of apnea and hypopnea per hour of sleep (apnea–hypopnea index).

Management

- All patients with OSA should be educated on lifestyle changes such as a lateral sleeping position, avoidance of alcohol or sedative medications, and weight loss.
- Continuous positive airway pressure (CPAP) during sleep should be offered to all patients diagnosed with OSA who are having symptoms.
- Surgery (tonsillectomy, uvulopalatopharyngoplasty, tracheostomy) is reserved for patients who fail or cannot tolerate CPAP and lifestyle modifications.

UPPER RESPIRATORY TRACT DISEASES

ACUTE COUGH

General Facts

- Cough is a common presenting complaint of patients.
- Acute cough is defined as a cough of <3 weeks' duration and is most commonly caused by the postnasal drip associated with the common cold.
- See Table 10-5 for causes of acute cough.

CONQUER THE WARDS!

UACS, asthma, and GERD account for the vast majority of causes of chronic cough in nonsmokers with normal CXR, who are not on angiotensin-converting enzyme (ACE) inhibitors.

TABLE 10-5. Causes of Acute Cough	
Prevalence	**Cause**
Very common	Postnasal drip (due to common cold, acute bacterial sinusitis, allergic rhinitis, environmental irritant rhinitis)
Common	COPD exacerbation Pneumonia Asthma
Less common	Pertussis Congestive heart failure Aspiration syndromes Pulmonary embolism

TABLE 10-6. Causes of Chronic Cough	
Prevalence	**Causes**
Common	UACS Asthma GERD
Less common	Chronic bronchitis Bronchiectasis Postinfectious cough (pertussis)
Uncommon	Bronchogenic carcinoma ACE inhibitors
Rare in adults	Psychogenic cough

ACE, angiotensin-converting enzyme; *GERD*, gastroesophageal reflux disease; *PNDS*, postnasal drip syndrome.

CHRONIC COUGH

General Facts

- Defined as a cough of >3 weeks' duration.
- Common causes include upper airway cough syndrome (UACS) or postnasal drip, asthma, and gastroesophageal reflux disease (GERD), among other causes (Table 10-6).

UPPER AIRWAY COUGH SYNDROME

General Facts

- UACS, also known as postnasal drip syndrome, is thought to be the single most common cause of both acute and chronic cough.
- UACS may be caused by a mucous hypersecretory phenotype that develops following chronic exposure of the respiratory tract to particulate matter, allergens, irritants, and pathogens. The mechanical action of secretions dripping into the hypopharynx triggers the cough reflex.
- All causes of rhinosinusitis can cause postnasal drip and cough.

Clinical Features

- Cough, more on lying down and more at night when the patient sleeps.
- Nasal discharge or nasal obstruction.
- Dripping sensation or tickle in the throat; drainage may be present on the posterior pharyngeal wall.

Management

- **UACS** is treated with a second-generation antihistamine (e.g., cetirizine) and a decongestant.
- Intranasal corticosteroids are used in cases where UACS is secondary to allergic rhinitis or symptoms are more persistent.

SINUSITIS

General Facts

- Sinusitis is a common cause of UACS and cough. It is also associated with allergic rhinitis, dental infections, foreign body or tumor, cystic fibrosis, and asthma.
- Acute sinusitis is a bacterial infection that usually involves an obstructed maxillary sinus, whereas chronic sinusitis is the persistence of sinus inflammation for ≥3 months.

Clinical Features

- Purulent nasal discharge and sinus pain worse on bending forward are the hallmark clinical findings.
- Fever can occur in severe cases.
- On physical exam, assess for tenderness to percussion over sinuses.

Diagnostic Workup

- Transillumination of the sinuses with a flashlight can show asymmetries.
- CT scan is extremely sensitive but is not specific to sinusitis, and many false positives occur. CT scan should be reserved for hospitalized patients or for the diagnosis of chronic sinusitis.
- Severe sinusitis can cause complications in surrounding tissues, such as orbital cellulitis; epidural, subdural, or cerebral abscess; and dural sinus venous thrombosis.

Management

- **Acute sinusitis:** Routine treatment with antibiotics is *not* indicated. If initial symptomatic treatment with antihistamines and antiinflammatory medications is not effective, nasal corticosteroids should be tried.
- If severe symptoms persist or there are indications of spreading infection, antibiotics are started and should be directed against the most likely bacterial organisms: *Streptococcus pneumoniae, Haemophilus influenzae,* and *Moraxella catarrhalis.* Treatment involves amoxicillin or TMP-SMZ or amoxicillin–clavulanic acid for 1 to 2 weeks.
- **Persistent chronic sinusitis** may require subspecialist involvement for prolonged antibiotics or surgical interventions to improve drainage.

CONQUER THE **BOARDS!**

UACS was previously known as postnasal drip syndrome. This will help you remember that a dripping sensation or tickle in the throat may be present.

INTERSTITIAL LUNG DISEASE

General Facts

- A group of diverse disorders involving the parenchyma of the lung that cause alveolitis, interstitial inflammation, or fibrosis.
- Interstitial lung disease (ILD) can be secondary to other diseases (see Table 10-7—these are the most commonly seen and it is not an exhaustive list) or idiopathic (called idiopathic interstitial pneumonia).
- Secondary causes can be categorized as follows:
  - Infectious: Usually seen in immunocompromised patients.
  - Occupational and environmental exposures: Most common identifiable causes.
  - Medications.
  - Rheumatic diseases: Most are common with ILD.
- **Idiopathic interstitial pneumonia** is characterized by infiltration of the interstitial compartment with inflammatory cells. Table 10-8 presents the three major types (chronic fibrosing, acute/subacute fibrosing, and smoking related) and some of their features. However, there continues to be debate among experts whether these distinct types are truly different or just a spectrum of disease. Further, there may also be a familial component to each, although the vast majority of patients with idiopathic interstitial pneumonia have no familial component (> 80%).

CONQUER THE **BOARDS!**

Indications for antibiotics are limited. Antibiotics for sinusitis are mainly reserved for severely symptomatic cases.

TABLE 10-7. Pneumoconiosis

Occupational and Environmental Exposures		Radiographically disease tends to be predominately upper zone except for asbestos
Silicates	Silica ("silicosis") Asbestos ("asbestosis") Mica (K and Mg aluminum silicates) Beryllium ("berylliosis")	asbestosis is typically found in lower lungs; other silicates in mid and upper, outer
Carbon	Coal dust ("coal worker's pneumoconiosis") Graphite	
Metals	Tin Aluminum Iron ("arc welder's lung")	
Inhaled organic dusts	Farmer's lung Bird fancier's disease Synthetic dusts (fiber lung – nylon, acrylic)	Farmers' lung is reaction to mold in crops Bird Fancier's Disease is from bird excrement/waste
Medications (common drugs that cause ILD)	**Antibiotics** Ethambutol, nitrofurantoin **Antiinflammatory** Azathioprine Cyclophosphamide Methotrexate Rituximab Sulfasalazine **Antiarrhythmic** Amiodarone	

(Continued)

TABLE 10-7. Pneumoconiosis (*Continued*)

	Chemotherapy and radiation Bleomycin Melphalan Etoposide Paclitaxel Thalidomide **Illicit drugs** (cocaine, heroin, talc)	
Rheumatic diseases	SLE Systemic scleroderma Rheumatoid arthritis Polymyositis/dermatomyositis Mixed connective tissue disease Sarcoidosis Vasculitis Granulomatosis with polyangiitis Eosinophilic granulomatosis with polyangiitis Goodpasture disease Amyloidosis	 Lower lung fields Lower lung fields
Infections	Fungal disease Coccidioidomycosis Cryptococcosis *Pneumocystis jirovecii* Atypical pneumonias Viral pneumonias HIV	

HIV, human immunodeficiency virus; *SLE*, systemic lupus erythematosus.

CONQUER THE BOARDS!

CHARTS cause fibrosis in upper lung zones:

- Coal worker's pneumoconiosis
- Histiocytosis, Langerhans cell; hypersensitivity pneumonitis (chronic)
- Ankylosing spondylitis
- Radiation (usually unilateral, radiation for breast cancer)
- Tuberculosis
- Silicosis, sarcoidosis (chronic)

I SOAR can cause fibrosis in lower lung zones:

- UIP
- Systemic sclerosis
- Others (e.g., drug induced)
- Asbestosis
- Rheumatoid arthritis

TABLE 10-8. Idiopathic Interstitial Lung Disease

Idiopathic Disease	Typical Characteristics
Chronic Fibrosing	
Idiopathic pulmonary fibrosis/ usual interstitial pneumonia (UIP)	■ Fifth or sixth decade of life, male > female incidence ■ Slowly progressive dyspnea and nonproductive cough ■ Likely not inflammatory but a **primary fibroblastic proliferation and fibrogenesis problem.** ■ **Computed tomography (CT):** • **Peripheral and bibasilar reticular opacities with honeycombing** in lower lung fields ■ **Path:** Heterogenous appearance with normal lung alternating with interstitial inflammation (lymphocytes, plasma cells) and fibrotic zones with collagen. Honeycomb changes seen ■ **Treatment:** Pirfenidone (antifibroblastic agent), nintedanib (tyrosine kinase inhibitor). Lung transplant is an option ■ **Prognosis:** 10-year survival 25%
Nonspecific interstitial pneumonia (NSIP)	■ **Presentation:** Often more subacute than UIP with fevers and signs of connective tissue disease ■ **Associated** with connective tissue disease (CTD), HIV, and hypersensitivity pneumonitis, which is often seen in toxic exposures ■ **CT:** Similar to UIP, but unlike UIP can have areas of organizing pneumonia

(*Continued*)

TABLE 10-8. Idiopathic Interstitial Lung Disease (*Continued*)

Idiopathic Disease	Typical Characteristics
Acute/Subacute Fibrosing	
	■ **Path:** Interstitial mononuclear inflammatory cells with or without fibrosis ■ **Treatment:** Glucocorticoids are usually used, but azathioprine and mycophenolate mofetil can also be used. NSIP patients are candidates for **lung transplant.** ■ **Prognosis:** Much better than UIP. Up to 75% recover
Cryptogenic organizing pneumonia (COP)	■ Subacute presentation with fever, nonproductive cough, and dyspnea heralded by a flulike illness ■ **CT:** Extensive areas of patchy air-space consolidation representing organizing pneumonia ■ **Path:** Intraluminal plugs (fibroblasts) of inflammatory debris in small airways and alveolar ducts ■ **Treatment:** Glucocorticoids, azathioprine and/or cyclophosphamide ■ **Prognosis:** Majority of patients see recovery with medical treatment
Acute interstitial pneumonia (AIP)	■ Acute and rapidly progressive symptoms and is very similar to adult respiratory distress syndrome (ARDS), except no preceding catastrophic event ■ **Chest x-ray (CXR) and CT:** Show diffuse opacities ■ **Path:** Extensive interstitial fibroblast proliferation and diffuse alveolar damage ■ **Prognosis:** Very poor with high mortality
Smoking Related	
Desquamative interstitial pneumonia (DIP)	■ >90% are smokers, usually 40 to 50 years old ■ **CT:** • Less severe than UIP • **Ground-glass opacities (no reticular opacities)** • **Minimal fibrotic changes** • **Path:** Striking feature is numerous mononuclear cells in the distal air spaces (smoker's macrophages) • **Treatment/Prognosis:** Smoking cessation is key. Can be treated with glucocorticoids, azathioprine, or cyclophosphamide • **Prognosis:** 10-year survival >70%
Respiratory bronchiolitis interstitial lung disease (RB-ILD)	■ **Path:** Pigmented macrophages in the respiratory bronchiole lumens ■ Difficult to differentiate this from DIP and so are often seen as similar diseases

Clinical Features

- **History:**
  - Classic findings are dyspnea (chronic, progressive), exercise intolerance, nonproductive cough, and tachypnea.
  - Attention should also be paid to history of smoking, medication use, occupational and environmental exposures, and family history of ILD.
- **On examination**
  - End-inspiratory dry "Velcro" type crackles can be heard.
  - In more severe cases, clubbing of digits can be found and signs of pulmonary hypertension, such as splitting of heart sounds and lower extremity edema, can be found too.
  - It is also important to look for extrapulmonary evidence for systemic diseases associated with ILD (see Table 10-8).

Diagnostic Workup

Initial workup for patients suspected to have ILD includes the following:

- **Labs:** Other than the usual labs like complete blood count (CBC) and complete metabolic panel to assess for liver and kidney disease, screening for rheumatologic diseases is warranted:
  - Antinuclear antibodies (ANA), rheumatoid factor, and cyclic citrullinated peptide antibodies. Further testing for other autoimmune disorders should be based on these initial tests and the initial history and physical examination.
- **Imaging:**
  - **Chest x-ray (CXR)** is usually done first and will show a reticular or nodular pattern. However, many patients with ILD will have a normal CXR.
  - **High-resolution CT** is the diagnostic modality of choice for ILD and should be obtained on all patients suspected of having this condition.
- **PFTs** should also be obtained and mostly demonstrate restrictive abnormalities and reduced gas transfer (high DL_{co}).
- **Lung biopsy**: Diagnosis of ILD can usually be made based on these tests, but bronchoalveolar lavage and biopsy may need to be done to further delineate the cause of ILD.

Management

- **Secondary ILD:** Removal/cessation of exposure to known environmental causes and treatment of underlying disease.
- All patients should receive supportive care with supplemental oxygen as needed.
- **Idiopathic ILD:** Steroids (possibly in combination with cyclophosphamide or azathioprine) and lung transplant are the only definitive treatments.

Environmental Lung Diseases/Pneumoconiosis

Following are some more details on the environmental exposures that cause ILD. Of note, **hypersensitivity pneumonitis** is often caused by these same environmental exposures, and high-resolution CT can look very similar to ILD. One common distinguishing factor of hypersensitivity pneumonitis is >20% lymphocytes on bronchoalveolar lavage, but often lung biopsy is the only definitive way to tell the difference.

- **Asbestosis:** A diffuse ILD caused by dust from mineral silicates. Asbestos exposure is associated with an increased risk of **mesotheliomas** (also lung cancers). Smokers with asbestos exposure are particularly at a high risk for developing lung cancer.
- **Silicosis:** Nodular fibrosis of the lung caused by exposure to silica dust, sand blasting, or the manufacture of abrasive soaps. These patients are at a greater risk of developing pulmonary tuberculosis (TB) disease.
- **Coal worker's pneumoconiosis:** An occupational hazard of ~50% of all coal miners; they develop progressive, massive fibrosis, usually involving the upper lung fields.
- **Byssinosis (cotton dust exposure):** Patients experience "chest tightness" with an associated decrease in FEV_1 with exposure to cotton dust. Clinically behaves like COPD. Treatment is to wear protective equipment and to use bronchodilators.
- **Farmer's lung:** A *hypersensitivity pneumonitis* caused by exposure to spores of thermophilic actinomycetes. Thought to be associated with a suppressor T-cell defect and is immunoglobulin G (IgG) mediated. Symptoms include fever, chills, cough, and dyspnea, and episodes occur more frequently during wet weather. Treat with steroids, and avoid exposure. Long-term complications include pulmonary fibrosis and weight loss.

CONQUER THE **BOARDS!**

A farmer presents with fever, cough, and difficulty breathing after several days of filling his silo with grain. *Think: Hypersensitivity pneumonitis from farmer's lung.*

CRITICAL CARE

RESPIRATORY FAILURE

General Facts

- Respiratory failure is due to a breakdown in the natural gas exchange mechanisms involving arterial oxygen, carbon dioxide, or both.
- Failure to maintain adequate oxygen in the blood is known as **hypoxemic respiratory failure**, whereas a failure to exchange carbon dioxide leading to rises in serum CO_2 levels is called **hypercapnic respiratory failure**.

Clinical Features

- Respiratory failure can cause SOB and altered mentation.
- Hypoxemia or hypercapnia can lead to acid–base disturbances and electrolyte imbalances.
- Hypercapnia can manifest with somnolence and worsening mentation.

Diagnostic Workup (see figure 10-2)

- When suspected clinically or via SPO_2, the most important test to perform is an ABG. This will show the level of arterial O_2 and CO_2, hence determining whether hypoxic respiratory failure, hypercapnic respiratory failure, or both are present (Figure 10-2).
- Hypercapnic respiratory failure can be caused by a variety of conditions that can affect the mechanics of CO_2 exchange. Pulmonary conditions such as COPD can cause CO_2 retention. Extrapulmonary conditions such as diaphragm neuromuscular abnormalities or neurologic causes (Guillain–Barré syndrome, myasthenia gravis, cerebrovascular accident [CVA]) that can have an effect on pulmonary mechanics can cause hypercapnia.

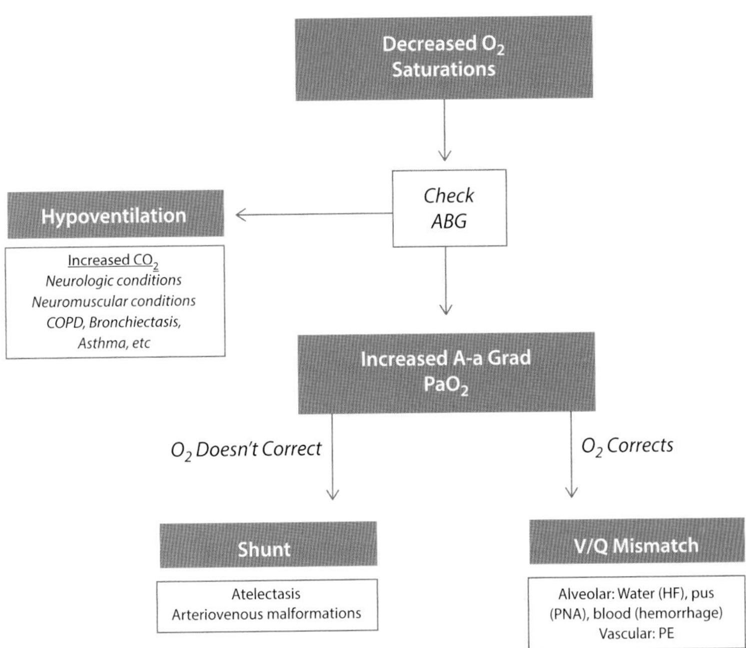

FIGURE 10-2. Workup of respiratory failure.

- Hypoxia can occur via shunting or ventilation and perfusion (V/Q) mismatch. Shunting, such as arteriovenous malformations, typically does not correct with supplemental O_2, whereas mismatches in V/Q tend to improve with supplemental O_2. V/Q mismatches include pneumonia, pulmonary edema, or diffuse alveolar hemorrhage (Figure 10-3).

Management

- Supportive care with supplemental oxygen or noninvasive or invasive mechanical ventilation can help provide immediate benefits while pursuing workup and management of the underlying cause.

MECHANICAL VENTILATION

When to Intubate and Start

- The need for mechanical ventilation requires careful clinical judgment.
- Failure to protect the airway, severe hypoxia, severe hypercapnia, acid–base consequences of respiratory abnormalities, and increased work of breathing are all indications for intubation (Figure 10-3).
- Early identification of patients that may have impending respiratory failure is also important. Concerning findings in an ABG or abnormal vital signs may suggest future need for intubation, including:
  - PaO_2/FiO_2 <300 to 200
  - Increased $Paco_2$ + tachypnea
  - RR >30 to 35
  - PaO_2 <50 on 50% or greater FiO_2
  - $Paco_2$ >55 lung function (i.e., no COPD, fibrotic lung disease)
  - pH <7.3
  - Use of accessory muscles
- In select cases, positive-pressure ventilation (usually with bilevel positive airway pressure [BiPAP]) may provide adequate support and delay or defer the need for mechanical ventilation.

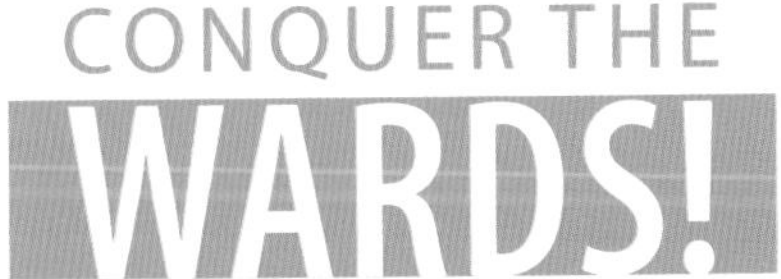

Contraindications for the use of positive-pressure ventilation include excess secretions or inability to protect the airway.

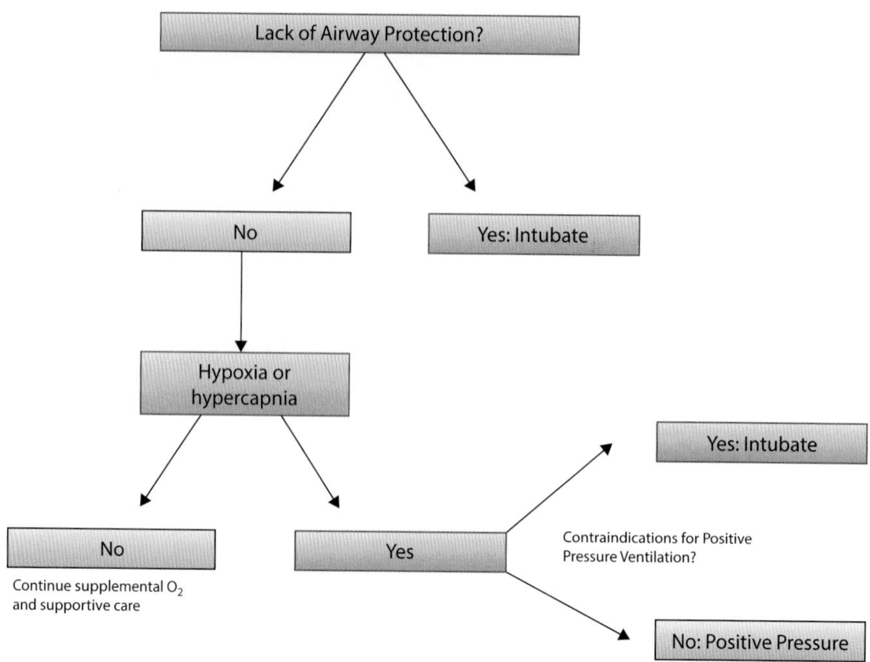

FIGURE 10-3. Management of respiratory failure

Ventilator Modes

- **Assist control** delivers a minimum set number of breaths, which are delivered no matter if the patient triggers a breath or not. The ventilator in this mode can be set to volume control (set the volume of air given with each breath) or pressure control (set amount of pressure given with each breath). If the patient initiates a breath, the full amount of volume or pressure is given every time. This is the most supportive mode.
- **Synchronized intermittent mandatory ventilation** delivers a minimum number of supported breaths synchronized with the patient's efforts. Additional patient-initiated breaths are not ventilator supported, and the patient must overcome resistance of the ventilator circuit during spontaneous breaths.
- **Pressure support** is a setting where the ventilator supports patient-initiated breaths with a set inspiratory pressure, which is usually lower, allowing for the patient to breathe more on their own. This modality can be used to assess the ability to breathe and for weaning from the ventilator.
- **CPAP** is a setting where the patient breathes spontaneously while the ventilator maintains constant airway pressure, usually just to overcome the resistance of the ventilator circuit (about 5 cm water).

Ventilator Variables

- FiO_2 is the fraction of inspired oxygen.
- PEEP is the positive end-expiratory pressure. This is used to help prevent alveolar collapse and increase oxygenation.
- Inspiratory time or normal I:E ratio is approximately 1:2. It can be controlled on a mechanical ventilator for the management of obstructive diseases. For example, with asthma you may need to increase the expiratory time.
- Peak inspiratory pressure is determined by large airway resistance and compliance and may indicate obstruction (e.g., mucous plug) or a leak in the ventilator.

- The plateau pressure is pressure at the end of inspiration, when flow has ceased, and is dependent on the lung parenchyma. Increased plateau pressure suggests decreased flexibility of the lung tissue, known as lung compliance. This can be seen when alveoli are full of fluid (adult respiratory distress syndrome [ARDS], pneumonia).

Ventilator Management

- Always ask yourself what the underlying need for mechanical ventilation is. For patients with hypoxia, management of the FiO_2 based on ABG results is key. Patients with hypercapnia will require management of ventilation and gas exchange.
- Troubleshoot low pO_2 by increasing FiO_2 and potentially increasing PEEP as well in order to recruit more alveoli.
- Troubleshoot a high pCO_2 by increasing the minute ventilation. This is done by changing the tidal volume or respiratory rate.
- Remember to always monitor the effectiveness and safety of mechanical ventilation with daily ABGs, CXRs, and frequent vital signs. Any change should prompt repeat ABG testing and modification of the mechanical ventilation settings accordingly.
- Daily chest imaging is needed to assess for complications such as pneumothorax or migration of the endotracheal tube (ET).
- Daily sedation holidays and daily assessments for weaning off the ventilator are also important. If failure to wean occurs, think of causes that may contribute to failure of weaning trials. The rapid-shallow breathing index and other formulas can help you identify patients that are ready for extubation.

CONQUER THE **WARDS!**

Fail to wean:
Fluid overload:
Airway resistance
Infection
Low O_2
Thyroid
Oxygen
Wheezing
Electrolytes
Antiinflammatory needed (steroids)
Neuromuscular disease.

ACUTE RESPIRATORY DISTRESS SYNDROME

General Facts

- A condition that results from diffuse alveolar damage leading to increased permeability of alveolar capillaries, causing cellular exudative fluid to fill alveoli.
- ARDS can be caused by direct (aspiration, pneumonitis, pneumonia) or indirect injury (shock, sepsis, severe pancreatitis, transfusion-associated lung injury) that can cause increased pulmonary permeability and inflammation.

CONQUER THE **WARDS!**

Always think of ARDS in patients with acute bilateral infiltrates, noncardiogenic edema, and hypoxia.

Diagnostic Workup

- A clinical evaluation based on the Berlin definition will help you discern if ARDS is present. An **ABG** is necessary to obtain an accurate Pao_2. The Berlin definition includes acute onset of reduced oxygenation (Pao_2/Fio_2 <300 for mild; moderate <200; severe <100), bilateral infiltrates without alternative explanation, and noncardiogenic pulmonary edema. Note the Fio_2 in these equations is expressed as a decimal form (40% oxygen is 0.40 Fio_2).
- **Chest imaging via CXR or CT** will help define the extent of bilateral pulmonary infiltrates present.

CONQUER THE **WARDS!**

Treatment for ARDS is mostly supportive. A research network called ARDSNet has developed guidelines to help clinicians. These are available online with pocket cards that are easy to print.

Management

- O_2 treatment does not improve hypoxia in ARDS. Fluid-filled, consolidated, or collapsed alveoli lead to effective arteriovenous shunting.

- Supportive strategies include aggressive fluid management, the ARDSNet protocol for mechanical ventilation management, and other interventions such as prone position and paralysis.
- Treatment usually involves hemodynamic support and treatment of the underlying disease.
- Overall has a high mortality and very little evidence that any treatments change this.

HIGH-YIELD LITERATURE

Thompson BT, Bernard GR. ARDS Network (NHLBI) studies – Successes and challenges in ARDS clinical research. *Crit Care Clin*. 2011;27(3):459-468.

SHOCK

- Shock is a state of tissue hypoxia due to hypotension and tissue hypoperfusion. It can be due to cardiogenic, septic, hypovolemic, or distributive (allergic or neurogenic) causes.
- Distributive shock can occur due to severe allergic reactions or due to spinal trauma.
- Hypovolemic shock can occur due to severe blood loss or fluid losses.
- Cardiogenic shock can occur in the setting of an acute myocardial infarction (MI) or severely decompensated heart failure.
- Septic shock occurs in the setting of infection with a severe systemic inflammatory response.
- Cardiogenic, hypovolemic, and septic shock can be differentiated by assessing pulse pressures, capillary refills, volume status, and overall history and clinical context (Figure 10-4).

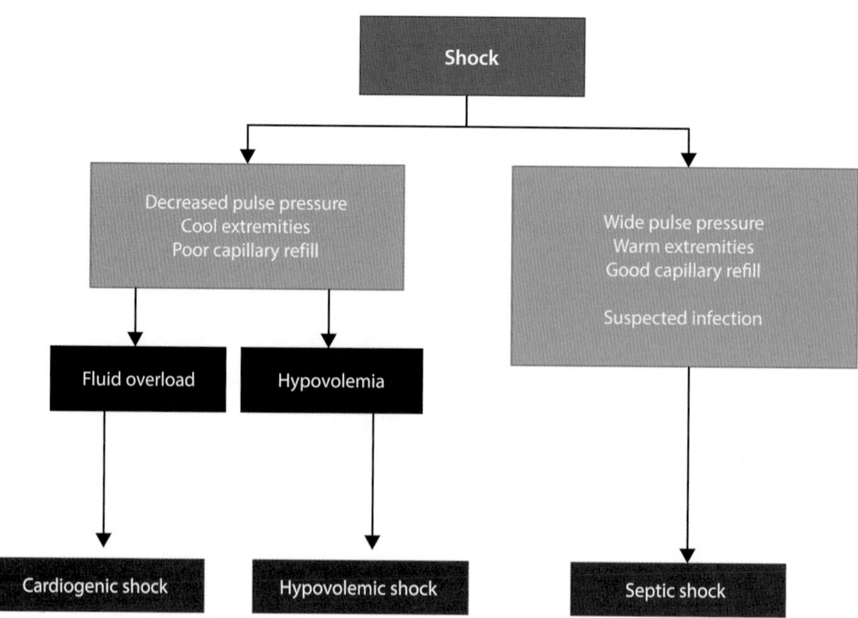

FIGURE 10-4. Types of shock.

Clinical Features

- Regardless of cause, patients will have hypotension and signs of hypoperfusion and end-organ damage.
- Signs of end-organ damage include altered mental status, renal failure, transaminitis, and cold extremities.
- Lactic acidosis from tissue hypoperfusion may lead to respiratory compensation. Respiratory muscles demand more oxygen in a low oxygen state, which may then lead to respiratory failure.

Diagnostic Workup

- **Lactic acid** should always be checked and is a good measure of tissue hypoperfusion and should be ordered to help follow improvement.
- Always obtain an **ECG**, as cardiogenic shock from acute MI is a medical emergency and will require cardiac catheterization.
- **Blood cultures** and an infectious workup should be pursued if there is any sign of infection or clinical suspicion for infection.
- **Review medication lists** and make sure no new medications have been added that can lower blood pressure or cause anaphylaxis.

Management

- Treat the underlying cause.
- See Cardiogenic Shock and Sepsis and Shock sections.

SEPSIS AND SEPTIC SHOCK

- Sepsis is an inflammatory state that can occur with severe infections, resulting in capillary leak and shock.
- The definitions of sepsis have evolved over the past 30 years. Understanding current and prior definitions is useful, as the terminology is sometimes used interchangeably in hospitals.
- The first consensus definition of sepsis (Sepsis-1) involved a spectrum of infection with severe inflammatory response syndrome (SIRS), sepsis, severe sepsis, and septic shock. Severe sepsis was defined as SIRS + infection + tissue hypoperfusion that was responsive to fluids, whereas septic shock implied the need for vasopressors (Figure 10-5).
- Due to the limitations of SIRS and Sepsis-1, multiple other consensus definitions have been made. The latest definition (Sepsis-3) uses the sequential organ failure assessment (SOFA) or the quick SOFA (qSOFA)

CONQUER THE WARDS!

qSOFA is a simple tool.

- Altered mental status
- Low BP
- RR >22

If you have two of these, your qSOFA is positive.

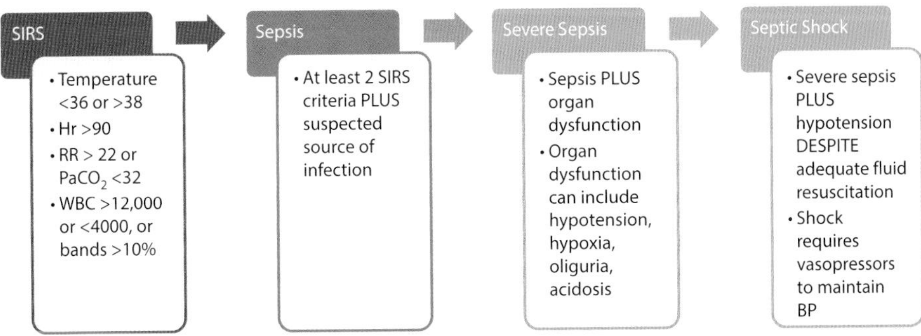

SIRS
• Temperature <36 or >38
• Hr >90
• RR > 22 or PaCO2 <32
• WBC >12,000 or <4000, or bands >10%
Sepsis
• At least 2 SIRS criteria PLUS suspected source of infection
Severe Sepsis
• Sepsis PLUS organ dysfunction
• Organ dysfunction can include hypotension, hypoxia, oliguria, acidosis
Septic Shock
• Severe sepsis PLUS hypotension DESPITE adequate fluid resuscitation
• Shock requires vasopressors to maintain BP

FIGURE 10-5. Spectrum of sepsis and septic shock.

to determine or screen for tissue hypoperfusion. Severe sepsis is no longer in use, as the term is considered redundant. It has been replaced by the term sepsis (positive qSOFA), and septic shock remains a shock state with vasopressor needs.

Diagnostic Workup

- Obtain broad laboratory workup, including CBC, chemistries, and LFTs to assess for any signs of organ dysfunction, including renal and liver abnormalities.
- **Lactic acid** is needed to both diagnose and treat tissue hypoperfusion.
- Obtain two blood cultures and culture each central venous catheter if present.
- Consider obtaining a urine culture and urinalysis, especially in patients who cannot report urinary symptoms due to altered mentation.
- **CXR** to assess for infiltrates.

Management

- The goals of care are to treat the underlying cause (antibiotics, source control), aggressive hydration (intravenous fluids [IVF]), and vasopressors if needed toward a goal mean arterial pressure of >65.
- Immediate broad-spectrum antimicrobials should be started within 1 hour of recognition. Delays can increase mortality. Always start broad and modify later based on further clinical and microbiologic data.
- Aggressive hydration is the key management intervention with either crystalloids or colloids. This usually means use of 1-L boluses.
- Monitor hemoglobin (HGB) and transfuse if <7, as this will help with oxygen delivery.
- Vasopressor management will start with norepinephrine. Other vasopressors (vasopressin) are added if the patient reaches the maximum dose of norepinephrine.
- The use of corticosteroids is controversial. May not have a mortality benefit in all scenarios. Always check cortisol levels if shock is refractory.
- Monitor cardiac function and need for cardiac inotropes.

CARDIOGENIC SHOCK

General Facts

- Cardiogenic shock occurs when cardiac abnormalities affect the ability of tissues to receive adequate perfusion.
- Acute MI, acute decompensated heart failure (ADHF), valvular rupture, and other cardiac conditions can lead to poor cardiac function and shock.

Clinical Features

- Similar to other shock states; signs of tissue hypoperfusion will occur, including oliguria, cold extremities, and altered mental status.
- Specific causes may have other symptoms, such as chest pain for MI, progressive lower extremity (LE) edema for ADHF, and new or worsening murmurs for valvular disorders.

Diagnostic Workup

- **ECG** should be obtained immediately to rule out any new acute MI. ST elevations, new left bundle branch block (LBBB), and other abnormalities should prompt immediate cardiac catheterization.

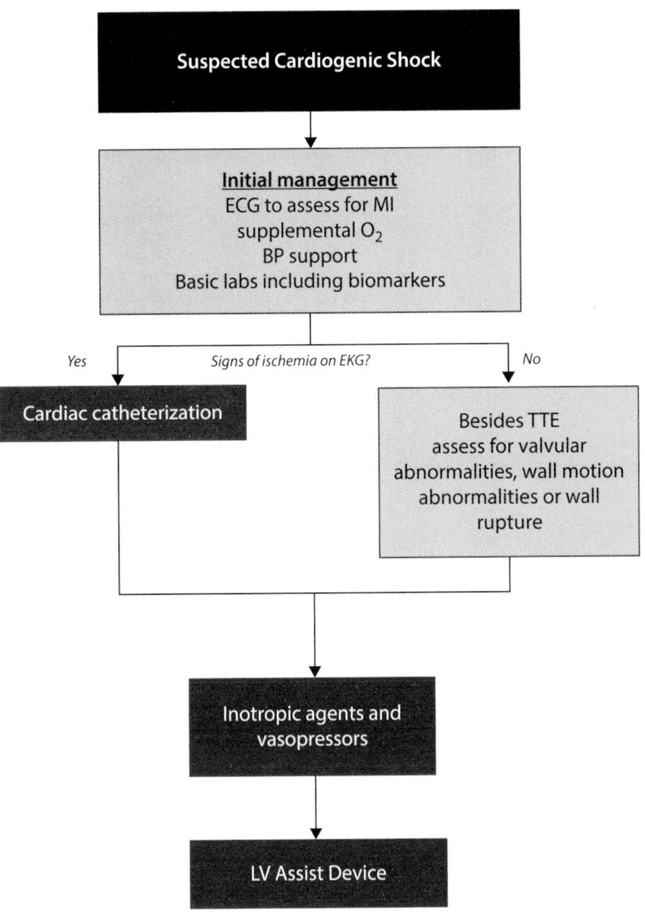

FIGURE 10-6. Cardiogenic shock.

- **Bedside echocardiography** should be performed to assess cardiac output and look for any new valvular abnormality.

Management

- ICU or coronary care unit (CCU) admission for continuous vital signs, telemetry, and intensive nursing care is needed. Depending on the cause of the cardiogenic shock, the following interventions may be needed:
  - Inotropic medications (e.g., dobutamine).
  - Vasopressors.
  - Intraarterial balloon pumps and left ventricular assist devices.
- Treatment of the underlying cause, such as immediate cardiac catheterization for acute MI, should be pursued (Figure 10-6).
- Cardiothoracic surgery may be needed for structural valvular abnormalities or papillary muscle rupture.

HEMOPTYSIS

- Coughing up of blood due to bleeding from the lower respiratory tract.
- See Table 10-9 for a list of causes.
- **Massive hemoptysis** is any amount of bleeding causing clinical impairment of respiratory function. There is no consensus volume that defines this, but more than 100 to 200 mL of **bright red blood** in a 24-hour period is concerning.

TABLE 10-9. Causes of Hemoptysis

Incidence	Cause
Common	Epistaxis (most common) Bronchitis and bronchiectasis (second most common) Lung cancer Tuberculosis Pneumonia Pulmonary embolism Coagulopathy Congestive heart failure
Rare	Pulmonary hypertension Vasculitis Collagen vascular disease Pulmonary arteriovenous malformation Granulomatosis with polyangiitis Goodpasture syndrome Trauma Foreign body

CONQUER THE **BOARDS!**

A patient presents with hemoptysis, sinusitis, and glomerulonephritis. On physical exam, you notice a "saddle-nose" deformity. *Think: Granulomatosis with polyangiitis.* **Next step:** Send for circulating antineutrophil cytoplasmic antibody (ANCA).

Diagnostic Workup

- Clinical evaluation and quantification of blood is key.
- Workup includes **BOTH** CT (to identify cause) and bronchoscopy (to localize).

Management

- Supplemental oxygen as needed.
- Position patient with bleeding side down to reduce risk of aspiration.
- Suppression of cough reflex (i.e., codeine) can be helpful.
- Patients with massive hemoptysis need immediate intubation with large-bore ET tube (8 or larger if possible) and endobronchial treatments such as cold saline or epinephrine. Bronchial artery embolization may be needed.

CONQUER THE **BOARDS!**

A patient presents with dyspnea, hemoptysis, and acute renal failure. *Think: Goodpasture syndrome.* **Next step:** Send for anti-glomerular basement membrane antibodies.

PULMONARY EMBOLUS

General Facts

- **Definition:** Obstruction of the pulmonary artery or its branches with material outside the lung (thrombus, air, tumor, or fat). Most commonly due to thrombus dislodging or migration of a deep venous thrombus from the extremities.
- Pulmonary embolism (PE) is often categorized into hemodynamically stable or unstable PE.
  - **"Massive" PE** = hemodynamically unstable (hypotension) PE.
  - **"Submassive" PE** = hemodynamically stable but with signs of right ventricular strain on echocardiogram or ECG.
  - "Low-risk" PE = hemodynamically stable with no signs of right ventricular strain.
- Very large PEs that impede blood flow in both the right and left pulmonary arteries are called **saddle emboli.**
- Risk factors for venous thromboembolism (VTE) include immobilization (long flights, surgery, fracture), hypercoagulability (malignancy, pregnancy, genetic), or medications (oral contraceptives, tamoxifen).

CONQUER THE **WARDS!**

If a patient has hypoxia with a normal CXR, consider a PE.

Wells Score	
3	Clinical Signs and Symptoms of DVT?
3	PE Is #1 Diagnosis, or Equally Likely
1.5	Heart Rate > 100?
1.5	Immobilization at least 3 days, or Surgery in the Previous 4 weeks
1.5	Previous, objectively diagnosed PE or DVT?
1	Hemoptysis?
1	Malignancy w/ Treatment within 6 mo, or palliative?
	Patient has none of these

Score <2	Score <2-6	Score >6
Low probability	Intermediate probability	High probability

FIGURE 10-7. Diagnostic workup of pulmonary embolism.

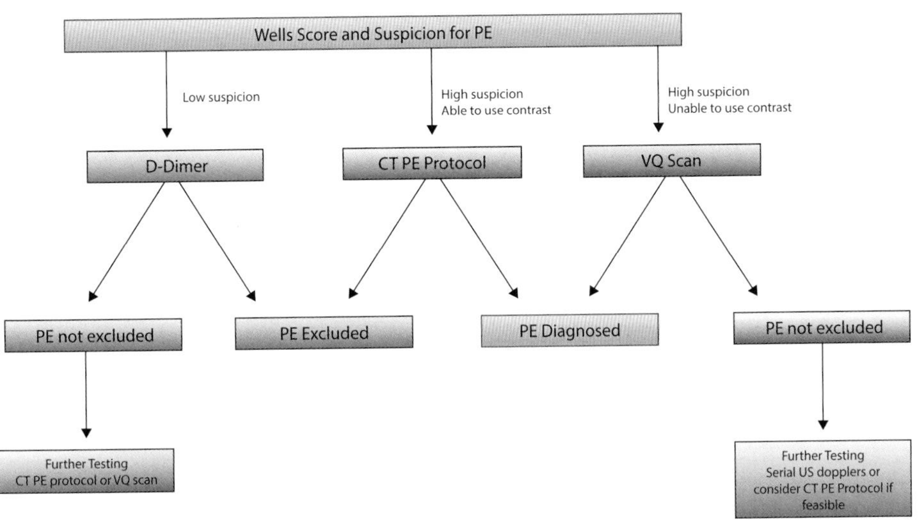

FIGURE 10-8. Diagnostic workup of pulmonary embolism.

CONQUER THE **BOARDS!**

Know these key findings on chest imaging:

Westermark sign: Oligemia seen on the CXR distal to the PE. (Rare finding in the times of CT angiograms; however, a favorite topic on rounds with attendings).

Hampton's hump: Wedge-shaped infiltrate seen on CXR.

Clinical Features

No sign or symptom is specific for PE.

- Sinus tachycardia (most common rhythm disturbance), dyspnea, cough, tachypnea, pleuritic chest pain, hemoptysis, and hypoxia can all be present.
- **Wells score** is an evidence-based score to help you calculate the probability of a PE. Look for clinical signs and symptoms of deep vein thrombosis (DVT), heart rate >100, immobilization at least 3 days or surgery in the previous 4 weeks, previous objectively diagnosed PE or DVT, hemoptysis, and history of malignancy to help you calculate the Wells score (Figure 10-7).

CONQUER THE **WARDS!**

If a patient with a known or suspected PE has ECG findings consistent with right ventricular strain or hypotension, consider fibrinolytics.

Diagnostic Workup (see table 10-10)

- The probability of a PE based on your Wells score can help guide your diagnostic workup.
- A patient with low or moderate probability for a PE can undergo noninvasive testing first, such as a D-dimer. If negative, PE is effectively ruled out. However, a positive test should prompt better testing such as a CT with contrast (Figure 10-8).

CONQUER THE **WARDS!**

There are a lot of great web-based calculators that will help you calculate the Wells score. Do an internet search and find your favorite one!

TABLE 10-10 Diagnostic options for PE and DVT

Helical (spiral) CT	Also called CTPA (CT of pulmonary arteries); to look for embolus in the pulmonary vasculature. Most common. Fast and convenient, fairly sensitive. Downside: IV contrast can damage kidneys and can miss peripheral PEs.
Pulmonary angiogram	The gold standard for detection of PE. Very sensitive. Downside: Invasive test.
Ventilation-perfusion scan (V/Q scan)	To look for perfusion defects at site of PE. Does not affect kidneys. Okay for pregnant patients. Downside: long test and not useful in patients with underlying lung disease.
Lower extremity Dopplers	To detect DVT— a positive test will make one more suspicious of PE if symptoms are present.

- **Other tests that should be considered to evaluate for right ventricular (RV) strain:**
  - **ECG:** All patients with PE or suspected PE should have an ECG. Look for signs of RV strains such as S wave in lead I and Q and inverted T waves in lead III; when found, this is a characteristic sign (S1Q3T3 is the mnemonic).
  - **B-Natriuretic peptide:** If it is high can indicate RV strain.
  - **Echocardiogram**: This should be obtained in any patient who is hemodynamically unstable or who has a large tumor burden on CT scan.

Management

- Immediate anticoagulation is warranted. Severity of disease will help define therapeutic modality, admission to the hospital or to the ICU.
- For ambulatory patients with minimal symptoms and low risk for PE, low-molecular-weight heparin (LMWH) or direct oral anticoagulants (DOACs) can be used without admission to the hospital. Patients with more severe disease or comorbidities will require observation in the hospital.
- Massive PE or submassive PE will require ICU admission and possible thrombolytic therapy. In these cases heparin drips are the anticoagulation of choice because many of the studies with LMWH and DOAC excluded massive or submassive PE patients. Thrombolysis can be done via interventional pulmonary angiography or via embolectomy.
- Chronic anticoagulation can be achieved with warfarin, LMWH, or new oral anticoagulants such as apixaban or rivaroxaban. Duration of therapy will depend on whether risk factors and if any prior thrombi have occurred.
- If a PE or DVT occurred after a reversible risk factor or was provoked, duration can be 3 to 6 months. A second event, unprovoked event, or history of malignancy will require lifelong anticoagulation.

CONQUER THE BOARDS!

Angiography is the gold standard in the diagnosis of:

- Deep vein thrombosis
- Dissecting aortic aneurysm
- Ischemic bowel syndrome
- Pulmonary embolism

CONQUER THE WARDS!

Clinical signs and symptoms of DVT:
PE is #1 diagnosis OR equally likely
Heart rate >100
Immobilization at least 3 days OR surgery in the previous 4 weeks
Previous, objectively diagnosed PE or DVT
Hemoptysis
Malignancy with treatment within 6 months or palliative

HIGH-YIELD LITERATURE

Wells PS, Anderson DR, Rodger M, et al. Excluding pulmonary embolism at the bedside without diagnostic imaging: Management of patients with suspected pulmonary embolism presenting to the emergency department by using a simple clinical model and D-dimer. *Ann Intern Med*. 2001;135(2):98-107.

PULMONARY HYPERTENSION

General Facts

- Pulmonary hypertension (pHTN) is an increase in pressures in the pulmonary vasculature.
- pHTN is defined by a mean pulmonary artery pressure above 25 mm Hg at rest.
- pHTN can be due to primary disease or secondary to other causes (Table 10-11).

Clinical Features

- SOB and dyspnea on exertion are the hallmarks of pHTN.
- Right-sided heart failure can occur, with peripheral edema and abdominal distension.
- The World Health Organization (WHO) classifies patients as Class I if asymptomatic, Class II if symptoms occur with ordinary activities of daily living, Class III if symptoms occur with minimal activity, and Class IV if symptomatic at rest.

Diagnostic Workup

- If you suspect a patient has pHTN, the initial test is transthoracic echocardiography (TTE). Echocardiography can estimate pressures and identify patients with increased pressures. The exact mm Hg may be overestimated
- A right heart catheterization (RHC) with measurement of pressures is the gold standard and must be done to confirm pHTN and can also guide therapy. Often during a RHC, calcium channel blockers or other vasodilators can be injected to see if pulmonary pressures decrease.
- Workup for secondary causes should be based on risk factors and suspicion. Generally this workup would include:
  - ANA to screen for connective tissue diseases and HIV (Workup Group 1).
  - Echocardiogram (Workup Group 1 and 2).

TABLE 10-11. Classification of Pulmonary Hypertension

Group 1: Primary pHTN	Group 2: Left Heart Disease	Group 3: Lung Disease or Hypoxia	Group 4: Chronic Thromboembolic Disease	Group 5: Unclear or Multifactorial Causes
Idiopathic pHTN Familial pHTN Associated with connective tissue disease HIV Schistosomiasis Congenital heart disease	Atrial or ventricular dysfunction Left-sided heart failure Left-sided valvular disease	COPD ILD OSAHS Chronic hypoxia	Multiple PE events Hypercoagulable states with multiple PEs	Sarcoidosis Histiocytosis Thyroid disease Sickle cell disease

COPD, chronic obstructive pulmonary disease; *HIV*, human immunodeficiency virus; *ILD*, interstitial lung disease; *OSAHS*, obstructive sleep apnea–hypopnea syndrome; *PE*, pulmonary embolism; *pHTN*, primary hypertension.

- PFTs (Workup Group 3) and sometimes a sleep study if there are risks for OSA.
- CT pulmonary angiogram to rule out thromboembolic disease and ILD (Workup Group 3 and 4).

Management

- Supportive care with oxygen and diuretics will help improve quality of life.
- Patients that respond to vasodilator testing on RHC can be treated with oral calcium channel blockers (CCBs).
- If there is no sustained response to CCBs, other treatment modalities such as PDE-5 inhibitors (sildenafil, vardenafil), prostanoids (epoprostenol, treprostinil), or endothelin receptor antagonists (bosentan, ambrisentan) can be used alone or in combination.
- Secondary causes should be treated, such as anticoagulation for chronic thromboembolic pulmonary hypertension (CTEPH) and management of any underlying cardiac or pulmonary disease.

DISEASES OF THE PLEURA

PLEURAL EFFUSION

Abnormal accumulation of fluid within the space between the parietal and visceral pleural membranes of the lungs. Pleural effusion is classified as transudative or exudative.

- **Transudative** pleural effusions are due to:
  - Increased hydrostatic pressure as in heart failure.
  - Decreased oncotic pressure, as in nephrotic syndrome.
- **Exudative** pleural effusions are due to increased capillary permeability, usually secondary to an inflammatory process.

Diagnostic Workup

- Any unilateral pleural effusion of unclear etiology should generally be tapped for diagnostic pleural fluid analysis (Figure 10-9).

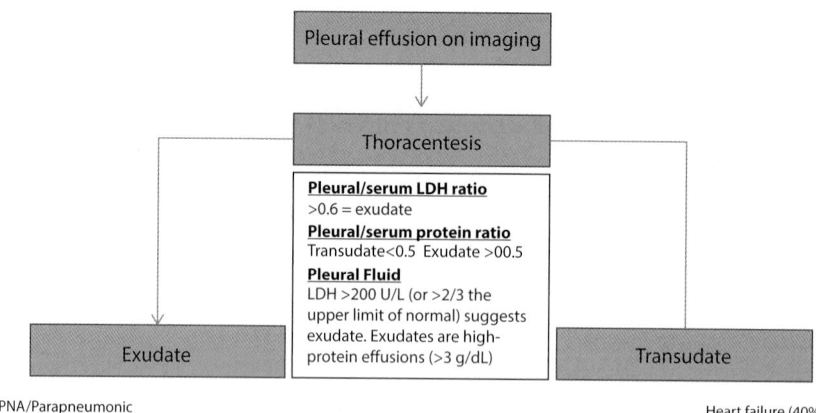

FIGURE 10-9. Pleural effusions.

- Any pleural fluid should be analyzed for total and differential cell count, protein, glucose, lactate dehydrogenase (LDH), and pH (if there is suspicion of empyema) (Table 10-12).
- **Light criteria** *(learn this for exam):* The effusion is an **exudate** if **one** or more of the following is present:
    - Ratio of pleural to serum protein >0.5.
    - Ratio of pleural to serum LDH >0.6.
    - Pleural fluid LDH more than two-thirds upper normal limit of serum LDH.

Common Associations (see table 10-13)

- **Parapneumonic effusion:** As the name suggests, it should be suspected if an effusion develops in the setting of a pneumonia. Any parapneumonic effusion is an exudate, with a high neutrophil count.
    - A "simple" parapneumonic effusion can become "complex" and "complicated." If any of the following is present, it should be considered an empyema:
        a. pH <7.2, glucose <40 mg/dL, LDH >1000.
        b. Positive Gram stain or culture, which also means the effusion is an empyema.
    - Complicated parapneumonic effusions and empyemas can also become loculated.

TABLE 10-12. Biochemical Characteristics and Causes of Pleural Effusions

Gross Blood	Low Glucose	High Amylase
■ Tumor (breast cancer, lung cancer, lymphoma) ■ Pulmonary infarction ■ Hemothorax: Defined as pleural fluid hematocrit >50% of serum hematocrit; causes include trauma and aortic dissection	■ Complicated parapneumonic effusion and empyema ■ Rheumatoid arthritis (glucose extremely low, usually <15 mg/dL) ■ Tumor ■ Tuberculosis	■ Pancreatitis ■ Renal failure ■ Tumor ■ Esophageal rupture: High salivary amylase is useful in diagnosis; surgical emergency with high mortality if not treated immediately

TABLE 10-13. Other Tests That Can be Ordered on Pleural Fluid

Disease	Diagnostic Pleural Fluid Tests
Malignancy	Positive cytology
Lupus pleuritis	Pleural fluid serum ANA >1.0
Tuberculous pleurisy	Positive AFB stain and culture ADA
Esophageal rupture	High salivary amylase, pleural fluid acidosis (often as low as 6.00)
Chylothorax	Triglycerides (>110 mg/dL); lipoprotein electrophoresis (chylomicrons)
Hemothorax	Hematocrit (pleural fluid/blood >0.5 g/dL)
Urinothorax	Creatinine (pleural fluid/serum >1.0 mg/dL)
Extravascular migration of central venous catheter	Observation (milky if lipids are infused); pleural fluid/serum glucose >1.0 mmol/L

ADA, adenosine deaminase; *AFB*, acid-fast bacillus; *ANA*, antinuclear antibodies.

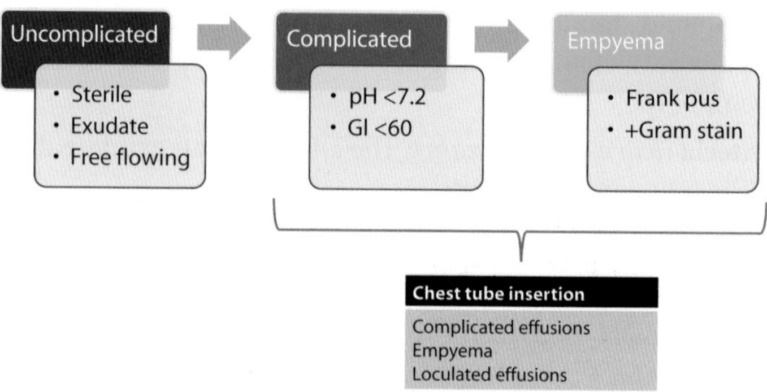

FIGURE 10-10. Management of pleural effusions.

Management

- After a diagnostic thoracentesis is performed, treatment of the underlying cause is key.
- Indications for chest tube placement will depend on the complexity of the effusion, presence of loculations, or pus (Figure 10-10).
- Complex effusions with loculations that do not fully resolve with chest tube placement will need cardiothoracic surgery assessment for possible video-assisted thoracoscopy surgery (VATS).

HIGH-YIELD LITERATURE

Light RW, Macgregor MI, Luchsinger PC, Ball WC Jr. Pleural effusions: The diagnostic separation of transudates and exudates. *Ann Intern Med*. 1972;77(4):507-513.

Light RW, Erozan YS, Ball WC Jr. Cells in pleural fluid. Their value in differential diagnosis. *Arch Intern Med*. 1973;132(6):854-860. 2018;391(10115): P31-40.

PNEUMOTHORAX

General Facts

- A pneumothorax occurs when there is air in the pleural space. It can be a primary spontaneous pneumothorax, or it can be secondary to other causes.
  - Primary spontaneous pneumothorax occurs in a person with normal lungs, whereas secondary spontaneous pneumothorax occurs in patients who have underlying lung disease.
- Spontaneous pneumothorax affects approximately 20,000 persons annually, usually from rupture of a subpleural bleb or pleural necrosis due to lung disease.

A 20-year-old tall man arrives complaining of sudden onset of severe shortness of breath and pleuritic chest pain. *Think: Primary spontaneous pneumothorax.*

Clinical Features

- Chest pain, dyspnea, hyperresonance, or decreased breath sounds on affected side.
- Tracheal deviation *away* from affected side (in tension pneumothorax).

Diagnostic Workup

- Upright CXR is ~83% sensitive; demonstrates an absence of lung markings where the lung has collapsed.

Management

- 100% oxygen can help oxygenate and helps with resorption of pneumothorax.
- For pneumothoraxes >20% of lung volume or with symptoms, perform intervention to remove air (needle aspiration if stable, chest tube placement if unstable).
- Pleurodesis to adhere the visceral and parietal pleura in cases of recurrent pneumothorax or persistent air leak.

MEDIASTINITIS

General Facts

- Inflammation in the mediastinum that can be due to inflammation or infection. Inflammatory causes can include autoimmune conditions, trauma, or surgery. Infectious causes can be due to esophageal perforation, tuberculosis (TB), histoplasmosis, or inhalational anthrax.

Clinical Features

- Fever and dyspnea can develop.
- Severity will depend on the underlying cause, with esophageal perforation as an example of an acute surgical emergency, while histoplasmosis and tuberculosis are chronic inflammatory conditions.

Management

- Correction of underlying cause.

PNEUMOMEDIASTINUM

General Features

- Air in the esophagus typically means rupture of a surrounding organ has occurred. Esophageal rupture is the first possibility to be considered (often associated with left hydropneumothorax).
- **Boerhaave syndrome:** Ruptured esophagus from violent retching. Associated with very high mortality if not identified and managed surgically.
- Rupture of alveolus, bronchus, or trachea can also cause pneumomediastinum.

Physical finding in pneumomediastinum:

Hamman sign: A crunching sound occurring with the heartbeat.

Treatment

- Requires surgical intervention to repair any ruptures.

Lung Cancer

General Facts

- Leading cause of cancer death in both men and women in the United States.
- Cases have been decreasing in men, but increasing in women.
- Smoking is by far the most important causative factor in the development of lung cancer.
- Passive smoke exposure, radon gas exposure, asbestos, arsenic, and nickel exposure are other common risk factors.

Types

- **Small cell lung cancer (SCLC):**
  - Typically in a central location.
  - SCLC is sensitive to chemotherapy, and surgery is *not* indicated as first-line therapy.
  - SCLC has poor prognosis with high recurrence after initial response to chemotherapy.
  - **Two-stage system:**
    a. Limited disease: Tumor confined to ipsilateral hemithorax and nodes. **Treatment:** Chemotherapy and radiation to lung and prophylactically to cranium. For some patients surgical resection is possible if the tumor is small.
    b. Extensive disease: Tumor in contralateral thorax, distant metastases, pericardial effusion, or pleural effusion (even if on the same side). **Treatment:** Chemotherapy alone.
  - SCLC has a rapid doubling time, so patients must receive chemotherapy quickly after diagnosis.
- **Non–small cell lung cancer:**
  - Includes squamous cell and adenocarcinoma. Tissue diagnosis must include enough tissue for molecular testing, as this determines the ability to use immunotherapy.
  - Treated with surgery if early stage, and combination of chemotherapy, radiation, and surgery at later stages. Prognosis varies with stage.

A 61-year-old heavy smoker presents with shoulder pain, ptosis, and anhidrosis. What does he have? Pancoast tumor (metastasis to supraclavicular lymph node in lung cancer).

Clinical Features

- Cough, hemoptysis, dyspnea, weight loss, and malaise.
- Symptoms from mediastinal involvement either from spread of the tumor or large mediastinal lymphadenopathy include hoarseness (recurrent laryngeal nerve paralysis), dysphagia, and superior vena cava syndrome.
- Associated (paraneoplastic) syndromes (see Table 10-14).

Chronic cough is the most common symptom of lung cancer.

Management

- The two main types of lung cancer, small cell and non–small cell cancer, have different responses to radiotherapy, chemotherapy, and surgery (see Table 10-15). Generally, small cell is always treated with chemotherapy and never surgery; non–small cell is treated with surgery if cancer is local +/– chemotherapy and immunotherapy.

TABLE 10-14. Syndromes Associated with Lung Cancer

Horner syndrome	Sympathetic nerve paralysis produces enophthalmos, ptosis, miosis, and ipsilateral anhidrosis.
Pancoast syndrome	Superior sulcus tumor injuring the eighth cervical nerve and the first and second thoracic nerves and ribs, causing shoulder pain radiating to the arm.
Superior vena cava syndrome	Tumor causing obstruction of the superior vena cava and subsequent venous return, producing facial swelling and plethora, cough, headaches, epistaxis, and syncope. Symptoms worsened with bending forward and on awakening in the morning.
Syndrome of inappropriate antidiuretic hormone (SIADH)	Ectopic antidiuretic hormone release in the setting of plasma hypo-osmolarity, producing hyponatremia without edema. Seen in small cell lung cancer.
Eaton–Lambert syndrome	Presynaptic nerve terminals attacked by antibodies, decreasing acetylcholine release. Treated by plasmapheresis and immunosuppression; 40% associated with small cell lung cancer, 20% have other cancer, 40% have no cancer.
Trousseau syndrome	Venous thrombosis associated with metastatic cancer.
Parathyroid hormone (PTH)–like hormone	Results in high calcium, low phosphate; seen in squamous cell lung cancer.

TABLE 10-15. Distinction Between Small and Non–Small Cell Lung Cancer

Characteristic	Small Cell Lung Cancer	Non–Small Cell Lung Cancer
Histology	Small, dark nuclei; scant cytoplasm	Copious cytoplasm, pleomorphic nuclei.
Ectopic peptide production (causing paraneoplastic syndromes)	■ ACTH—causes a Cushing syndrome ■ ADH—causes SIADH (low Na^+) ■ Eaton–Lambert syndrome ■ Gastrin—can cause stomach ulcer ■ Calcitonin—can cause low Ca^+ ■ ANF	■ PTHrP (PTH-% related peptide). Presents with hypercalcemia. Classically in squamous subtype.
Response to radiotherapy	80%–90% will shrink	30%–50% will shrink
Response to chemotherapy	Very responsive to chemotherapy	Somewhat responsive to chemotherapy
Surgical resection	Not indicated	For stages I, II, IIIA
Included subtypes	Small cell only	Adenocarcinoma, squamous cell, large cell
Five-year survival rate, all stages	50%	10% in later stages; up to 90% in early stages

ACTH, adrenocorticotropic hormone; *ADH*, antidiuretic hormone (also known as arginine vasopressin [AVP]); *ANF*, atrial natriuretic factor; *PTH*, parathyroid hormone.

CHAPTER 11 DERMATOLOGY

OVERVIEW OF HIGH-YIELD TOPICS IN DERMATOLOGY

DESCRIBING SKIN LESIONS

- **Primary skin lesions** develop as a direct result of a dermatologic or systemic disease process. This is the primary manifestation of the disease within the skin. An accurate description of these lesions requires knowledge of basic dermatologic nomenclature (Table 11-1).
- **Secondary skin lesions** evolve from primary lesions or as a consequence of the patient's interactions with primary lesions, such as scratching (Table 11-2) (Figures 11-1 and 11-2).
- Topical steroids are the cornerstone of therapy for many dermatologic conditions. There are multiple different topical formulations and potencies (Table 11-3).

TABLE 11-1. Definitions of Primary Skin Lesions

Macule	A flat, nonpalpable area of skin discoloration (vitiligo, cafe au lait spot).
Papule	An elevated, palpable solid area of skin <0.5 cm diameter (acne, lichen planus).
Plaque	An elevated area of skin >2 cm diameter that has a larger surface area compared to its elevation above the skin (psoriasis, seborrheic keratosis).
Wheal	An elevated, rounded or flat-topped area of dermal edema that disappears within hours (urticaria).
Vesicle	A circumscribed, elevated, fluid-containing lesion of <0.5 cm diameter (varicella zoster).
Bullae	A circumscribed, elevated, fluid-containing lesion of >0.5 cm diameter (pemphigus vulgaris).
Pustule	A circumscribed, elevated, pus-containing lesion (acne, erythema nodosum).
Nodule	An elevated, palpable solid lesion >0.5 cm diameter (nodulocystic acne, erythema nodosum).
Petechiae	A red-purple nonblanching macule <0.5 cm diameter, usually pinpoint in size (meningococcemia).
Purpura	A red-purple nonblanching macule >0.5 cm diameter (Henoch-Schönlein purpura).
Telangiectasia	A blanchable dilated blood vessel (rosacea, cirrhosis, Osler-Weber-Rendu).

TABLE 11-2. Definitions of Secondary Skin Lesions

Scale	An accumulation of dead, exfoliating epidermal cells (Figure 11.1).
Crust	Dried serum, blood, or purulent exudate that accumulates on the skin surface (scab) (Figure 11.2).
Erosion	A superficial loss of epidermis, leaving a denuded, moist surface; heals without scarring because it does not penetrate through the dermal-epidermal junction.
Excoriation	A linear erosion produced by scratching.
Ulcer	A loss of epidermis extending into the dermis; heals with scarring because it penetrates into dermis.
Scar	Replacement of normal skin with fibrous tissue as a result of healing.
Atrophy	Thinning of skin.
Lichenification	Thickening of epidermis with accentuation of normal skin markings.

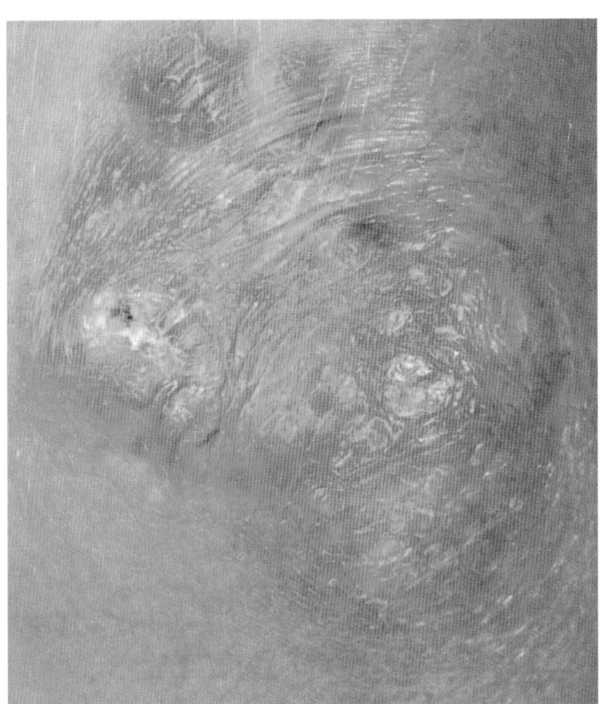

FIGURE 11-1. Scale. (Source: https://images.app.goo.gl/vogb6dKZEEvj8Beq8.)

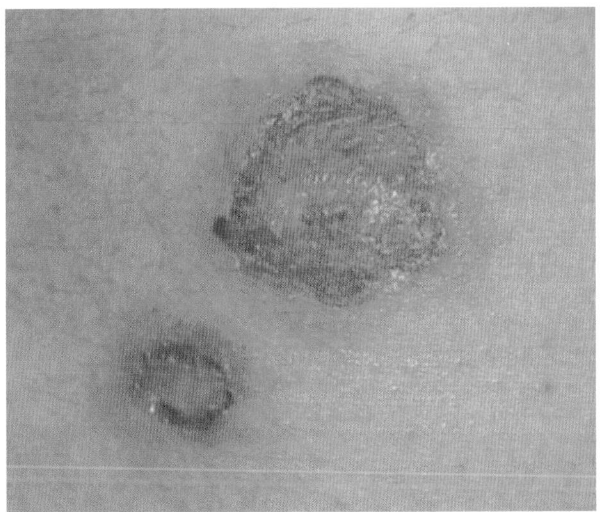

FIGURE 11-2. Crust. (Source: https://images.app.goo.gl/Cz1A7cqsNn83Yq857.)

TABLE 11-3. Topical Steroid Potency

Potency	Topical Steroid
Low	Hydrocortisone 0.5%–1% Desonide 0.05% Fluocinolone 0.01%
Medium	Hydrocortisone 0.2% Triamcinolone 0.1% Fluocinolone 0.025
High	Betamethasone 0.05% Triamcinolone 0.1%

IMMUNE-MEDIATED DISEASES ASSOCIATED WITH SKIN FINDINGS

IMMEDIATE TYPE I HYPERSENSITIVITY REACTIONS (IGE MEDIATED)

General Facts

- **Immunoglobulin E (IgE) and mast cell mediated** (immunologic reaction mediated) characterized by vasodilation and transudation of fluid.
- **Pathophysiology:** As the antigen binds to IgE on the mast cell surface, the mast cell degranulates and releases histamine and prostaglandin, causing vasodilation, increased capillary permeability, and smooth muscle contraction.

CONQUER THE **BOARDS!**

A deficiency of C1 esterase can cause hereditary angioedema.

Clinical Features

- **Urticaria** (hives/wheals): Leakage of plasma into the dermis causes a swelling after exposure to allergen. Wheals usually last <24 hours and may recur on future exposure to the antigen.
- **Angioedema:** A deeper involvement of subcutaneous tissues with less demarcated swelling, usually characterized by swelling of the eyelids, lips, and tongue (see Figure 11-3). Angioedema has 2 types: mast cell mediated and bradykinin mediated.
- **Anaphylaxis** is the most severe systemic form of type I hypersensitivity reaction, characterized by bronchoconstriction and hypotension.

CONQUER THE **WARDS!**

ACE inhibitors are a common cause of angioedema. It a bradykinin-induced angioedema, which is not associated with urticaria or systemic allergic reaction. Treatment includes airway support and discontinuing the medication. Steroids and antihistamines are typically not effective.

Management

- Antihistamines (H_1 and H_2 blockers) primarily for urticarial disease.
- Corticosteroids can be used for more severe cases.
- Airway protection may be needed for severe angioedema with life-threatening airway compromise.
- Epinephrine can be used for anaphylaxis (Figure 11-3).

HYPERSENSITIVITY (LEUKOCYTOCLASTIC) VASCULITIS

- **Definition:** A group of vasculitides where immune complexes lodge in small blood vessels, resulting in inflammation; fibrinoid necrosis; and painful, palpable purpura.

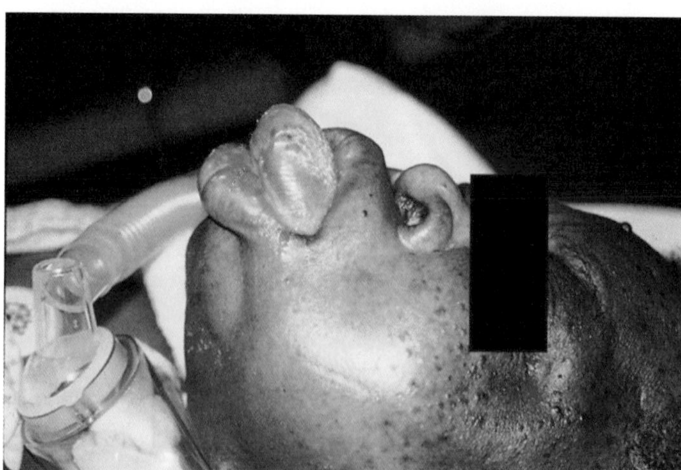

FIGURE 11-3. Angioedema. Note severe tongue, lip, and peri-orbital swelling. In addition, patient has a tracheostomy to maintain the airway. (Reproduced, with permission, from Knoop KJ, Stack LB, Storrow AB, et al. *Atlas of Emergency Medicine*, 3rd ed. New York: McGraw-Hill, 2010: 112. Photo contributor: W. Brian Gibler, MD.)

- Common causes:
  - Infection – such as Henoch-Schönlein (immunoglobulin A vasculitis) due to a streptococcal infection and penicillin use. Small-vessel vasculitis with purpura of lower extremities, buttocks, and immunoglobulin A (IgA) deposits in glomeruli.
  - Medications: Sulfonamides, penicillin, cephalosporins, phenytoin, and allopurinol are common.
  - Connective tissue disorders (systemic lupus erythematosus [SLE], Sjögren syndrome, rheumatoid arthritis, Wegener granulomatosis).
  - Neoplasms: Rare cause less than 5% of all patients with vasculitis.

CONQUER THE **BOARDS!**

Think of IgA vasculitis/HSP in cases with palpable purpura, arthritis, arthralgia, abdominal pain, and renal disease.

Clinical Features

- Pruritus and pain, associated with fever and malaise.
- **"Palpable purpura"** – multiple, scattered, **nonblanchable** red papules distributed over lower extremities, arms, and buttocks (see Figure 11-4).
- May be crusted due to necrosis of tissue overlying the blood vessel.

Diagnostic Workup

- Biopsy of the affected lesion, preferably one that has been present for approximately 24 hours. Prior to that may only show neutrophils, and after about 48 hours it may only show necrosis.

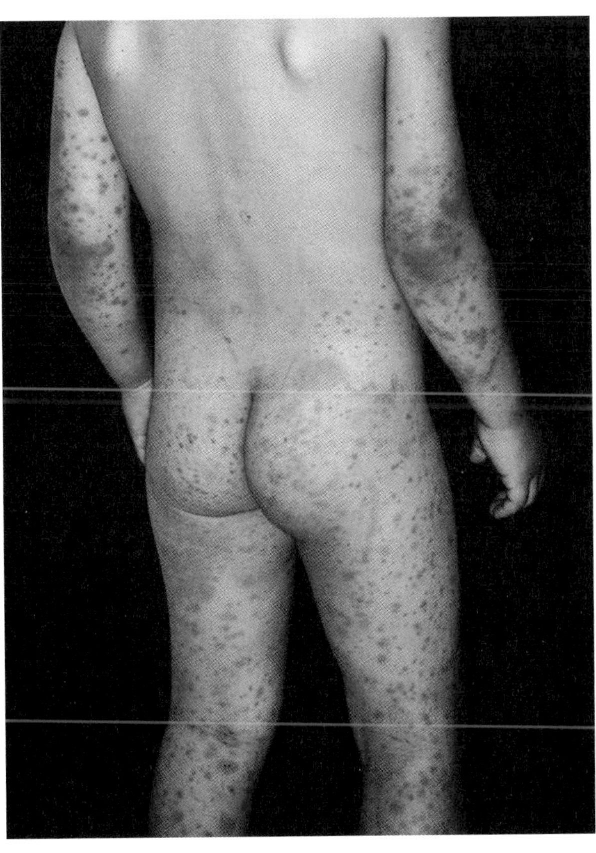

FIGURE 11-4. Henoch-Schönlein purpura. (Reproduced, with permission, from Knoop KJ, Stack LB, Storrow AB, et al. *Atlas of Emergency Medicine,* 3rd ed. New York: McGraw-Hill, 2010: 361. Photo contributor: Kevin J. Knoop, MD, MS.)

Management

- Eliminate and/or treat causative agent.
- Systemic corticosteroids/immunosuppressive agents.

CONQUER THE WARDS!

Think of allergic conditions when you see the **allergic triad:**
-**A**topic dermatitis
-**A**llergic rhinitis
-**A**sthma

ATOPIC DERMATITIS/ECZEMA

General Facts

An acute or chronic relapsing pruritic type I **(IgE) immediate hypersensitivity** inflammatory reaction where scratching and rubbing lead to further lichenification of the skin (often described as the "itch that rashes").

Risk Factors

- Family history.
- History of allergies.
- Asthma.
- Increased IgE .

CONQUER THE BOARDS!

Remember, atopic dermatitis has these key affected areas:
FACE
Flexor surfaces get **A**dults.
Children get **E**xtensor surfaces.

Exacerbating Factors

- Scratching.
- **Stress.**
- Infection, wool, skin dehydration, pregnancy, menstruation, and foods (milk, eggs), and symptoms are usually worse in winter.
- Usually improves with age.

Clinical Features

- Pruritus, typically involving the flexor surfaces or extensor surfaces.
- **Infantile eczema:** Red, exudative, crusty, and oozy lesions primarily affecting the face (cheeks) and extensor surfaces; spares diaper area; may clear by 2 years of age.
- **Juvenile and adult eczema:** Dry, lichenified pruritic plaques distributed over flexural areas (antecubital, popliteal, neck).
- Secondary bacterial and viral infections with *Staphylococcus,* herpes simplex virus, and molluscum contagiosum can occur.

Diagnostic Workup

- Mainly a clinical diagnosis with thorough history and physical examination.

Management

- Topical corticosteroids are the mainstay of therapy, along with lubrication of dry skin with emollients.
- Education and counseling to avoid scratching, as this will provoke the rash.

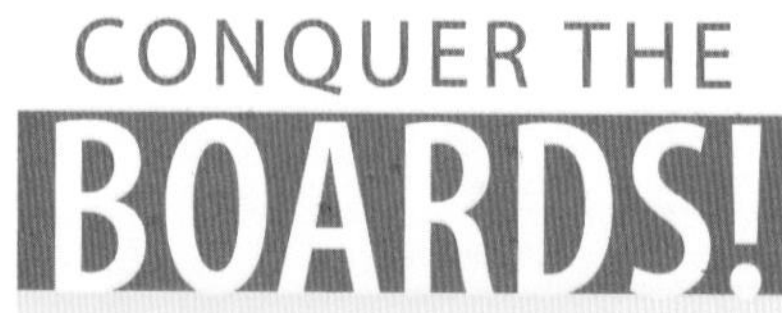

ACD is a T-cell-mediated, delayed-type hypersensitivity response.

ALLERGIC CONTACT DERMATITIS

General Facts

- Dermatitis resulting from skin contact with a substance causing a delayed (type IV) hypersensitivity immune response.
- Triggers include poison ivy, oak, and sumac; nickel commonly found in jewelry; and formaldehyde, rubber, and chemicals in shoes.

Clinical Features

- Intensely pruritic rash with linear, papular, erythematous lesions with **distinct margins in the distribution of the exposure** (for example, if allergic to watch band, there is a bandlike rash in the same spot around the wrist).

Diagnostic Workup

- Clinical diagnosis, with focus on exposure history.
- Patch testing can be used to confirm the diagnosis.

Management

- Avoidance of allergen exposure is key.
- If exposure occurs and allergic contact dermatitis (ACD) ensues, topical or systemic steroids/antihistamines can help mitigate the symptoms.

CONQUER THE WARDS!

The distribution of ACD: Lesions are typically localized to skin areas that come in contact with the allergen, most commonly the face, hands, feet, and lips.

IRRITANT CONTACT DERMATITIS

General Facts

- Dermatitis resulting from exposure to substances that cause physical, mechanical, or chemical irritation to the skin.
- Triggers include common exposures after daily repetitive use of substances such as soapy water, cleansers, and rubbing alcohol.

Clinical Features

- Erythematous, pruritic chapped skin; dryness; fissuring.
- Most commonly affects hands.

Diagnostic Workup

- Clinical diagnosis with emphasis on exposure history.
- Patch testing may be necessary to differentiate from allergic contact dermatitis.

Management

- Goal is to restore normal epithelial barrier and then protect.
- Key strategies include decreased exposure to soap and water and emollients.
- Severe cases may need topical corticosteroids.

MISCELLANEOUS INFLAMMATORY CONDITIONS

PITYRIASIS ROSEA

General Facts

A common self-limiting eruption of a single **herald patch** (see Figure 11-5) followed by a generalized secondary eruption within 2 weeks.

- The rash lasts around 2 to 6 weeks.
- Herpes simplex virus type 7 is suspected.
- Affects children and young adults, primarily ages 10 to 40.
- Clusters of cases in spring and fall.

CONQUER THE WARDS!

A young person presents with a pruritic, spotted rash on the trunk that began as one solitary larger patch. *Think: Pityriasis rosea.*

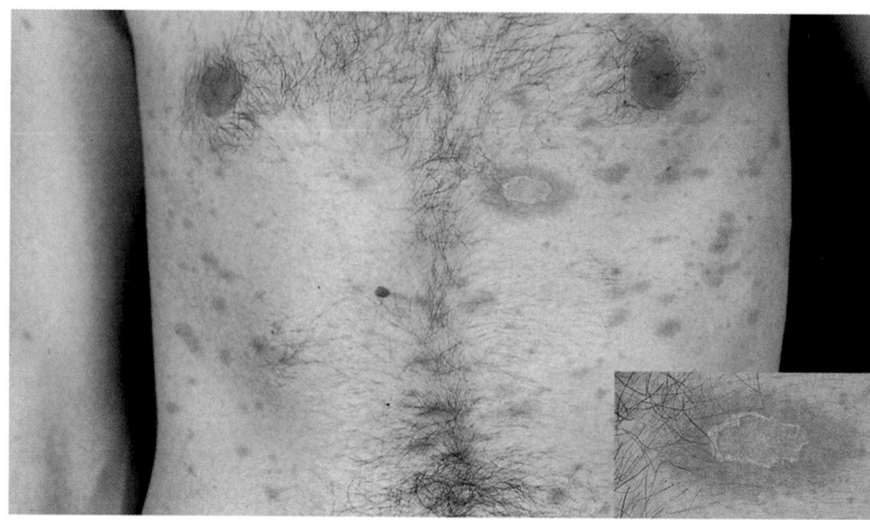

FIGURE 11-5. Pityriasis rosea. Papules and small erythematous plaques; note herald patch, an erythematous plaque with scale in central portion of lesion and collarette on border. (Reproduced, with permission, from Wolff K, Johnson RA, Suurmond D. *Fitzpatrick's Color Atlas & Synopsis of Clinical Dermatology,* 5th ed. New York: McGraw-Hill, 2005: 119.)

Clinical Features

- Mild pruritus (present in 75% of cases).
- A 2- to 10-cm solitary, oval erythematous **herald patch** with a collarette of scale precedes the generalized eruption in 80% of patients.
- Within days, multiple smaller pink, oval, scaly patches appear over trunk and upper extremities.
- Secondary eruption occurs in a **Christmas tree** distribution, oriented parallel to the ribs.
- May have prodrome of headache, fever, and malaise.

Diagnostic Workup

- Clinical diagnosis.

Management

- Symptomatic management with topical steroids, antihistamines for pruritis.
- Ultraviolet B (UVB) phototherapy or sunlight can help.

Common Questions on Rounds:
When does the rash of pityriasis rosea usually resolve?
What virus has been linked to pityriasis rosea?

CONQUER THE WARDS!

As no treatment shortens the disease course of PR, reassurance and patient education on clinical length and spontaneous resolution are important.

PSORIASIS

General Facts

- Chronic, noninfectious hyperproliferative inflammatory disorder characterized by **thick adherent scales**. The chronic inflammation causes increased epidermal cell proliferation, forming thick, adherent scales.
- Often presents with multiple exacerbations and remissions.
- Risk factors include trauma, infection, emotional stress, and drugs (lithium, beta blockers, iodine, and antimalarials).

CONQUER THE WARDS!

A 35-year-old man presents with salmon-colored papules covered with silvery white scale on his scalp, elbows, and knees. *Think: Psoriasis.*

Clinical Features

- Mild pruritus along with well-demarcated, thick, **"salmon-pink" plaques** with an adherent silver-white scale.
- Lesions are usually distributed bilaterally over the **extensor surface** of extremities, often on elbows and knees, and trunk and scalp.
- **Nails** are commonly involved:
  - Pitting of nails.
  - Oil spots (yellow-brown spots under nail plate).
  - Onycholysis (separation of distal nail plate from nail bed).
  - Subungual hyperkeratosis (thickening of epidermis under nail plate).
- **Koebner phenomenon** – Lesions occurring at sites of injury
- **Auspitz sign** – Pinpoint capillary bleeding occurs if scale is removed.
- Associated with numerous systemic diseases, including cardiovascular, hypertension (HTN), diabetes mellitus (DM), autoimmune disease, malignancy, inflammatory bowel disease (IBD), etc.
- **Complications:**
  - Ocular complications include blepharitis, conjunctivitis, and uveitis.
  - Psoriatic arthritis, a destructive arthritis of the distal interphalangeal joints of the hands and feet (rheumatoid factor).

Management

- For **mild disease**, topical medications such as steroids, tar, anthralin, or calcipotriene.
- For **severe disease:** Systemic therapy—usually phototherapy or immunosuppressants (UVB phototherapy, PUVA [psoralen + ultraviolet A], retinoids, methotrexate, cyclosporine, infliximab).

ERYTHEMA NODOSUM

General Facts

- An inflammatory disorder of **subcutaneous fat (panniculitis)** characterized by painful, erythematous nodules on the lower legs.
- Causes include:
  - Idiopathic.
  - Infection (strep, tuberculosis, histoplasmosis, coccidiomycosis).
  - Medications (sulfonamides, oral contraceptives).
  - Autoimmune (commonly seen in sarcoid and IBD).
  - Malignancy (lymphoma and leukemia are most common).
  - Pregnancy.

Clinical Features

- Painful nodules scattered over lower legs, bilaterally but not symmetrically (see Figure 11-6).
- Can be associated with fever, malaise, and arthralgias.

Management

- Usually resolves spontaneously in a couple of weeks
- Removal or treatment of underlying cause is key.
- Nonsteroidal antiinflammatory drugs (NSAIDs), potassium iodide, and steroids can be used to reduce symptoms.

CONQUER THE WARDS!

A 23-year-old woman presents with a cough, and a chest x-ray shows mediastinal lymphadenopathy. She has painful nodules on the skin of the tibia. *Think: Erythema nodosum as a manifestation of sarcoidosis.*

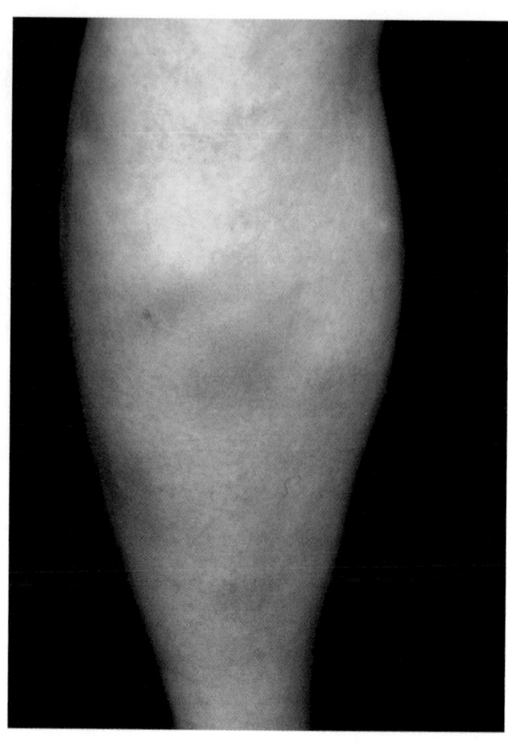

FIGURE 11-6. **Erythema nodosum.** (Reproduced, with permission, from Wolff K, Johnson RA, Suurmond D. *Fitzpatrick's Color Atlas & Synopsis of Clinical Dermatology*, 5th ed. New York: McGraw-Hill, 2005: 149.)

CONQUER THE WARDS!

Target lesions are the characteristic finding of EM.

CONQUER THE BOARDS!

HSV is the most frequent infectious agent associated with EM.

CONQUER THE WARDS!

Think of allergic conditions when you see the **allergic triad:**
-**A**topic dermatitis
-**A**llergic rhinitis
-**A**sthma

CONQUER THE BOARDS!

Stevens-Johnson syndrome and toxic epidermal necrolysis are severe variants of erythema multiforme that are potentially life threatening.

ERYTHEMA MULTIFORME

General Facts

- A general name used to describe an immune complex–mediated hypersensitivity reaction to different causative agents, usually infections.
- Erythema multiforme (EM) can be caused by medications (penicillins, sulfonamides, barbiturates, NSAIDs, thiazides, phenytoin), viruses (usually herpes simplex virus, but also hepatitis A and B), bacteria (*Streptococcus, Mycoplasma*), fungi, malignancy, radiotherapy, or pregnancy.

Clinical Features

- Although characterized by **target lesions**, multiforme refers to the wide variety of lesions that may be present, including papules, vesicles, and bullae (see Figure 11-7).
- Affected sites include dorsa of hands, palms and soles, penis (50%), feet, and face.

Management

- Discontinue offending agent and treat any underlying infections (e.g., oral acyclovir to prevent herpes outbreak).

STEVENS-JOHNSON SYNDROME AND TOXIC EPIDERMAL NECROLYSIS

General Facts

- Stevens-Johnson syndrome (SJS) and toxic epidermal necrolysis (TEN) are considered by many to be part of the same spectrum of disease, with SJS being the less severe condition.

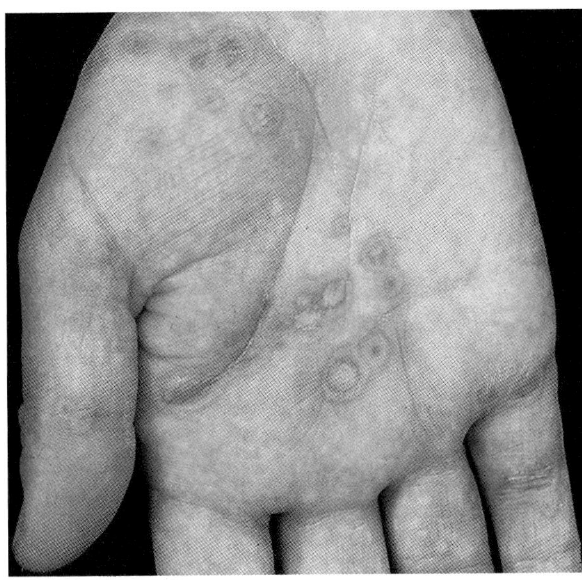

FIGURE 11-7. **Erythema multiforme.** (Reproduced, with permission, from Wolff K, Johnson RA, Suurmond D. *Fitzpatrick's Color Atlas & Synopsis of Clinical Dermatology*, 5th ed. New York: McGraw-Hill, 2005: 141.)

- **SJS** is defined as skin detachment in <10% of the body surface area. Mucous membranes are affected in over 90% of patients, usually in 2 or more distinct sites (ocular, oral, and genital). (see figure 11-8)
- Ocular involvement may result in scarring, corneal ulcers, or uveitis; 5% mortality. May evolve to TEN.
- **TEN** involves widespread full-thickness necrosis of skin covering >30% of body surface area. Mucous membranes are also involved in over 90% of cases.
- **SJS/TEN** overlap involves skin detachment of 10% to 30% of body surface area with mucous membrane involvement.

CONQUER THE **BOARDS!**

Stevens-Johnson syndrome and toxic epidermal necrolysis can be distinguished by body surface area affected:
SJS: <10%
SJS-TEN overlap: 10%–30%
TEN: >30%

Clinical Features

- Prodrome of fever and influenza-like symptoms.
- Pruritus, pain, tenderness, and burning.
- Classic targetlike lesions symmetrically distributed on dorsum of hand, palms, soles, face, and knees. Many cases have mucosal lesions—painful erythematous erosions on lips, buccal mucosa, conjunctiva, and anogenital region.
- Initial **target lesions** can become confluent, erythematous, and tender, with bullous formation and subsequent loss of epidermis.
- Epidermal sloughing may be generalized, resembling a second-degree burn, and is more pronounced over pressure points.
- **Nikolsky sign** (sloughing of skin with gentle pressure).

CONQUER THE **WARDS!**

SJS: < 10% body involvement
TEN: >30% body involvement
SJS-TEN overlap: 10%–30% body involvement

Diagnosis

Biopsy.

Complications

- Secondary skin infections.
- Fluid and electrolyte abnormalities.
- Dehydration.
- Death (30% mortality).

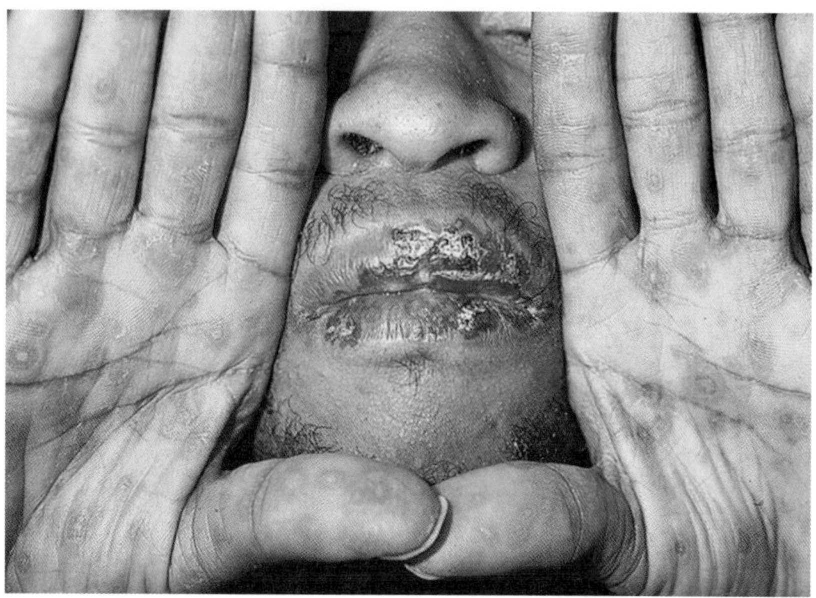

FIGURE 11-8. **Oral and Hand Manifestations of Stevens Johnson Syndrome**

Management

- Removal and/or treatment of causative agent (suppressive therapy with acyclovir to prevent recurrences of herpes simplex virus).
- Hospitalization for severe disease, fluids, and steroids.
- In general, SJS/TEN needs tertiary-level care at a center with a burn unit. A multidisciplinary team with intensive care, dermatology, and ophthalmology may be warranted.

HIGH-YIELD LITERATURE

Stern RS, Divito SJ. Stevens-Johnson syndrome and toxic epidermal necrolysis: Associations, outcomes, and pathobiology – Thirty years of progress but still much to be done. *J Invest Dermatol.* 2017;137:1004.

LICHEN PLANUS

General Facts

- A chronic inflammatory condition that affects skin, nails, hair, and mucous membranes.
- Lichen planus (LP) is thought to be an autoimmune condition and can overlap with lupus.
- The estimated prevalence worldwide is in the range of 0.2% to 5%.
- It is more common in females, with a ratio of 3:2.
- Most cases are diagnosed between the ages of 30 and 60.

Clinical Features

- LP primarily affects the dorsal hands, flexural wrists and forearms, trunk, anterior lower legs, and oral mucosa.
- Violaceous papules and plaques with overlying, reticulated, fine white scale (Wickham striae) are characteristic.

Diagnostic Workup

- Skin biopsy can find parakeratosis, acanthosis of the epithelium, saw-toothed rete ridges, and liquefaction degeneration of the basal layer.
- A thorough history is necessary to assess for underlying undiagnosed autoimmune disease.

Management

- Corticosteroids are the cornerstone of management. Topical steroids can be used first, with systemic steroids reserved for severe cases.

ROSACEA

General Facts

- Rosacea is a chronic condition that affects the skin and blood vessels in the face, nose, and forehead.
- The etiology is not known, but a family history carries a higher risk, and certain triggers such as alcohol, sun exposure, stress, alcohol, and caffeine can worsen the condition.
- The condition is more common in women, particularly those of Caucasian descent.

Clinical Features

- Redness; small and superficial dilated blood vessels on facial skin.
- Typical areas with rosacea include the face, nose, and forehead.

Diagnostic Workup

- Clinical diagnosis.

Management

- Behavioral modification to reduce stress and avoid inciting factors such as sunlight, alcohol use, and other dietary restrictions can help.
- Oral antibiotics such as doxycycline are sometimes used and are thought to reduce inflammation in affected tissues.
- Laser therapy can help cauterize abnormal blood vessels.

DECUBITUS ULCERS

General Facts

- Any pressure-induced ulcer that occurs secondary to external compression of the skin, resulting in ischemic tissue necrosis; may extend to underlying subcutaneous tissue, muscle, joints, or bones.
- Many patients who develop these are in the hospital.
- Risk factors include immobility, malnutrition, elderly, diabetes, and decreased level of consciousness.

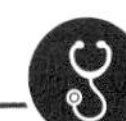

Decubitus ulcers develop over bony prominences: sacrum, ischial tuberosities, iliac crests, greater trochanters, heels, elbows, knees, and occiput. Can develop at any site that can be compressed against a hard surface.

Clinical Features

- Stage **I**—nonblanching erythema of intact skin.
- Stage **II**—partial-thickness skin loss involving epidermis and/or dermis (superficial ulcer).

- Stage **III**—full-thickness skin loss involving epidermis and dermis (deep, crateriform ulcer). May involve damage to subcutaneous tissue, extending down to but not through fascia.
- Stage **IV**—full-thickness skin loss with extensive damage to muscle, bone, or other supporting structures.
- Complications can include osteomyelitis, bacteremia, and sepsis.

Management

- **Prophylaxis:** Mobilizing patients as soon as possible, repositioning patients every 2 hours, pressure-reducing devices (foam, air, or liquid mattresses), and correction of nutritional status.

TABLE 11-4. Fever and Rash–Commonly Tested Infectious Causes

Disease	Etiology	Skin Findings	Rash Characteristics	Other Clinical Findings
Measles	Paramyxovirus	Blanching erythematous maculopapular rash that becomes confluent.	Rash starts at hairline and behind ears → centrifugally to face → neck/trunk, extremities.	Koplik's spots, fever, cough, coryza, conjunctivitis.
Rubella	Rubella virus	Similar to measles but patient doesn't look as "sick."	By second day, facial exanthem fades.	Prominent postauricular, posterior cervical lymph nodes.
Varicella (chickenpox)	Varicella-zoster virus	Pruritic vesicular lesions in successive crops; vesicles evolve to pustules and crust over time.	First lesions begin on face/scalp → trunk/back.	Herpes zoster (shingles): painful vesicular lesions; does not cross midline.
Erythema infectiosum (fifth disease)	Parvovirus B19	Erythematous macules and papules giving lacy "reticulated" appearance.	"Slapped cheek" in children.	
Roseola infantum ("exanthem subitum")	HHV-6, HHV-7	Multiple blanchable macules and papules trunk → extremities (after high fever prodrome).	Rash spares face.	Primarily in infants. High fever 3–4 days prior to appearance of rash.
Infectious mononucleosis	Epstein-Barr virus	Generalized maculopapular rash in 100% of patients with administration of ampicillin/amoxicillin.		Splenomegaly.
Scarlet fever	Group A *Streptococcus*	Coarse, erythematous, blanching rash; circumoral pallor; strawberry tongue; linear petechiae in skin folds (pastia's lines).	Rash fades in several days → desquamation of skin.	Rash appears 1–3 days after strep pharyngitis.
Acute rheumatic fever	Group A *Streptococcus*	Erythema marginatum (transient macular rash with central clearing found on proximal extremities).	Subcutaneous nodules on bony prominences.	

- **Local wound care is an important part of management.** Proper cleansing with mild agents, moisturizing to maintain hydration and promote healing, and use of topical creams to promote healing and prevent progression.
- Debridement of necrotic tissues and placement of flaps and skin grafts may be needed for advanced ulcers.
- Infected ulcers will need antibiotics in addition to debridement and local wound care.

SHINGLES

SHINGLES (HERPES ZOSTER)

General Facts

- An acute dermatomal viral infection caused by reactivation of latent varicella-zoster virus that has remained dormant in a sensory root ganglion (see table 11-4).
- The virus travels down the sensory nerve, resulting initially in dermatomal pain, followed by skin lesions.
- Usually occurs in people >50 or immunocompromised.
- Skin lesions are vesicles located unilaterally along the dermatome that ultimately crust over (see figure 11-9).

Clinical Features

- Neuropathic pain involving 2 to 3 contiguous dermatomes without crossing the midline.
- Dissemination with multiple dermatomes and large body surface area involvement can occur in immunocompromised hosts.
- Lesions typically have vesicles and evolve toward crusting. Once lesions are all crusted, the patient is no longer considered infectious (Figure 11-9).
- End-organ damage can occur, including ocular or hepatic involvement.
- **Postherpetic neuralgia** (more common in the elderly and may persist for weeks to years after infection).
- **Herpes zoster ophthalmicus:** Lesions on nasal tip or eye indicate zoster involvement of the nasociliary branch of the ophthalmic nerve, resulting in uveitis, conjunctivitis, retinitis, optic neuritis, or glaucoma. An ophthalmic consult is necessary.
- **Ramsay Hunt syndrome:** Lesions on external surface of ear or auditory canal indicate zoster involvement of facial and auditory nerve, resulting in facial paralysis, hearing loss, changes in taste perception, ear pain, and vertigo.

Diagnostic Workup

- **Typically a clinical diagnosis.**
- Confirmation via polymerase chain reaction (PCR) testing of fluid within vesicles can be done.
- **Tzanck preparation** can reveal multinucleated giant cells and culture of lesions, but is rarely done.

Management

- **Oral:** Antivirals (valacyclovir, famciclovir).
- **Intravenous (IV) antivirals for end-organ disease or disseminated disease.**
- **Pain control with analgesics and gabapentin.**

CONQUER THE **BOARDS!**

Patient >50 years old who presents with a painful rash in a small distribution on only one side of their body. Consider treatment for herpes zoster.

CONQUER THE **WARDS!**

Varicella-zoster virus is contagious when vesicles are present. Can also be spread via respiratory route. Those exposed without immunity are at risk of developing primary varicella (chickenpox).

CONQUER THE **WARDS!**

Herpes zoster is a clinical diagnosis, and treatment is most efficacious if started within 72 hours of rash onset.

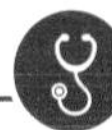

Patients with herpes zoster can infect nonimmune contacts with chickenpox. Exposed nonimmune contacts should be treated with varicella-zoster immune globulin (VZIG).

CONQUER THE **WARDS!**

Multiple treatment options require close monitoring of pregnancy status due to toxicity. Sexually active females of childbearing age on isotretinoin require monthly follow-up and 2 forms of birth control while taking this medication.

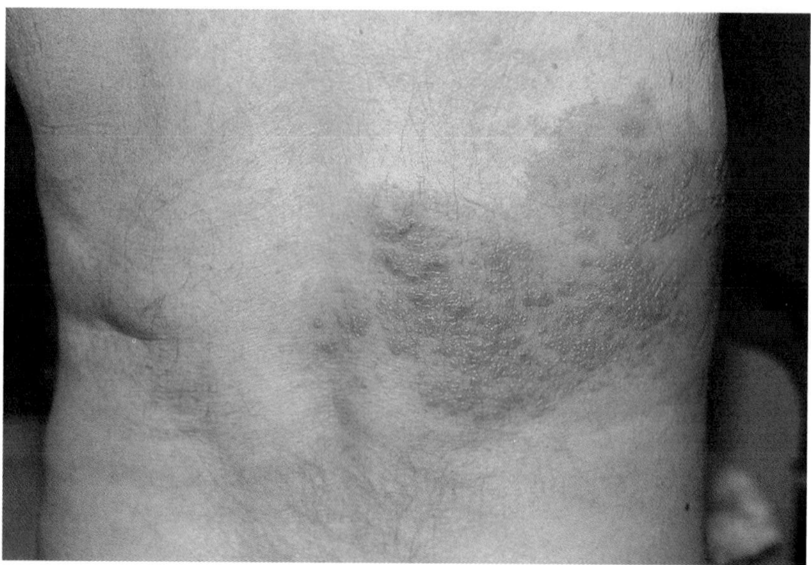

FIGURE 11-9. Unilateral dermatomal rash seen in shingles

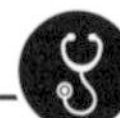

Meningococcemia is fatal if untreated. Treat empirically prior to completion of tests if suspected on clinical grounds.

CONQUER THE BOARDS!

Young, otherwise healthy patient who lives in crowded living space such as dorm or barracks. The patient will present with fever, headache, and rash. Start antibiotics promptly. Crowded living situations are a risk factor for meningococcemia.

CONQUER THE WARDS!

Patients with suspected meningitis will often be started on steroids with initial treatment of meningitis. Once *Neisseria* meningitis is identified, steroids can be held, as no clinical benefit has been shown as with other etiologies of meningitis.

MENINGOCOCCEMIA (*NEISSERIA* MENINGITIS)

General Facts

- A potentially fatal disease resulting from meningococcal bacteremia, usually affecting children 6 months to 1 year old, asplenic, or complement-deficient patients.

Clinical Features

- Acutely ill patient often with discrete **pink macules, papules,** and **petechiae,** which can be distributed over the trunk, extremities, and palate (Figure 11-10).
- With fulminant disease, patients have **purpura,** ecchymosis, and a confluent area of gray-black necrosis.
- Signs of meningeal irritation (e.g., nuchal rigidity).
- Complications include meningitis (50% to 90%) and **Waterhouse-Friderichsen syndrome** (fulminant meningococcemia with adrenal hemorrhage).

Diagnostic Workup

- Blood cultures reveal meningococci.
- Cerebrospinal fluid (CSF) culture is usually positive.
- PCR testing of urine, throat, or rectum can yield positive for *Gonorrhea.*

Management

- Admission to intensive care unit.
- Vancomycin and ceftriaxone IV at first clinical suspicion of meningococcemia.
- Prophylaxis is indicated for household contacts and individuals with intimate contacts. Medical personnel who have had contact with oral secretions will require prophylaxis as well.

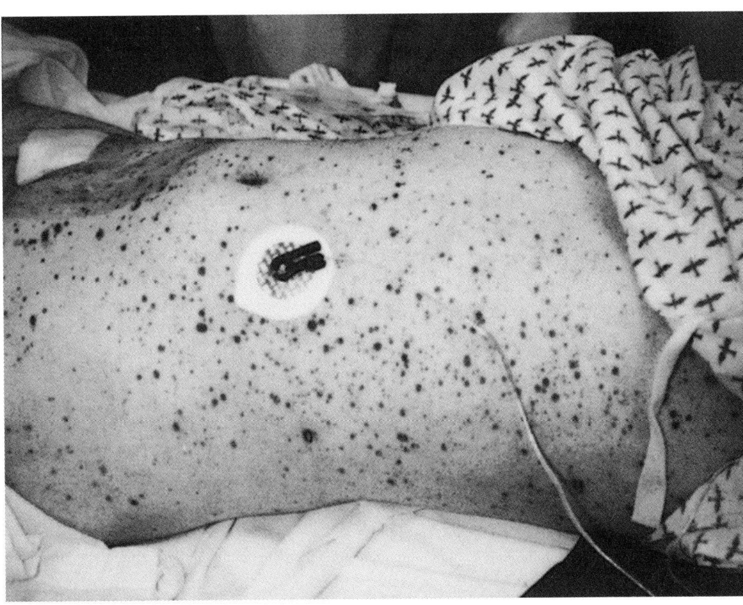

FIGURE 11-10. **Skin findings in disseminated Meningococcus**

ACNE VULGARIS

General Facts

- Inflammation of pilosebaceous units of certain areas of the body, including face, trunk, upper arms, and upper back caused by *Propionibacterium acnes* within the follicle.
- Typically seen in adolescents and up to 25 years.
- **Comedones** are the result—open (blackheads) and closed (whiteheads).
- Nodules or cysts are seen in more severe cases.

Management

- Goal is to remove plugging and treat infection (combination treatment is best).
- **Mild:** Topical antibiotics (clindamycin, erythromycin), benzoyl peroxide, topical retinoids.
- **Moderate:** Consider adding oral antibiotic (e.g., minocycline) or oral contraceptives in females.
- **Severe:** Isotretinoin (Accutane).

SEBORRHEIC KERATOSIS

- The most common benign tumor of the elderly.
- Develops from proliferating epidermal cells.
- Appears as waxy, stuck-on, tan-brown, verrucous lesions.
- **Sign of Leser–Trelat** is the association of multiple seborrheic keratoses with internal malignancy, usually adenocarcinoma of the gastrointestinal tract. No treatment is necessary.

CONQUER THE **BOARDS!**

Seborrheic keratosis is a common finding in elderly patients. But when presented with a patient who reports multiple seborrheic keratosis lesions developing over a short period (~3 to 6 months), evaluation for remote-site malignancy should be initiated.

CONQUER THE WARDS!

Patients with a history of basal cell carcinoma are at increased risk of subsequent lesions. Approximately 40% of patents will have another lesion within 5 years. Surveillance is critical.

SKIN CANCERS

BASAL CELL CARCINOMA

- The **most common** type of skin cancer due to a malignancy of the epidermal basal cells.
- Basal cells invade locally but almost never metastasize.
- Usually affects ages >40 years. Fair skin with chronic sun exposure or radiation therapy is a common risk factor.
- Diagnosed with biopsy and treated with excision.

A 47-year-old white man presents with pearly, painless, ulcerated nodules with **overlying telangiectasias**. *Think: Basal cell carcinoma.*

Clinical Findings

- **Nodular type:** A single translucent, **"pearly,"** waxy nodule or papule with **telangiectasias** and a **rolled border,** distributed on the face and neck.
- **Superficial spreading type:** Multiple erythematous scaly plaques with a well-defined border distributed primarily on the trunk; no relation to sun exposure.
- **Sclerosing type:** Yellowish white sclerotic waxy plaques with poorly defined borders, resembling scar tissue or morphea.
- **Pigmented type:** May have any of the previous characteristics with pigmentation and is easily confused with malignant melanoma.

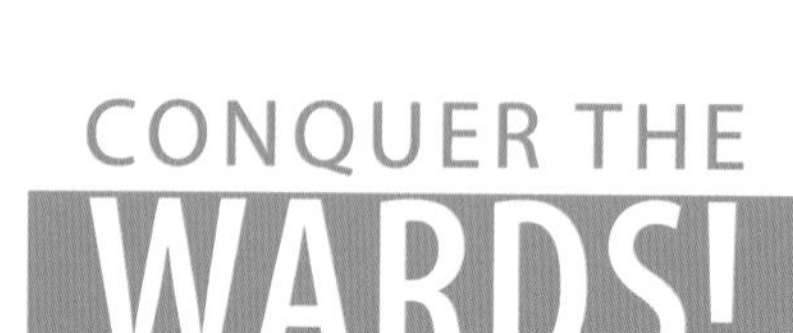

Test

Dysplastic nevus is a premalignant precursor to malignant melanoma.

CONQUER THE BOARDS!

Skin cancer is the most common type of cancer in humans. Malignant melanoma accounts for ~2%, but accounts for most deaths.

SQUAMOUS CELL CARCINOMA

- A tumor of malignant keratinocytes accounting for the second most frequent type of skin cancer.
- Growth may be from an **actinic keratosis** or de novo.
- Related to sun exposure, radiation exposure, immunosuppression, human papillomavirus, and xeroderma pigmentosum.

Clinical Findings

- An erythematous scaling plaque that may be eroded or ulcerated with crust.
- Usually on sun-exposed area of lips, cheeks, ears, and scalp.
- Biopsy reveals malignant keratinocytes invading the dermis with keratin pearls.

Management

- Excision or radiation if surgery cannot be done.

MALIGNANT MELANOMA

General Facts

- Melanoma is the malignant proliferation of melanocytes (pigment cells).
- It is the deadliest skin cancer.

- It may arise from normal-appearing skin (70%) or from a preexisting melanocytic nevi (mole) (30%).
- **Prognosis is based on the thickness of the primary tumor,** measured histologically according to the depth of invasion from the surface to the deepest part of the tumor (Breslow classification) or according to the depth of penetration in relation to the different layers of the dermis (Clark classification).
- Risk factors include sun exposure, fair skin, and family history.

Clinical Features

- **Superficial spreading melanoma:** Accounts for 70% of melanomas; characterized by horizontal growth. May develop as a new mole or as a change in a preexisting mole. It appears as an elevated plaque with irregular borders and variegated colors, but evolves into a nodule with bleeding and ulceration.
- **Nodular melanoma:** Characterized only by a vertical growth. Develops as a blue, gray, or black papule or nodule that may ulcerate or bleed. Associated with a poor prognosis because it metastasizes early.
- **Lentigo maligna melanoma:** Accounts for 10% of melanomas and occurs on sun-exposed areas of the skin in elderly patients. A slow-growing macule that gradually forms irregular borders, indistinct edges, or variable shades of color. May be present for years as a macule (lentigo maligna) before the development of melanoma.
- **Acral lentiginous melanoma:** Accounts for <5% of melanomas and is most common in individuals with increased skin pigment. Develops as a flat, variably pigmented macule on the palms, soles, and nail beds that enlarges peripherally and then becomes nodular.

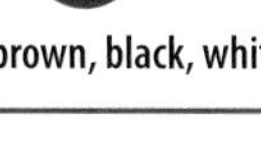

Melanomas can be brown, black, white, or blue.

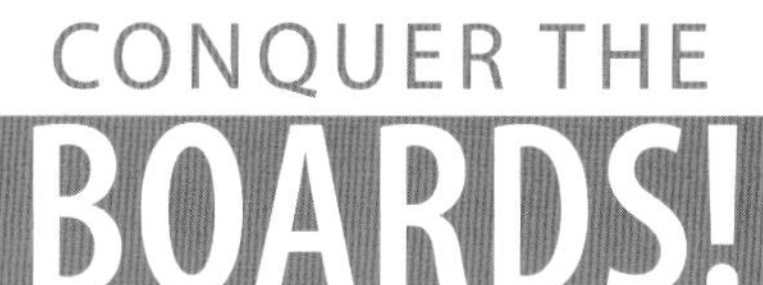

Suspicious features of malignant melanoma include the ABCDEEs:
Asymmetry
Border (irregular)
Color (variegated and mottled)
Diameter (>0.6 cm)
Elevation
Enlargement

Management

- Surgical excision with margins of at least 1 cm, depending on the depth of lesion for local disease.
- Interferon may be added in high-risk patients as adjuvant therapy.

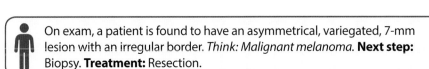

On exam, a patient is found to have an asymmetrical, variegated, 7-mm lesion with an irregular border. *Think: Malignant melanoma.* **Next step:** Biopsy. **Treatment:** Resection.

CHAPTER 12 PSYCHIATRY

OVERVIEW OF HIGH-YIELD TOPICS IN BASICS OF MENTAL HEALTH IN THE PRIMARY CARE CLINIC

With national limitations in access to psychiatry services (due to insufficient numbers of practicing psychiatrists), the role of screening, diagnosis, and first-line treatment often falls to primary care physicians in the clinic. Depression, generalized anxiety disorder, and panic disorder are the most common psychiatric diseases diagnosed and treated in primary care clinics. Patients with severe depression or anxiety, refractory depression or anxiety, or mental health conditions such as schizophrenia and bipolar disorder should be referred for psychiatric evaluation.

DEPRESSION

Epidemiology and Screening

- The lifetime prevalence of major depression in the United States has been found to be as high as 17%, and the annual prevalence rate is nearly 7%.
- Rates of depression are higher in patients with chronic medical illness (~25% lifetime risk).
- Risk factors include prior episodes, family history, female gender, poor social support, life stressors, childhood traumas, chronic medical illnesses, and a history of substance use.
- The U.S. Preventive Services Task Force (USPSTF) recommends screening all patients during routine visits.
- Use the PHQ-2 to screen, with a positive answer to either question indicating possible depression and the need to follow up. The 2 questions are: "During the last month, have you often been bothered by feeling down, depressed, or hopeless?" and "During the last month, have you often been bothered by having little interest or pleasure in doing things?"
- After an initial positive PHQ-2 screen, proceed to a full PHQ-9 to evaluate for the presence of depression and assess severity.

> **CONQUER THE WARDS!**
>
> Though we should screen all patients, you should especially consider screening patients with fatigue, chronic pain, insomnia, or otherwise unexplained symptoms.

Diagnostic Criteria

The Diagnostic and Statistical Manual of Mental Disorders (DSM-5) diagnostic criteria for depression are as follows:

- Five or more of the following symptoms (SIG E CAPS) must be present during the same 2-week period, with one of the symptoms being either depressed mood or loss of interest or pleasure.
  - Sleep (hypersomnia or insomnia).
  - Interest (loss of interest or pleasure in activities).
  - Guilt (worthlessness).
  - Energy (fatigue).
  - Concentration.
  - Appetite (up or down) or weight (loss or gain).
  - Psychomotor agitation or retardation.
  - Suicidal ideation.
- Symptoms cause significant distress.
- Episode is not attributable to medical condition or substance use.
- No other psychiatric disorder is present that better explains the symptoms.
- No history of a manic or hypomanic episode.

> **CONQUER THE WARDS!**
>
> For the precise diagnostic criteria, see the DSM-5. The PHQ-9 is based on these 9 symptoms and is the tool most providers use in clinic to diagnose and assess disease. severity.

Principles of Initial Treatment

The goal of therapy is to restore baseline functionality.

- Screen ALL patients for suicidality (passive or active).
- Options include psychotherapy and pharmacotherapy, with the evidence suggesting that combination therapy (both psychotherapy and pharmacotherapy) is superior to either option alone.
- For pharmacotherapy, selective serotonin reuptake inhibitors (SSRIs) are generally the first-line therapy, but with no evidence to support one particular agent (recent meta-analyses have found conflicting results). There is no evidence that initial therapy with multiple agents achieves superior outcomes. Other options include atypical agents (bupropion, mirtazapine), serotonin modulators (trazodone), tricyclics, and monoamine oxidase inhibitors (MAOIs).
- The choice of initial therapy should be individualized, considering potential drug–drug interactions, patient preference, cost/availability, and side effect profiles.
- Electroconvulsive therapy (ECT) can be used in very refractory cases.

CONQUER THE WARDS!

Though there is no specific data indicating these must be the first-line choices, the most commonly prescribed first-line SSRIs in the United States are sertraline, citalopram, and escitalopram.

ANXIETY DISORDER

General Facts

- Inappropriate experience of worry/fear and its physical manifestations unequal to the magnitude of the perceived stressor.
- Symptoms occur more days than not and interfere with daily functioning.
- Symptoms are not attributable to another mental disorder, medical condition, or substance abuse.
- Diagnosis is based on clinical presentation and DSM criteria

Subtypes

- Generalized anxiety disorder.
- Panic disorder.
- Obsessive-compulsive disorder.
- Others (not be addressed in this book):
  - Phobias.
  - Selective mutism.
  - Adjustment disorder.

CONQUER THE WARDS!

Generally speaking, patients who have typical and recurrent panic attacks can be diagnosed with having panic disorder without an extensive workup, but brief consideration should be given to the potential disease mimics.

CONQUER THE BOARDS!

Excessive and persistent worrying is pathognomonic for GAD.

GENERALIZED ANXIETY DISORDER

General Facts

- Excessive worrying lasting >6 months unrelated to specific situation or event associated with somatic symptoms.

Clinical Features

- Excessive, persistent worry that is difficult to control.
- Symptoms lasting >6 months.
- Associated with 3 or more somatic symptoms:
  - Restlessness.
  - Fatigue.

CONQUER THE WARDS!

Effectiveness of SSRIs should be seen approximately 4 to 6 weeks after initiating treatment.

- Difficulty concentrating.
- Irritability.
- Muscle tension.
- Disturbed speech.

Differential Diagnosis

- Depression with anxiety.
- Panic disorder.
- Adjustment disorder.
- Substance use disorder.

Management

Short-Term Therapy

- Benzodiazepines can be used for immediate symptom relief.
- Should be tapered as soon as possible due to high risk of tolerance and dependence.

Long-Term Therapy

- The first step is to assess the degree of disability or impairment to determine the need for medical treatment.
- Options include **psychotherapy** (cognitive-behavioral therapy [CBT]) or **pharmacotherapy**, or a combination of the 2.
- The decision to start CBT is largely based on patient preference and resource availability.
- **First-line pharmacotherapy:** SSRIs or serotonin-norepinephrine reuptake inhibitors (SNRIs) are first-line, with the decision between agents made on the drug's side effect profile, drug–drug interactions, and patient preference.
- **Second-line pharmacotherapy:** For patients on medical therapy with only a partial response to SSRI or SNRI therapy, buspirone can be added as an adjunct (but is generally not used as monotherapy, given its limited efficacy).
- Benzodiazepines can be a potentially useful adjunct, but have numerous potential side effects that limit their long-term use, including the risk of dependence or abuse, rebound after discontinuation, and worsening of any depressive symptoms. As such, they are generally reserved for more refractory cases.

CONQUER THE **BOARDS!**

When choosing medical therapy for generalized anxiety disorder and panic disorder, antidepressants (SSRIs or SNRIs) are always first-line therapy, NOT benzodiazepines or buspirone.

CONQUER THE **WARDS!**

You can augment the effect of SSRIs with the addition of buspirone.

PANIC DISORDER

Clinical Features and Diagnosis

- Panic attacks generally present with acute-onset, intense episodes that can last minutes to an hour. In a panic disorder, the patient experiences recurrent episodes.
- Diagnostic criteria for a panic attack include an abrupt surge of intense fear or discomfort peaking within a minute, during which time at least 4 of the following occur: palpitations, sweating, shaking, shortness of breath, choking/gagging sensations, chest pain, nausea or abdominal pain, dizziness or lightheadedness, chills or hot flashes, paresthesias, depersonalization (being detached from oneself), fear of losing control or "going crazy," or fear of dying.

CONQUER THE **WARDS!**

Perioral and/or acral paresthesias, when present, are fairly specific to panic attacks.

- A diagnosis of panic disorder implies a history of recurrent panic attacks, with attacks followed by a month or more of persistent concern or worry about future attacks and with attacks not attributable to other psychiatric disorders, substance use, or chronic medical conditions.

Differential Diagnosis

The differential diagnosis can be quite wide, depending on the predominant symptom that the patient is describing, but considerations should include:

- Substance use disorders.
- Other anxiety disorders (generalized anxiety disorders, phobia, social anxiety).
- Cardiac conditions (angina, arrhythmias).
- Pulmonary conditions (pulmonary embolism, chronic obstructive pulmonary disease [COPD], asthma).
- Hyperthyroidism.
- Pheochromocytoma.

Principles of Initial Treatment

- **First-line therapy** generally consists of SSRIs or SNRIs, generally at lower doses than used in the management of depression or **CBT**. There is no evidence for one over another.
- **Other options: Tricyclic antidepressants (TCAs)** are also a possible option, though they have more side effects, which can prove limiting. **Benzodiazepines** can be a useful adjunct, as they are effective and quick acting, though there is potential for abuse. They are often prescribed along with an antidepressant early in treatment to hasten response, but can be used long term in selected patients.

CONQUER THE **WARDS!**

Patients may present to other physicians for complaints (e.g. dermatology office for symptoms related to excessive handdwashing).

CONQUER THE **BOARDS!**

OCD can be difficult to distinguish from other psychiatric disorders; however, OCD must include intrusive thoughts, images, or urges, along with repetitive behaviors.

OTHER COMMON PRIMARY CLINIC PSYCHIATRIC DISORDERS

OBSESSIVE-COMPULSIVE DISORDER

General Facts

- Characterized by obsessions and/or compulsions that lead to significant distress in social or personal areas.
- Typically begins in adolescence/early adulthood.
- Has higher rates of coexisting psychiatric disorders than in the general population.

Clinical Features

- **Obsessions**: Persistent, unwanted, and intrusive ideas, thoughts, impulses, or images that lead to marked anxiety or distress (fear of contamination, fear of harm to oneself or others).
- **Compulsions**: Repeated mental acts or behaviors that neutralize anxiety from obsessions (handwashing, elaborate rituals, counting, excessive checking).
- Patients recognize the behaviors are excessive and irrational.

Management

- **CBT** using exposure and desensitization is first-line and recommended first over pharmacotherapy.
- **Pharmacotherapy:** First-line agents include SSRIs, clomipramine; second-line are SNRIs.

HIGH-YIELD LITERATURE

American Psychiatric Association (APA). Practice guideline for the treatment of patients with obsessive-compulsive disorder.

World Federation of Societies of Biological Psychiatry (WFSBP). Guidelines for the pharmacological treatment of anxiety disorders, obsessive-compulsive disorder and posttraumatic stress disorder in primary care.

POST-TRAUMATIC STRESS DISORDER

General Facts

- Stress disorder triggered by a traumatic experience.
- Follows exposure to an extreme, life-threatening traumatic event, such as combat, witnessing a violent crime, or assault, that evoked intense fear, helplessness, or horror.

Clinical Features

- Symptoms last longer than 1 month.
- Re-experiencing of the event (nightmares).
- Avoidance of stimuli associated with the trauma.
- Numbed responsiveness.
- Arousal (hypervigilance).

Management

- **Pharmacotherapy**
  - Short-term: Target anxiety with beta-blockers and alpha-2-agonists (clonidine).
  - Long-term: First-line are SSRIs, but adding buspirone, TCAs, and MAOIs can be helpful.
- **Psychotherapy and support groups** are important adjuncts to pharmacotherapy.

CONQUER THE WARDS!

Generally speaking, patients who have typical and recurrent panic attacks can be diagnosed with having panic disorder without an extensive workup, but brief consideration should be given to the potential disease mimics.

CONQUER THE WARDS!

Studies showed that CBT is more effective than SSRIs alone in the treatment of OCD.

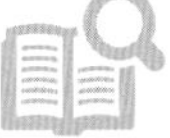

HIGH-YIELD LITERATURE

Stein MB, Sareen J. Generalized anxiety disorder. *N Engl J Med*. 2015;373:2059.

Baldwin DS, Polkinghorn C. Evidence-based pharmacotherapy of generalized anxiety disorder. *Int J Neuropsychopharmacol* 2005; 8:293.

DISORDERS THAT SHOULD BE REFERRED TO PSYCHIATRY

BIPOLAR DISORDERS

General Facts

- Bipolar disorders are a group of mood disorders that are characterized by distinct episodes of mania or hypomania with or without distinct episodes of depression.

CONQUER THE WARDS!

Military veterans, refugees, and traumatically injured civilians are at increased risk of PTSD.

CONQUER THE BOARDS!

A diagnosis of PTSD is made only after a month has passed since the traumatic event; symptoms occurring less than this should be diagnosed as acute stress disorder.

CONQUER THE BOARDS!

DIGFAST for Recall of Mania/Hypomania Symptoms:

Distractibility
Impulsivity/Indiscretions
Grandiosity
Flight of ideas (racing thoughts)
Activities (increased, may be dangerous)
Sleeplessness
Talkativeness (pressured speech; loud, rapid speech)

CONQUER THE WARDS!

Notice an abrupt onset of manic symptoms in a patient without a psychiatric history? Work through medical, neurologic, and psychiatric differentials. Particularly consider **intoxication.**

CONQUER THE BOARDS!

A patient presenting with manic symptoms including psychosis does not have bipolar disorder II. Psychotic symptoms **only** occur in mania, not hypomania.

- The hallmark of bipolar disorders is prolonged (at least several days) mood episodes; however, the variability in presentation makes diagnosis challenging.
- Psychosis may co-occur during a manic or depressive episode. Onset is typically in the late teens to early twenties.
- Comorbidities are common, substance use disorders are seen in as many as 60% of patients, and anxiety disorders are seen in as many as 50% of patients.
- Suicide risk is high in patients with bipolar disorder, and almost half of all patients will attempt suicide at least once in their lives.

Clinical Features

- **Mania:** Elevated, expansive, or irritable mood; increased activity; and decreased sleep with severe impact on daily functioning. Lasts at least 1 week.
- **Hypomania:** Elevated or irritable mood, increased activity, and decreased sleep with mild to moderate impact on daily functioning. Lasts at least 4 days.
- **Depression:** Episode of major depression that is discrete in length, may have abrupt onset and offset.

Subtypes (Table 12-1)

- Bipolar I disorder.
- Bipolar II disorder.
- Cyclothymic disorder.
- Unspecified bipolar disorder.

TABLE 12-1. DSM-5 Criteria for Bipolar Disorders I and II

	Bipolar Disorder I	Bipolar Disorder II
Manic episode	Yes	No
Hypomanic episode	Common but not required	Yes
Major depressive episode	Usual but not required	Yes

BIPOLAR DISORDER I

General Facts

- Severe chronic mood disorder with distinct episodes of mania, hypomania, and usually depression.
- Most patients (>70%) have psychotic features when manic. Average age at onset is 18.

Clinical Features

- At least one episode of mania is necessary for diagnosis.
- Major depressive episodes are typical but not needed for diagnosis.

Management

- Patients with bipolar disorder I may require intermittent hospitalization.
- Many are able to return to fully functional levels between mood episodes.
- Pharmacotherapy includes (Table 12-2):

  First line: Mood stabilizers (usually lithium) with an antipsychotic. Valproate is also commonly used as a mood stabilizer.

  Second line: Switching antipsychotics and in refractory cases, ECT.
- Antidepressants can be considered in resistant cases with depression, but only after the patient has been started on a mood-stabilizing medication.

TABLE 12-2. Medications for Bipolar Disorder	
Mood Stabilizers	**Antipsychotics**
Lithium Lamotrigine Divalproex/valproate Carbamazepine Oxcarbazepine	Aripiprazole Asenapine Chlorpromazine Clozapine Haloperidol Lurasidone Olanzapine Paliperidone Quetiapine Risperidone Ziprasidone

BIPOLAR DISORDER II

General Facts

- Chronic mood disorder characterized by at least one hypomanic episode and at least one major depressive episode.
- Typically patients have had recurrent depressive and hypomanic episodes.

Clinical Features

- Hypomanic episodes must be noticeable by others but **not** severe enough to cause social or occupational impairment and **not** severe enough to result in hospitalization.
- Higher mood episode frequency than bipolar disorder I with multiple and unpredictable episodes of both severe depression and hypomania.

Management

- May require psychiatric hospitalization during episodes of severe depression.
- Treatment options are similar to bipolar disorder I, with mood stabilizers and antipsychotics as the mainstay of treatment. However, generally monotherapy is used with either a mood stabilizer or antipsychotic.

CONQUER THE WARDS!

Patients with bipolar disorder II typically present during an episode of major depression. Consider bipolar disorder in patients with severe depression, as they are unlikely to initially recognize hypomania.

CYCLOTHYMIC DISORDER

General Facts

- Chronic, fluctuating mood disorder lasting at least 2 years with several periods of hypomanic symptoms and depressive symptoms without a distinct hypomanic or major depressive episode.

Clinical Features

- Criteria for mania, hypomania, or major depression have never been met.
- Symptoms are not attributable to a medical comorbidity or medication side effect.
- Symptoms cause clinically significant impairment.

Management

- Many patients diagnosed with cyclothymia will subsequently develop bipolar disorder I or II.
- Treatment is similar to that of bipolar disorder I and II, and the current mood episode should direct medication choice, including:
  - Mood stabilizers.
  - Antidepressants.
  - Antipsychotic medications.
- Psychotherapy

CONQUER THE WARDS!

Serotonin reuptake inhibitors are not contraindicated in patients with bipolar disorder. There is a risk of mood switching to mania, which is greater in bipolar disorder I than bipolar II, but this risk can be minimized with a mood stabilizer.

HIGH-YIELD LITERATURE

Grande I, Berk M, Birmaher B, Vieta E. Bipolar disorder. *Lancet.* 2016;387:1561-1572.

PSYCHOTIC DISORDERS

General Facts

- **Definition:** Psychosis can be seen as a loss of contact with reality, and the hallmarks of psychotic disorders are hallucinations and delusions.
  - **Hallucinations** are perceptions one has when awake without stimuli. Auditory hallucinations are the most common in psychosis, followed by visual.
  - **Delusions** are fixed, false beliefs not typical of the person's cultural background. They can be bizarre (i.e., implausible) or nonbizarre. The most common theme of delusions is persecutory (e.g., believing you're being monitored by the FBI), but there are many other themes (e.g., grandiose, referential, somatic, religious, nihilistic, erotomanic).
  - Other symptoms of psychosis include **disorganized speech** (ranging from tangentiality to word salad), **disorganized behavior** (serious impairment in goal-directed behavior, including unpredictable agitation, catatonia, or incoherent behavior), and **negative symptoms** (particularly blunted emotional expression and avolition, but also anhedonia, paucity of thought/speech, and social withdrawal).
- **Causes:** The differential diagnosis for psychosis is very broad, with many potential medical causes. Psychosis may be due to a primary psychotic disorder (listed next) or due to secondary causes leading to delirium. For example:
  - Neurologic disease (traumatic brain injury [TBI], seizures, cerebrovascular accident [CVA], dementias, Huntington or Parkinson disease).
  - Substances (both prescribed medications and drugs of abuse).
  - Medical illnesses such as infection, hepatic or uremic encephalopathy, endocrine disorders, and autoimmune disorders.

CONQUER THE **WARDS!**

All types of hallucinations can be present in primary psychotic disorders. However, olfactory, gustatory, and tactile hallucinations are more common in neurologic disorders, or may be substance-induced.

Subtypes

- Schizophrenia spectrum (schizophreniform disorder, schizophrenia).
- Brief psychotic disorder.
- Delusional disorder.
- Schizoaffective disorder.
- Major depressive disorder with psychotic features.
- Bipolar disorder with psychotic features.

SCHIZOPHRENIA SPECTRUM

General Facts

- Psychotic syndrome lasting at least 1 month (schizophreniform) or 6 months (schizophrenia). Usual onset is early twenties in men, late twenties in women.
- Schizophrenia has approximately a 1% lifetime prevalence worldwide.
- Females and males have a similar prevalence, but often less severe presentation in women.

Clinical Features

- Two or more of the following (including at least one of a, b, or c):
  a. Delusions.

b. Hallucinations.
c. Disorganized speech.
d. Grossly disorganized or catatonic behavior.
e. Negative symptoms.

- No major depressive, manic, or mixed episodes during this time.
- Length of illness.
  a. Schizophreniform disorder: lasts between 1 month and 6 months.
  b. Schizophrenia: lasts at least 6 months.

Management

- Patients with schizophrenia may require intermittent hospitalization, but frequently are able to thrive in the community.
- They frequently benefit from team-based approaches to care, such as **assertive community treatment** (ACT), which involves a multidisciplinary team going to meet the patient to ensure high-quality, comprehensive care. This is on top of antipsychotic medications, psychotherapy (particularly CBT), and psychosocial intervention (social skills training and family psychoeducation) (Table 12-3).

CONQUER THE BOARDS!

The only antipsychotic with strong evidence suggesting it is more effective than the others is clozapine. However, it has significant side effects and requires frequent and lifelong monitoring of ANC due to risk of neutropenia.

TABLE 12-3. Antipsychotic Treatment for Schizphrenia

First-Generation Antipsychotics ("Typicals")	Second-Generation Antipsychotics ("Atypicals")
Chlorpromazine (Thorazine) Fluphenazine (Prolixin) Haloperidol (Haldol) Loxapine (Loxitane)	Aripiprazole (Abilify) Asenapine (Saphris) Clozapine (Clozaril) Lurasidone (Latuda) Olanzapine (Zyprexa) Paliperidone (Invega) Quetiapine (Seroquel) Risperidone (Risperdal) Ziprasidone (Geodon)

HIGH-YIELD LITERATURE

Lehman AF, Lieberman JA, Dixon LB, et al. *Practice Guideline for the Treatment of Patients with Schizophrenia*. 2nd ed. New York, NY: American Psychiatric Association; 2010. Available online at https://psychiatryonline.org/pb/assets/raw/sitewide/practice_guidelines/guidelines/schizophrenia.pdf.

BRIEF PSYCHOTIC DISORDER

General Facts

- A short-term "psychotic break" lasting less than one month, often secondary to an acute stressor.

Clinical Features

- One or more of the following: delusions, hallucinations, or disorganized speech.
- May include grossly disorganized or catatonic behavior.
- Lasts less than 1 month and must resolve completely.

Management

- May require psychiatric hospitalization if the patient presents risk of harm to self or others; otherwise, may be appropriate for outpatient management.
- **Short-term pharmacotherapy:** Antipsychotics (first- or second-generation).

CONQUER THE WARDS!

Notice abrupt-onset psychotic symptoms in a patient without a psychiatric history? Work through medical and neurologic differentials, particularly **delirium.** These causes are especially likely in the elderly.

- Removal of stressor (if applicable).
- **Long-term therapy:** If secondary to a stressor, targeted psychotherapy may be helpful in addressing this and preventing relapse.

DELUSIONAL DISORDER

General Facts

- Characterized by one or more delusions, with no other signs/symptoms of psychosis.

Clinical Features

- One or more delusions for at least 1 month.
- Never met symptom criteria for schizophrenia (i.e., no hallucinations, disorganized speech, etc.).
- No obviously odd/bizarre behavior nor marked impairment in function *aside from the impact of the delusions.*

Management

- Often does not respond to inpatient psychiatric care and may be better served by outpatient care so long as the patient doesn't present a risk of harm to themselves or others.
- Antipsychotics, although not particularly effective (50% remission rate).
- CBT.

> CONQUER THE **BOARDS!**
>
> The way to distinguish schizoaffective disorder from a mood disorder with psychotic features is easy. In **bipolar disorder** or **major depressive disorder** with psychotic features, the *mood disorder* comes first, and the psychosis is only secondary to the mood episode. In **schizoaffective disorder**, the *schizo* comes first: thus, they're psychotic sometimes without mood symptoms.

MIXED AFFECTIVE/PSYCHOTIC DISORDERS

These include schizoaffective disorder, bipolar disorder with psychotic features, and major depressive disorder with psychotic features.

SCHIZOAFFECTIVE DISORDER

- Simultaneously meets criteria for a major mood episode (manic or depressed) AND the symptom criteria for schizophrenia.
- Has delusions or hallucinations for at least 2 weeks WITHOUT mood symptoms.
- Spends most of the time in a major mood episode (manic and/or depressed).
- Bipolar type: Has had a manic episode (may also have had depressive episodes).
- Depressive type: Has only had depressive episodes.

MOOD DISORDER WITH PSYCHOTIC FEATURES

General Facts

- Meets criteria for a major mood episode (manic or depressive).
- Has delusions and/or hallucinations during the course of the mood episode.
- Does NOT have psychotic symptoms outside of a mood episode.

Management

- Although there are multiple opinions on the appropriate treatment of mixed affective/psychotic disorders, generally the gold standard of care is to treat both the mood disorder and the psychotic disorder, requiring more than one medication.

- Antipsychotics.
- Mood stabilizers (for bipolar disorder/type).
- Antidepressants (for depressive disorder/type).

SUBSTANCE-RELATED DISORDERS

General Facts

- **Substance-related disorders** include substance use disorders and substance-induced disorders.
  - Substance use disorders: The common feature among substance use disorders is an individual's continued use of the substance despite significant problems related to its use, including impaired control, social impairment, risky use, tolerance, and withdrawal. Intense cravings can lead to repeated relapses and continued drug use and abuse.
  - Substance-induced disorders include intoxication and withdrawal, with specific clinical features depending upon the substance used and/or abused.

Clinical Features

- Regardless of substance of choice, the problematic use of the substance must cause clinically significant impairment by at least 2 of the following criteria, within a 12-month period:
  - The substance is taken in larger quantities and over longer periods of time.
  - There is a persistent desire to use or difficulty cutting down on use.
  - Time is spent dedicated to acquiring the substance of choice.
  - Substance use interferes with work, school, or home.
  - Continues substance use despite negative social and interpersonal consequences.
  - Withdrawal from activities due to substance use.
  - Substance use in risky or dangerous environments.
  - Substance use is continued despite recognized negative physical and psychological effects.
  - Cravings.
  - Tolerance.
  - Withdrawal.

Management

- Management depends on the substance used, the risks associated with acute intoxication and/or withdrawal from that substance, and the clinical recommendations for treatment related to that specific substance.
- The Substance Abuse and Mental Health Services Administration (SAMHSA) recommends screening, brief intervention, and referral to treatment (SBIRT) for recognition of substance use disorders by primary care providers.
- Interventions and referrals may differ based on the substance abused, especially with regard to pharmacologic treatments; however, there is significant overlap in nonpharmacologic treatment recommendations.

The following sections discuss the most commonly abused substances: tobacco, alcohol, opioids, and sympathomimetics.

CONQUER THE **BOARDS!**

CAGE is used to screen for alcohol abuse and alcohol use disorder:

Cut—Do you ever feel you should cut back on drinking?

Annoyed—Do you ever feel **annoyed** when others question your drinking?

Guilty—Do you ever feel **guilty** for your drinking?

Eye-opener—Do you ever need an **eye-opener** in the morning?

CONQUER THE BOARDS!

For smoking cessation on the shelf exam, choose behavioral therapy PLUS either varenicline OR **2** forms of nicotine replacement therapy (patch and a short-acting agent for PRN use).

TOBACCO USE

Epidemiology

- About 1 in 6 adult Americans uses tobacco products.
- Smoking is the leading preventable cause of mortality.
- On surveys, nearly two-thirds of smokers say they want to quit, and nearly half of all smokers report a quit attempt in the last year. However, only ~5% of smokers who make an unaided attempt to quit are still abstinent at 1 year.

Complications of Tobacco Use

- Increases risk of death (cardiac, pulmonary, cancer).
- Malignancy: Increases risk of numerous types of cancer, including lung cancer, head and neck cancer, bladder cancer, esophageal/gastric/colon cancer, and pancreatic cancer.
- Cardiovascular: Premature atherosclerosis, coronary artery disease, stroke, and peripheral vascular disease.
- Pulmonary: Chronic cough, COPD, and increased risk of pulmonary infections.

Barriers to Quitting

- One of the main barriers to quitting is the addictiveness of nicotine and the withdrawal symptoms. Symptoms peak in the first 3 days of cessation and subside over several weeks and can include appetite changes, weight gain, mood changes, irritability, insomnia, difficulty concentrating, and restlessness.
- Another barrier to quitting is social triggers. Patients need to identify their triggers and reshape their habits.

SMOKING CESSATION COUNSELING (THE 5 A'S)

- **ASK**: Ask all patients about tobacco use (in all forms, including secondhand smoke).
- **ADVISE**: Advise all tobacco users of the harms of smoking and benefits to quitting in clear and brief language. There is high-quality evidence that interventions <5 minutes have effectiveness in improving quit rates.
- **ASSESS**: Assess readiness to change.
  - Precontemplation: Not ready to quit.
  - Contemplation: Considering a quit attempt.
  - Preparation: Actively planning a quit attempt.
  - Action: Actively involved in a quit attempt.
  - Maintenance: Achieved smoking cessation.
- **ASSIST**: If the patient is contemplative (or at stages beyond), provide assistance. This may include 1) setting a quit date, 2) addressing barriers to quitting, 3) discussing potential effects of quitting (both withdrawal symptoms and long-term benefits), 4) discussing behavioral interventions to overcome barriers, and 5) discussing pharmacologic agents to increase success rates.
- **ARRANGE**: Arrange short-term follow-up with the patient within 1 to 2 weeks of the quit date.

Behavioral and Pharmacotherapy for Smoking Cessation

- Therapy for smoking cessation generally consists of behavioral therapy PLUS either A) 2 forms of nicotine replacement therapy or B) varenicline, with single-agent nicotine replacement therapy or bupropion being other options.

- **Behavioral therapy**: Effective, especially when paired with pharmacologic agents. If no office-based therapy is available, referral to free telephone quitlines (1800-QUIT-NOW in the United States) or online resources can be helpful.
- **Nicotine replacement therapy (NRT)**: The patch is main long-acting option, with short-acting options including lozenge, gum, spray, or tablets. Will generally pair a patch to control baseline nicotine withdrawal symptoms with a short-acting agent to control cravings on an as-needed (PRN) basis.

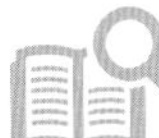

HIGH-YIELD LITERATURE

E-cigarettes vs. Nicotine replacement therapy for smoking cessation:

In this small RCT, e-cigarettes resulted in significantly better smoking cessation outcomes than other forms of nicotine-replacement therapy.

Hajek P, Phillips-Waller A, Przulj D, et al. A randomized trial of e-cigarettes versus nicotine-replacement therapy. *N Engl J Med.* 2019;380:629-637.

- **Varenicline**:
  - Mechanism: Partial agonist of the alpha-4 beta-2 nicotinic receptor, which works to partially stimulate the receptor and decrease symptoms from nicotine withdrawal and blocks nicotine from tobacco smoke from binding to the receptor.
  - Reduces cravings and withdrawal symptoms.
  - Will generally start varenicline and then have patient set tobacco quit date around 1 week later.
  - Side effects: Initial concerns for neuropsychiatric and cardiovascular effects have not been borne out in the literature. Does increase risk of headaches, insomnia, and vivid dreams.
- **Bupropion:**
  - Mechanism: Enhances central nervous system (CNS) noradrenergic and dopaminergic release.
  - Contraindicated in patients with seizure disorder, as it reduces seizure threshold.
  - Side effects: Insomnia, agitation, dry mouth, headache.
- **Electronic cigarettes (E-cigarettes):**
  - Not traditionally recommend by physicians, but many patients use them or may ask you about them. Emerging data (see later) suggest these may play an important role in smoking cessation.
  - E-cigarettes contain nicotine, ethylene glycol, and flavorings, so the patient still ingests nicotine but avoids many of the toxic constituents of cigarette smoke.
  - The benefits and harms of e-cigarettes are not well-understood, but are widely thought to be significantly less risky than usual cigarettes, so may be an option for patients who will consider them but are not willing to stop using nicotine products.

CONQUER THE WARDS!

Although the CAGE questionnaire has a long history of being taught to medical students, it has poor data to support its use, relatively poor performance in real-world settings (especially in women), and is less commonly used than other screening tools.

HIGH-YIELD LITERATURE

Smoking cessation agents and risk of neuropsychiatric side effects

Anthenelli RM, Benowitz NL, West R, et al. Neuropsychiatric safety and efficacy of varenicline, bupropion, and nicotine patch in smokers with and without psychiatric disorders (EAGLES): A double-blind, randomised, placebo-controlled clinical trial. *Lancet*. 2016;387(10037):2507-2520.

ALCOHOL USE DISORDER

Consequences of Alcohol Use

Alcohol use has numerous potentially harmful effects, including:

- CNS: Cerebellar dysfunction, memory issues.
- Cardiovascular: Hypertension, stroke, cardiomyopathy, coronary artery disease.
- Gastrointestinal: Pancreatitis (acute and chronic), chronic liver disease and cirrhosis, gastroesophageal reflux disease (GERD), esophagitis, peptic ulcer disease (PUD).
- Endocrine: Accelerated bone loss, hypogonadism.
- Malignancy: Oral cancer, head and neck cancers, laryngeal cancer, esophageal/gastric/colon cancer, pancreatic cancer, liver cancers, and breast cancer.

Screening for Alcohol Use Disorder and Diagnosis

- Recommended limits of alcohol use are no more than 5 drinks/day and no more than 14 drinks/week on average for men and no more than 3 drinks/day and no more than 7 drinks/week on average for women.
- Numerous screening and diagnostic tools exist (some are reviewed next), but most often will begin with initial question of how often a patient has exceeded the previously noted limits.
- Other tools used in clinical practice include the AUDIT-C (3 items) (Table 12-4), AUDIT (10 items), or CAGE (4 items).
- The DSM-5 diagnostic criteria require the presence of 2 of 11 symptoms in the past year. Dependence and tolerance are 2 of these symptoms, and

Table 12-4. AUDIT-C Questionnaire for Detecting Alcohol Use Disorder

Question	Scoring (Points)				
	1	2	3	4	5
How often do you have a drink containing alcohol?	Never	Monthly or less	2–4 times per month	2–3 times per week	4 or more times per week
How many standard drinks containing alcohol do you have on a typical day?	1 or 2	3 or 4	5 or 6	7–9	10 or more
How often do you have 6 or more drinks on one occasion?	Never	Less than monthly	Monthly	Weekly	Daily or almost daily

Maximum score of 12. A score ≥4 in men or ≥3 in women is considered positive.

together can clinch the diagnosis but are NOT required to diagnose alcohol use disorder.

Outpatient Management of Alcohol Use Disorder

- The main decision is whether patients should undergo psychosocial counseling, pharmacologic management, or both. Patients with more mild alcohol use disorder may only require counseling or support groups such as Alcoholics Anonymous (AA).
- First-line medication options include naltrexone or acamprosate. Other agents with some evidence supporting their use include disulfiram, topiramate, and gabapentin.
  - Naltrexone: Available in oral and injectable formulations. Blocks the mu-opioid receptor and can reduce cravings. Generally thought to be the most effective option. Can cause transaminitis, so liver function tests (LFTs) should be periodically monitored.
  - Acamprosate: Mechanism not entirely clear, but works to reduce craving. Must be taken 3 times daily, which may limit adherence. Less effective than naltrexone.
  - Disulfiram: Inhibits aldehyde dehydrogenase and prevents alcohol's metabolism, resulting in accumulation of acetaldehyde and accompanying sweating, flushing, nausea, and vomiting. Only to be used in very motivated patients who will take the medication daily.

Management of Alcohol Withdrawal

- **General management**: Many patients require hospitalization. Replete thiamine before giving glucose and folate to patient.
- Withdrawal syndromes can vary from mild anxiety and tremor, to alcohol withdrawal seizures, to delirium tremens (Figure 12-1).
- **Alcohol withdrawal can be life-threatening and should be aggressively treated with benzodiazepine tapers**. Usual onset is 12 to 24 hours after the last drink.
- Data are superior for symptom-triggered therapy using a symptom score (such as Clinical Institute Withdrawal Assessment [CIWA] (Figure 12-2)), but many hospitals use long-acting benzodiazepines such as chlordiazepoxide with a slow taper.

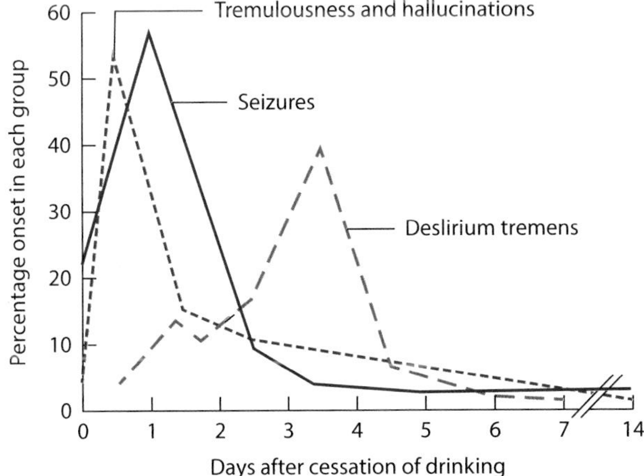

FIGURE 12-1. Timeline of Alcohol Withdrawal Symptoms. (From Simon RP, Aminoff MJ, Greenberg DA: Clinical Neurology, 10th ed. Copyright © McGraw-Hill Education. All rights reserved. Figure created using data from Victor M, Adams RD. The effect of alcohol on the nervous system. Res Publ Assoc Res Nerv Ment Dis. 1952;32: 526-573.)

Patient: ______________________ Date: __________ Time:____:____

Pulse or heart rate, taken for one minute:________ Blood pressure: ___/___

Nausea and vomiting. Ask 'Do you feel sick to your stomach? Have you vomited?"
Observation:
0—No nausea and no vomiting
1—Mild nausea with no vomiting
2—
3—
4—Intermittent nausea with dry heaves
5—
6—
7—Constant nausea, frequent dry heaves, and vomiting

Tremor. Ask patient to extend arms and spread fingers apart.
Observation:
0—No tremor
1—Tremor not visible but can be felt, fingertip to fingertip
2—
3—
4—Moderate tremor with arms extended
5—
6—
7—Severe tremor, even with arms not extended

Paroxysmal sweats
Observation:
0—No sweat visible
1—Barely perceptible sweating; palms moist
2—
3—
4—Beads of sweat obvious on forehead
5—
6—
7—Drenching sweats

Anxiety. Ask "Do you feel nervous?"
Observation:
0—No anxiety (at ease)
1—Midlity anxious
2—
3—
4—Moderately anxious or guarded, so anxiety is inferred
5—
6—
7—Equivalent to acute panic states as occur in severe delirium or acute schizophrenic reactions

Agitation
Observation:
0—Normal activity
1—Somewhat more than normal activity
2—
3—
4—Moderately fidgety and restless
5—
6—
7—Paces back and forth during most of the interview or constantly thrashes about

Tactile disturbances. Ask 'Do you have you any itching, pins and needles sensations. burning. or numbness, or do you feel like bugs are crawling on or under your skin?"
Observation:
0—None
1—Very mild itching, pins and needles sensation, burning, or numbness
2—Mild itching, pins and needles sensation, burning, or numbness
3—Moderate itching, pins and needles sensation, burning, or numbness
4—Moderately severe hallucinations
5—Severe hallucinations
6—Extremely severe hallucinations
7—Constant nausea, frequent dry heaves, and vomiting

Auditory disturbances. Ask 'Are you more aware of sounds around you? Are they harsh? Do they frighten you? Are you hearing anything that is disturbing to you? Are you hearing things you know are not there?"
Observation:
0—Not present
1—Very mild harshness or ability to frighten
2—Mild harshness or ability to frighten
3—Moderate harshness or ability to frighten
4—Moderately severe hallucinations
5—Severe hallucinations
6—Extremely severe hallucinations
7—Continuous hallucinations

Visual disturbances. Ask "Dose the light appear to be too bright? Is its color different? Dose it hurt your eyes? Are you seeing anything that is disturbing to you? Are you seeing things you know are not there?"
Observation:
0—Not present
1—Very mild sensitivity
2—Mild sensitivity
3—Moderate sensitivity
4—Moderately severe hallucinations
5—Severe hallucinations
6—Extremely severe hallucinations
7—Continuous hallucinations

Headache, fullness in head. Ask "Dose your head feel different/ Does it feel like there is a band around your head?"
Do not rate for dizziness or lightheadness: otherwise, rate severity.
0—Not present
1—Very mild
2—Mild
3—Moderate
4—Moderately severe
5—Severe
6—Very severe
7—Extremely severe

Orientation and clouding of sensorium. Ask "What day is this? Where are you? Who am I?"
Observation:
0—Orientated and can do serial additions
1—Cannot do serial additions or is uncertain about date
2—Date disorientation by no more than two calendar days
3—Date disorientation by more than two calendar days
4—Disorientated for place and/or person

Total score: ________ (maximum - 67) Rater's initials ________

FIGURE 12-2. Alcohol Withdrawal Assesment Scoring Guidelines (CIWA-Ar)

- **Alcohol withdrawal seizures**: Generally occur 12 to 48 hours after the last drink. Should treat with more aggressive use of agents for alcohol withdrawal (benzodiazepines, phenobarbital, and/or propofol) rather than use of antiepileptics.
- **Delirium tremens**: Occurs in about 5% of patients, and untreated can result in a mortality rate of almost 30%. Clinical syndrome of hallucinations, disorientation, tachycardia, diaphoresis, hypertension, and hyperthermia in the setting of alcohol cessation. Requires intensive care unit (ICU) level of care for treatment escalation.

HIGH-YIELD LITERATURE

Standing benzodiazepines vs. Symptom-triggered benzodiazepine use in alcohol withdrawal:

Saitz R, Mayo-Smith MF, Roberts MS, Redmond HA, Bernard DR, Calkins DR. Individualized treatment for alcohol withdrawal: A randomized, double-blind controlled trial. *JAMA.* 1994;272(7):519.

- Refractory alcohol withdrawal (refractory to benzodiazepine therapy) necessitates ICU-level monitoring, airway protection, and potential adjunctive use of medications such as phenobarbital or propofol.

OPIOID USE DISORDER

Epidemiology and Pharmacology

- Over the last decade in the United States, there has been a significant rise in the use of both heroin and illicit prescription medications.
- Opioids are now the most common cause of drug overdose death in the United States.

Clinical Manifestations

- During acute intoxication, can see significant sedation with associated slurring of speech. On examination, may see miosis (constricted pupils). Those with chronic use may have have a normal examination.
- Health consequences of long-term opioid use include risk of overdose (including respiratory depression and death), opioid-induced constipation, opioid-induced hyperalgesia (paradoxical increase in pain and sensitivity), and any consequences of the route of administration (e.g., endocarditis or infections such as HIV or hepatitis C or B if injecting).

Screening in the Clinic and Diagnosis of Opioid Use Disorder

- All patients with medical conditions that may have been acquired through opioid use (endocarditis, HIV or hepatitis C or B) should be screened.
- Many clinics have adopted universal screening protocols, given the significant increase in rates of opioid use throughout the United States.
- There is no single accepted screening technique—options include the Rapid Opioid Dependence Screen or the DAST-10.

Treatment of Acute Intoxication or Overdose

- The main concern is for mental and respiratory status. Need high index of suspicion in patients without known opioid use disorder.
- Once opioid toxicity is suspected, prompt attention should be paid to the patient's airway and breathing. Naloxone should be given intravenously. If excess naloxone is given, withdrawal may be precipitated, which should be closely monitored (and not empirically treated with opioids). Multiple dose of naloxone may be required, depending on the opioid used by the patient.

Treatment of Opioid Withdrawal Syndromes

- Clinical features: Agitation, restlessness, diarrhea, nausea/vomiting, rhinorrhea, myalgias and joint pains, and piloerection.
- Opioid withdrawal can produce significant symptoms and should be treated to prevent relapse, but generally will not result in death even if untreated, except in rare circumstances.
- Management may include opioid agonist therapy (methadone, buprenorphine), benzodiazepines, and/or clonidine. Other symptom-driven treatments may also be useful.

Treatment in the Outpatient Setting

- Focus in the clinic should be on harm reduction—aiming for long-term abstinence but ensuring patients are using safely if they are not ready to quit. Harm reduction interventions may include needle exchange programs, never using opioids alone, and developing an overdose plan.

> **CONQUER THE WARDS!**
>
> Given that there is no universally recommended screening tool for opioid use disorder, ask your clinic preceptor what the clinic uses. If they don't have a good answer, consider using the Rapid Opioid Dependence Screen.

- Prescribe intranasal naloxone for PRN use on themselves or friends to all patients whether they are currently abstinent or not.
- Refer interested patients for pharmacologic therapy with either methadone (as part of a supervised methadone maintenance program) or buprenorphine–naloxone (prescribed by primary care physicians if they have applied for a waiver).

SYMPATHOMIMETICS

Mechanism and Pharmacology

- Enhances monoamine neurotransmitter (dopamine, norepinephrine, serotonin) activity in the CNS and peripheral nervous system (PNS) by blocking reuptake pumps.
- Cocaine base ("crack" or "freebase") can be smoked but not injected.
- Cocaine salt cannot be smoked, but is readily injected (intravenously or subcutaneously) or insufflated ("snorted") through the nose.
- Intended effects for patients include increased energy, alertness, and sociability, along with feelings of euphoria. However, there are numerous short- and long-term consequences to use.

Cocaine Intoxication (Acute and Chronic)

- CNS: Increased risk of seizure or stroke.
- Cardiovascular system: Premature atherosclerosis, hypertension, tachycardia, myocardial infarction, cardiomyopathy, myocarditis.
- Pulmonary system: Shortness of breath, wheezing, "crack lung" (acute pulmonary syndrome with fever, hypoxia, diffuse alveolar infiltrates, and respiratory failure).

Management of Acute Cocaine Intoxication

- Initial attention to vital signs (hyperthermia), airway, breathing, and circulation.
- Use benzodiazepines to control excess sympathetic discharge and anxiety.
- Treat organ-specific toxicity. Avoid beta blockade (due to risks of unopposed alpha-adrenergic activity), and consider alpha blockade with agents such as phentolamine for refractory hypertension. Optimal management strategies for "crack lung" are unclear, and efforts should focus on supportive respiratory care.

Cocaine Withdrawal

- Symptoms are bothersome but rarely medically serious.
- Symptoms include depression, anxiety/agitation, cravings, and sleep changes.

Long-Term Management of Cocaine Use Disorders

- Referral to long-term counseling and support groups. Only psychological interventions have shown consistent and long-term improvements in abstinence rates.
- Numerous agents have been examined with varying degrees of data, including dopamine agonists, long-acting amphetamines, and bupropion, but patients should be referred to physicians with experience in addiction medicine.

HIGH-YIELD LITERATURE

Kelber HD, Weiss RD, Anton Jr AF, et al. *Practice Guideline for the Treatment of Patient with Substance Use Disorders*. 2nd ed. New York, NY: American Psychiatric Association; 2010. Available online at https://psychiatryonline.org/pb/assets/raw/sitewide/practice_guidelines/guidelines/substanceuse.pdf.

McIntyre JS, Charles SC, Anzia DJ, et al. *Treating Substance Use Disorders: A Quick Reference Guide*. New York, NY: American Psychiatric Association; 2006. Available online at https://psychiatryonline.org/pb/assets/raw/sitewide/practice_guidelines/guidelines/substanceuse-guide.pdf.

Table 12-5. Intoxication Treatment

Substance	Intoxication Symptoms	Treatment
Alcohol	Mood lability, aggression, slurred speech, incoordination, unsteady gait, nystagmus, impairment in attention, memory difficulties, stupor	
Cannabis	Conjunctival injection, pupil constriction, increased appetite, dry mouth, tachycardia, euphoria, paranoia, anxiety, impaired motor coordination, social withdrawal, impaired short-term memory, nausea, vomiting	Antipsychotic medications for severe psychosis.
Phencyclidine/ hallucinogens	Hypertension, tachycardia, horizontal nystagmus, disconjugate gaze, ataxia, diminished pain response, dysarthria, muscle stiffness, hallucinations, delusions, disorientation, seizures, hyperacusis	Benzodiazepines, antihistamines, antihypertensives, and antipsychotics.
Opioids	Euphoria, respiratory depression, drowsiness, slurred speech, impaired attention and memory, miosis, psychomotor retardation	Naloxone to reverse severe respiratory depression. Repeat every 3 minutes until respiratory depression is reversed.
Inhalents	Dizziness, euphoria, ataxia, confusion, tremor, slurred speech, lethargy, incoordination, tachycardia, arrhythmia, wheezing, dyspnea	
Sedative/ hypnotic	Mood lability, aggression, slurred speech, incoordination, unsteady gait, nystagmus, impairment in attention, memory difficulties, stupor	Flumazenil for acute benzodiazepine intoxication.
Stimulants	Euphoria, anxiety, tics, increased sociability, tachycardia, pupillary dilation, hypertension, nausea, vomiting, sweating, chills, psychomotor agitation, confusion, arrhythmias, hallucinations	Antihypertensives, benzodiazepines, and antipsychotics.

CONQUER THE WARDS!

Use the Clinical Institute Withdrawal Assessment (CIWA) tool to monitor alcohol withdrawal severity. CIWA components include rating nausea/vomiting, tremor, sweating, anxiety, agitation, tactile disturbances, auditory disturbances, visual disturbances, headache, and orientation.

Use the Clinical Opiate Withdrawal Scale (COWS) to monitor for opiate withdrawal severity. COWS components include rating heart rate, sweating, restlessness, pupil size, muscle/joint aches, runny nose or tearing, GI distress, tremor, yawning, anxiety, and gooseflesh skin.

CHAPTER 13 GASTROENTEROLOGY AND HEPATOLOGY

OVERVIEW OF HIGH-YIELD TOPICS IN GASTROENTEROLOGY AND HEPATOLOGY

VASCULAR PROBLEMS OF THE ABDOMEN

ABDOMINAL AORTIC ANEURYSM

General Facts

- Abdominal aortic aneurysms (AAAs) are the most common site of atherosclerotic aneurysms and most commonly affect men.
- Dilation of the abdominal aorta usually involves the infrarenal arteries.
- It is important to identify AAA, as they can leak or rupture, resulting in a life-threatening emergency.

Clinical Features

- Usually asymptomatic unless there is a leak or rupture.
- If ruptured:
  - Hypotension.
  - Abdominal or back pain.
- **Risk factors:**
  - Smoking.
  - History of atherosclerosis.
  - Abdominal trauma.
  - Size >5 cm associated with 20% to 40% 5-year risk of rupture.

Physical Exam Findings

- Vitals: If ruptured, you may see hypotension and tachycardia.
- Abdominal exam: Pulsatile mass in the abdomen (easier to identify in thinner patients).

Diagnostic Workup

Diagnosis is based on imaging. Preferred imaging modalities depend on whether you are screening for an AAA in a patient with risk factors or pursuing a diagnosis of a ruptured AAA for someone who is acutely ill.

- **Angiogram is the gold standard** for the diagnosis of AAA. But often, it is easier and more practical to obtain **magnetic resonance imaging (MRI) or computed tomography (CT) with intravenous (IV) contrast** as the initial test if you are worried about a ruptured AAA.
- **Abdominal ultrasound:**
  - All men between the ages of 65 and 75 who have ever smoked should get a one-time screening with an abdominal ultrasound. This is the preferred initial modality, given its lower cost.
  - If the AAA appears large or complicated, then an angiogram or cross-sectional imaging test, as mentioned earlier, can be performed to further characterize the AAA and assist with preoperative planning.

Management

- **Ruptured AAA:**
  - Emergent surgical consultation for possible repair.
  - IV access and type and screen so that blood transfusions and fluids can be given quickly to prevent hemorrhagic shock from blood loss.
- **Medical management:**
  - **Asymptomatic patients with AAA <5.5 cm** can be managed conservatively with medical management.
  - This is aimed at the risk factors mentioned earlier. Controlling hyper-

tension, smoking cessation, and treating coronary artery disease are the mainstays of medical management.
- Ultrasound every 6 to 12 months for surveillance should be performed to ensure the AAA is not growing rapidly, as this is a risk factor for rupture.

- **Surgical management:**
  For the following patients because of high risk for rupture:
  - **AAA diameter >5.5 cm.**
  - Rapidly progressive (>0.5 cm growth in 6 months or 1 cm in a year).
  - Symptomatic (abdominal pain or limb ischemia, which can result in claudication).

ACUTE MESENTERIC ISCHEMIA

General Facts

- Mesenteric ischemia occurs when there is interruption of intestinal blood flow to the intestinal blood supply.
- Ischemia of the superior mesenteric artery (SMA) affects the jejunum, ileum, and right colon, while the inferior mesenteric artery (IMA) affects the left colon and rectum.
- There are 2 types of mesenteric ischemia: acute and chronic.
  1. **Acute mesenteric ischemia** results from an abrupt interruption of the blood supply, usually from an embolus or in the setting of thrombus, and is a surgical emergency.
  2. **Chronic mesenteric ischemia** results from slow narrowing of vessels due to atherosclerosis and results in episodic, postprandial symptoms, often in the setting of weight loss, which are not life threatening. The focus for the remainder of this section will be on acute mesenteric ischemia.

Clinical Features

Patients with acute mesenteric ischemia usually present with acute onset of abdominal pain, nausea, vomiting, and sometimes rectal bleeding. The following are risk factors for acute mesenteric ischemia and should raise suspicion of this diagnosis in any patient:

- Atherosclerosis.
- Hypertension.
- Diabetes.
- Atrial fibrillation (can lead to embolic obstruction of the artery).
- Hypotension.
- Heart failure, which leads to a low-flow state.
- Hypercoagulability.

Physical Exam Findings

- **Severe abdominal pain out of proportion to the exam** is the hallmark of acute mesenteric ischemia. The patient may be screaming in pain but their abdomen is soft without peritoneal signs.
- **Rectal exam**: May see rectal bleeding, though this isn't always the case.

Diagnostic Workup

- **Elevated lactic acid:** Laboratory workup may show a metabolic acidosis from an elevated lactic acid level.

- **Imaging** must be done to confirm the diagnosis. A **CT angiography (CTA) of the abdomen** should be obtained if acute mesenteric ischemia is suspected. Like many vascular problems, conventional angiography is the gold standard if cross-sectional imaging is not diagnostic.

Management

Acute mesenteric ischemia is a life-threatening emergency, and the goal of treatment is to restore blood flow to the intestines before ischemia leads to necrosis of the bowel. Emergent surgery consult should be obtained for revascularization. Occasionally, anticoagulation may be started and the patient observed if they are a poor surgical candidate or are clinically stable.

ESOPHAGEAL DISORDERS

ESOPHAGEAL DYSPHAGIA

General Facts

- Dysphagia can be either **oropharyngeal** or **esophageal**.
- **Esophageal dysphagia** usually occurs due to either a **structural pathology** or from a **motility disorder**. This is opposed to **oropharyngeal dysphagia**, which occurs in the setting of oral intake and results from the inability to transfer a food bolus from the oropharynx to the esophagus. Oropharyngeal dysphagia is often from a structural problem or neuromuscular etiology (such as stroke).
- Two common motility disorders you may encounter include **achalasia**, a neurogenic disorder with impaired relaxation of the lower esophageal sphincter (so food can't get through), and **diffuse esophageal spasm**, which results from frequent nonperistaltic contractions (often causes chest discomfort).
- Esophageal dysphagia will be the focus of the remainder of this section. The most common causes are listed below in table 13-1.

Table 13-1. Common Causes of Dysphagia

Oropharyngeal Dysphagia	Esophageal Dysphagia
Neurologic pathology	Peptic stricture
Stroke	Severe GERD
Parkinson disease	Esophageal cancer
ALS and myasthenia gravis	Eosinophilic esophagitis
Zenker diverticulum	Motility disorder
Head and neck cancer	Achalasia
Cervical web	Diffuse esophageal spasm
	Scleroderma
	Zenker diverticulum

ALS, amyotrophic lateral sclerosis; *GERD*, gastroesophageal reflux disease.

Clinical Features

- Progressive esophageal dysphagia that worsens over time is suggestive of a **structural pathology**, and the most worrisome etiology is a tumor (adenocarcinoma or squamous cell carcinoma), especially in the setting of weight loss. Esophageal webs and Schatzki rings are other common noncancerous etiologies.
- **Intermittent dysphagia** to both solids and liquids suggests a **motility disorder**, such as achalasia or diffuse esophageal spasm.
- Patients may also complain of chest pain, nausea, vomiting, and/or weight loss.

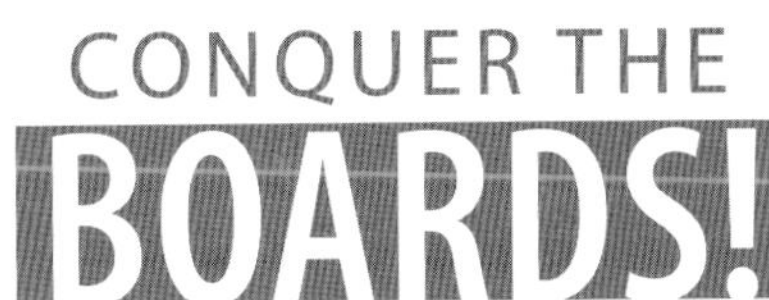

Dysphagia, esophageal webs, and iron deficiency anemia → *Think: Plummer–Vinson syndrome!*

Diagnostic Workup

- **Upper endoscopy:** This is the first test in the workup for dysphagia because it allows direct visualization of the esophagus and allows a gastroenterologist to obtain biopsies of tissue if a cancer is found.
- **Barium esophagram** is also a common test that can be performed in order to provide a roadmap of esophageal anatomy and can also provide limited motility information. This may be a preferred test if the patient is unable to undergo endoscopic evaluation based on their preference or clinical stability (See Figure 13-1 and 13-2).
- **Esophageal manometry** is performed for patients that have a suspected motility disorder.

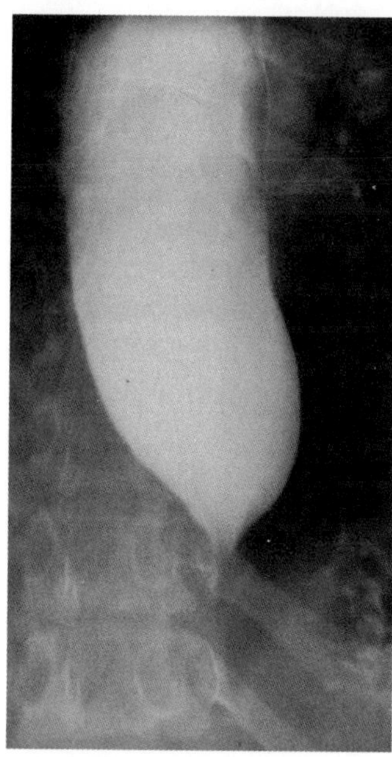

FIGURE 13-1. Barium esophagram in a patient with achalasia demonstrating a dilated esophagus with a sharply tapered "bird's beak" narrowing.

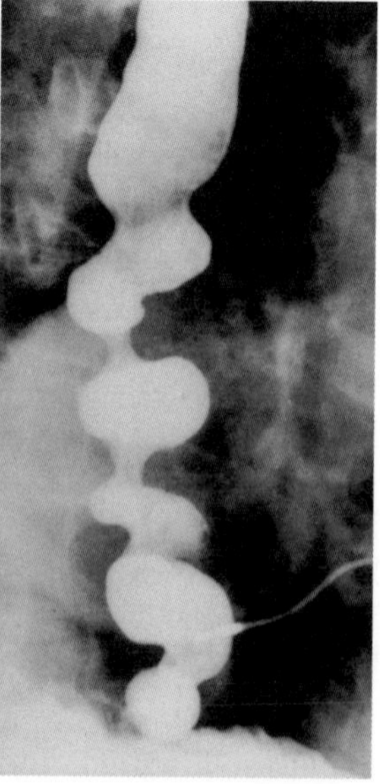

FIGURE 13-2. Barium esophagram in a patient with diffuse esophageal spasm demonstrating the characteristic "corkscrew" pattern.

Management

Management is aimed at the underlying pathology.

- **Esophageal strictures** can be dilated endoscopically by a gastroenterologist.
- **Cancers** can be treated accordingly through chemotherapy, radiation, or surgery.
- **Achalasia**: Has a variety of management options, including endoscopic dilation or botulinum toxin injection, as well as endoscopic and surgical myotomy.
- **Diffuse esophageal spasm** is often treated with calcium channel blockers (diltiazem) or peppermint oil.
- **Zenker diverticulum**: Outpouching due to a defect in the muscular wall of the posterior hypopharynx. In addition to dysphagia (oropharyngeal or esophageal), halitosis, regurgitation, and aspiration can occur. Diagnosis is seen on barium swallow, and management is surgical cricopharyngeal myotomy.

Common Question on Rounds

What is the difference between dysphagia and odynophagia?

Dysphagia is a sensation of food being "stuck," while odynophagia is pain with swallowing.

ESOPHAGITIS

General Facts

- Esophagitis is inflammation of the esophagus. There are a variety of causes, which correspond to certain patient risk factors.
- Odynophagia, or painful swallowing, is often seen with infectious causes of esophagitis. This is in contrast to the symptom of dysphagia mentioned earlier, which is a feeling of food or liquid getting "stuck" in the throat.
- **Common Differential Diagnosis of Esophagitis:**
  - Infectious (cytomegalovirus [CMV], herpes simplex virus [HSV], *Candida* most commonly), especially in immunosuppressed patients (patients with HIV or receiving chemotherapy).
  - Acid reflux.
  - Eosinophilic esophagitis.
  - Radiation.

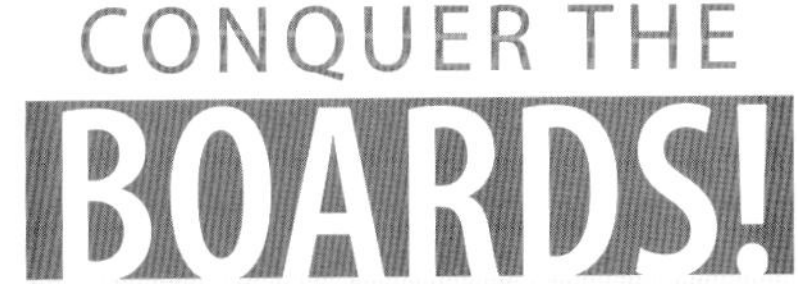

A young male with asthma who presents with a food impaction → *Think: Eosinophilic esophagitis!*

Clinical Features

- Odynophagia, often with infectious causes or radiation.
- Dysphagia.
- Chest pain.
- Anemia or overt gastrointestinal (GI) bleeding if severe.
- May be asymptomatic.

Physical Exam Findings

If you suspect a patient has esophagitis, it is extremely important to closely examine the mouth, as oral thrush is highly suggestive of *Candida*-related esophagitis. You may see melena on the rectal exam in severe cases.

CONQUER THE WARDS!

Dysphagia or odynophagia with oral thrush? Treat for *Candida*. No need for an endoscopy if patients improve!

Diagnostic Workup

- **Upper endoscopy** is the gold standard because it allows direct visualization of the esophagus and allows a gastroenterologist to obtain biopsies of tissue and ulcers.
  - CMV and HSV cause ulcers, and viral inclusions will be seen on biopsies.
  - *Candida*-related esophagitis is demonstrated by white plaques with yeast or pseudohyphae on biopsy.
  - Eosinophilic esophagitis will demonstrate an increased number of eosinophils (>15 per high power field) in the distal and proximal esophagus on biopsy.
- **Barium esophagram** is also a common test performed, but this will not provide a specific diagnosis.

Management

Management is aimed at the underlying pathology.

- HSV and CMV: Acyclovir or ganciclovir.
- *Candida* esophagitis: Fluconazole.
- Reflux esophagitis: Acid suppression with proton pump inhibitors are used for reflux esophagitis.
- Eosinophilic esophagitis: Proton pump inhibitors are also first-line treatment along with topical steroids and dietary modification for patients that do not respond.
- Radiation esophagitis: There is no direct treatment for this, and treatment focuses on symptom control. Swallowed viscous lidocaine can be used to ameliorate the symptoms of odynophagia. It can also be used in any of the other causes of esophagitis.

ESOPHAGEAL RUPTURE

General Facts

Esophageal perforation or rupture can be related to esophagitis, but it is a separate pathology that is a medical emergency.

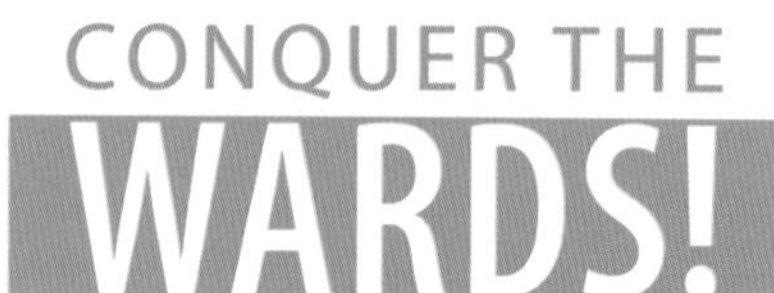

Patients who have repeated episodes of nonbloody emesis who suddenly develop hematemesis → *Think: Mallory–Weiss tear!*

- **Differential Diagnosis of Esophageal Perforation:**
  - Boerhaave syndrome (full-thickness tear; its precursor can be a Mallory–Weiss tear, which is a *partial*-thickness tear).
  - Iatrogenic trauma (during endoscopy, esophageal dilation, tube placement).
  - Foreign body or food impaction.

Clinical Features

- Severe chest pain.
- Dyspnea.
- Inability to tolerate secretions, spitting up saliva (seen in food impaction).

Physical Exam Findings

- **Subcutaneous emphysema**: You can palpate the skin of the anterior upper body and feel the trapped air underneath the skin.
- **Hammon crunch** is a "crunching sound" auscultated in the precordium suggesting mediastinal emphysema. This is rarely seen but often asked on rounds.
- **Decreased breath sounds** at the bases or dullness to percussion suggesting a pleural effusion.

Diagnostic Workup

Chest x-ray (CXR) is often obtained first and can reveal nonspecific findings of pleural effusion, mediastinal widening, subcutaneous emphysema, or hydropneumothorax. However, to definitively diagnose an esophageal leak, you should obtain a **contrast esophagram or CT of the chest with oral contrast**. A water-soluble contrast agent should be used instead of barium, because barium can cause an inflammatory reaction if it leaks out and contacts the pleura. If a pleural effusion is sampled, a **high amylase level** is suggestive of an esophageal perforation.

Management

- Management is aimed at closure of the perforation, which can be done surgically or sometimes endoscopically.
- Antibiotics should be used for 1 to 2 weeks (piperacillin and tazobactam cover most enteric gram-negative and anaerobic organisms) and monitored closely.
- Patients with food impactions should receive an emergent endoscopy to remove the food bolus in order to prevent an esophageal perforation from happening.

Common Question on Rounds

What is the difference between a Mallory–Weiss tear and Boerhaave syndrome?
A Mallory–Weiss tear is a partial-thickness esophageal tear, while Boerhaave syndrome refers to a full-thickness perforation.

GASTROESOPHAGEAL REFLUX DISEASE

General Facts

- GERD is the reflux of acidic gastric contents into the esophagus. The primary mechanism that allows this to happen is relaxation of the lower esophageal sphincter.
- **Risk factors** for GERD are:
  - Hiatal hernia.
  - Delayed gastric emptying or gastroparesis.
  - Alcohol.
  - Cigarette smoking.
  - Coffee.
  - Chocolate.
  - Hormones (estrogen, progesterone).
  - Central obesity.

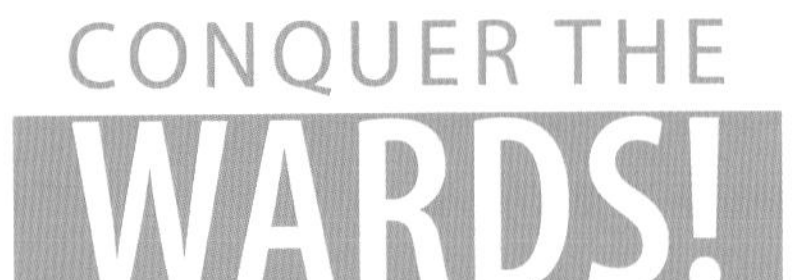

The 3 most common cause of chronic (often nocturnal) cough are GERD, asthma, and postnasal drip.

Clinical Features

- Substernal burning pain.
- Dysphagia (if peptic stricture develops).
- Sour taste in mouth (water brash).
- Cough.
- Hoarseness.

Diagnostic Workup

- Often, no diagnostic workup is required, and patients can undergo lifestyle modification or be started on a trial of proton pump inhibitors (PPIs) to see if symptoms resolve.
- If any alarm symptoms are present (nonresponse to PPI, weight loss, new onset in older patient, anemia, overt GI bleeding), an endoscopy should be performed to rule out other pathologies such as ulcers or cancer.

Management

- **Lifestyle modification** is the first-line treatment. This includes elevating the head of the bed, discontinuing foods that may decrease lower esophageal tone, weight loss if indicated, and avoiding meals and snacks less than 3 hours before bed.
- **Primary pharmacologic management** if lifestyle modifications don't work within 8 weeks includes H2 blocker or PPI. In general, a "step-up" approach to secretory inhibition can be utilized, using H2 blockers as first-line and transition to PPI if breakthrough symptoms continue to occur. Use the lowest dosages, up to twice daily, that control symptoms.
- **Nonresponders:** Patients who do not respond to high-dose PPI therapy within 6 to 8 weeks or obese men over age 50 (risk factor for Barrett esophagus) may be considered for endoscopy (EGD) for evaluation of any structural pathology. Surgical correction with Nissen fundoplication can be considered in certain patients who fail pharmacotherapy.

Complications

Complications of GERD include:

- **Esophagitis** due to prolonged exposure of the distal esophagus to gastric contents.
- **Peptic strictures** (approximately 10% of patients).
- **Barrett esophagus** can occur in long-standing reflux, especially in males with central obesity. This is a transformation of the normal squamous epithelium of the lower esophagus to columnar epithelium, which resembles the stomach lining. This mucosal change can be precancerous and requires close surveillance endoscopies by a gastroenterologist. Therefore, esophageal adenocarcinoma is another rare complication.

CONQUER THE WARDS!

Esophageal cancer? Upper two-thirds of the esophagus: usually squamous. Lower third: usually adenocarcinoma.

Common Question on Rounds

Is there any literature suggesting complications of chronic PPI use in certain patients?

Chronic PPI use has been associated with:

- *Clostridium difficile* infection.
- Hypomagnesemia.
- Renal insufficiency.

Bone fractures, dementia, and pneumonia have been linked to chronic PPI use, but more robust studies are needed to determine causality.

In general, PPIs should be used at the lowest dose and shortest duration needed to minimize these potential risks.

DISORDERS OF THE STOMACH

PEPTIC ULCER DISEASE

General Facts

- Peptic ulcer disease (PUD) consists of **gastric ulcers (GUs)** and **duodenal ulcers (DUs)**.
- **Gastritis** refers to nonspecific acute or chronic inflammation of the stomach lining and is a histologic diagnosis, meaning it is seen on biopsy.
- A brief review of gastric physiology will aid in better understanding the risk factors for the development of PUD.
  - Gastrin is made by G cells in the antrum of the stomach, and this stimulates the parietal cells to secrete **hydrochloric acid** into the gastric lumen via a proton pump (parietal cells are also stimulated by histamine and acetylcholine).
  - Gastrin also stimulates secretion of **bicarbonate** into the protective mucous gel that lines the stomach. Bicarbonate secretion is conversely inhibited by nonsteroidal antiinflammatory drugs (NSAIDs) and alcohol. The mucosal gel layer is promoted by prostaglandin E and impaired by NSAIDs and steroids.
- **Risk factors:**
  - *Helicobacter pylori* infection (produces urease, breaking down the gastric mucosal layer).
  - NSAID use (inhibits production of prostaglandin, which helps produce the mucosal barrier of the stomach).
  - Older age.
  - Cigarette smoking.
  - Alcohol, which inhibits bicarbonate secretion.

Clinical Features

- Burning, gnawing, epigastric pain.
- There is a classic teaching that GU pain is exacerbated by food, while DU pain is typically relieved by food. However, this is frequently not the case in patients.
- Iron-deficiency anemia.
- GI bleeding possible (melena or hematochezia/hematemesis if brisk bleeding).
- Gastric outlet obstruction (can occur if ulcers are near the pylorus).

Diagnostic Workup

- **Endoscopy:** PUD can only be diagnosed via upper endoscopy. Biopsies should be performed to test for *H. pylori* infection, and patients should be treated if they test positive. It is important to note that *H. pylori* infection is common in the general population and infection doesn't always lead to PUD.
- Diagnosing *H. pylori* can be done via the following:
  - Urea breath test: Radiolabeled urea is given orally, and *H. pylori* break it down to produce CO_2 and ammonia. The CO_2 can be detected in breath samples. False positives are uncommon, but false negatives can be seen in patients taking PPIs, so they should be stopped before the test.

- Stool antigen: Possibly the most cost-effective option, with similar sensitivity and specificity as breath testing. PPIs should be discontinued for 2 weeks prior to testing to prevent false-negative results.
- Endoscopic biopsy: During an EGD, biopsies of the stomach mucosa can be sent to test for *H. pylori*.
- Serology: Serologies for *H. pylori* do little to distinguish prior vs. active infection and have limited utility in practice and are therefore not generally recommended.

Management

Treatment depends on the risk factors or cause.

- **PPI:** All patients benefit from a PPI, and it should be continued for at least 6 weeks.
- ***H. pylori* infection:** Patients with *H. pylori* infection should be treated with quadruple therapy (e.g., PPI, amoxicillin, tetracycline, bismuth). Triple therapy with amoxicillin, clarithromycin, and PPI used to be the gold standard, but given the high rates of clarithromycin resistance in the population, quadruple therapy is now recommended as first-line.
- **Lifestyle modifications:** Patients should be counseled on smoking cessation and alcohol cessation and to avoid NSAIDs.
- **Follow-up EGD:** Should be performed after a 4- to 6-week course of PPI therapy in most patients with GUs. If ulcers do not resolve, repeat biopsies should be done.

Complications

The 2 major complications of PUD are:

- **Bleeding** (20% incidence): Bleeding will be evident by melena, or if brisk bleeding is occurring, it can manifest as hematochezia or hematemesis (see later section on GI bleeding).

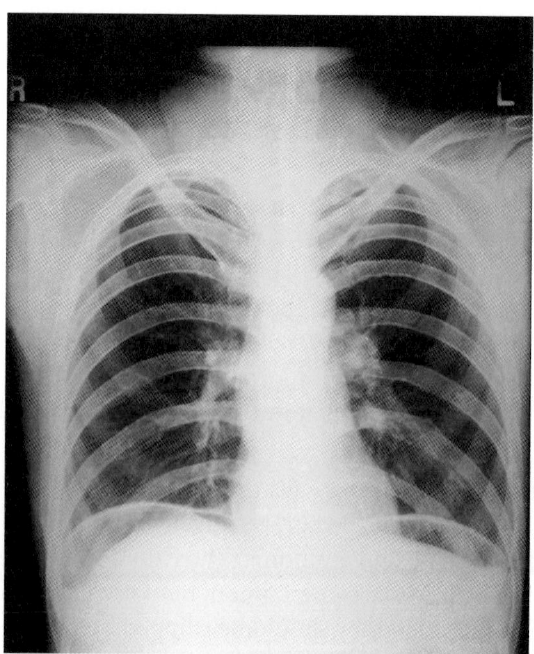

FIGURE 13-3. Upright chest film in a patient with a perforated duodenal ulcer, showing free air underneath both hemidiaphragms.

- **Perforation** (7% incidence): Perforation can occur if the ulcer erodes through the serosal layer and is manifested by severe abdominal pain, free air on x-ray, and peritoneal signs (guarding and rebound tenderness). A caveat to this is if an ulcer perforates the posterior duodenum, it may not result in free air because the duodenum is retroperitoneal. Any perforated PU is a surgical emergency.

Complications of chronic gastritis: Chronic gastritis can lead to atrophy of the parietal cells, leading to a decreased production of intrinsic factor and subsequent malabsorption of vitamin B_{12}. This is called pernicious anemia. Chronic gastritis can also lead to intestinal metaplasia of the gastric mucosa, which can be a precursor to gastric cancer.

Other Causes of PUD

Zollinger–Ellison Syndrome (ZES) or Gastrinoma

- This is a gastrin-secreting neuroendocrine tumor in or near the pancreas.
- The **triad of PUD, gastric acid hypersecretion, and a highly elevated gastrin level** (>1000 pg/mL) can confirm the diagnosis.
- Diarrhea is the most common initial presenting symptom.
- Diagnosis can be performed with a **secretin stimulation test**. Normally , secretin will inhibit G-cell release of gastrin, leading to a decrease in gastrin levels. However, in a patient with a gastrinoma, secretin paradoxically stimulates gastrin release, leading to a rise in serum gastrin.

CONQUER THE BOARDS!

ZES is associated with multiple endocrine neoplasia type 1 (MEN1). All patients should be screened for hyperparathyroidism with a parathyroid hormone (PTH) level.

Gastric Cancer

- A repeat endoscopy should be performed after a 4- to 6-week course of PPI therapy in most patients with GUs.
- Ulcers that do not resolve with acid suppression or treatment of *H. pylori* should be biopsied again to ensure they are not cancerous (adenocarcinoma or lymphoma).

DISORDERS OF THE PANCREAS

ACUTE PANCREATITIS

General Facts

- Acute pancreatitis is inflammation of the pancreas due to parenchymal autodigestion of proteolytic enzymes. In more severe cases, this is associated with systemic inflammatory response syndrome (SIRS), which can progress to multiorgan failure and acute respiratory distress syndrome.
- There are several different etiologies of acute pancreatitis, but by far the most common are alcohol and gallstones.
- **Etiologies of acute pancreatitis:**
  - Gallstones.
  - Alcohol.
  - Less common etiologies:
    - Drugs: Thiazides, azathioprine, antiretrovirals, estrogen, angiotensin-converting enzyme (ACE) inhibitors.
    - Hypertriglyceridemia.
    - Autoimmune.
    - Neoplasm.

- Complication of endoscopic retrograde cholangiopancreatography (ERCP).
- Idiopathic.

Clinical Features

- **Classic (typical) symptoms:**
  - Severe epigastric pain that radiates to the back.
  - Improved when sitting up and leaning forward.
  - Worsened with meals.
- Nausea and vomiting.
- Low-grade fever.
- **Physical exam:**
  - Epigastric or upper quadrant tenderness that radiates to back, guarding but no rebound.
  - **Pulmonary exam**: May hear decreased breath sounds at the bases or dullness to percussion suggesting a pleural effusion in severe pancreatitis.
  - **Skin exam**: Grey–Turner sign (bruising of the flank) and Cullen sign (periumbilical bruising) suggest hemorrhagic pancreatitis.

Diagnostic Workup

- To diagnose acute pancreatitis, you need to meet 2 of the following 3 criteria:
  - Typical associated abdominal pain.
  - Serum lipase value greater than 2 to 3 times the upper limit of normal. Amylase is commonly sent but is not necessary, as lipase is more specific for pancreatitis.
  - Radiographic findings (typically CT with contrast) of pancreatitc inflammation.
- **Imaging:** Imaging is not necessary to diagnose acute pancreatitis, but imaging to rule out causes is often done. **An abdominal ultrasound** is generally performed to assess for gallstones as a risk factor, especially when liver enzymes are elevated. **A CT scan** can be performed if patients do not improve after a few days or clinical status worsens to look for pancreatic necrosis, which would then possibly require surgical intervention.
- **Serum IgG4 level:** If no clear etiology is found and autoimmune pancreatitis is in the differential, you can send for a serum IgG4 level, but it is not routinely sent on initial presentations.
- There are several severity scores for pancreatitis mortality, all of which utilize various demographic and laboratory data and have online calculators. Well-known scoring systems include the Ranson criteria, Bedside Index for Severity in Acute Pancreatitis (BISAP) and Acute Physiology and Chronic Health Evaluation II (APACHE II) score.

Management

IV hydration: The hallmark of treatment is IV hydration. This is incredibly important, and patients should get a bolus of several liters of IV fluid at diagnosis and be continued on a high rate of maintenance fluids during the first 24 to 48 hours of diagnosis.

CONQUER THE WARDS!

The most reliable marker of pancreatitis mortality is blood urea nitrogen (BUN). It should trend downward with appropriate fluid management.

- **Nutritional status:** Another important concept is optimizing nutritional status. Classic teaching had kept patients nothing by mouth (NPO) for days until their pain completely resolved, and their diet was advanced very slowly from clear liquids to solid foods. Now, we know that patients with mild pancreatitis should be started on a low-fat diet (fat may stimulate the pancreas to work harder) as soon as they have an appetite. Patients who are critically ill from pancreatitis should have a nasogastric tube placed and started on enteral nutrition once stabilized.

- **Antibiotics are not indicated** for most patients with acute pancreatitis and are only used for complications of the disease, including infected necrosis (more on this later).

Complications

Pseudocyst:

- Pancreatic pseudocysts are encapsulated collections of fluid that can form adjacent to the pancreas several weeks after an episode of acute pancreatitis.
- These are often incidentally seen on imaging.
- They do not need any specific treatment unless they are large and symptomatic (abdominal pain, or causing obstructive symptoms such as nausea and early satiety, in which case they can be drained via interventional radiology or surgery).

Walled-off necrosis:

- Necrotizing pancreatitis can leave behind a collection of necrotic material that can become infected. When this happens, the patient will usually develop a new fever or worsening leukocytosis several days after presentation, which should prompt you to start antibiotics (usually a carbapenem, given its ability to penetrate the pancreas) and get a CT scan with IV contrast.
- These necrotic collections can become encapsulated, which is called walled-off necrosis. The treatment for this is necrosectomy, or debridement, which can be performed by skilled endoscopists or surgeons.

Splenic vein thrombosis:

- A general rule of thumb is that any significant visceral inflammation that is near a vein can lead to thrombosis. As such, sometimes patients with pancreatitis can develop splenic vein thromboses.
- These can lead to the formation of gastric varices, but not esophageal varices.
- No specific treatment is generally indicated for isolated splenic vein thrombosis.

Ileus:

- Just like local inflammation, this can result in thrombosis; it can also cause dysmotility of the nearby small bowel loops and result in an ileus.
- Abdominal x-ray will show a "sentinel loop," which is a distended small bowel loop. There also may be an air–fluid level on x-ray.

Common Question on Rounds

When should we consider feeding the patient with acute pancreatitis?
As soon as the patient has an appetite and pain is controlled.

HIGH-YIELD LITERATURE

Lactated Ringer's is the fluid of choice in acute pancreatitis:

Wu BU, Hwang, JQ, Gardner TH, et al. Lactated Ringer's solution reduces systemic inflammation compared with saline in patients with acute pancreatitis. *Clin Gastroenterol Hepatol*. 2011;9(8):710.

Blood urea nitrogen predicts mortality:
Wu BU, Johannes RS, Sun X, et al. Early changes in blood urea nitrogen predict mortality in acute pancreatitis. *Gastroenterology*. 2009;137(1):129.

CHRONIC PANCREATITIS

General Facts

- After repeated insults to the pancreas, such as in acute pancreatitis, the inflammation over time can cause scarring and pancreatic duct obstruction, which leads to chronic pancreatitis.
- Unlike acute pancreatitis, chronic pancreatitis may have a subclinical course where it goes unnoticed until the disease progresses.
- Though both acute and chronic pancreatitis can cause abdominal pain, chronic pancreatitis can lead to malabsorption because the exocrine function of the pancreas is impaired.
- **Common causes of chronic pancreatitis:**
  - Alcohol abuse (70% to 80%) is the most common cause.
  - Hereditary pancreatitis.
  - Cystic fibrosis.

Clinical Features

- Severe epigastric pain that radiates to the back, worsens with meals.
- Steatorrhea (*exocrine* dysfunction leads to malabsorption).
- Hyperglycemia (*endocrine* dysfunction in severe cases).

Diagnostic Workup

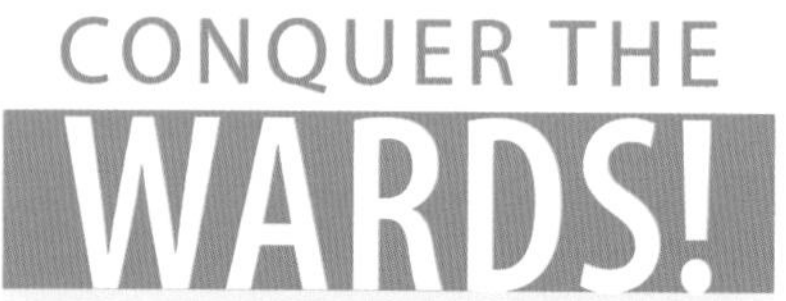

MRCP = imaging test great for visualizing the bile and pancreatic ducts

ERCP = endoscopic procedure that allows therapeutic interventions but may be a more invasive way to get similar diagnostic information

- **CT scan** is usually the first imaging done in the workup. If pancreatic calcifications are seen on imaging, the diagnosis is confirmed.
- **Magnetic reasonance choalngiopancreatography (MRCP)** will often be done after CT scan or in conjunction with a CT scan. It allows for better visualization of the pancreatic ducts and can also be performed with secretin administration to evaluate pancreatic exocrine function.
- **ERCP** is another option if imaging is inconclusive. **An ERCP** is an endoscope inserted through the mouth into the duodenum. A smaller scope is then inserted through the ampulla of Vater of the common bile duct, allowing visualization (by injecting dye) of the pancreatic duct, hepatic duct, common bile duct, duodenal papilla, and gallbladder. ERCP can be interventional as well as diagnostic. Stones can be removed from the bile or pancreatic ducts, obstructed ducts can be stented, and biopsies can be performed.
- **Other tests:**
  - **Stool tests** like elevated fecal fat or low fecal elastase can help support the diagnosis.
  - **Hemoglobin A_{1C}**, as patients may suffer from diabetes due to loss of the pancreas's ability to produce and release insulin.
  - **Vitamin levels**: Without the pancreas releasing digestive enzymes, patients develop fat-soluable vitamin malabsoprtion (vitamins A, D, E, K).

Management

- **Lifestyle modifications:** Patients should abstain from alcohol and cigarette smoking and minimize intake of fatty foods.
- **Pancreatic enzyme supplements:** Patients with malabsorption should be started on pancreatic enzyme supplements. There is also some evidence that enzyme replacement may help with pain symptoms.
- **Surgery:** Gastroenterologists can perform certain maneuvers through ERCP or endoscopic ultrasound (EUS) for advanced management. Surgery is usually reserved for refractory symptoms.

DISORDERS OF THE LIVER

ACUTE PANCREATITIS

General Facts

- The liver has many important functions, including:
  - Glucose homeostasis.
  - Urea cycle.
  - Vitamin storage.
  - Detoxification of many endogenous and exogenous substances.
  - Synthesis of plasma proteins, bile acids, coagulation factors, and lipids.
- Liver function tests (LFTs) are a group of laboratory tests that generally comprise the aspartate aminotransferase (AST), alanine aminotransferase (ALT), bilirubin, alkaline phosphatase, and gamma-glutamyl transferase (GGT). In actuality, these tests are not reliable predictors of liver function but are more representative of injury patterns.
- More accurate assessments for liver *function* can be inferred from the **prothrombin time** (elevated in dysfunction from impaired synthesis of coagulation factors) and **albumin** (decreased in poor function as the liver synthesizes this).
- The major types of liver injury are outlined here and in Table 13-2:
  - **Hepatocellular injury** is transaminase-predominant and suggests injury to the liver parenchyma.

Table 13-2. Liver Injury Patterns

Test	Hepatocellular Injury	Cholestatic Injury	Mixed Injury
AST/ALT	↑↑↑	Slightly elevated↑	↑ or ↑↑
Alkaline Phosphatase	↑	↑Very elevated↑	↑ or ↑↑
Bilirubin	↑	↑↑Normal to very elevated	↑ or ↑↑
		Variably elevated	
GGT	↑	↑Very elevated	↑ or ↑↑
Differential Diagnosis	Viral hepatitis Ischemia Wilson disease Autoimmune hepatitis Nonalcoholic steatohepatitis (NASH) Drug induced	Acute cholangitis Primary biliary cirrhosis (PBC) Primary sclerosing cholangitis (PSC) Infiltrative processes (cancer, amyloid) Drug induced	Viral hepatitis Autoimmune hepatitis Alcoholic hepatitis Drug induced

ALT, alanine transaminase; *AST*, aspartate transaminase; *GGT*, gamma-glutamyl transpeptidase.

- **Cholestatic injury** is predominately alkaline phosphatase with conjugated hyperbilirubinemia and suggests obstruction, as seen in choledocholithiasis, primary sclerosing cholangitis (PSC), and primary biliary cirrhosis (PBC).

- **Higher indirect to direct bilirubin ratio:** The differential would include hemolysis or Gilbert syndrome (harmless, common defect in bilirubin conjugation).
- **High alkaline phosphatase** is nonspecific and elevated in bone disease and pregnancy. An elevated **GGT** helps point toward the liver being the source of a patient's elevated alkaline phosphatase.

ACUTE LIVER FAILURE

General Facts

- Acute liver failure is diagnosed in patients with the following:
  - Acute hepatocellular injury.
  - Coagulopathy (international normalized ratio [INR] >1.5).
  - Encephalopathy in the absence of preexisting liver disease or cirrhosis.
- Besides encephalopathy, patients will complain of change in skin, urine, and stool color due to the increase in bilirubin.

Differential Diagnosis

The differential diagnosis for acute liver failure is broad; common etiologies include:

- Acetaminophen overdose (most common in the United States).
- Viral hepatitis.
- Drug induced (other than acetaminophen) – worldwide, antibiotics are the most common cause.
- Alcoholic hepatitis.
- Autoimmune hepatitis.
- Wilson disease.
- Hepatic ischemia: This is usually due to hypoperfusion from another underlying condition such as septic shock, cardiogenic shock, or hypovolemic shock.
- Budd–Chiari (see later).
- Acute fatty liver of pregnancy.

Diagnostic Workup

- **Thorough history:** All patients with acute liver failure should have a thorough history focusing on any medications, drugs, or risk factors for hepatitis A, B, C, and D.
- **Laboratory tests:** All patients should receive a laboratory workup for the common liver diseases mentioned earlier:
  - Acetaminophen level.
  - Alcohol level.
  - Urine toxicology.
  - Viral hepatitis serologies:
    - A, B, C, and E
    - CMV, HSV, and Epstein–Barr virus (EBV) polymerase chain reaction (PCR)
  - Autoimmune workup:

    - Antinuclear antibodies (ANA).
    - Anti-smooth muscle antibodies (ASMA).
    - Immunoglobulin G (IgG) level.
  - Ceruloplasmin for Wilson disease.
  - Iron, ferritin, and total iron binding capacity (TIBC) for hemochromatosis.
- **Right upper quadrant (RUQ) ultrasound with Doppler** to look for clot and evaluate liver morphology.
- **Ammonia and phosphorous level:** Mortality in acute liver failure comes from cerebral edema, which correlates with the degree of encephalopathy. This is one of the few clinical circumstances where a serum ammonia level is useful and can be trended to correlate with the degree of cerebral edema. As the liver regenerates, phosphorus is used up, so patients that have low phosphorus levels can be an encouraging sign.

Management

- Treatment of acute liver failure includes reversing the underlying cause medically, if possible, or liver transplantation.
- Patients should be monitored in the liver transplant center, often in the intensive care unit (ICU) setting, with frequent neurologic checks.
- Vitamin K IV or subcutaneously can be given in an effort to reverse any nutritional component of INR elevation.
- For acetaminophen overdose, *N*-acetylcysteine is the antidote (IV drip over several hours) and should be started immediately if there is a concern for this, and sometimes is started while workup for causes continues.
- With regard to liver transplantation, if the patient is a transplant candidate, they are listed in the United Network for Organ Sharing (UNOS) as "Status 1A" and are placed at the top of the waiting list in their region.

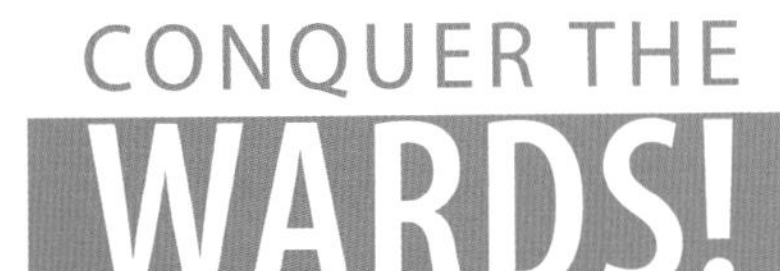

Acetaminophen overdose is a common cause of acute liver failure. Be sure to start *N*-acetylcysteine IV and refer to a transplant center.

Common Question on Rounds

What prognostic criteria are used to help identify patients who are likely to benefit from transplantation in acute liver failure (ALF)?

- King's College criteria is used in ALF to predict who needs referral for urgent transplantation. There are 2 sets of criteria: one for acetaminophen and one for nonacetaminophen ALF. Both include major and minor criteria. The major criteria for acetaminophen-induced ALF is an arterial pH <7.3. For nonacetaminophen ALF, the major criteria is an INR >6.5.

VIRAL HEPATITIS

General Facts

- Several viral infections can cause liver damage, but we will focus on the more common etiologies here, which are:
  - Hepatitis A, B, C, D, and E.
  - CMV.
  - HSV.
  - Varicella-zoster virus (VZV).
  - EBV.

Clinical Features

- RUQ pain.
- Nausea, vomiting, malaise, fever.
- Jaundice.
- Diarrhea (hepatitis A and E).

Physical Exam Findings

- Jaundice and conjunctival icterus.
- Posterior cervical lymphadenopathy.
- RUQ tenderness without rebound or guarding.
- Hepatomegaly.
- Splenomegaly.

HEPATITIS A/HEPATITIS E

General Facts

- Both are RNA viruses.
- Spread by fecal-oral route.
- Incubation period: 15 to 50 days.
- Hepatitis E virus can cause chronic hepatitis in immunocompromised patients and has a high rate of fulminant liver failure in pregnant patients.

Diagnostic Workup

- Anti–hepatitis A virus (HAV) or Anti–hepatitis E virus (HEV) IgM: Positive indicates acute infection.
- Anti-HAV IgG: Immunity from prior infection or vaccination.

Management

- Self-limited, supportive care.

Prevention

- Improved hygiene practices.
- If exposed to HAV: Can administer immunoglobulin.
- Give **HAV vaccination** to all patients with:
  - Chronic liver disease.
  - Travel to high-risk countries.
  - High-risk behaviors for transmission: Travel to areas with poor sanitation, contact with another person with hepatitis A, homosexual activity in men, exposure to daycare centers, and illicit drug use.

HEPATITIS B/HEPATITIS D

General Facts

- Hepatitis B is a DNA virus (the only one).
- Hepatitis D ("delta") is an RNA virus that requires coinfection with hepatitis B virus (HBV) for replication.
- HBV is spread by percutaneous or mucous membrane exposure to blood, semen, and saliva. hepatitis D virus (HDV) is spread as a coinfection (at the same time as HBV) or as a superinfection (in someone who was already infected with HBV).

- HBV and HDV coinfected patients have more severe disease.
- Incubation period: 45 to 160 days.
- Less than 10% of infected adults (but 90% of neonates) will develop chronic hepatitis.
- Infection carries a risk of developing hepatocellular carcinoma (HCC), even in noncirrhotic patients.

Diagnostic Workup

- See Table 13-3 for more thorough description of the various HBV serologies, but quick rules:
  - HB Surface Ag: Means infection is present.
  - Anti-HB Core IgM: Acute infection (window period).
  - Anti-HB Core IgG: Past or present infection.
  - Anti-HB Surface IgG: Past infection or vaccination (indicates immunity).
  - Anti-HDV IgM: Acute coinfection.
- You can also send PCR tests for the quantity of viral DNA/RNA for HBV/HDV, respectively.

Table 13-3. Hepatitis B Markers

Disease State	Marker	Approximate Time from Exposure to Detection in Serum	Explanation
Early infection	HBcAg (hepatitis B core antigen)	Never detectable	Intracellular antigen expressed in infected hepatocytes; not detectable in the serum.
Acute infection	Anti-HBc IgM	1.5–6 months	Window period (there can be a several-week gap between the disappearance of HB-sAg and the appearance of anti-HBs in the serum, during this time infection can be detected with anti-HBc IgM).
Active hepatitis or carrier	HBsAg	1–6 months	Viral protein coat.
High infectivity, chronic hepatitis	HBeAg	1–4 months	Indicates ongoing viral replication.
Low infectivity	Anti-HBe	4 months to years	Present in acute phase.
Immunity (past infection or vaccine)	Anti-HBs IgG	6 months to years	In serum after disappear-ance of HBsAg.
Remote infection	Anti-HBc IgG	6 months to years	Remains detectable longest.

Management

- For HBV: Entecavir or tenofovir is preferred; lamivudine is less favorable due to increasing viral resistance.
- For HDV: Interferon-alpha.
- Hepatocellular screening for certain populations of patients:
  - Family history of HCC.
  - Asian males >40 years, females >50 years.
  - All Africans and African Americans.

Prevention

- Exposed newborn: Give hepatitis B immune globulin (HBIG) and HBV vaccine.
- Adult exposure: HBV vaccination; can give HBIG if <7 days from exposure.
- Give HBV vaccination to all patients with chronic liver disease or those who have high-risk behaviors for transmission.
- By preventing HBV, you prevent the infectious ability of HDV.

HEPATITIS C

General Facts

- RNA virus, several genotypes.
- Spread by blood and bodily fluid contact (prior blood transfusions, tattoos, IV drugs).
- HBV and HDV coinfected patients have more severe disease.
- Incubation period: 15 to 160 days.
- Higher risk of developing chronic hepatitis (70% to 80%) compared to HBV in adults.

Diagnostic Workup

- Anti–hepatitis C virus (HCV) IgG:
  - First-line test for **chronic HCV**, not for acute HCV.
  - Either prior exposure to the virus or active infection.
  - Not a protective antibody (unlike in HAV and HBV).
- PCR for HCV RNA:
  - If the previous antibody test is positive, this test should be sent.
  - A positive viral load indicates active infection; a negative viral load in the setting of anti-HCV IgG indicates a cleared infection.
  - PCR should also be sent if you suspect **acute HCV**, as it can take up to 12 weeks to develop the IgG antibody after inoculation.

Management

- Direct-acting antivirals:
  - Ledipasvir–sofosbuvir is commonly used, but it is important to note that many regimens are selected based on the genotype and comorbidities of the patient.
- Interferon and ribavirin are used as adjuncts in certain patients.
- Acute infection can clear spontaneously in some patients, so it is not unreasonable to monitor for spontaneous viral clearance in patients that are not at high risk of transmission and patients that do not have another underlying liver disease.

Prevention

- No vaccination or immune globulin available, though luckily current treatment regimens have high rates of remission or sustained virologic response.
- Patients can be reinfected after cure, so be sure to counsel against high-risk behaviors.

ACUTE ALCOHOLIC HEPATITIS

General Facts

- Alcohol ingestion can lead to acute inflammation of the liver called acute alcoholic hepatitis.
- Patients usually have a long-standing history of years of heavy alcohol use.
- There is a range of how sick patients can be who develop this, but it can have a very high morbidity and mortality if severe.

Clinical Features

- **Genitourinary:** Fatigue and fever.
- **GI:** RUQ pain and abdominal distention that can be severe enough to mimic an acute abdomen, ascites.
- **Skin and eyes:** Jaundice and conjunctival icterus.
- Lower extremity edema.
- **Neurologic:** Encephalopathy and asterixis.

Diagnostic Workup

- There is no specific test for the diagnosis of acute alcoholic hepatitis. Patients will have an acute liver injury with the following labs:
  - AST:ALT ratio greater than 2:1.
  - Increased bilirubin and GGET.
  - Increased INR.
  - Leukocytosis, elevated mean corpuscular volume (MCV), and fevers, which is different from alcohol-induced cirrhosis.
- **Abdominal ultrasound** should be obtained to assess for hepatomegaly, ascites, and rule out biliary obstruction. If ascites is present, it should be sampled to ensure there is no spontaneous bacterial peritonitis (SBP).
- **Viral hepatitis** should be ruled out with serologic testing.
- **Liver biopsy:** This is the gold standard for diagnosis but it is rarely needed; if it is performed you will see neutrophil-rich steatohepatitis, hepatocyte ballooning, and Mallory–Denk bodies on histology.

Management

- **Steroids:** After infection has been ruled out with blood cultures, oral steroids can be considered.
  - First you must calculate the **discriminant function (DF)**, a formula based on prothrombin time and bilirubin.

$$\text{DF} = 4.6 \times (\text{PT} - \text{control PT}) + \text{serum TB})$$

  - If the DF >32 then steroids can be started.
  - **Lille Model Score**, which calculates survival probability, should be computed based on laboratory data on day 1 and day 7 of steroid therapy to ensure that the patient is benefiting from them; if not, steroids should be stopped.
  - Otherwise, patients should complete a 6-week course of steroids which includes a 2-week taper.
- **Manage complications of advanced liver disease:** In addition to considering steroids, patients should be managed for complications of advanced liver disease, including ascites, edema, and encephalopathy. If

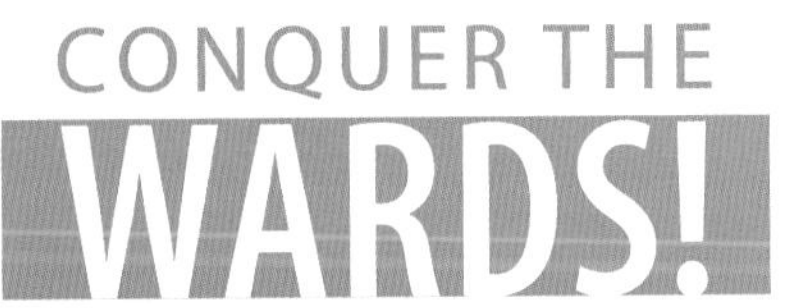

The AST/ALT in acute alcoholic hepatitis is rarely >300 U/L.

patients do not respond to steroids or have a high Model for End-Stage Liver Disease (MELD) score, they should be referred to a liver transplant center. It is imperative that patients are counseled on complete alcohol abstinence. Folate and thiamine supplementation are given to prevent vitamin deficiencies that pertain to chronic alcohol consumption.

NONALCOHOLIC STEATOHEPATITIS

- **Histologically** looks exactly like alcoholic hepatitis, but patients have no history of alcohol use and it does not present acutely.
- **Diagnosis:** It is diagnosed clinically in patients without significant alcohol use who have hepatic steatosis and liver injury without another cause. Patients are usually asymptomatic and have mild elevations in their AST and ALT. For definitive diagnosis, it requires a liver biopsy, but that is often unnecessary.
- **Risk factors**. Risk factors include obesity, diabetes, and hypertriglyceridemia.
- **Treatment:** The cornerstone of treatment is weight loss. Vitamin E in nondiabetics and pioglitazone are the only approved medications that can be used as adjuncts, and many clinical trials are ongoing.
- **Prognosis:** Nonalcoholic steatohepatitis (NASH) usually has a benign course but can eventually lead to cirrhosis over time.

Common Question on Rounds

When would you consider steroids for someone with acute alcoholic hepatitis?
If someone has a discriminant function >32 and he or she has been ruled out for infection.

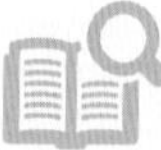

HIGH-YIELD LITERATURE

The STOPAH trial, comparing prednisolone and pentoxifylline:

Thursz MR, Richardson P, Allison M, et al. Prednisolone or pentoxifylline for alcoholic hepatitis. *N Engl J Med.* 2015;372(17):1619-1628.

Data behind the Lille Score:

Louvet A, Naveau S, Abdelnour, M, et al. The Lille model: A new tool for therapeutic strategy in patients with severe alcoholic hepatitis treated with steroids. *Hepatology.* 2007;45(6):1348-1354.

METABOLIC LIVER DISEASES

General Facts

- The 3 most common metabolic disorders that lead to liver disease are:
  - Hereditary hemochromatosis.
  - Alpha-1 antitrypsin (A1AT) deficiency.
  - Wilson disease.
- **Hereditary hemochromatosis** is a disorder that results in increased intestinal absorption of iron, which then deposits in various places in the body due to iron overload. The most common subtype is the HFE gene associated type, which results in the mutation of C282Y. It has a predominance in Caucasian males of middle age. Women tend to present later in life because menstruation serves as a form of iron loss.

- **A1AT deficiency** is a disorder where A1AT is misfolded and retained in the liver, causing hepatocyte damage. A1AT is a protease inhibitor of elastase/proteinase and is also a cause of emphysema.
- **Wilson disease** results in a defect of copper transportation, resulting in less copper excretion into bile. In addition to the liver, copper can be deposited in the basal ganglia, which gives rise to some of the neuropsychiatric symptoms.
- All 3 metabolic liver diseases are autosomal recessive, and all result in a mineral or protein abnormally accumulating in parts of the body. Over time, the liver can become cirrhotic due to ongoing damage in which case liver transplantation can be considered.

Clinical Features

The clinical features of Hereditary Hemochromatosis, A1AT Deficiency and Wilson disease are very different. (See Table 13-4)

Table 13-4. Associated Signs, Symptoms, or Exam Findings

Hereditary Hemochromatosis	A1AT Deficiency	Wilson Disease
Bronzing of skin	Cerebral aneurysm	Neuropsychiatric symptoms
Hypogonadism	Ulcerative panniculitis	Choreiform movements
Cardiomyopathy		Kayser–Fleischer rings in cornea
Diabetes mellitus		
Arthropathy		

Diagnostic Workup

Hereditary Hemochromatosis

- **Screening test**: Transferrin saturation >45%, and serum ferritin should be elevated as well (typically >400 ng/mL).
- **Diagnosis:** In these patients, an HFE gene test should be performed to look for the C282Y mutation. If the mutation is confirmed, the diagnosis is made. Subsequently, liver biopsy can be considered in certain patients at risk for advanced fibrosis (ferritin >1000, age >40, abnormal LFTs).

CONQUER THE **WARDS!**

Although unrelated to this section, an elevated stool A1AT is diagnostic of protein-losing enteropathy: a cause of chronic diarrhea.

A1AT Deficiency

- **Screening test**: Serum A1AT level.
- **Diagnosis:** If the A1AT level is low (it can be falsely low, as it is also an acute-phase reactant), you then send gene testing for PiZZ (homozygous) or PiMZ (heterozygous). This confirms the diagnosis, but liver biopsy can be performed, which will show periodic acid–Schiff (PAS)–positive, diastase-resistant globules.

CONQUER THE **BOARDS!**

Acute liver failure, low alkaline phosphatase, Coombs-negative hemolytic anemia = Wilson disease.

Wilson Disease

- **Screening test:** Low ceruloplasmin level (<20 mg/dL).
- **Diagnosis:** Definite diagnosis requires several elements of supporting data, which can include neuropsychiatric symptoms, urinary copper collection of >100 mcg over 24 hours, Kayser–Fleischer rings, or liver biopsy.

Management

Hereditary Hemochromatosis

Phlebotomy every 7 to 14 days is the cornerstone of treatment, with the goal of reaching a hematocrit >30% and ferritin of 50 ng/mL. Phlebotomy improves cardiac disease, diabetes, and bronzing of the skin but does not reverse the arthropathy, hypogonadism, or cirrhosis.

A1AT Deficiency

There is no specific treatment for liver disease related to A1AT deficiency. Patients should be screened for HCC and may eventually need liver transplantation if cirrhosis develops. If the liver is transplanted, this is curative and it will not recur.

Wilson Disease

Chelation therapy with trientine or D-penicillamine.

CIRRHOSIS

General Facts

- Chronic hepatic injury and inflammation stimulate the production of fibrosis, and cirrhosis occurs when the degree of liver fibrosis (staged from 0 to 4, with 4 being cirrhosis) advances to a point where liver function is impaired along with findings of portal hypertension.
- Common etiologies include viral hepatitis, steatohepatitis (alcohol- or nonalcohol-related fatty liver disease), autoimmune liver disease, PSC, primary biliary cholangitis (PBC), hemochromatosis, cardiac disease, Wilson disease, and A1AT deficiency.
- Regardless of the etiology, patients who develop cirrhosis can develop similar complications of portal hypertension. Major complications of portal hypertension include thrombocytopenia and leukopenia from splenic sequestration, esophageal varices, and ascites.
- A patient progresses from "compensated" to "decompensated" cirrhosis if he or she experiences any of the following: ascites, hepatic encephalopathy, or a variceal bleed.

Clinical Features

Signs and symptoms:

- Jaundice, pruritis (increased bilirubin).
- Bleeding (decreased clotting factors, thrombocytopenia).
- Anorexia, fatigue, nausea, vomiting.
- Encephalopathy.

Physical Exam Findings (See PE Section for Further Details)

- **HEENT**: Conjunctival icterus, temporal muscle wasting.
- **Chest**: Gynecomastia.
- **Abdominal**: Fluid wave from ascites, caput medusae, splenomegaly.
- **Extremities**: Lower extremity edema.
- **Skin**: Jaundice, spider angiomas, palmar erythema.
- **Neurologic**: Encephalopathy and asterixis.

Diagnostic Workup

- Cirrhosis should be suspected in patients with a clear history of chronic liver disease who develop synthetic dysfunction (prothrombin time elevation, hypoalbuminemia) or evidence of portal hypertension (thrombocytopenia, varices, ascites)
- **MR elastography and ultrasound:** Liver biopsy continues to be the gold standard in diagnosis; however, this is not always necessary now that we

have validated noninvasive fibrosis assessment tools (transient elastography via ultrasound or MR elastography).

- **MELD:** The MELD score and Child–Turcotte–Pugh score can help prognosticate patients with cirrhosis. The MELD score is calculated from the patient's INR, bilirubin, creatinine, and sodium values. The MELD score is currently used to help allocate organs to patients listed for liver transplantation. Patients with acute liver failure are at the top of the list, regardless of MELD score.
- **Serum–ascites albumin gradient (SAAG):** Patients can develop ascites as a complication of portal hypertension, but there are other etiologies that lead to ascites as well, such as heart failure, nephrotic syndrome, pancreatitis, and malignancy. The SAAG is a useful test in assessing new-onset ascites.

$$\text{SAAG} = \text{Serum Albumin} - \text{Ascites Albumin}$$

A SAAG >1.1 signifies portal hypertension, while a SAAG <1.1 is usually due to another etiology.

Management

- Management of cirrhosis is essentially management of the complications of cirrhosis (see later). It also includes alcohol cessation, avoiding hepatotoxins, avoiding shellfish (specifically raw oysters, which can harbor *Vibrio vulnificus* and cause liver failure), and making sure patients receive vaccinations for HAV, HBV, pneumococcus, and influenza.
- Patients who have decompensated cirrhosis (among other special situations) are candidates for liver transplantation, given their risk of mortality over time. Their priority on the transplant waiting list is dictated by their MELD score. After transplantation, patients will need to be on lifelong immunosuppression to prevent graft rejection.

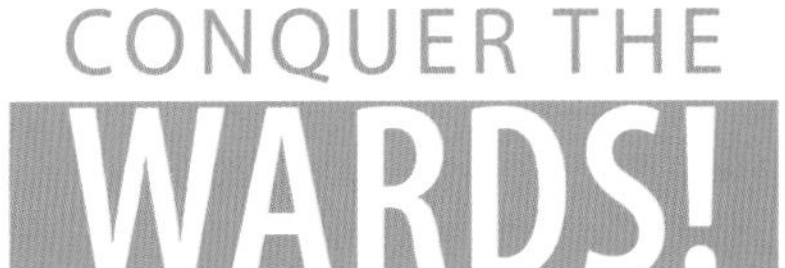

Patients with cirrhosis can take acetaminophen, just make sure it's less than 2000 mg/day.

Complications

Varices

- Varices occur in the setting of portal hypertension and can develop in a variety of places but most commonly in the esophagus, stomach, or rectum.
- Varices can bleed, and their risk of doing so correlates with their size and degree of portal hypertension.
- **Acute variceal bleeding:** Managed similar to other causes of GI bleeding (see later). The blood loss from a variceal bleed can be life threatening and is a medical emergency. A GI consult should always be called if a variceal bleed is suspected.
- **Chronic management:**
  - **Upper EGD**: All patients diagnosed with cirrhosis should have an upper endoscopy performed to screen for esophageal varices, and periodically thereafter.
  - **Prevention**: Nonselective beta-blockers (nadolol, propranolol, carvedilol) can be used to prevent variceal bleeds in patients with varices.
  - **A transjugular intrahepatic portocaval shunt (TIPS)** may be needed if endoscopic attempts are unsuccessful. TIPS is the creation of a channel between the hepatic vein and the intrahepatic portion of the portal vein by interventional radiology. It is used in cirrhotic patients with refractory variceal bleeds and ascites as a bridge to transplant.

Ascites/Lower Extremity Edema

- Ascites can be diagnosed on exam (positive fluid wave or shifting dullness test) or imaging such as ultrasound or CT scan.
- **Diagnosis:** Ascites from portal hypertension will show:
  - **High SAAG** (>1.1).
  - **Low protein** (serum protein less than 2.5 g/dL).
- **Treatment:**
  - Sodium-restricted diet (less than 2000 mg a day).
  - Diuretics: Furosemide and spironolactone together at a 20/50 ratio is typical.
  - In patients who do not respond to diuretics, large-volume paracentesis can be performed.
  - If frequent paracenteses are needed, patients may be considered for TIPS.

Spontaneous Bacterial Peritonitis (SBP)

- An infection in the ascites of a cirrhotic patient caused by translocation of bacteria from the intestine into ascitic fluid, resulting in peritonitis.
- Fever and abdominal pain can be present.
- You should have a very low threshold to perform a diagnostic paracentesis in a hospitalized cirrhotic person with ascites, as patients can decompensate quickly in the setting of untreated SBP.
- **Diagnosis** is made with a polymorphonuclear cell count >250 cells/microliter in the ascitic fluid or positive ascites culture.
- **Treatment** generally consists of a cephalosporin for enteric gram-negative coverage, as well as life-long prophylactic antibiotics, given the high risk of recurrence.

CONQUER THE WARDS!

The most common organism in SBP: *Escherichia coli.*

Hepatic Encephalopathy

- This is a (usually) reversible change in sensorium.
- The exact pathways aren't fully understood, but this is thought to occur due to increased exposure to ammonia and altered neurotransmission.
- **Diagnosis:** This is a clinical diagnosis, as ammonia levels are not sensitive or specific. The severity of encephalopathy can range from minimal sleep–wake disturbance all the way to coma. Asterixis (flapping of hands with outstretched arms) may be seen on exam.
- **Treatment** is lactulose (acidifies ammonia, preventing absorption and promoting its excretion in stool) and rifaximin (kills urea-producing bacteria in the gut). However, there is often some other precipitant (e.g., infection, bleeding, toxin) that will also need to be treated, so it is important to rule out these causes of hepatic encephalopathy.
- Of note, patients who undergo TIPS are at risk of developing worsening encephalopathy.

Hepatorenal Syndrome

- **Definition:** The development of acute renal injury in patients with advanced hepatic disease.
- **Diagnosis:** Hallmarks include a low urine sodium <20 mEq/L, hyponatremia, and hypotension. Patients should undergo a volume challenge (generally with IV albumin) to exclude pre-renal causes of renal injury before making the diagnosis.

- **Treatments** are currently limited, but include IV albumin, midodrine, and octreotide.

Hepatopulmonary Syndrome

- **Definition:** This results from vasodilation of the pulmonary vascular bed in cirrhotic patients leading to a ventilation–perfusion mismatch.
- Patients will have platypnea (shortness of breath [SOB] when sitting up and improved when supine) and orthodeoxia (decrease in oxygen saturation while upright).
- **Diagnosis:** Low PaO_2 on arterial blood gas, combined with either a bubble echocardiogram (agitated saline is administered and the visualization of bubbles can signify shunting) or pulmonary angiogram.
- **Treatment:** The only cure is liver transplantation.

Hepatocellular Carcinoma

- All patients with cirrhosis are at risk of developing HCC.
- They should undergo ultrasound examination, triple-phase CT, or MRI every 6 months to screen for this.

PORTAL HYPERTENSION

Cirrhosis is not the only cause of portal hypertension. Two common causes are discussed here.

Portal Vein Thrombosis/Budd–Chiari Syndrome

- Thrombosis in the portal vein occludes blood flow to the liver, and when this occurs the backup of blood can increase portal vein pressures and lead to complications of portal hypertension (varices and ascites).
- **Diagnosis:** Doppler ultrasound imaging or contrast-enhanced CT will diagnose the vascular occlusion.
- **Treatment** includes anticoagulation, vascular stenting, or TIPS.

Congestive Heart Failure (CHF)

- Portal hypertension from CHF is most often seen in right-sided heart failure, where back pressure leads to portal hypertension and congestive hepatopathy.
- **Diagnosis:** Ascites can develop, which will have **high SAAG** >1.0 like in cirrhotic ascites, but also **high protein** in the ascites >2.5 g/dL (this distinguishes ascites from liver cirrhosis).

Common Questions on Rounds:

How do you calculate a SAAG?
SAAG = Albumin concentration of serum – Albumin concentration of ascites

What physical exam findings do you expect to see in someone with cirrhosis?
Spider angiomata, temporal muscle wasting, gynecomastia (males), palmar erythema, jaundice, caput medusae.

LIVER ABSCESSES

General Facts

- Liver abscesses are the most common type of visceral abscess.
- They most commonly affect the right lobe of the liver, probably because it receives more of the blood flow.
- Symptoms are nonspecific, and usually manifest as fever and RUQ abdominal pain.

Etiologies

- Pylephlebitis (often manifests as a portal vein thrombus with sepsis).
- Biliary tract disease (gallstones, malignant obstruction).
- Surgical or penetrating wounds.
- Hematogenous seeding from the systemic circulation.

Common Microorganisms

Most are polymicrobial; common organisms include:

- *Enterobacter, Escherichia coli, Enterococcus, Pseudomonas aeruginosa.*
- *Staphylococcus aureus, Streptococcus pyogenes.*
- *Klebsiella pneumoniae* – most common in Asia.
- *Candida* – can be seen in neutropenic patients.
- Tuberculosis – often initial cultures are negative, since this is difficult to culture.
- *Entamoeba histolytica* – endemic to India, Africa, Central/South America.
- *Echinococcus* – can result in multiloculated cysts.

Diagnostic Workup

- **CT with contrast** is usually the most helpful study to characterize liver abscesses.
- **Serologies:** *Echinococcus* and *E. histolytica* can be diagnosed with serology as well.

Management

Treatment depends on the size, location, and symptoms.

- **Large abscesses** may require drainage with interventional radiology or even surgical excision plus antibiotics guided by drainage cultures.
- **Small abscesses**: Drainage may not be possible. Empiric antibiotics with amoxicillin–clavulanate or a fluoroquinolone and metronidazole for several weeks may be needed.
- *Echinococcus* is treated with albendazole.
- *E. histolytica* is treated with metronidazole and paromomycin.

DISORDERS OF THE BILIARY TREE

CHOLELITHIASIS AND CHOLECYSTITIS

General Facts

- Bile is produced in the liver and stored in the gallbladder where it is acidified and concentrated.

- The presence of fat and amino acids in the proximal duodenum causes the release of cholecystokinin, which stimulates gallbladder contraction.
- **Cholelithiasis** is the term for gallstones, whereas **choledocholithiasis** refers to gallstones in the bile duct. There are 3 types of gallstones:
  - **Cholesterol stones** are the most common and can be seen in obesity or rapid weight loss, oral contraception, and ileal disease.
  - **Pigmented stones** are often seen in hemolysis or sickle cell disease.
  - **Mixed stones** are a mixture of the cholesterol and pigmented stones.
- Gallstones are common, and they don't always cause problems. However, gallstones can cause pain if they transiently obstruct the cystic duct; this pain is called biliary colic. If the cystic duct remains obstructed, it can lead to cholecystitis, which is gallbladder inflammation, which can perforate if untreated.

Clinical Features

- **Biliary colic** can be described as RUQ pain that lasts between 2 and 6 hours, usually worse after meals, and associated with a crescendo-decrescendo intensity.
- Cholecystitis is characterized by RUQ pain that does not improve and may be associated with fever.
- Nausea and vomiting can occur in both.
- Risk factors for cholelithiasis (**the 5 Fs**):
  - Female sex.
  - Fat (obesity).
  - Fertile (multiparity).
  - Forty (age >40).
  - Family history.
- **Physical exam:**
  - Positive Murphy sign (arrest of inspiration while palpating the RUQ).
  - Rebound tenderness.

Diagnostic Workup

- **RUQ ultrasound:** If there is suspicion for cholelithiasis or cholecystitis , an RUQ ultrasound is the test of choice and the first imaging test that should be ordered. Ultrasound findings of gallstones, gallbladder wall thickening, and pericholecystic fluid have a positive predictive value >90% for cholecystitis.
- **Hepatobiliary iminodiacetic acid (HIDA) scan:** If cholecystitis is suspected but ultrasound is not diagnostic, a HIDA scan is performed. During a HIDA scan, technetium 99m–labeled iminodiacetic acid is injected intravenously and taken up by hepatocytes. Normally, the gallbladder should be visualized within 1 hour; if it is not visualized, this is diagnostic of cholecystitis.
- **Lab tests:** In addition to these imaging studies, LFTs and lipase should be checked to rule out an acute hepatitis (AST/ALT elevation), biliary obstruction (conjugated hyperbilirubinemia and alkaline phosphatase elevation), or pancreatitis. In cholecystitis, an elevated white blood cell count with increased polymorphonuclear neutrophils (PMNs) can be seen as well.

Management

- **Antibiotics** (usually a second- or third-generation cephalosporin) should be given to all patients suspected of having cholecystitis while imaging is obtained.

CONQUER THE BOARDS!

Common biliary bugs:

E. coli, Klebsiella, Enterococcus, Bacteroides

- **Cholecystectomy** is the definitive management for biliary colic and cholecystitis. Elective surgery can be performed for biliary colic, especially if it is recurrent. Urgent surgery should be performed for all patients with cholecystitis in order to prevent gallbladder perforation and peritonitis.
- **Cholecystostomy tube:** If a patient is too sick to undergo surgery, interventional radiology can place a cholecystostomy tube to decompress the gallbladder. This tube connects the gallbladder to an external bag that drains bile.

Complications

- **Gallstone ileus**: This occurs if a large gallstone gets impacted and fistulizes (forms a communication) with the intestine, where it then enters and can then cause a bowel obstruction. Diagnosis is usually made with CT, and treatment is surgical.
- **Mirizzi syndrome**: This occurs when an impacted gallstone in the cystic duct extrinsically obstructs the common bile duct that drains the liver. If the common bile duct is obstructed, ascending cholangitis can develop (more on this in the next section). This is diagnosed with ultrasound or MRCP and treatment is surgical.

Other Types of Cholecystitis

- **Acalculous cholecystitis:** This is cholecystitis in the absence of gallstones. Makes up 5% to 10% of cases of cholecystitis. Usually occurs in seriously ill patients (e.g., trauma, burn victims). Additional risk factors include older age, diabetes, major surgery, and HIV. Associated with more rapid clinical deterioration and increased morbidity and mortality. Patients are often too sick to undergo surgery, so cholecystostomy tubes are typically placed to decompress the gallbladder.

Common Question on Rounds

What patient demographic is at risk of developing cholelithiasis?
Obese females of child-bearing age.

ASCENDING CHOLANGITIS

General Facts

This refers to inflammation and infection of the biliary outflow tract. It is commonly caused by a stone (choledocholithiasis), stricture, or tumor. When the biliary system becomes infected without the ability to drain, the patient can become septic and decompensate quickly. This is a medical emergency.

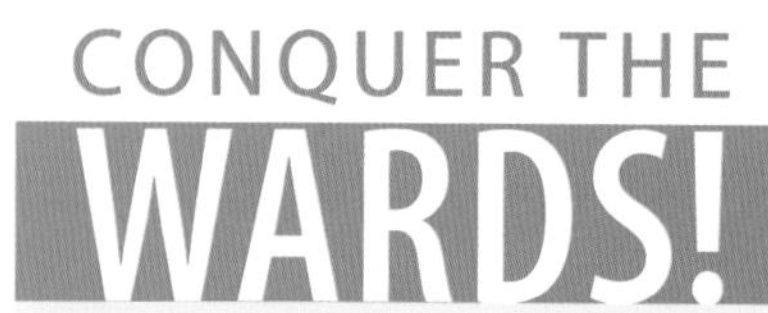

Charcot triad: RUQ pain, jaundice, fever

Reynolds pentad (add): Hypotension, altered mental status

Clinical Features

- RUQ pain, jaundice, fever (all 3 found in ~25% of patients).
- Hypotension, altered mental status (worse prognosis if these are present).

Physical Exam Findings

- Vitals: Fever, tachycardia +/− hypotension.
- HEENT exam: conjunctival icterus.
- Abdominal exam: RUQ pain without rebound or guarding.
- Skin exam: Jaundice.
- Neurologic exam: +/− Confusion.

Diagnostic Workup

Patients will have a conjugated hyperbilirubinemia and elevated alkaline phosphatase consistent with a cholestatic liver injury pattern. They will likely have more mild elevation in AST/ALT. Imaging should start with a RUQ ultrasound, which should show intrahepatic biliary dilation and possibly stones in the common bile duct (extrahepatic duct). If the imaging is inconclusive, an MRCP is the next study of choice. An ERCP is both diagnostic and therapeutic, but invasive, and would be done after confirmation of the diagnosis of ascending cholangitis.

Management

All patients should be resuscitated with fluids and started on broad-spectrum antibiotics to cover gram-negatives. Patients with ascending cholangitis should undergo ERCP to decompress the biliary system for definitive source control. Through ERCP, the gastroenterologist can remove obstructing stones, perform a sphincterotomy to allow bile easier passage into the duodenum, and place stents for benign or malignant strictures. If patients are too unstable to undergo an ERCP, interventional radiology can place percutaneous drainage catheters into the biliary system for decompression.

Common Questions on Rounds

What is Charcot's triad? Reynold's pentad? What is their significance?
Refer to the symptoms/signs of acute cholangitis and offer prognostication.
Charcot's triad: fever, RUQ pain, jaundice.
Reynold's pentad: The first 3 plus hypotension and confusion (worse prognosis).

PRIMARY SCLEROSING CHOLANGITIS

General Facts

PSC is a chronic progressive disorder of the intrahepatic and extrahepatic biliary tree, characterized by inflammation and fibrosis. This results in biliary strictures that can precipitate bacterial cholangitis (as noted earlier). This disease is predominant in males and has a strong association with inflammatory bowel disease (IBD), ulcerative colitis more so than Crohn disease. It is a risk factor for cholangiocarcinoma (cancer of the biliary tree). Patients with PSC can develop liver cirrhosis.

Clinical Features

- May be asymptomatic early in disease course.
- Pruritis, jaundice, and fatigue are the most common symptoms.

Diagnostic Workup

Patients will have a conjugated hyperbilirubinemia and elevated alkaline phosphatase on routine labs. A GGT should be drawn to confirm the increased alkaline phosphatase is from a biliary source. GGT is specific for a biliary source of alkaline phosphatase, which is consistent with a cholestatic liver injury pattern. The alkaline phosphatase can also be elevated in diseases of the bone (e.g., Paget disease, bone metastases).

PSC that affects the medium and larger bile ducts can be diagnosed with MRCP. If it is only affecting the smaller bile ducts, a liver biopsy may be needed (onion-skin fibrosis seen on histology). ERCP can also diagnose PSC (you'll see a "string-of-beads" appearance on cholangiogram), but this is not the first-line test, given its invasiveness. Patients may have positive antibodies for perinuclear antineutrophil cytoplasmic antibodies (p-ANCA), but this is nonspecific.

Management
Unfortunately, there are no medical treatments for PSC that have shown consistent benefit. Ursodeoxycholic acid is a synthetic bile acid that decreases the cholesterol content of bile and may help with the pruritis that patients can experience.

Patients who develop symptomatic strictures may undergo ERCP for stricture dilation or stenting. Given its association with IBD, all patients with PSC should undergo colonoscopy at the time of diagnosis. If IBD is diagnosed, they undergo annual colonoscopy for cancer screening; otherwise, every 5 years. If PSC progresses into end-stage liver disease or decompensated cirrhosis, a liver transplant evaluation should be performed.

Complications
Cholangiocarcinoma: This refers to cancer of the bile ducts, and PSC is a major risk factor for this, but it can occur in the absence of PSC as well. Patients present with jaundice and weight loss. Diagnosis starts with a contrast-enhanced MRCP, and a serum CA 19-9 level will be elevated. Tissue diagnosis is confirmatory but not always indicated and depends on the clinical situation. It can be obtained by cytology brushings during ERCP or with biopsy. Surgical resection is the only curative option, and liver transplantation can also be considered in highly selective patients. The prognosis is overall poor, with 5-year survival rates for localized disease being around 13% to 24%.

Ascending cholangitis: See prior section on this. Repeated episodes of cholangitis can be an indication for liver transplantation.

PRIMARY BILIARY CHOLANGITIS

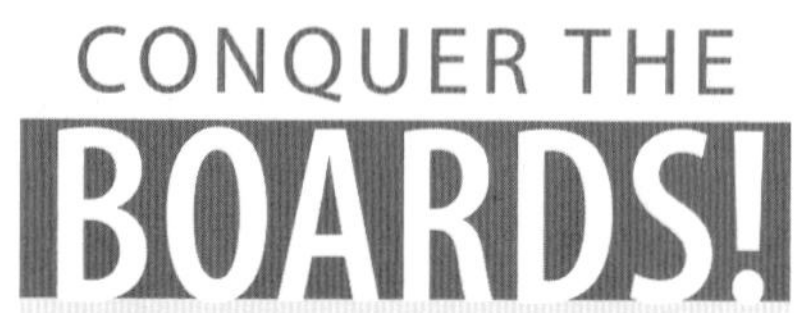

PSC: Young men with IBD

PBC: Older women with autoimmune disease

General Facts
PBC is an autoimmune disease causing destruction of the intrahepatic bile ducts. It was formerly known as primary biliary cirrhosis. This disease is predominant in females and has a strong association with other autoimmune diseases (Sjögren syndrome, scleroderma, thyroid disease). Patients with PBC, like PSC, can develop liver cirrhosis.

Clinical Features

- Pruritis.
- Fatigue.
- Jaundice as the disease progresses.

Physical Exam Findings

- HEENT: Xanthelasmas (cholesterol deposits on medial aspect of eyelids) may be present.
- Skin exam: Xanthomas (cholesterol deposits in skin) may be present, excoriations from itching.

Diagnostic Workup
Patients will generally have an elevated alkaline phosphatase and GGT as the first clue to diagnosis. If suspected, an antimitochondrial antibody (AMA) should then be sent. The majority of patients are positive for AMAs (90%

sensitive). There are no diagnostic imaging findings. If the diagnosis is still in question, liver biopsy can be performed.

Management

Ursodeoxycholic acid is first-line therapy and may slow progression of the disease. However, over a third of patients will not respond to this therapy. In these patients, obeticholic acid can be used, which is a synthetic bile acid and agonist of the farnesoid X nuclear receptor (FXR). FXR activation inhibits bile acid synthesis from cholesterol. Liver transplant is the only cure and is recommended in patients with end-stage liver disease. Patients should be screened for fat-soluble vitamin deficiencies (vitamin A, D, E, K). They should also be screened for osteoporosis, hypercholesterolemia, and thyroid disease.

Common Question on Rounds:

Which antibody is often positive in PBC?
AMA

DISORDERS OF THE COLON

DIVERTICULAR DISEASE

General Facts

Diverticulosis is an acquired condition of the colon in which saclike protrusions of the colonic mucosa herniate through a defect in the muscle layer (where nutrient arteries insert). They are most common in the sigmoid colon, as this is the narrowest area of the colon and is subject to high pressures. Diverticulosis occurs with increasing frequency as patients age, and there is an association with a low-fiber diet but it is unclear if this is causal. Though diverticulosis is common in the general population, it usually does not cause symptoms. The 2 major, separate complications to know about are **diverticular bleeding** and **diverticulitis**, which will be the focus of this section. Diverticular bleeding occurs when there is erosion through one of the feeding blood vessels causing severe, painless rectal bleeding. This is the most common cause of lower GI bleeding in patients over 60. Diverticulitis, on the other hand, occurs when the diverticulum gets impacted and inflammation or infection occurs. This causes abdominal pain without profuse rectal bleeding.

Clinical Features

- Uncomplicated diverticulosis: Asymptomatic.
- Diverticulitis: Abdominal pain (most often in left lower quadrant [LLQ]), fever.
- Diverticular bleeding: Painless rectal bleeding.

Physical Exam Findings

- Vitals: Hypotension, tachycardia (if bleeding); fever (if diverticulitis).
- Abdominal exam: LLQ pain, with or without rebound or guarding (if diverticulitis).
- Rectal exam: Bright red blood or maroon stool (in diverticular bleeding).

Diagnostic Workup

Uncomplicated diverticulosis is most commonly noted as an incidental finding during colonoscopy. It may also be seen if significant on CT scan.

CONQUER THE WARDS!

Diverticulosis is more common in the left colon, but bleeding is more common from the right colon due to the thinner colonic wall.

Diverticular bleeding: Suspect this in any older patient who is presenting with significant lower GI bleeding. Initial management is often with a CT angiogram to localize a culprit bleeding vessel to embolize and a GI consult for possible colonoscopy.

Diverticulitis: Diagnosed with CT with IV and oral contrast. This will show an inflamed diverticula, pericolic fat stranding, or complications of diverticulitis such as abscess or obstruction.

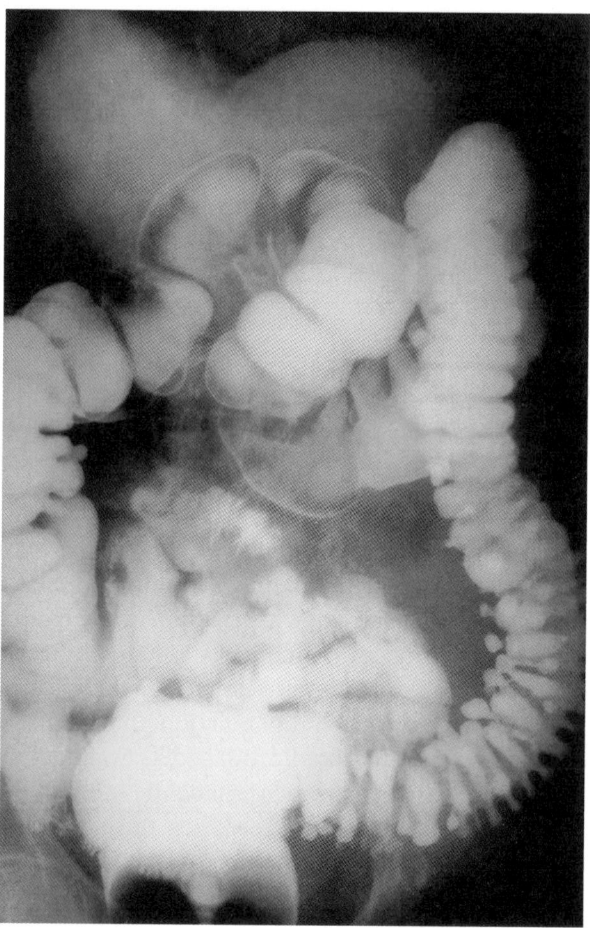

FIGURE 13-4. Barium study in a patient with diverticulosis demonstrates many small contrastfilled outpouchings mostly in the sigmoid colon.

Management

Diverticular bleeding: Initial management should be fluid resuscitation, establishing large-bore IV access, and close monitoring. If a culprit vessel is found on angiogram, it can be embolized by interventional radiology. If a culprit vessel is seen on colonoscopy, it can be treated endoscopically. In refractory cases where embolization or colonoscopy has failed, surgical colectomy may be needed, though this is rare. Fortunately, diverticular bleeding often resolves without intervention.

Diverticulitis: Initial management should be fluids and pain control, and patients should be started on antibiotics and kept NPO if severe. Antibiotic choice should cover gram-negative anaerobes, particularly *E. coli, Klebsiella, Enterobacter, Bacteroides,* and *Enterococcus* (typically ciprofloxacin and metronidazole). Patients should not undergo colonoscopy in the acute setting due to the risk of perforation from the inflammation. However, they should be considered for colonoscopy 6 to 8 weeks after diagnosis, as diverticulitis is sometimes provoked in the setting of underlying colon cancer.

Complications

Complications of diverticulitis: In severe diverticulitis, perforation can occur, causing peritonitis and sepsis. Colonic fistulas can also form from colonic inflammation adhering to another organ, such as the bladder (which will cause fecaluria) or the vagina (causing fecal vaginal discharge). Strictures can also appear after the inflammation subsides, which can cause a large-bowel obstruction. The management for all these complications is surgical. Complicated diverticulitis can also cause abscess formation in the area of the initial attack. Depending on the size of the abscess, in addition to antibiotics, it may require draining by interventional radiology or surgical management.

Segmental colitis associated with diverticulosis (SCAD): This can be found on colonoscopy where there is inflammation surrounding the diverticula. It presents similar to IBD. This can cause abdominal pain, cramping, and diarrhea. Treatment is antibiotics, 5-ASA, or immunosuppressive agents.

Common Question on Rounds

What is the most common cause of lower GI bleeding in the older adult?
Diverticular bleeding

CLOSTRIDIUM DIFFICILE COLITIS

General Facts

C. difficile is a spore-forming anaerobe that can be normally found in the GI tract. Its overgrowth is inhibited by competing gut flora. When it is made possible for overgrowth to occur, such as with antibiotic exposure, which selectively eradicates its competitors, *C. difficile* can cause inflammation and damage to the colonic mucosa through release of exotoxins. This form of colitis is also termed pseudomembranous colitis. In addition to antibiotic use, outpatient or inpatient health care exposure is another risk factor for developing this disease.

Clinical Features

- Diarrhea, usually watery and nonbloody.
- Crampy abdominal pain.
- Fever.
- Leukocytosis often rapidly rising. Think *C. difficile* when the white count is above 20,000.

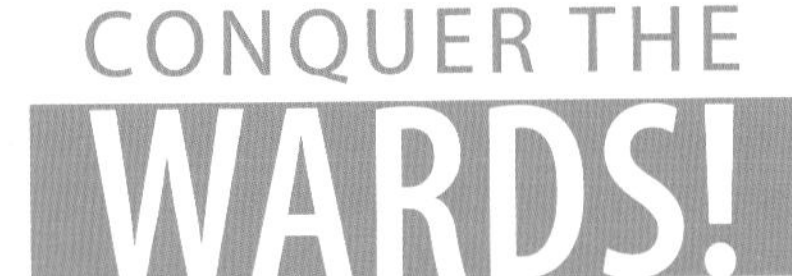

Recent antibiotic use is a common precipitating risk factor for developing *C. difficile* colitis!

Physical Exam Findings

Abdominal exam:

- Hyperactive bowel sounds.
- Diffuse abdominal pain without rebound or guarding.
- Abdominal distention with hypoactive bowel sounds is concerning for toxic megacolon (a complication we will discuss later).

Diagnostic Workup

C. difficile colitis is a clinical diagnosis in a patient with symptomatic diarrhea, confirmed by a **stool test** for its associated antigen and toxin. Colonoscopy is not needed or recommended for diagnosis, but pathognomonic findings include yellowish membranous plaques (pseudomembranes) adherent to the colonic mucosa.

Management

The first-line treatment for all patients is vancomycin given orally. Offending antibiotics should be discontinued, if possible. In patients with recurrent episodes of *C. difficile* colitis, they should be considered for a fecal microbiota transplantation.

Complications

Toxic megacolon: This is a dreaded complication if the inflammation from the infection spreads through all layers of the colonic wall. Patients will develop abdominal distention and severe pain, and may even become constipated. Imaging will show colonic dilation and may show "thumbprinting" (bowel-wall edema). There is a high mortality with this. In addition to close monitoring and serial abdominal exams, patients will need surgical consultation for possible colectomy.

CONQUER THE WARDS!

Recent antibiotic use is a common precipitating risk factor for developing *C. difficile* colitis!

Common Questions on Rounds

What are some risk factors for developing *C. difficile* colitis?
Recent antibiotic use, health care setting exposure such as hospital admission, advanced age, IBD.

What laboratory values help you determine how severe someone's *C. difficile* infection is?
Serum creatinine >1.5 mg/dL or a white blood cell (WBC) >15,000 cells/mL are indicative of a severe infection.

HIGH-YIELD LITERATURE

Fecal microbiota transplantation for recurrent infection

Van Nood E, Vrieze A, Nieudworp, M, et al. Duodenal infusion of donor feces for recurrent *Clostridium difficile. N Engl J Med.* 2013;368(22):407-415.

IRRITABLE BOWEL SYNDROME

General Facts

Irritable bowel syndrome (IBS) is a functional bowel disorder with an alteration of intestinal motility and visceral hypersensitivity that causes changes in bowel habits and discomfort. It is a common outpatient GI diagnosis, typically presenting in younger patients, and is more common in females. It is associated with stress.

Clinical Features

- Abdominal pain related to defecation (may improve or worsen).
- Change in stool frequency.
- Change in stool consistency.

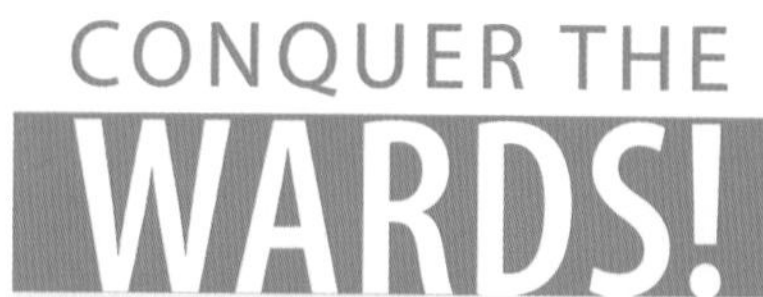

Mimics of IBS:

Inflammatory bowel disease, celiac disease, lactose intolerance, microscopic colitis, laxative abuse

Physical Exam Findings

- Abdominal exam: Hyperactive bowel sounds are possible, mild abdominal tenderness also possible but no rebound or guarding, abdomen should be soft.

Diagnostic Workup

The formal diagnostic criteria are the Rome IV Diagnostic Criteria, which are based on the patient's symptoms; however, it is important to realize that IBS is a diagnosis of exclusion. Laboratory workup for electrolyte abnormalities, iron deficiency, celiac disease, inflammatory markers (erythrocyte sedimentation rate [ESR] or C-reactive protein [CRP]), and stool tests for infection should be performed to support the absence of another disease process. Colonoscopy is not needed for initial diagnosis unless there are other red flags such as rectal bleeding, need for colon cancer screening, or persistent symptoms despite therapy.

Management

Treatment can be complicated and tailored to the individual patient. All patients should be reassured. Other useful adjuncts include dietary modification (low "FODMAP" diet), fiber, antidepressants, and psychotherapy. A diet containing fermentable oligosaccharides, disaccharides, monosaccharides, and polyols (FODMAPs) can be poorly absorbed in certain patients. These sugars remain in the intestinal lumen where bacteria can rapidly ferment the compounds and release gas in the process. This gas can cause bloating and abdominal discomfort.

INFLAMMATORY BOWEL DISEASE

General Facts

IBD is an autoimmune-mediated, chronic inflammation affecting the GI tract. Both are more common in Caucasians and those with an Ashkenazi Jewish background. Peak incidence occurs in ages 15 to 35 and can run in families. There are 2 major types:

- Crohn disease (CD): It can affect **any part** of the GI tract, from the mouth to anus. The inflammation with CD is also transmural, meaning it affects all mucosal layers, which allows for formation of fistulae and abscesses.
- Ulcerative colitis (UC): UC **only affects the colon** and only the mucosal layer. UC always progresses from the rectum and ascends more proximally to the cecum.

CD that affects a significant portion of the colon and UC harbor an increased risk of colon cancer.

Clinical Features

Crohn's Disease and Ulcerative Colitis each have distinct clinical features and pathology (See Table 13-5 and 13-6). There are also typical extraintestinal manifestations of IBD that are important to know. (See Table 13-7)

Table 13-5. Signs and Symptoms

Crohn Disease	Ulcerative Colitis
Diarrhea +/– blood	Bloody diarrhea
Obstructive symptoms (nausea, vomiting)	**Tenesmus**
Perianal fistula	**Urgency**
Anemia, fatigue, fever	Anemia, fatigue, fever

Table 13-6. Pathology

Crohn Disease	Ulcerative Colitis
Affects any part of the GI tract (mouth to anus)	Affects colon only
Transmural inflammation with granulomas	Mucosal inflammation only
Skip lesions (interspersed normal and affected bowel)	**Contiguous inflammation** without skip lesions
Rectum can be spared	**Rectum involved**
Cigarette smoking risk factor for disease activity	Cigarette smoking is not a risk factor
Fistulas or abscesses possible	No fistulas or abscesses generally seen

Table 13-7. Extraintestinal Manifestations of Inflammatory Bowel Disease (Occurs in 20% of Patients)		
Eye involvement	Uveitis Episcleritis	CD > UC Uveitis, erythema nodosum, and colitic arthritis are commonly seen together.
Dermatologic	Erythema nodosum Pyoderma gangrenosum Aphthous ulcers	CD, especially in children > UC Parallels disease course (gets better as IBD improves) UC > CD May or may not follow disease course CD
Arthritis	Colitic arthritis Ankylosing spondylitis	CD > UC Parallels disease course 30 times more common in UC Unrelated to disease course
Hematologic	Anemia Thromboembolism	UC = CD UC = CD
Hepatobiliary	Fatty liver Hepatitis Cholelithiasis Primary sclerosing cholangitis	UC = CD UC = CD UC = CD
Renal	Secondary amyloidosis → renal failure	UC > CD CD Unrelated to disease course

Physical Exam Findings

- HEENT: Aphthous ulcers (in CD), uveitis, episcleritis.
- Abdominal exam: Abdominal pain, if localized in right lower quadrant (RLQ) think CD; a distended abdomen can be possible in small bowel obstruction (CD) or toxic megacolon (UC).
- Rectal exam: Perianal fistulae (in CD).
- Skin: Pyoderma gangrenosum, erythema nodosum.

Diagnostic Workup

Colonoscopy to the terminal ileum with biopsies is needed to confirm the diagnosis. If the findings on colonoscopy are suggestive of IBD (erythematous friable mucosa, ulceration), CT or MR enterography should be obtained to rule out extracolonic CD. This can demonstrate fistulae, abscesses, or small-bowel strictures. UC won't show these features. Inflammatory markers with ESR, CRP, or fecal calprotectin can be useful to trend response to treatment.

Management

The management of IBD is complex and individualized to the patient. Classes of medications that are used include aminosalicylates (5-ASAs), corticosteroids, immunomodulators (azathioprine, 6-mercaptopurine, methotrexate), and biologic medications. Biologic medications include tumor necrosis factor (TNF)-alpha inhibitors (many including infliximab and adalimumab), integrin inhibitors (vedolizumab), and interleukin (IL)-12/IL-23 inhibitors (ustekinumab). The goal of treatment is mucosal healing in order to prevent complications and disease progression. Patients should be followed closely by a gastroenterologist to determine when colonoscopy is needed to check if therapies are working and also for dysplasia surveillance to prevent colon cancer.

CONQUER THE WARDS!

Chronic scarring of the colon from healed inflammation can lead to retraction and loss of haustra; this is called "lead pipe colon."

CONQUER THE WARDS!

In fistulizing forms of Crohn disease, avoid steroid use and choose a TNF-alpha inhibitor.

In refractory cases, surgical colectomy can be curative for UC. There is no curative surgery for CD, since it can affect any part of the GI tract, but it is sometimes needed regardless to manage complications.

In hospitalized patients presenting with a flare of IBD, stool studies, including *C. difficile* testing, should be sent, and if negative IV corticosteroids can be considered.

Complications

Abscess, Fistula: This can happen with CD. Treatment is antibiotics and drainage of abscess, if possible (surgically or through interventional radiology). Perianal fistulas can sometimes be managed by surgical seton placement.

Stricture: Inflammatory strictures are typically a presenting symptom in small-bowel CD, where a patient may present with a small-bowel obstruction. Strictures can also occur in CD at surgical anastomoses after a resection is performed.

Intestinal perforation: Though rare, this can occur if inflammation is severe and untreated with UC and CD. Treatment would be antibiotics and surgical consultation.

Toxic megacolon: Similar to *C. difficile* colitis, this can happen in severe colitis from UC.

Common Questions on Rounds:

What complications happen in CD that generally do not happen in UC?
Fistulae, abscess, small-bowel obstruction.

What should be done before starting steroids in the hospitalized patient with an IBD flare?
Rule out *C. difficile* infection.

HIGH-YIELD LITERATURE

Combination therapy for Crohn's disease

Colombel JF, Sandborn, Reinisch W, et al. Infliximab, azathioprine, or combination therapy for Crohn's Disease. *N Engl J Med*. 2010;362(15):1383-1395.

COLORECTAL CANCER

General Facts

Colon cancer is the second most common cause of cancer death in the United States. Most cases are thought to arise from precancerous polyps called adenomas.

Clinical Features

- **Signs and symptoms:**
  - Iron-deficiency anemia (associated symptoms of pallor, fatigue).
  - Overt rectal bleeding or occult bleeding in stool.
  - Constipation.
  - Change in stool caliber.
  - Weight loss.

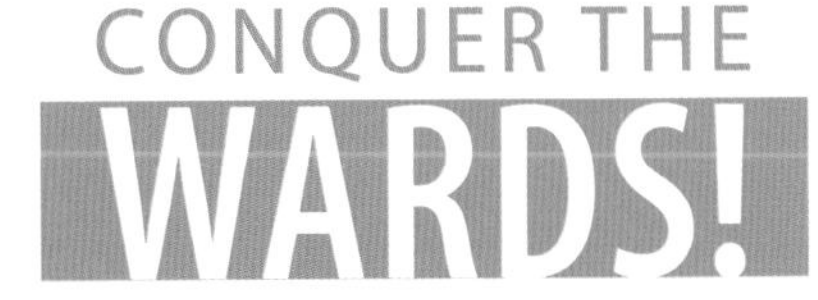

Steptococcus bovis bacteremia is associated with colon cancer.

- **Risk factors:**
  - Older age.
  - Personal or family history of colon adenomas or colon cancer.
  - Long-standing IBD.
  - Hereditary colon cancer syndromes (more on this later).

Physical Exam Findings

- Often no localizing findings until more advanced.
- Abdominal exam: Abdominal distention and pain if patient has progressed to large-bowel obstruction.
- Rectal Exam: Guaiac positive stool or overt bleeding (rare).

Diagnostic Workup

Screening (USPSTF Recommendations 2016)

There are many different methods to screen patients for colon cancer. Screening should start at age 50, unless the patient has additional risk factors such as a family history of colon adenomas or cancer. Screening patients above age 75 is an individualized decision at the discretion of the primary care physician and should be considered if the patient's overall health is good with a life expectancy >10 years, or if prior colonoscopy findings showed high-risk lesions such as cancer or adenomatous polyps. The screening test of choice should be chosen based on shared decision-making with each patient (See table 13-8).

Table 13-8.

Screening Test	Screening Interval	Notes
Stool tests:		
Fecal occult blood test (FOBT)	Annually	Does not require bowel preparation, anesthesia, or transportation to the exam.
Fecal immunochemical test (FIT)	Annually	
FIT-DNA	Every 1–3 years	
Radiology test:		
Computed tomographic (CT) colonography	Every 5 years	Lacks procedural risk of colonoscopy, but still requires bowel preparation, and extracolonic incidental findings may be found.
Endoscopic tests:		
Colonoscopy	Every 10 years	Screening and diagnostic management of positive results can be performed at same time. Long interval for negative screening exams. Requires bowel preparation, anesthesia, and transportation to exam. Preferred for irritable bowel disease (IBD) patients or hereditary cancer syndromes.
Flexible sigmoidoscopy	Every 5 years	Has fallen out of favor in the United States, as it does not visualize the right colon.
Flexible sigmoidoscopy + FIT	Flexible sigmoidoscopy every 10 years; FIT annually	Has fallen out of favor in the United States, as it does not visualize the right colon.

Diagnosis

Colonoscopy is the test of choice to diagnose colon cancer in the setting of a positive screening test, as it allows direct visualization and the ability to sample the tumor for a tissue diagnosis. Labs often demonstrate iron-deficiency anemia from occult blood losses over time. Carcinoembryonic antigen (CEA) can be elevated as well, but is not used as a screening test, but rather trended postoperatively after a resection to monitor for cancer recurrence. Abnormal LFTs can indicate liver metastases.

Figure 13-5 shows an "apple-core lesion" with a colonic stenosis on barium enema. Nonspecific, but think of colon cancer. This visually helps demonstrate how colon cancer can sometimes lead to obstructive symptoms.

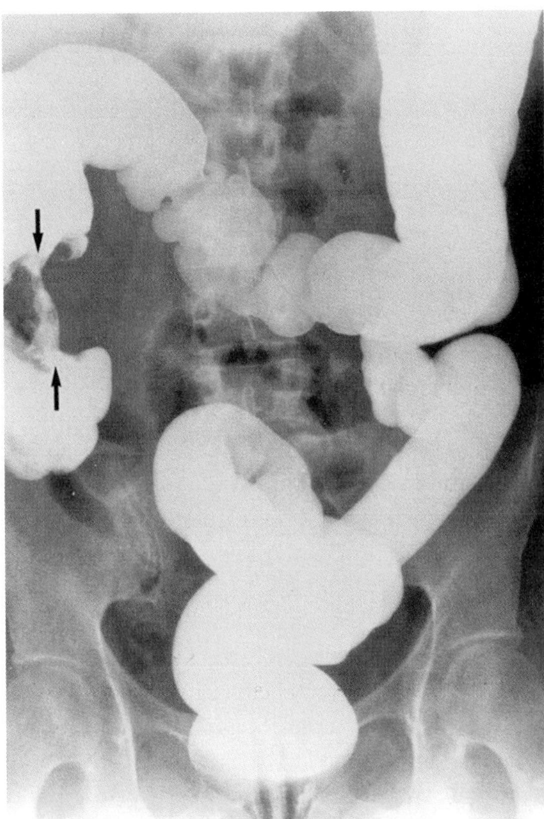

FIGURE 13-5. Barium study in a patient with colon cancer demonstrates an "apple core"–shaped filling defect at the site of a circumferential neoplasm. (Reproduced, with permission, from Schwartz SI, Fischer JE, Spencer FC, Shires GT, Daly JM. *Schwartz's Principles of Surgery,* 7th ed. New York: McGraw-Hill, 1998: 1347.)

Dukes and TNM are both staging systems for colon cancer. TNM is preferred (see Table 13-9).

Table 13-9. TNM Staging (Preferred)

Tis	Carcinoma in situ.
T1	Tumor invades submucosa.
T2	Tumor invades muscularis propria.
T3	Tumor invades through the muscularis propria into the subserosa, pericolic or perirectal tissues.
T4	Tumor directly invades other organs or structures.

Table 13-9. TNM Staging (Preferred) (Continued)

NX	Regional nodes cannot be assessed.
N0	No positive nodes.
N1	Metastasis in 1–3 regional lymph nodes.
N2	Metastasis in 4 or more regional lymph nodes.
MX	Distant metastasis cannot be assessed.
M0	No distant metastasis.
M1	Distant metastasis.

Stage 0	Tis	N0	M0
Stage I	T1–2	N0	M0
Stage IIA	T3	N0	M0
Stage IIB	T4	N0	M0
Stage IIIA	T1–2	N1	M0
Stage IIIB	T3–4	N1	M0
Stage IIIC	Any T	N2	M0
Stage IV	Any T	Any N	M1

Management

Colon polyps can be removed at the time of colonoscopy. Hyperplastic polyps are benign and do not increase the risk of colorectal cancer. Adenomatous polyps (tubular, tubulovillous, and villous adenomas) are precancerous. The time interval to undergo repeat surveillance colonoscopy should be shortened depending on the size and number of adenomas seen. Large adenomas (>1 cm) or >3 adenomas generally warrant a 3-year interval, 1 to 3 adenomas generally warrant a 5-year interval, and if no polyps or only hyperplastic polyps are seen 10 years is appropriate.

Chemotherapy, radiation, and surgery are used to manage colorectal cancer. Radiation is generally reserved for rectal cancer. Many early stage (stage I to II) cancers can be cured with surgery alone. Stage III cancers can be treated with resection and adjuvant chemotherapy (5-year survival 40% to 60%). Stage IV is metastatic disease, usually treated with chemotherapy only, but can resect lesions if they are symptomatic (5-year survival <10%). Colonoscopy should be performed 6 to 12 months after surgical resection to exclude synchronous lesions.

Complications

Iron-deficiency anemia: This develops in the setting of chronic, occult blood loss.

Large-bowel obstruction: This can occur if the cancer extends into the colonic lumen and causes a blockage. Patients will present with abdominal distention, pain, nausea, and obstipation. There is a risk for colonic perforation. Treatment is either surgical or endoscopic colonic stent placement.

Hereditary Colon Cancer Syndromes

- **Familial adenomatous polyposis (FAP):** Autosomal dominant condition in which thousands of adenomatous polyps appear throughout the colon by age 25. Most untreated patients develop colon cancer by age 40. Treatment is a prophylactic total colectomy. Two subsets of FAP include:
  - **Gardner syndrome:** Characterized by supernumerary teeth, osteomas, and fibrous dysplasia of the skull.
  - **Turcot syndrome:** Associated with brain tumors.

- **Lynch syndrome:** Also known as hereditary nonpolyposis colon cancer (HNPCC). Autosomal dominant condition with defect in DNA mismatch repair genes. Often multiple other primary cancers in the family (gynecologic, renal, small bowel, among others). Diagnostic criteria include the Amsterdam criteria, where 3 or more associated cancers are present in a patient's family, one of whom is a first-degree relative of the other 2, affecting 2 or more generations, with one person before age 50.

Peutz–Jeghers syndrome: Polyposis of the small intestine (hamartomas) with multiple pigmented melanin macules in the oral mucosa. Also associated with breast and pancreatic cancer.

HIGH-YIELD LITERATURE

Time intervals for polyp surveillance after initial colonoscopy:

Lieberman DA, Rex DK, Winawer SJ, et al. Guidelines for colonoscopy surveillance after screening and polypectomy: A consensus update by the US Multi-Society Task Force on Colorectal Cancer. *Gastroenterology*. 2012;143(3):844-857.

Multitarget stool DNA testing:
Imperiale TF, Ransohoff DD, Itzkowitz SH, et al. Multitarget stool DNA testing for colorectal-cancer screening. *N Engl J Med*. 2014;370:1287-1297.

NEUROENDOCRINE TUMORS

General Facts

- Neuroendocrine tumors (NETs) arise from ectodermal stem cells in the gut, usually in the ileum or appendix. These are commonly called "carcinoid" tumors, but this term can be confusing and has fallen out of favor.
- These are slow-growing tumors and can cause symptoms if they secrete various neurotransmitters/hormones such as serotonin [5-HT], bradykinin, and histamine.
- Though slow growing, they can still metastasize to the lymph nodes, lung, or liver.
- Most are idiopathic, but can be associated with multiple endocrine neoplasia type I (MEN type I).
- Prognosis is determined by the size and location of the primary tumor and presence or absence of metastases.

Clinical Features

- They are often found incidentally.
- **Carcinoid syndrome**, which is associated with metastatic NETs that originate in the gut and often involve the liver: Diarrhea (serotonin), flushing (bradykinin), wheezing (histamine), cardiomyopathy (classically right heart involvement).
- Bowel obstruction or appendicitis from tumor growth.

Diagnostic Workup

Urine 5-hydroxyindoleacetic acid (5-HIAA) as an initial test and **abdominal CT** to look for mass.

Management

- Somatostatin (octreotide) can improve symptoms and slow tumor growth.
- Radiotherapy and surgical management can be used for localized management.

Complications

Carcinoid crisis: Triggered by tumor manipulation during surgery or endoscopy, which leads to a massive release of neurotransmitters/hormones, which can cause hemodynamic instability. Octreotide should be given before these procedures for patients with a history of carcinoid syndrome.

Bowel obstruction: Caused by tumor growth in the intestines.

OVERT GASTROINTESTINAL BLEEDING

General Facts

- Overt GI bleeding refers to macroscopic bleeding, as evident by visualized blood. Occult GI bleeding is microscopic bleeding that can cause anemia over time.
- Overt GI bleeding can be life threatening in the acute setting and is the focus of this section.
- **Upper GI bleeding** refers to bleeding above the ligament of Treitz.
- **Lower GI bleeding** refers to bleeding starting from the ileocecal valve. Anything in between refers to small-bowel bleeding.

CONQUER THE **WARDS!**

Not all black stool is GI bleeding!

Iron or bismuth consumption can turn stool black.

Epistaxis or gum bleeding can lead to melena.

Clinical Features

- Overt bleeding:
  - Upper GI source:
    - Hematemesis (bright red blood in vomit).
    - Coffee-ground emesis (old, brown, digested blood; nonspecific).
  - Upper or lower GI source:
    - Melena (black, tarry stool, only requires 50 cc of blood).
    - Hematochezia (bright red blood).
- Orthostasis (lightheadedness with supine to upright positioning) or syncope if significant blood volume is lost.

Differential Diagnosis

The differential diagnosis for GI bleeding is broad. Table 13-10 presents some representative examples, with the most common in bold for each anatomic distribution.

CONQUER THE **WARDS!**

CBC in acute hemorrhage will not affect true severity of bleed, since it takes time for concentrations to change.

Diagnostic Workup

- **History and physical:** Thorough history and physical, including **a rectal exam.**
- **Labs:**
  - **Complete blood count (CBC)** (noting any change from baseline Hgb).
  - INR.
  - Type and screen.
  - Basic chemistries should be sent.
- **Nasogastric lavage**, a technique performed by placing a nasogastric tube and irrigating the stomach, assessing for aspiration of bloody contents;

Table 13-10. Differential Diagnosis for GI Bleeding

UGIB	LGIB	Small Bowel
Peptic ulcer	**Diverticulosis**	**Angioectasia**
Esophageal or gastric varices	Hemorrhoids	IBD
Esophagitis	Angioectasia	NSAID ulceration
Angioectasia	Ischemia	Henoch–Schonlein purpura
Portal HTN gastropathy	Post-polypectomy bleeding	Meckel diverticulum
Dieulafoy lesion	Dieulafoy lesion	Dieulafoy lesion
GAVE	IBD	Osler–Weber–Rendu
Mallory–Weiss tear	Stercoral ulcer	Amyloidosis
Marginal ulcer	Cancer	
Hemobilia	Rectal varices	
Hemosuccus pancreaticus	Radiation proctopathy	

HTN, hypertension; *IBD*, inflammatory bowel disease.

has fallen out of favor, since this does not rule out an upper GI bleed if negative.

- **EGD and colonoscopy:** Endoscopic evaluation is a cornerstone of the diagnostic and therapeutic management of GI bleeding.
  - If **melena, hematemesis, or coffee-ground emesis** is the chief complaint, this indicates an upper source. EGD is performed first to look for an upper GI source of bleeding, and if this is unrevealing then a colonoscopy is done.
  - If **hematochezia** is the chief complaint, this generally reflects a lower GI source and colonoscopy is done first.
  - However, it is important to note that brisk upper GI bleeding (usually in the setting of hemodynamic instability) can lead to hematochezia, while slow lower GI bleeding can lead to melena.
  - If EGD and colonoscopy are both unrevealing, a small-bowel evaluation with capsule endoscopy is done.
  - If EGD, colonoscopy, and capsule endoscopy are negative, then a **tagged red blood cell (RBC) scan or CT angiography** are other useful diagnostic adjuncts if patients continue to bleed without an endoscopic source identified.

CONQUER THE WARDS!

Blood is broken down and reabsorbed in the proximal intestine. Therefore, a BUN:Cr ratio >30 is suggestive of an UGIB.

Management

- Initial management is medical stabilization with 2 large-bore IVs, fluids, and blood products if needed. Target a hemoglobin >7 in most patients.
- **Upper GI bleeding**: Patients should be started on IV PPI therapy.
- **Variceal bleeding**: In patients with cirrhosis, they should also be started on:
  - Octreotide infusions to decrease portal hypertension AND
  - Antibiotics for SBP prophylaxis.
- **EGD and colonoscopy:** Endoscopic evaluation is a cornerstone of the diagnostic and therapeutic management of GI bleeding. During EGD and colonoscopy, there are tools that gastroenterologists can employ to stop

various types of bleeding, such as clip placement, epinephrine injection, and thermal coagulation (using argon or bipolar current).

- If melena, hematemesis, or coffee-ground emesis are the chief complaint, this indicates an upper source. EGD is performed first to look for an upper GI source of bleeding and if this is unrevealing then a colonoscopy is done.

- **Prognosis** is dependent on endoscopic appearance. The Forrest Classification helps provide prognostic information on rebleeding risk (without intervention) in peptic ulcers based on their endoscopic appearance (see Table 13-11). Generally patients with Forrest Class 1 (A and B) and Class 2 (A and B) are monitored for several days post-endoscopy, even with intervention, due to high rates of rebleeding. Forrest Class 2 C and 3 are safely discharged home.

Table 13-11. Endoscopic Predictors of Recurrent Peptic Ulcer Hemorrhage (Forrest Class)

Forrest Class	Endoscopic Finding	Approximate Rebleeding Risk
1A	Active spurting vessel	90%
1B	Oozing	50%
2A	Visible vessel, not oozing	30%
2B	Adherent clot	20%
2C	Flat pigmented spot	8%
3	Clean base ulcer	5%

Common Question on Rounds:

What transfusion strategy do we utilize for someone presenting with a GI bleed?
We target a hemoglobin >7 g/dL (see High-Yield Literature box).

HIGH-YIELD LITERATURE

Transfusion goals in acute upper GI bleeding:

Villaneuva C, Coloma Abosch, A, et al. Transfusion strategies for acute upper gastrointestinal bleeding. *N Engl J Med.* 2013;368:11-21.

DIARRHEA

History and Associated Differential Diagnoses

The differential for diarrhea is broad, and a thorough history is key. When taking a history, it is helpful to categorize diarrhea in terms of **duration** and **stool character** to help narrow your differential diagnosis.

Duration

Acute diarrhea is defined as diarrhea lasting less than 2 weeks. The majority of acute diarrheal episodes are due to an infectious source and are self-limited.

The history is very important in helping narrow down the cause, and the most important aspects to ask about are:

- Signs of volume depletion:
  - Orthostatic hypotension, decreased skin turgor, lightheadedness.
  - These would likely require IV fluids +/– admission.
- Stool character: The volume, frequency, and, most importantly, the presence of blood in the stool can narrow the differential for the infectious case of the diarrhea:
  - Large-volume stool: Diarrhea originates from the small bowel.
  - Frequent, small-volume stool: Diarrhea originates from the large bowel.
  - Inflammatory signs (fever, bloody or mucoid stools) point to the following bacteria:
    - ***Campylobacter***: Association with Guillain–Barre syndrome.
    - *Yersinia*: Can mimic CD.
    - ***Shigella.***
    - ***Salmonella***: raw eggs, uncooked chicken.
    - **Enterohemorrhagic** *E. coli*: Shiga toxin–producing *E. coli* O157:H7, associated with hemolytic uremia syndrome.
- **Food history**: Type of food ingested can lead to a particular bacteria, and the timing of the onset of symptoms is helpful.
  - <6 hours: Suggests preformed toxin of *S. aureus* or *Bacillus cereus.*
  - 8 to 16 hours: Suggests *Clostridium perfringens.*
  - >16 hours: All other causes.
- Common infectious causes of acute diarrhea (<2 weeks) (most often an infectious source):
  - Common infections:
    - Noninvasive bacterial (nonbloody):
      - Enterotoxigenic *E. coli* (ETEC): Most common cause of traveler's diarrhea.
      - *S. aureus*: Quick onset, more vomiting than diarrhea, associated with mayonnaise.
      - *B. cereus*: Associated with reheated rice.
      - *C. perfringens.*
      - ***C. difficile.***
      - *Vibrio cholerae*: Spoiled shellfish.
    - Invasive bacterial (bloody):
      - ***Campylobacter***: Association with Guillain–Barre syndrome.
      - *Yersinia*: Can mimic CD.
      - ***Shigella.***
      - **Salmonella**: Raw eggs, uncooked chicken.
      - **Enterohemorrhagic** *E. coli*: Shiga toxin–producing *E. coli* O157:H7, associated with hemolytic uremia syndrome.
      - *Vibrio parahaemolyticus.*
    - Viral:
      - Affecting colon: CMV – in immunocompromised patient, adenovirus.
      - Rotavirus, norovirus (most common), small bowel.
    - Protozoa (can also be chronic).
      - *Giardia lamblia, Entamoeba histolytica*, cryptosporidium, microsporidium, *Cyclospora*, *Cystoisospora* (common in AIDS).

Chronic diarrhea (>4 weeks): The differential here is broader and will need to rely on more historical clues such as the stool character.

CONQUER THE WARDS!

Stool Osmotic Gap =

290 – 2 (Fecal Na + K)

- **Stool character**
- Inflammatory:
  - Mucosal irritation and inflammation with results in bloody stool or visible mucus
  - Examples: Invasive infection or IBD.
- Secretory:
  - Oversecretion of water by the small and large bowel.
  - Watery diarrhea that persists in times of fasting (waking up in middle of night).
  - Stool osmotic gap <50.
  - Examples: Noninvasive infections, neuroendocrine tumors (gastrinoma, VIPoma), hyperthyroidism, microscopic colitis, nonosmotic laxatives.
- Osmotic:
  - Ingestion of nonabsorbable solutes.
  - Watery diarrhea associated with meals.
  - Stool anion gap >100.
  - Examples: Lactose intolerance, osmotic laxatives.
- Malabsorptive:
  - Problem with digestion (i.e., lack of digestive enzymes) or transport (i.e., problem with small-bowel mucosa) of nutrients.
  - Associated with meals, similar to osmotic diarrhea.
  - Greasy, foul-smelling stools; steatorrhea; sometimes with visible oil droplets (signifying fat malabsorption).
  - Can get vitamin (A, D, E, K, B_{12}) or iron deficiency.
  - Examples and brief highlights:
    - **Celiac sprue**: Autoimmune condition affecting the small bowel triggered by gluten. Associated with dermatitis herpetiformis. Small-bowel biopsies will show atrophy and flattening of the villi. Treatment is a gluten-free diet or steroids in severe disease.
    - **Tropical sprue**: Similar to celiac (also has flattening of intestinal villi), its cause is unknown but thought to be from an infection endemic to the Caribbean. Associated with megaloblastic anemia (B_{12} deficiency). Treatment is vitamin B_{12} and folate supplementation in addition to tetracycline.
    - **Whipple disease**: Caused by *Tropheryma whippelii*, most often in white males, that can have multiorgan involvement (including the central nervous system). Small-bowel biopsies show PAS-positive macrophages in the laminal propria. Treatment is ceftriaxone IV followed by TMP-SMX.
    - **Protein-losing enteropathy:** Failure of plasma proteins (albumin and gamma globulin) to be reabsorbed and subsequently excreted from the GI tract. Associated with increased lymphatic pressure or lymphatic obstruction (such as CHF, cancer) or mucosal injury (IBD or celiac). Patients can develop anasarca from protein loss. Diagnose with A1AT levels in the stool. Treatment is targeted to the underlying cause.
    - **Chronic pancreatitis:** Discussed previously.
- **Pertinent past medical history**
  - Food intake prior to onset.
  - Sick contacts.
  - Travel history.
  - Any GI-related surgery.

- Medications.
- Recent antibiotic use.

Diagnostic Workup

Acute diarrhea doesn't necessarily require diagnostic workup if symptoms are mild. If symptoms are severe (fever or volume depletion or hospitalization), then workup is as follows:

- **Stool testing:** The first tests to send are stool WBC, bacterial culture, *C. difficile* stool testing, and ova and parasites, since the vast majority of acute diarrheal illnesses are infectious.

Chronic diarrhea workup starts with the same infectious workup as earlier. If that is negative, then additional testing based on the patient's presentation and history is warranted.

- **Stool electrolytes** to calculate the stool anion gap (290- 2(Fecal Na + K)).
- **Fecal fat measurements or fecal elastase** (both abnormal in pancreatic exocrine insufficiency).
- **Endoscopy for biopsies** of the small bowel and colon (needed to diagnose microscopic colitis, CMV, or IBD).

For celiac disease, the initial workup can show a positive anti-tissue transglutaminase IgA antibody (TTG-IgA), but small-bowel biopsies showing flattened villi confirm the diagnosis. Antigliadin and antiendomysial antibodies are also associated with celiac disease. Associated with HLA-DQ2/DQ8 (common in the general population, but if patients test negative for both haplotypes, this will rule out celiac disease).

CONQUER THE WARDS!

In patients with IgA deficiency, their TTG-IgA may be falsely negative and therefore doesn't rule out celiac disease.

The D-xylose test is rarely used in clinical practice, but it demonstrates important concepts in small-bowel malabsorption that are often tested on board exams. During the test, a patient is given D-xylose orally. D-xylose is a simple carbohydrate that requires small-bowel transport, but not digestive enzymes, to be absorbed. Therefore, if there are adequate amounts in the blood and urine, this demonstrates adequate small-bowel absorption. Low levels indicate a problem with small-bowel mucosal transport. A course of antibiotics can be given to treat for small intestinal bacterial overgrowth (SIBO), but if excretion is still not normal, think of malabsorption due to a luminal pathology such as celiac disease.

Management

Patients need to be assessed for dehydration and start oral or IV rehydration and electrolyte replacement depending on the severity of volume depletion. Patients may need inpatient evaluation if they are hypotensive, febrile, elderly, or appear ill. If patients are moderately to severely ill with a presumed infectious diarrhea, stool should be sent for culture and ova and parasites, with empiric treatment using a fluoroquinolone such as ciprofloxacin or azithromycin. Antimotility agents (loperamide) are an option in noninfectious diarrhea. Otherwise, the management depends on the etiology of the diarrhea. Pancreatic exocrine insufficiency is treated with pancreatic enzyme supplementation, IBD is treated with immunotherapy, and microscopic colitis is treated by avoiding culprit medications (PPI, NSAIDs) and budesonide or bismuth.

CHAPTER 14 NEPHROLOGY/ ACID–BASE DISORDERS

OVERVIEW OF HIGH-YIELD TOPICS IN NEPHROLOGY

ACUTE KIDNEY INJURY

General Facts

Definition: The Kidney Disease Improving Global Outcomes (KDIGO) definition of acute kidney injury (AKI):

- Increase in serum creatinine by ≥0.3 mg/dL within 48 hours.
- Increase in serum creatinine by ≥1.5 times baseline if known over 7 days.
- Urine volume <0.5 mL/kg/h for 6 hours (oliguria).

Etiology

Accurate diagnosis of all etiologies of AKI requires a thorough history and physical examination (Figure 14-1):

1. Pre-renal AKI.
2. Intrinsic renal AKI.
3. Postrenal AKI.

PRE-RENAL AKI

General Facts

- **Definition of pre-renal AKI**: AKI in which kidney glomerular and tubular functions remain intact but there is impaired *kidney perfusion.*
- **Causes of pre-renal AKI:**
  - Absolute decrease in blood volume.
    - Volume depletion.

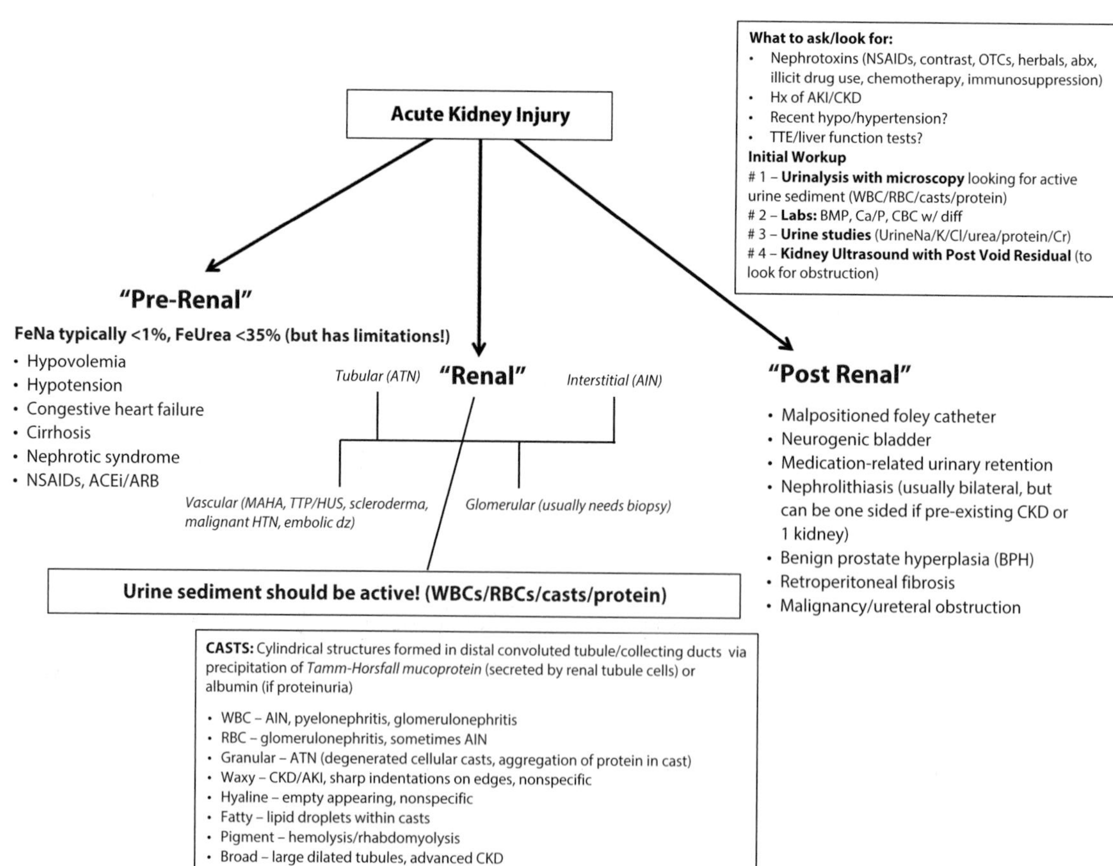

FIGURE 14-1. Differential Diagnosis for Acute Renal Failure

    - Gastrointestinal (GI) losses: Nausea, vomiting, diarrhea.
    - Kidney losses: Polyuria, diuretics.
  - Hemorrhage.
- Reductions in kidney perfusion due to edematous states.
  - Congestive heart failure (CHF) (cardiorenal syndrome [CRS]) – low-flow state.
  - Cirrhosis (hepatorenal syndrome [HRS]).
- Drugs that affect glomerular hemodynamics:
  - Decrease **afferent** arteriolar dilatation: Nonsteroidal antiinflammatory drugs (NSAIDs) or calcineurin inhibitors.
  - Decrease **efferent** arteriolar constriction: Angiotensin-converting enzyme (ACE) inhibitors or angiotensin receptor blockers (ARBs).

Diagnostic Workup

If the history and physical are consistent with a possible pre-renal AKI, the following labs should be obtained:

- **Basic metabolic panel:** In pre-renal states, look for aBUN: Cr ratio >20:1.
- **Urine sodium:** A urine sodium<20 mEq/L suggests a pre-renal state
- **Urine osmolality:** Urine osmolality >500 mOsm/kg or urine osmolality greater than plasma osmolality indicates a pre-renal state.
- **Calculate FeNa** (fractional excretion of sodium) or **FeUrea** (fractional excretion of urea).
  - **FeNa** is the most widely used but it is not accurate when patients are using diuretics. In those cases, you can use **FeUrea**. In addition, both the FeNa and FeUrea have several limitations and should be used with caution. To calculate the fractional excretion of Na or urea, use the following formula and substitute sodium or urea for X:

    (Urine X * Serum Creatinine) / (Urine Creatinine * Serum X) * 100%

  - **Interpretation of FeNa:**
    - <1% – pre-renal.
    - 1%–2% – pre-renal or acute tubular necrosis (ATN).
    - > 2% – ATN.
  - **Interpretation of FeUrea:**
    - <35% – pre-renal.
    - 35%–50% – pre-renal or ATN.
    - >50% – ATN.

Treatment

- All patients should have **intake and output** strictly monitored and **daily weights.**
- **Depends on etiology!**
  - **Hypovolemic**: Intravenous fluids. Find and reverse the underlying cause of hypovolemia. Pre-renal AKI reverses relatively quickly with fluids in hypovolemia. Prolonged pre-renal AKI can lead to tubular damage.
  - **CRS: Diuretics** relieve venous congestion to improve kidney perfusion and improve cardiac output if in cardiogenic shock. Sometimes dobutamine drips are used in these situations.
  - **HRS:** Some evidence for **midodrine** and **octreotide** to improve kidney perfusion and combat splanchnic vasodilation, though definitive treatment is liver transplant.

RENAL (INTRINSIC) AKI

General Facts

Definition of renal AKI: AKI in which there is injury to part of the kidney parenchyma.

Etiologyl

- Glomerular diseases: Nephritic and nephrotic syndromes (see Glomerular Disorders" section).
- Interstitial diseases: Acute interstitial nephritis.
  - Classically, described with presence of fever, rash, eosinophilia, and eosinophiluria but these features are not commonly seen.
  - Causes:
    - Autoimmune diseases: Sjögren disease, sarcoidosis.
    - Medications: β-lactam antibiotics, NSAIDs, proton pump inhibitors (PPIs)
- Tubular disease: ATN
  - Ischemic: Hypotension from any cause leads to impairment of kidney perfusion and tubular necrosis.
  - Sepsis: Mediated by both hypotension and inflammation and cytokine-induced injury.
  - Toxic (common causes):
    - **Contrast:** IV contrast for computed tomography (CT) scan and cardiac catheterization. **Note: Urine sodium can often be <20 mg/dL.**
    - **Antibiotics:** Aminoglycoside antibiotics, vancomycin commonly.
    - **Rhabdomyolysis:** Myoglobinuria (look for elevated creatine kinase levels).
    - **Severe hemolysis** causing hemoglobinuria.

Diagnostic Workup

- BUN: Cr ratio 10:1 or 15:1.
- Urine sodium >20 mEq/L or FeNa≥1% or FeUrea ≥35%.
- Urine sediment:
  Tubular injury: Muddy brown granular casts.
  Interstitial injury: White blood cells (WBCs), WBC casts.
  Glomerular injury: "Glomerular Disorders" section.

Treatment

- Remove the inciting agent or treat underlying cause (i.e., immunosuppressants if primary glomerular disease, antibiotics and volume repletion if septic and hypotensive, withdrawal of offending agent if suspicion for drug-induced acute interstitial nephritis [AIN]).

CONQUER THE BOARDS!

A patient is being treated for an infection with penicillin and now presents with acute kidney injury several days after the initiation of antibiotic therapy. The urine sediment reveals numerous white blood cells and white blood cell casts. *Think: Acute interstitial nephritis and stop the antibiotic.*

CONQUER THE WARDS!

Don't order a test to look for urine eosinophils to confirm acute interstitial nephritis (AIN), as this test has both low sensitivity and specificity.

CONQUER THE BOARDS!

Your patient is found down after several days and has acute kidney injury, hyperkalemia, and a markedly elevated creatinine kinase (CK) level. *Think: Rhabdomyolysis.*

POSTRENAL AKI

General Facts

Definition: AKI from the obstruction of urinary outflow tracts.

Clinical settings for postrenal AKI: Think anatomy. Urine flows from kidney to ureters to bladder then to urethra.

Ureter Obstruction

- Retroperitoneal fibrosis.

- Obstructing kidney stones. (With normal kidney function, AKI unlikely unless bilaterally obstructing stones. However, if kidney function is impaired at baseline, one-sided obstruction may lead to AKI, as contralateral kidney is unable to compensate).

Bladder

- Neurogenic bladder (i.e., diabetic nephropathy, paralysis, anticholinergics, antihistamines).
- Bladder, urologic, or cervical tumor.

Urethra

- Malpositioned Foley catheter.
- Benign prostatic hypertrophy (BPH), prostate cancer.

Diagnostic Workup

- **Physical exam**: Lower abdominal palpation to look for distended bladder.
- **Renal ultrasound** is the image of choice because of the speed of obtaining it. But CT scan is also reasonable, especially if nephrolithiasis is a concern and can better delineate masses.
- **Hyperkalemia** is common due to the development of a type 4 renal tubular acidosis (RTA) in postrenal AKI.

Treatment

- **Find the level of the obstruction and relieve it!**
  - **Foley:** If the obstruction is at the level of the bladder or distal to it, place a temporary Foley catheter until more definitive treatment can be done to remove the obstruction.
  - **Percutaneous nephrostomy** (cannulation of renal pelvis resulting in flow of urine directly from kidney into an external bag) if obstruction is above bladder or unable to bypass with Foley catheter.
- **Postobstructive diuresis:** After relief of the obstruction, look out for postobstructive diuresis (mild to severe polyuria).
  - Solute diuresis from urea in AKI and sodium thought to be due to tubular dysfunction and washout of the medullary gradient.
    - Replace urinary losses with 0.45% NaCl (half normal saline), as urine in postobstructive diuresis will be hypotonic.
    - Vital signs as well as chemistries should be checked often, as various electrolyte abnormalities may result (i.e., hyperNa, hypoK, hypoMg, hypoCa).

General Guidelines to Investigate the Etiology of Acute Kidney Injury

1. Thorough history and physical exam. Are there recent medication or toxin exposures or relevant family history? How is their oral intake? Do they have an infection?
2. Urinalysis with microscopy: Presence of cells or protein may lead to a diagnosis such as glomerular disease (nephritic or nephrotic syndrome), interstitial disease, or urinary tract infection.
3. Examine the urine sediment. Looking at the urine sediment under a microscope may reveal casts or cells that may help narrow down your differential diagnosis (i.e., muddy brown casts are seen in ATN).
4. Calculate the fractional excretion of sodium. What does this tell you about the patient's effective circulating volume? Try the FeUrea if the patient is on diuretics.

CONQUER THE WARDS!

Palpate the lower abdomen to look for a distended bladder on physical exam. A bedside ultrasound can also confirm the presence of a distended bladder and lead to a quick diagnosis of obstructive uropathy. Treatment is placement of a Foley catheter.

CONQUER THE WARDS!

High urine output after obstruction relief is described as postobstructive diuresis. Urine output should be replaced with hypotonic fluid to prevent volume depletion. Electrolytes should be monitored and replaced often.

5. If you suspect urinary obstruction, check a kidney ultrasound to look for hydronephrosis or dilation or the calyces.

GLOMERULAR DISORDERS

NEPHROTIC SYNDROME

General Facts

Definition: Constellation of the following symptoms:

- Proteinuria >3 to 3.5 g/day.
- Serum albumin <3.5 f/dL.
- Edema.
- Hyperlipidemia.

Pathophysiology

- Glomerular filtration barrier defect leads to increased glomerular permeability to albumin, resulting in proteinuria and loss of albumin (hypoalbuminemia).
- **Hypoalbuminemia** leads to decreased plasma oncotic pressure, resulting in **edema**.
- Nephrotic syndrome also causes increased kidney sodium retention in collecting tubules, which leads to **edema**.
- **Hyperlipidemia** from decreased oncotic pressure from loss of albumin leads to increased hepatic lipoprotein synthesis.
- **Hypercoagulability** due to loss of clotting factors (e.g., antithrombin and plasminogen).

Common Causes

Table 14-1 lists causes of nephrotic syndrome in order of prevalence in the adult population

Primary Causes Of Nephrotic Syndrome

- **Focal segmental glomerulosclerosis (FSGS):**
  - **Most common cause** of idiopathic nephrotic syndrome in adults.
  - **Histopathology:** Glomerular scarring involving limited portion of glomeruli (segmental involvement).
  - **Causes:**
    1. Primary (idiopathic) : Often acute in onset as opposed to secondary, which has a slower onset.
    2. Secondary:
       - Viruses : HIV (collapsing variant), cytomegalovirus (CMV), Epstein–Barr virus (EBV), parvovirus.

Table 14-1. Causes of Nephrotic Syndrome

Primary	Secondary
Focal segmental glomerulosclerosis	Diabetes mellitus
Membranous nephropathy (MN)	Amyloidosis
Minimal change disease (MCD)	Systemic lupus erythematosus
	Hepatitis B or C, HIV, syphilis
	Malignancy (MN: solid tumors; MCD: hematologic malignancies)

- Drugs/toxins: Heroin, interferon, bisphosphonates, lithium, tacrolimus.
- Glomerular hyperfiltration injury: Morbid obesity, single kidney.
- Rare genetic disorders.

- **Complications:** Can lead to hypertension (HTN) and end-stage renal disease **(ESRD).**
- **Treatment:**
  - Idiopathic (primary) FSGS may include corticosteroids or cytotoxic therapy, as well as ACE inhibitors or ARBs.
  - Secondary FSGS: Need to treat the underlying disease.

- **Membranous nephropathy:**
  - **Common cause** of nephrotic syndrome in adults.
  - **Histopathology:** Caused by subepithelial immune complex deposition.
  - **Causes:** Can be **primary** (idiopathic) or **secondary:**
    - **Primary** membranous cause is found to be associated with phospholipase receptor antibody (PLA2R antibody).
    - **Secondary** membranous cause can be associated with:
      - Systemic lupus erythematosus.
      - Infection: Hepatitis B and syphilis most commonly. Rarely with hepatitis C, HIV.
      - Malignancy: Most commonly solid tumors (prostate, lung, breast, bladder, GI tract).
      - Medications: Penicillamine, NSAIDs.
  - **Treatment** of primary disease may include immunosuppressive medications (steroids with cytotoxic medications) and treatment of secondary disease is of underlying cause.

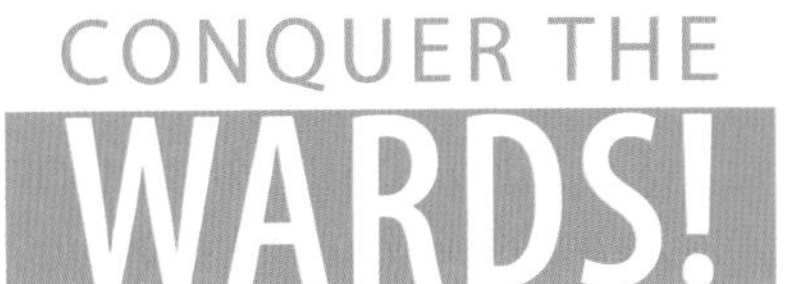

Rule of Thirds for membranous nephropathy prognosis:

One-third have spontaneous remission

One-third remain the same (do not progress or remit)

One-third progress to worsening chronic kidney disease

- **Minimal change disease** ("nil" disease, lipoid nephrosis):
  - **Most common cause of nephrotic syndrome in children** (80%).
  - Less common in adults (10% to 15% of idiopathic nephrotic syndrome).
  - **Histopathology:** Light microscopy is normal with "minimal change," but electron microscopy shows podocyte (subepithelial) foot process effacement.
  - **Treatment:** Often responds to steroid therapy; may need further immunosuppressives, including cytotoxics, in refractory or recurrent cases.
  - Less commonly progresses to advanced chronic kidney disease.

Secondary Causes of Nephrotic Syndrome

- **Diabetic nephropathy:** MOST COMMON secondary cause of nephrotic syndrome. Defined by the histopathology showing diffuse glomeruloscle. rosis and nodular glomerulosclerosis.
- **Amyloidosis:** Both AL (light chain) and AA (secondary amyloid from RA).
- Others: Lupus, infections (hepatitis B and C and HIV).

Diagnostic Workup

For all these patients a nephrology consult should be obtained to help tailor the workup, but following is a list of studies that should be considered.

- Random protein/creatinine ratio correlates closely with actual urine protein excretion.
- 24-hour urine for protein: Although the random protein/creatinine ratio is accurate, this is the gold standard.
- **Serologies:**
  - $HgbA_{1C}$.
  - Antinuclear antibodies (ANA).

- Complement (C_3 and C_4).
- Serum protein electrophoresis and urine protein electrophoresis.
- Hepatitis serologies, especially hepatitis B and C.
- HIV testing.
- Syphilis testing (rapid plasma reagin [RPR]).
- Cryoglobulins.

- **Kidney biopsy** will always be obtained in order to confirm the diagnosis. This is usually done by the nephrology consult service or, less commonly, by interventional radiology.

NEPHRITIC SYNDROME (GLOMERULONEPHRITIS)

General Facts

- Indicates glomerular inflammation and damage.

Clinical Features

- Hematuria (red blood cell [RBC] casts or dysmorphic RBCs) and/or mild proteinuria should raise suspicion for glomerulonephritis.
- AKI is often seen in glomerulonephritis, unlike nephrotic syndromes.
- Hypertension – acute onset or worsening of existing hypertension is seen in nephritic syndrome.

CONQUER THE BOARDS!

If a patient presents with hematuria immediately after an infection, think *IgA nephropathy*. If a patient presents 2 weeks after infection, think *postinfectious glomerulonephritis.*

Diagnostic Workup

- In general, the evaluation for etiologies of nephritic syndrome consists of serologies and lab tests that can help diagnose the following conditions.
- **Kidney biopsy** is ultimately necessary to make a definitive diagnosis.

Differential for Nephritic Syndrome

IgA Nephropathy (Berger Disease)

- **Most common** glomerulonephritis in the world.
- **Clinical presentations:** Often presents as gross hematuria with upper respiratory infection.
- **Histopathology:** On immunofluorescence: immune complex deposition of immunoglobulin A (IgA) in mesangial matrix ("mesangial hypercellularity").
- **Treatment:**
  - Conservative management with ACE inhibitors or ARBs in patients with normal kidney function and low-level proteinuria.
  - Corticosteroids in those with advancing kidney disease may be beneficial.

Postinfectious Glomerulonephritis

- Often associated with group A beta-hemolytic *Streptococcus* or *Staphylococcus* infection.
- **Clinical presentation:**
  - Presents 2 to 3 weeks after infection (e.g., pharyngitis or impetigo) with dark "coca-color" urine.
  - Usually reversible but occasionally progresses (children often have complete recovery).
- **Histopathology:** On immunofluorescence: granular immunoglobulin G (IgG) deposits, and on electron microscopy: subepithelial immune-complex deposits, or "humps," in basement membrane.
- **Clinical presentation:**

- Presents 2 to 3 weeks after infection (e.g., pharyngitis or impetigo) with dark "coca-color" urine
- Usually reversible but occasionally progresses (children often have complete recovery).

- **Workup:** Low complement levels; anti-streptolysin O (ASO) antibody titers can be helpful in diagnosis.
- **Treatment**:
  - Treat underlying infection.
  - Immunosuppressive drugs are ineffective.

Lupus Nephritis

- **Histopathology:**
  - **Endocapillary proliferation with immune complex depositions in subendothelial and mesangium.**
  - **Focal proliferative glomerulonephritis: <50% glomeruli involved.**
  - **Diffuse proliferative glomerulonephritis: >50% glomeruli involved.**
  - **Immunofluorescence: Involves all immunoglobulins and complements ("full house") immunostaining.**
- **Labs**: Low complements, positive ANA and anti-double-stranded DNA antibody.
- **Treatment: Steroid + cyclophosphamide or mycophenolate mofetil.**

Membranoproliferative Glomerulonephritis (MPGN)

- **Histopathology:** Deposition of immune complexes in **basement membrane**. Can see capillary walls with double contours (tram-track) appearance from interposition of mesangial cells into basement membrane.
- **Secondary** to hepatitis C or cryoglobulinemia, autoimmune disease, and monoclonal bone marrow disease.
- **Labs:** Low complement levels.
- **Treatment:** Treat the underlying disease.

Rapidly Progressive Glomerulonephritis (RPGN)

- Characterized by rapid decline in kidney function with nephritic syndrome (hematuria with RBC casts, proteinuria).
- With RPGN, often see crescents: proliferation of cells within Bowman capsule (include mononuclear phagocytes and glomerular epithelial cells).
- **Needs immediate diagnosis and treatment!**
- **Kidney prognosis of RPGN largely dependent on severity of kidney injury when treatment started.**

CONQUER THE **BOARDS!**

In 60% to 90% of patients, the anti-GBM Ab cross-reacts with pulmonary alveolar basement membranes—get both lung and kidney manifestations.

Classification of RPGN

Three categories of RPGN:

1. **Pauci-immune RPGN** (anti–neutrophil cytoplasmic antibody [ANCA]–associated vasculitis):
   - Most common cause of RPGN.
   - **Histopathology:** No immune complex deposits on biopsy.
   - **Labs: Positive ANCA** – serologic marker for pauci-immune RPGN associated with systemic small-vessel vasculitis.

- **Causes:**
  - Granulomatosis with polyangiitis (c-ANCA+).
  - Microscopic polyangiitis (p-ANCA+).
  - Eosinophilic granulomatosis with polyangiitis (Churg–Strauss) (negative ANCA or p-ANCA).
- **Treatment**: Steroids + cyclophosphamide or rituximab.

2. **Immune complex RPGN:**
   - **Histopathology:** Granular immune deposits on immunofluorescence.
   - **Causes:** Postinfectious glomerulonephritis, IgA nephropathy, MPGN, lupus nephritis, endocarditis.
   - **Lab: Low complement levels (except for IgA nephropathy).**
3. **Anti–glomerular basement membrane antibody (Ab) disease:**
   - **Histopathology:** Linear "ribbon-like" staining on immunofluorescence.
   - **Caused** by antibodies (usually IgG) against glomerular basement membrane.
   - **Ninety percent directed against the a-3 subunit of type IV collagen.**
   - **Goodpasture syndrome: Alveolar hemorrhage, glomerulonephritis, anti-GBM antibodies.**
   - **Treatment**: Steroids and cyclophosphamide, plasmapheresis.

CONQUER THE BOARDS!

Use **CAMPS** to remember the low-complement (C3, C4) kidney diseases:
Cryoglobulinemia (usually hepatitis C associated)
Atheroembolic disease
Membranoproliferative disorder
Postinfectious glomerulonephritis
Systemic lupus erythematosus (SLE)

Other Glomerular Diseases

- **Glomerular basement membrane diseases (often hereditary):**
  - Alport syndrome.
  - Thin basement membrane disease.

CHRONIC KIDNEY DISEASES

General Facts

Chronic kidney disease (CKD) can be staged by glomerular filtration rate (GFR) (see Table 14-2) or by proteinuria using the urine albumin–creatinine ratio (UACR) (see Table 14-3).

Etiology

- Often multifactorial!

Table 14-2. Staging by GFR

Stage	Glomerular Filtration Rate (GFR, cc/min/1.73 m^2)
1	≥90 with evidence of kidney damage (i.e., hematuria, proteinuria, genetic disease)
2	60–90 for more than 3 months
3A	45–59 for more than 3 months
3B	30–44 for more than 3 months
4	15–29 for more than 3 months
5/End-Stage Kidney Disease (ESKD)	<15 for more than 3 months

Table 14-3. Staging by Proteinuria

Stage	UACR
A1	**UACR <3 mg/g**
A2	**UACR 3–29 mg/g**
A3	**UACR >30 mg/g**

UACR, urine albumin–creatinine ratio.

CONQUER THE WARDS!

Anemia in patients with CKD is primarily due to erythropoietin deficiency and is treated to a target hemoglobin of 9 to 11 g/dL with erythropoiesis-stimulating agents (ESAs). Blood transfusions should be avoided in potential kidney transplant recipients to prevent antibody formation.

- **Diabetes mellitus and HTN** are the most common causes in the United States.
- Glomerular disease (nephritic and nephrotic syndromes; "Glomerular Disorders" section).
- Hepatorenal syndrome, cardiorenal syndrome.
- Tubulointerstitial diseases.
- Genetic diseases (i.e., polycystic kidney disease, Alport syndrome, variants of focal segmental glomerulosclerosis).
- Idiopathic.

Outpatient Management

- **Anemia:** Due to loss of erythropoietin, managed by monitoring and repletion of iron stores and erythropoiesis-stimulating agents (ESAs) when needed.
- **Secondary hyperparathyroidism:** See Hypocalcemia section.
- **Chronic metabolic acidosis:** Due to impaired proton excretion and ammoni agenesis. Oral bicarbonate supplementation to reach goal bicarbonate of >21 mg/dL to slow CKD progression and improve nutritional status and bone health.
- **Hyperkalemia:** As GFR decreases, urinary potassium excretion will decrease (this can be worsened by the use of ACE inhibitors and type 4 RTA in diabetic patients). Dietary restriction, loop diuretics, and kayexalate can be used to try to maintain normal potassium levels. Newer potassium-binding resins (i.e., patiromer) may also be used.

Treatment

- Unfortunately, limited options exist to slow progression of CKD. In addition to treatment of the underlying disease, ACE inhibitors may slow progression in patients with proteinuria, but watch for hyperkalemia as their CKD worsens.
- **Dietary modifications** may be helpful (decreased salt intake, limited protein intake in advanced CKD).
- **Preparation for kidney replacement therapy** (KRT) as GFR declines and drops below 20 cc/min/1.73 m^2 (this includes referral for kidney transplantation when appropriate, preparation for hemodialysis or peritoneal dialysis, or a plan for conservative management without renal replacement therapy [RRT]) (see Table 14-4).
- The decision to start RRT is not based on certain lab values. It is a clinical decision based on symptoms and labs. (See Table 14-5 on AEIOU for urgent indications for RRT.)

AUTOSOMAL DOMINANT POLYCYSTIC KIDNEY DISEASE

- Most often due to mutations in PKD1 (polycystin-1), less often PKD2. Those with PKD1 mutations will have faster progression to end-stage kidney disease (ESKD). Five percent of patients who initiate dialysis annually in the United States have underlying autosomal dominant polycystic kidney disease (ADPKD).
- Patients can present with flank pain or hematuria and are found to have enlarged kidneys and multiple cysts bilaterally (diagnostic criteria are

CONQUER THE WARDS!

Creatinine is mainly freely filtered by the glomerulus, with some secretion into the tubular lumen. Thus, it is used to estimate GFR (eGFR) but may be inaccurate if creatinine secretion is increased or decreased. Patients with low muscle mass will have an overestimation of GFR using creatinine, as their production of creatinine will be lower.

CONQUER THE WARDS!

Remember that GFR decreases exponentially with increases in creatinine. While an increase of the creatinine from 1 mg/dL to 2 mg/dL can represent a 50% decline in the GFR, an increase from 5 mg/dL to 6 mg/dL represents a very small change in the GFR.

CONQUER THE BOARDS!

Though chronic kidney disease often results in small, atrophic kidneys, large kidneys can be seen on kidney ultrasound in diabetic nephropathy, amyloidosis, polycystic kidney disease, and HIV-associated nephropathy (HIVAN).

Table 14-4. Kidney Replacement Therapies	
Kidney Replacement Therapy	**Features and Characteristics**
Hemodialysis (HD)	Can be performed as outpatient (in-center) three times/week or at home four to five times/week, requires vascular access (tunneled dialysis catheter or arteriovenous fistula/graft, which connects artery to vein). Treatment durations are typically 3–4 hours.
Continuous ambulatory peritoneal dialysis (CAPD) or **continuous Cycling peritoneal dialysis** (CCPD)	Performed at home using a PD catheter whose lumen rests in the peritoneal space. Hypertonic fluid is infused into the abdomen and then "urine" is manually drained after 4–6 hours or by an automatic cycler (the peritoneum serves as the dialysis). Fresh fluid is then again infused into the abdomen. Hypokalemia is common, and many patients have residual urine output.
Living or deceased donor kidney transplantation (LKT or DDKT)	In the United States, chronic kidney disease (CKD) patients can be placed on a waitlist for deceased donor kidney transplantation once the estimated glomerular filtration rate (eGFR) is less than 20 and they have completed the recipient evaluation. Thorough evaluations to assess potential kidney transplant recipients are done by kidney transplant centers.
Continuous renal replacement therapy (CRRT)	Performed in intensive care units, typically when the patient's hemodynamic status is tenuous. Modalities include continuous venovenous hemofiltration (CVVH), continuous venovenous hemodialysis (CVVHD), and continuous venovenous hemodiafiltration (CVVHDF).

CONQUER THE WARDS!

As CKD progresses, reductions in GFR dramatically impair clearance of insulin by the kidney. This may manifest as improved glycemic control.

Table 14-5. Indications for Urgent RRT

A-E-I-O-U

Acidosis (metabolic acidosis, refractory to medical therapy).

Electrolytes (most often potassium, refractory to medical therapy).

Ingestions (intoxication with a toxin that can be dialyzed, i.e., lithium, ethylene glycol, methanol, salicylates).

Overload (volume overload, refractory to diuretics).

Uremia (i.e., seizure, pericarditis, pruritus, altered mental status, uremic skin frost, metallic taste in mouth, anorexia, nausea/vomiting, platelet dysfunction).

CONQUER THE WARDS!

CKD patients may display isosthenuria, or the inability of the kidneys to concentrate urine. The urine specific gravity becomes fixed at 1.010.

based on age and the number of cysts or genetic testing). Family history is important!

- Other clinical manifestations include berry aneurysms (risk of subarachnoid hemorrhage), hepatic cysts, pancreatic cysts. and diverticula.
- Complications of polycystic kidneys are hypertension, recurrent urinary tract infections (UTIs), and kidney stones (calcium oxalate and uric acid stones).
- Treatment strategies include management of hypertension, adequate hydration, antidiuretic hormone (ADH) antagonists (i.e., tolvaptan) in select patients. A majority of patients will progress to ESKD and require dialysis and transplantation.

NEPHROLITHIASIS

General Facts

- **Definition**: Kidney and ureteral stones.
- Most are calcium-containing stones (80%), and stones tend to recur (15% at 1 year after first episode). Family history is also important! (see Table 14-6)

Table 14-6. Kidney stone types and features

Type of Stone	Shape	Unique Features or Risk Factors
Calcium oxalate	Envelope-shaped crystals or dumbbells (urine sediment)	1. Radiodense (seen on x-ray) 2. Associated with Inflammatory bowel disease (↑ oxalate reabsorption in bowel → increased calcium reabsorption) 3. Associated with hypercalcemia (primary hyperparathyroidism)
Calcium phosphate (less often than calcium oxalate)	Flat plates or rosettes (urine sediment)	High urine pH (>7) is a risk factor
Uric acid	Rhomboid or needle shaped (urine sediment)	1. Radiolucent (cannot see on x-ray) 2. Forms in low-pH urine (<5.5). 3. Risk factors: Gout, diabetes, and obesity
Struvite (**$MgNH_4PO_4$**)	Coffin lid shaped (urine sediment) "Staghorn calculi" (x-ray)	1. Common in *Klebsiella* or *Proteus* UTIs due to high urinary pH and urease. These bacteria *make urease* (cleaves urinary urea, yielding two molecules of ammonia, the conjugate base of ammonium).
Cystine	Hexagonal (urine sediment)	Pathognomonic for congenital cystinuria

UTI, urinary tract infection.

- Low fluid intake is a risk factor for ANY type of stone (warmer climate may also contribute).

Signs and Symptoms

- Severe, abrupt onset of colicky pain accompanied by nausea/vomiting that begins in the flank and may radiate toward the groin.
- Gross hematuria, urinary urgency may be present.
- If the stone is obstructing the collecting system, AKI and hydronephrosis may be present.

Diagnostic Workup

- **History:** The patient's presentation, prior history of kidney stones, and family history may help make the diagnosis of nephrolithiasis.
- **Urinalysis** may reveal the presence of hematuria (RBCs in the urine).
- **Radiographic studies:**
  - **Noncontrast abdominal CT** is the most sensitive, commonly used test to find small stones and hydronephrosis if present. This is first-line if you think the patient has a stone.
  - Plain abdominal film (kidney, ureter, bladder [KUB]) will reveal only radiopaque stones (not uric acid stones).
  - Kidney ultrasound can detect both stones and hydronephrosis if present (may miss small stones), so is usually not done if CT is available.

Treatment

In addition to pain control, the size of the stone and presence or absence of infection dictate further treatment.

- **Stones <10 mm should pass spontaneously**; alpha-blockers can be used to assist with passage of urine.
- **Stones >10 mm or patients with a UTI** should be referred for urologic evaluation. Options include decompression with a ureteral stent or percutaneous nephrostomy tube (for emergent decompression with sepsis due to UTI), extracorporeal shock wave lithotripsy (ESWL), or ureteroscopy.
- **Prevention:**
  - **Stone collection**, if possible, should be done and sent for composition analysis. Composition of the stone can help with preventive measures.
  - **24-hour urine collection** should be done in recurrent stone formers to look at urine volume and other parameters, including pH, calcium, citrate, and phosphate, as these results may also assist with preventive measures.

URINALYSIS INTERPRETATION

One of the most common tests to get in the hospital is a urinalysis. Table 14-7 lists information that will be helpful in interpreting a urinalysis. Urinalysis has 3 components:

Table 14-7. Interpretation of the Urinalysis

Finding	Significance
pH	In general, urine pH is variable. High urine pH (>7) may indicate urease-producing organisms (*Klebsiella, Proteus*) or type I renal tubular acidosis (RTA). Low urine pH (<5.5) may be present in type 4 RTA.
Specific gravity	High specific gravity (>1.010) may indicate hypovolemia and concentrated urine.
Protein	The urinalysis is more sensitive for albuminuria than other types of proteinuria (i.e., may not pick up immunoglobulins). Albuminuria suggests glomerular disease and podocyte injury. All types of proteinuria can be quantified with a 24-hour urine collection for protein, or a spot urine protein-to-creatinine ratio (UPCR) can be used.
Glucose	Glucosuria indicates either the presence of serum glucose >180 mg/dL or tubular dysfunction (i.e., proximal type 2 RTA).
"Blood"	Red or brown urine color will lead to a positive "blood" result and may indicate the presence of hemoglobin, myoglobin (rhabdomyolysis), red food (i.e., beets), or medications (i.e., rifampin). The presence of "blood" does NOT mean the presence of red blood cells (RBCs). If "blood" is detected, look at the microscopy results to see if RBCs are present.
Ketones	Ketonuria may be seen in diabetic/alcoholic/starvation ketoacidosis or isopropyl alcohol intoxication.
Nitrite	Presence indicates the possibility of nitrate-reducing bacteria (nitrate is reduced to nitrite).
Leukocyte esterase	Presence indicates white blood cells (pyuria, seen in acute interstitial nephritis or urinary tract infection).
Bilirubin	Indicates the presence of elevated bilirubin in the serum (i.e., liver disease, intravascular hemolysis).
Microscopic Examination	
Red blood cells	Hematuria (reported as cells seen per high power field) may indicate glomerulonephritis (if dysmorphic), tumor, trauma (e.g., due to Foley catheter), stones, kidney infarction, or malignant hypertension.
White blood cells	Pyuria (reported as cells seen per high power field) can be seen with urinary tract infection (UTI), acute interstitial nephritis ("sterile pyuria"), prostatitis, vaginitis.
Epithelial cells	Squamous epithelial cells (from the skin/urethra) or transitional epithelial cells (from the bladder) may be seen as a contaminant. The presence of renal tubular epithelial cells suggests acute tubular injury.
Casts	Urinary casts are formed in the distal convoluted tubule and the collecting duct via precipitation of Tamm–Horsfall protein secreted by the tubular cells. ■ RBC casts = possible nephritic syndrome and glomerulonephritis ■ White blood casts = possible acute interstitial nephritis (AIN) or UTI ■ Muddy brown granular casts = possible acute tubular necrosis (sepsis, hypoperfusion, vancomycin) ■ Hyaline casts: can be seen normally

1. Gross evaluation: Usually it will be reported as bloody, turbid, or cloudy. In general, whatever is seen grossly must correlate to rest of the urinalysis.
2. Urine dipstick.
3. Microscopic examination.

ACID–BASE DISORDERS

Understanding a patient's acid–base disorders can often provide important information about their clinical status and underlying diagnoses. Use the mnemonic pLACO to identify acid–base disturbances (Table 14-8).

General Principles

Before we get started on the mnemonic, a quick review of basic principles:

Chemistry 101: The Henderson–Hasselbach equation

$$HCO_3^- + H+ \rightarrow H_2CO_3^- \rightarrow H_2O + CO_2$$

$$pH = 6.1 + \log [(HCO_3)/(PCO_2 * 0.03)]$$

From this equation, **normal blood pH is calculated to be 7.4** and we can describe the four acid–base disorders:

- **Respiratory acidosis (acute or chronic):** Hypoventilation leads to increased CO_2.
  This shifts the equilibrium in the equation to the left, causing a rise in H^+ (and fall in pH) and a compensatory rise in bicarbonate (HCO_3^-).
- **Metabolic acidosis (gap or nongap):** An overall gain of acid and protons (H^+) causes a decrease in the pH. This shifts the equilibrium to the right, causing a fall in HCO_3^-.
- **Respiratory alkalosis (acute or chronic):** Hyperventilation leads to decreased CO_2.
  This shifts the equilibrium to the right, causing a fall in H^+ (thus a rise in pH) and a drop in HCO_3^-.
- **Metabolic Alkalosis:** An overall loss of protons causes the pH to rise. This shifts the equilibrium to the right, causing a rise in HCO_3^-.

Identify the Primary Acid–Base Disturbance (pLACO)

In order to identify the primary acid–base disturbance, you will need:

- **pH and CO_2** from an arterial blood gas **(ABG)**,which is obtained by drawing blood from the radial artery.
- **Serum bicarbonate** from a simple basic metabolic panel.

Table 14-8. Steps to Identify Acid–Base Disorders
p: Arterial pH <7.4 (acidemia) or pH >7.4 (alkalemia)
L: Labs
A: Anion gap
C: Compensation
O: Other process and osmolality

CONQUER THE WARDS!

Always look at a patient's albumin prior to calculating anion gap and correct a normal anion gap for the patient's serum albumin. For example , if the albumin is 2 g/L (normal is 3.5 to 5.0), the patient's normal anion gap is 5. If the albumin is normal, assume the anion gap is near 10.

Normal arterial pH is 7.4. If the pH is <7.4, or acidemic, the primary disorder is likely an acidosis. If the pH is >7.4, or alkalemic, the primary disorder is likely an alkalosis.

Often because ABGs require a physician to draw from the radial artery, patients will have venous blood gases drawn by nurses.

- In order to convert a venous pH to an arterial pH, add 0.04 to the venous pH.
- To estimate the arterial PCO_2, subtract 5 from the venous PCO_2.

Next, the PCO_2 and HCO_3 levels allow us to identify the primary disturbance. For example, a pH of 7.2 and a low serum bicarbonate level indicate a primary metabolic acidosis (Table 14-9).

Always Calculate the Anion Gap (pLACO)

The anion gap tells us about circulating anions that are not accounted for in the following equation:

$$\text{Anion gap} = \text{Major cations} - \text{Major anions} = [Na^+] - [Cl^-] - [HCO_3]$$

A patient's normal AG is determined by his or her serum albumin, the other major anion not included in the equation. The normal anion gap = (serum albumin)× 2.5. **For a patient with normal serum albumin, the normal AG is around 10.**

CONQUER THE BOARDS!

A high or elevated anion gap indicates the presence of additional circulating anions. These circulating anions consume bicarbonate and lead to anion gap metabolic acidosis (AGMA). For example, a patient with methanol poisoning develops an AGMA due to the metabolism of methanol to formic acid.

Elevated Anion Gap Acidosis

Table 14-10 lists the causes of an elevated anion gap. Another clue is to calculate **the osmolal gap**, which should be between 6 and 10 mOsmol/kg.

$$\text{Osmolal gap} = \text{Measured serum osmolality (from lab)} - \text{Calculated osmolality}$$

$$\text{Calculated serum osmolality} = 2{*}Na + BUN/2.8 + Glucose/18$$

High osmolal gap: If the osmolal gap is greater than 10, think glycols or methanol. Other iatrogenic causes are mannitol, glycine-based irrigants used in urologic surgery, or IV immunoglobulins.

Nongap Metabolic Acidosis

Nongap metabolic acidosis is caused by either GI or kidney losses. Use the **urine anion gap (UAG)** to distinguish between bicarbonate loss from the kidney (usually from RTA) or GI tract.

$$UAG = \text{urine } Na^+ + \text{urine } K^+ - \text{urine } Cl^-$$

Table 14-9. Acidosis vs Alkalosis

Primary Disorder	pH (Normal = 7.4)	PCO_2 (Normal = 35–45 mm Hg)	HCO_3 (Normal = 21–27 mEq/L)
Metabolic acidosis	↓	↓	↓
Respiratory acidosis	↓	↑	↑
Metabolic alkalosis	↑	↑	↑
Respiratory alkalosis	↑	↓	↓

Table 14-10. Etiologies of Anion Gap Metabolic Acidosis (GOLDMARK)

Cause	Acid	Notes
Glycols	Ethylene glycol: oxalic/glycolic acid Propylene glycol:lactic acid	Look for history of ingestion and an **elevated osmolal gap**!
Oxoproline	Oxoprolic acid	Chronic acetaminophen use
Lactate	Lactic acid	Elevated serum lactate due to hypoperfusion (type A) or impaired cellular metabolic/ischemia (type B)
D-Lactate	Lactic acid	Short bowel syndrome, gastrointestinal malabsorption
Methanol	Formic acid	**Elevated osmolal gap**, vision changes
Aspirin	Salicylic acid	AGMA and respiratory alkalosis
Kidney disease	Organic acids (sulfuric, phosphoric)	Elevated serum creatinine/BUN
Ketoacidosis	Acetoacetic/β-hydroxybutyric acid	Diabetic, alcoholic, or starvation-related ketoacidosis

AGMA, anion gap metabolic acidosis; *BUN*, blood urea nitrogen.

Table 14-11. Acid-Base Disorders

Primary Disturbance	How to Calculate Expected pCO_2 or HCO_3
Metabolic acidosis	Winter formula: Expected pCO_2, (within 2 mm Hg) = **1.5 * (HCO_3^-) + 8**
Metabolic alkalosis	For every ↑ in HCO_3 by 1, expected ↑ CO_2 by 0.06
Respiratory acidosis	**Acute (<2–3 days) : For** every 10 ↑ in CO_2, expected ↑ in HCO_3 by 1 **Chronic:** For every 10 ↑ in CO_2 expected ↑ in HCO_3 by 3
Respiratory alkalosis	**Acute (<2–3 days) :** For every ↓ in CO_2 by 10, **expected** ↓ in HCO_3 by 2 **Chronic:** For every ↓ in CO_2 by 10, expected ↓ in HCO_3 by 4

If the **UAG is positive**, think RTA. See later.
If the **UAG is neGUTive**, think GI or GUT losses.

Compensation (pLACO)

The body attempts to compensate for any primary acid–base disturbance. For metabolic disorders, compensation formulas will provide the expected pCO_2 if compensation has been achieved. Similar formulas for respiratory disorders will provide the expected HCO_3. Compensation formulas for all acid–base disturbances are listed in Table 14-11.

Look for a Third, or "Other," Disturbance and Check the Osmolal Gap (pLACO)

Up to 3 acid–base disturbances can be present at one time: 2 metabolic and 1 respiratory (we can only breathe rapidly or slowly). When an anion gap metabolic acidosis is present, we can use the "delta/delta" to uncover a second metabolic process that may be masked.

Delta/Delta

This means change, so look to see if the change in the serum bicarbonate is accounted for by the change in the anion gap, as each increase in the anion gap should consume 1 bicarbonate.

CONQUER THE WARDS!

When a metabolic acidosis is present, use the Winter formula to determine if respiratory compensation is present: **expected pCO_2 (within 2 mm Hg)** = 1.5 * (HCO_3^-) + 8. If the expected pCO_2 = 55 mm HG and the patient's pCO_2 is 40 mm Hg (less than the expected pCO_2), the patient has a metabolic acidosis and a respiratory alkalosis.

CONQUER THE WARDS!

Respiratory compensation, achieved by hyperventilation or hypoventilation, is fast and may occur in a matter of minutes. Metabolic compensation, achieved by the changes in bicarbonate reabsorption or generation by the kidney, is slower and can take 2 to 3 days. **If there is not appropriate compensation, there is a second acid–base disturbance. It is impossible to overcompensate or undercompensate.**

- **The delta/delta is actually the ratio between the change in the anion gap and the change in the bicarbonate (ΔAG/Δbicarbonate).**
- **ΔAG/Δbicarbonate = (patient's AG – normal AG) / (24 mEq/L – patient's bicarbonate).**
- If the ratio is near 1, then there is only one metabolic process: an anion gap metabolic acidosis.
- If the ratio is >2, the denominator (**Δbicarbonate)** is smaller than it should be. A second metabolic process is increasing the patient's bicarbonate, and this process is a **metabolic alkalosis.**
- If the ratio is <1, the denominator is larger than it should be. A second metabolic process is decreasing the patient's bicarbonate, and this is a **non–anion gap metabolic acidosis.**

CONQUER THE WARDS!

Type 3 RTA exists, but so rarely seen it is almost never discussed. It is a combination of type 1 and 2 in kids that is never seen now and in a rare inherited carbonic anhydrase II deficiency.

Putting It All Together

pLACO:

1. p: Is the pH acidemic or alkalemic?
2. L: Check the labs (HCO_3 and pCO_2). What is the primary acid–base disturbance?
3. A: Calculate the anion gap (Na – Cl – HCO_3). Is it elevated compared to the normal anion gap? The normal anion gap is near 10 if the albumin is normal.
4. C: Compensation. Choose the formula based on the primary disturbance and calculate the expected HCO_3 or pCO_2. Is there a second disorder?
5. O: Other and Osmolality. If there is an anion gap metabolic acidosis, calculate the "delta/delta." If it's not 1, what is the additional metabolic disorder (>2: metabolic alkalosis, <1: non–anion gap metabolic acidosis)?

Etiologies of Renal Tubular Acidosis

In a patient with a nongap metabolic acidosis and positive urine anion gap, you'll want to think about an RTA. Table 14-12 summarizes the 3 types.

Etiologies of Metabolic Alkalosis

- Causes of metabolic alkalosis can be differentiated based on the patient's volume status, urine chloride, and plasma renin activity (PRA).

Table 14-12. Types of Renal Tubular Acidosis (RTA)

Feature	Type 1 RTA	Type 2 RTA	Type 4 RTA
Problem	Impaired distal acidification	Proximal tubular bicarbonate wasting	True or pseudo hypoaldosteronism
Causes	**Autoimmune:** SLE, rheumatoid arthritis, Sjögren syndrome **Medications:** Lithium, amphotericin, topiramate	Multiple myeloma, heavy metals **Medications:** Tenofovir, cisplatin, acetazolamide, aminoglycosides	Diabetic nephropathy, obstructive uropathy **Medications:** ACEi, ARB, heparin, NSAIDs, spironolactone
Tubular cells involved	Type A intercalating cell (collecting duct)	Proximal tubular cells	Principal cell, type A intercalating cell (collecting duct)
Potassium	Low	Low to normal	High
Urine pH	>5.5	Variable	<5.5
Other features	Nephrolithiasis	Fanconi syndrome: Urinary wasting of HCO_3, K, glucose, phosphate, LMW proteins, citrate, uric acid	

ACEi, angiotensin-converting enzyme inhibitor; *ARB*, angiotensin receptor blocker; *LMW*, low molecular weight; *NSAID*, nonsteroidal antiinflammatory drug; *SLE*, systemic lupus erythematosus.

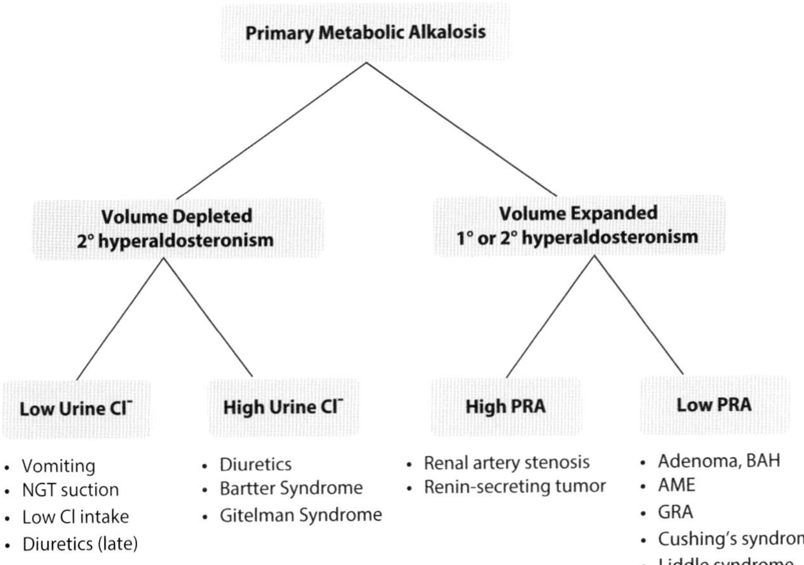

FIGURE 14-2. Differential Diagnosis of Primary Metabolic Alkalosis

- Other than chronic alkali ingestion, **all forms of metabolic alkalosis are states of hyperaldosteronism, as the action of aldosterone leads to expansion of effective circulating volume (ECV), urinary potassium loss, and reabsorption of bicarbonate.**
- Chronic or overingestion of antacids, milk, or bicarbonate tablets can also lead to metabolic alkalosis. Figure 14-2 summarizes the different etiologies (AME = apparent mineralocorticoid excess, seen with licorice ingestion; BAH = bilateral adrenal hyperplasia; NGT = nasogastric tube).
- The release of aldosterone can be in response to elevated renin levels (high PRA) or independent of renin (low PRA). Under normal conditions, renin secretion by the juxtaglomerular (JG) apparatus cells leads to convert angiotensinogen to angiotensin I and ultimately angiotensin II. Angiotensin II stimulates the release of aldosterone from the adrenal cortex and leads to systemic vasoconstriction.

Etiologies of Respiratory disturbances

Respiratory Acidosis: Decreased Minute Ventilation

- **Primary pulmonary diseases:**
  - Chronic obstructive pulmonary disease (COPD).
  - Alveolar infiltrates, most commonly PNA.
  - Pulmonary edema.
  - Restrictive lung disease.
  - Airway obstruction (foreign body, severe bronchospasm, laryngospasm)
  - Pneumothorax, flail chest.
- **Muscle and nervous system disorders**: Usually due to respiratory muscle weakness:
  - Myasthenia gravis (MG).
  - Muscular dystrophy.
  - Guillain–Barré syndrome.
  - Botulism, tetanus, organophosphate poisoning.
- **Decreased respiratory drive** (narcotic overdose, anesthesia, increased intracranial pressure).

CONQUER THE WARDS!

Respiratory disturbances are alterations in **minute ventilation (MV) = respiratory rate (RR) * tidal volume (TV).** If MV is increased or decreased, it is likely an increase or decrease in RR, TV, or both. For example, increased RR in anxiety leads to a respiratory alkalosis, while decreased TV in chronic obstructive pulmonary disease (COPD) leads to a respiratory acidosis.

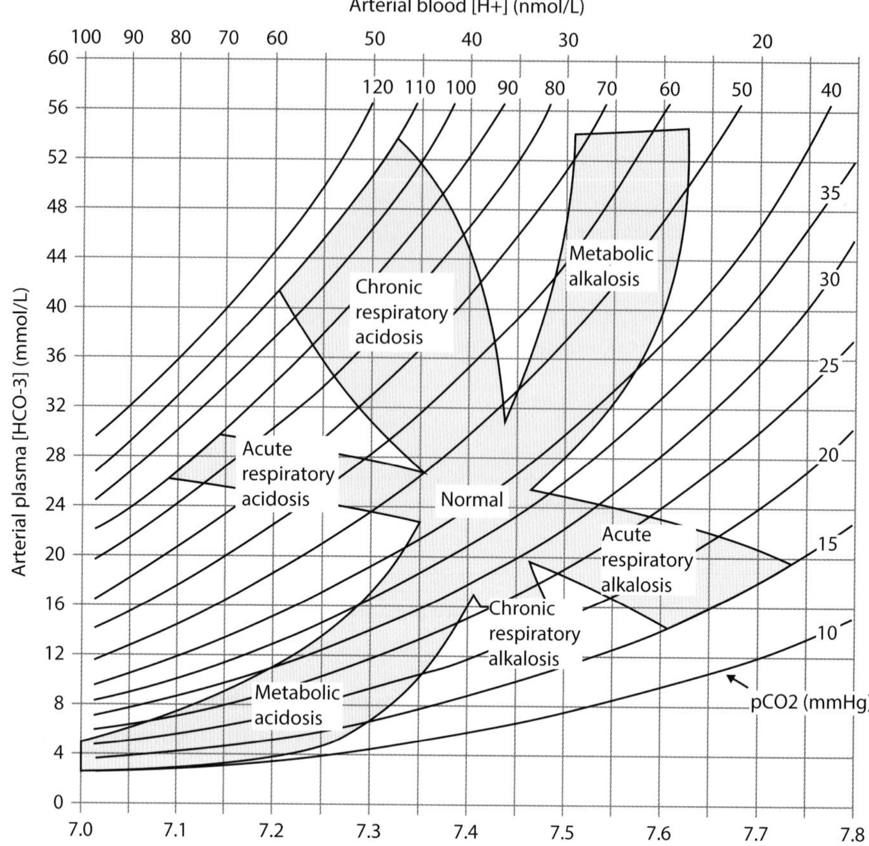

FIGURE 14-3. Acid-Base Disorders. (Used, with permission, from DuBose TD Jr: Acid-Base Disorders, in *Brenner and Rector's The Kidney*, 10th ed, Skorecki K, Chertow GM, Marsden PA, Taal MW, Yu ASL [eds]. Philadelphia: Saunders, 2016, p. 522.)

Respiratory Alkalosis: Increased Minute Ventilation

- Anxiety.
- Salicylates.
- **Infection:** Sepsis of any cause and often in patients with a pulmonary infection.
- Cerebrovascular accident (CVA).
- Pregnancy.
- Hyperthyroidism.

Finally, the acid–base nomogram (Figure 14-3) derived from the Henderson–Hasselbach equation can be helpful for identifying acid–base disturbances using the pH, bicarbonate, and pCO_2.

HYPOCALCEMIA

General Facts

- **Definition:** Low ionized calcium (<1.2 mmol/L) or serum calcium <8.5 mg/dL(after correction for albumin).
- **Correction for albumin:**
  - **For every decrease in serum albumin of 1.0 g/dL,** 0.8 mg/dL should be added to the serum calcium. For example, if the serum calcium is 8.0

mg/dL and the albumin is 3.0 g/dL (assume a normal albumin of 4.0 g/dL), then the corrected calcium is 8.0 + 0.8, or 8.8 mg/dL.
- For every **increase** in serum albumin of 1.0 g/dL, 0.8 mg/dL should be subtracted from serum calcium.
- Albumin is negatively charged and thus binds the positively charged calcium. Lower albumin levels result in higher unbound or free calcium levels, which is the most active form for calcium.

Etiology

- With calcium disorders, **think first about the parathyroid hormone (PTH)** and **1,25 OH**, which is **vitamin D (calcitriol, or activated vitamin D)**, as both help to maintain calcium homeostasis (See figure 14-4).
- **PTH** helps to **release calcium and phosphate from the bone and increases urinary absorption of calcium and excretion of phosphate**.
  - Stimulated by low free calcium and inhibited by increased free calcium levels.
  - Stimulates conversion of 25-OH vitamin D (calcidiol) to 1,25 dihydroxy vitamin D (calcitriol, activated vitamin D) in the kidney by 1 a-hydroxylase.
- **1,25 OH: vitamin D (calcitriol, or activated vitamin D) increases intestinal calcium absorption.**
- Following are some causes of hypocalcemia:
  - **Vitamin D deficiency** (intestinal malabsorption, cholestyramine, primidone, chronic kidney disease).
  - **Pseudohypoparathyroidism** (Albright's hereditary osteodystrophy) is end-organ resistance to PTH due to a defective PTH receptor.
  - **Toxins**: Fluoride, cimetidine, ethanol, citrate, phenytoin.
  - **Pancreatitis** (due to calcium deposition in an inflamed pancreas).
  - **Rhabdomyolysis, tumor lysis syndrome** (increased phosphate levels lead to formation of calcium–phosphate complexes, which decrease serum calcium levels).

CONQUER THE WARDS!

Secondary Hyperparathyroidism: Chronic kidney disease (CKD) can result in impaired conversion of calcidiol to calcitriol by the kidney, hypocalcemia, and ultimately elevated parathyroid levels. Increased phosphate levels in CKD (due to impaired urinary excretion) also drive release of parathyroid hormone (PTH). Elevated fibroblast growth factor-23 (FGF-23) in CKD patients also contributes to decreased calcitriol levels. This combination of hypocalcemia, hyperphosphatemia, and elevated PTH levels in patients with CKD is referred to as secondary hyperparathyroidism. Bone disease (i.e., osteomalacia, osteitis fibrosa cystica) can result in chronic bone turnover due to the persistent action of PTH. Adynamic bone disease (low bone turnover) may result if treatment leads to oversuppression of PTH.

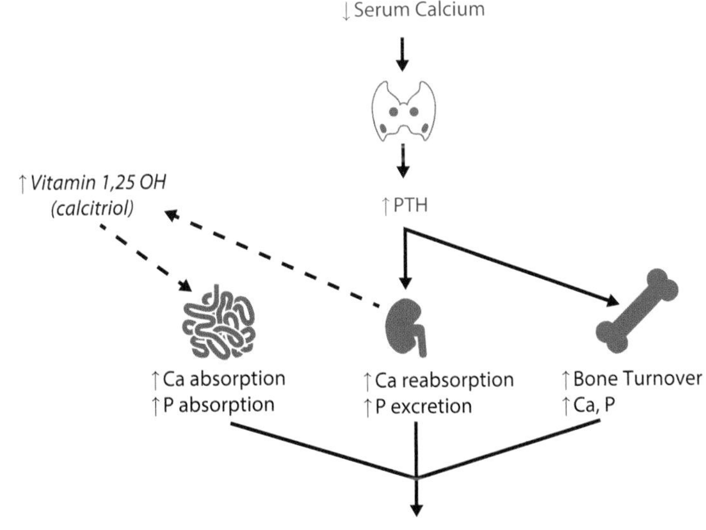

FIGURE 14-4. " Calcium Regulation" (Used, with permission, from DuBose TD Jr: Acid-base disorders, in *Brenner and Rector's The Kidney*, 10th ed, Skorecki K, Chertow GM, Marsden PA, Taal MW, Yu TD [eds]. Philadelphia: Saunders, 2016, p. 522.)

CONQUER THE WARDS!

Neck surgery, even long after the procedure, can be associated with postoperative hypoparathyroidism, usually due to ischemia of the parathyroid glands.

- **Severe magnesium deficiency** (magnesium is required for PTH secretion)
- **CKD** (secondary hyperparathyroidism).

Signs and Symptoms

- Circumoral paresthesia is usually the first symptom, followed by muscular tetany, which may be observed by looking for Chvostek and Trousseau signs:
  - **Chvostek sign:** Facial muscle spasm with tapping of the facial nerve.
  - **Trousseau sign:** Carpal spasm after occluding blood flow in forearm with blood pressure cuff.
- Acute, severe hypocalcemia may cause laryngospasm, seizures, confusion, or cardiovascular collapse with bradycardia and decompensated heart failure.

Diagnosis

- Clues to diagnosis can be provided by careful bedside evaluation: Evidence of prior neck surgery; evaluation of medications and medical history; and detailed family history looking for cases of hypocalcemia, hypoparathyroidism, or pseudohypoparathyroidism see table 14-3.
- Electrocardiogram (ECG) findings: Prolonged QT and ST intervals (peaked T waves are also possible, as in hyperkalemia).

Treatment

- **Symptomatic hypocalcemia:** Regardless of the etiology, IV hypocalcemia should be given.

CONQUER THE WARDS!

Tertiary Hyperparathyroidism: If CKD patients with secondary hyperparathyroidism develop hypercalcemia, it is called *tertiary* hyperparathyroidism and may require surgical removal of the parathyroid glands. This is caused by chronic low calcium causing severe hyperplasia of the parathyroid glands, and this leads to decreased responsiveness of the glands to high calcium.

Table 14-13. Main Etiologies of Hypercalcemia

PTH Mediated	Calcitriol Mediated	Non-PTH Mediated
1. Primary hyperparathyroidism* 2. Tertiary hyperparathyroidism 3. Zollinger–Ellison syndrome with MEN1 4. Ectopic PTH secretion (rare) 5. Lithium use	1. Excess vitamin D intake 2. Granulomatous disease: • Sarcoidosis • TB (increased 1-β hydroxylase activity) • Coccidioidomycosis	1. Multiple myeloma 2. PTH-related protein mediated** 3. Osteolytic metastases** 4. Increased bone turnover due to immobilization, hyperthyroidism 5. Excess intake or supplementation of calcium 6. Medications (most common) • Thiazides (increased urinary absorption) • Theophylline 7. Adrenal insufficiency

MEN, multiple endocrine neoplasia; *PTH*, parathyroid hormone; *TB*, tuberculosis.

*** Primary hyperparathyroidism:**

- May occur in conjunction with MEN 1 or 2A (all glands are hyperplastic) or in the setting of parathyroid adenoma.
- Usual presentation is asymptomatic hypercalcemia and hypophosphatemia (due to increased urinary excretion) noted on routine laboratory examination.

****Malignancy and hypercalcemia:**

- **Humoral hypercalcemia of malignancy:** Tumor production of PTH-related peptide (PTH-RP). PTH-RP is not detected by the usual PTH immunoassay, but has similar actions to endogenous PTH.
- **Local osteolytic hypercalcemia:** Malignant cells in multiple myeloma or solid tumors with bone metastases may cause osteoclast stimulation. Osteoclast-activating factors (OAFs) include RANK-ligand interleukins, transforming growth factors, and other cytokines.

CONQUER THE BOARDS!

Primary hyperparathyroidism (autonomous secretion of PTH by a parathyroid adenoma or due to parathyroid hyperplasia) is the most common cause of hypercalcemia in the outpatient setting. Malignancy is the most common cause in the inpatient setting (look for more severe hypercalcemia, usually greater than 13 mg/dL).

CONQUER THE WARDS!

Acute pancreatitis can be precipitated by hypercalcemia.

- **Asymptomatic hypocalcemia:**
  - For PTH deficiency:
    - Replacement therapy with calcidiol or calcitriol.
    - High oral calcium intake.
    - Thiazide diuretics are used to enhance urinary calcium reabsorption and prevent calcium-containing kidney stones.
  - Repletion of magnesium for hypomagnesemia
- For secondary hyperparathyroidism and CKD:
  - Calcidiol and calcitriol supplementation.
  - Calcium supplementation.
  - Dietary phosphate restriction.
  - Enteric phosphate binders.

HYPERCALCEMIA

General Facts

- **Definition:** Defined as high ionized calcium (>1.3 mmol/L) or high serum calcium >10.4 mg/dL (after correction for albumin) (see Table 14-13).

Etiology

- **Think first about the PTH** and **1,25 OH**, **vitamin D (calcitriol, or activated vitamin D)**, as both help to maintain calcium homeostasis.
- Main etiologies of hypercalcemia.
- Causes of hypercalcemia: **CHIMPANZEES**
  - **C**alcium supplementation.
  - **H**yperparathyroidism/**H**yperthyroidism.
  - **I**mmobility/**I**atrogenic.
  - **M**etastasis/**M**ilk alkali syndrome.
  - **P**aget disease.
  - **A**ddison disease/**A**cromegaly.
  - **N**eoplasm.
  - **Z**ollinger–Ellison syndrome.
  - **E**xcessive vitamin A.
  - **E**xcessive vitamin D.
  - **S**arcoidosis.

Signs and Symptoms

- Signs of volume depletion: Hypercalcemia-nduced nephrogenic diabetes insipidus (resistance to ADH) contributes to volume depletion.
- ECG findings: QT interval shortening and varying degrees of atrioventricular (AV) block.

Treatment

- **Isotonic fluids are first-line treatment.** If the patient develops signs of overload, **loop diuretics** can be given with volume repletion, but the first line of therapy is volume repletion!
- **Calcitonin** and **bisphosphonates** are used after intravenous fluids (IVF). They both inhibit osteoclasts.
- **Dialysis** can remove calcium in cases of severe or refractory hypercalcemia.

CONQUER THE WARDS!

Denosumab, a RANK-ligand and osteoclast inhibitor, can be used for the treatment of refractory hypercalcemia of malignancy.

CONQUER THE WARDS!

Classic signs of hypercalcemia: "Moans, bones, stones, groans, thrones" = mental status changes/ depression, bone pain, kidney stones, constipation, polyuria

CONQUER THE WARDS!

Hungry bone syndrome is the rapid transfer of calcium and phosphate into bones following removal of a hyperactive parathyroid nodule or parathyroid glands and can result in severe hypocalcemia.

CONQUER THE WARDS!

Phosphate is especially important for weaning patients off ventilators, since the diaphragm requires a lot of adenosine triphosphate (ATP) for energy.

- **Parathyroidectomy** is possible in cases of primary hyperparathyroidism. When surgery is not possible, cinacalcet (a "calcimimetic," which binds the calcium-sensing receptor) may be used to try to suppress PTH secretion.

HYPONATREMIA

General Facts

- Hyponatremia is a commonly seen disorder that requires prompt recognition and meticulous management to prevent neurologic sequelae. Hyponatremia is defined as a plasma Na^+ concentration <135 mEq/L.
- Hyponatremia occurs when there is an excess of water in relation to solute due to:
  - Most often: Inability to excrete water.
  - Less commonly: Excess water Ingestion.
  - Excretion of water is regulated by the activity of ADH. Thus, most commonly hyponatremia is the result of activity of ADH. ADH release leads to increased water reabsorption via aquaporin 2 (AQP2) in the distal nephron. ADH secretion may be "appropriate" (e.g., decreased effective circulating volume) or "inappropriate" (e.g., syndrome of inappropriate ADH [SIADH]).

Clinical Features

Usually more severe with acute hyponatremia (onset within 24 to 48 hours) or when Na drops below 120 mEq/L in chronic hyponatremia.

Symptoms of Acute Hyponatremia

- Earliest symptoms (Na between 125 and 130 mEq/L):
  - Nausea.
  - Malaise.
- Severe symptoms (Na drops below 120 mEq/L):
  - Fatigue, lethargy, obtundation, cerebral edema, seizures.
  - Coma **(most dreaded consequence of cerebral edema is cerebral herniation).**

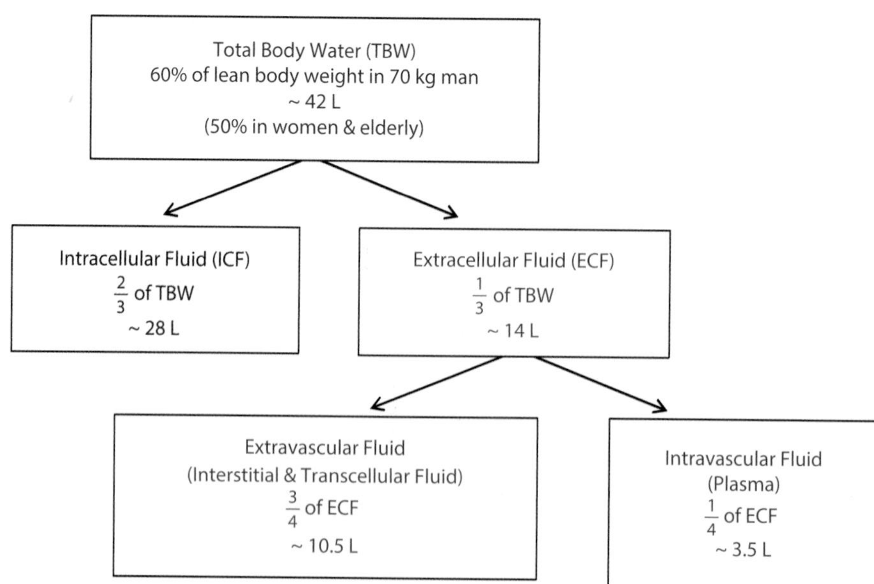

FIGURE 14-5. Body fluid compartments.

Symptoms of chronic hyponatremia include fatigue, memory loss, and falls.

Pathophysiology

- **ADH is often the driver of hyponatremia.** When ADH is present, aquaporins are inserted into the collecting duct of the nephron and allow for water reabsorption.
  - Stimuli for ADH release from the posterior pituitary are **high osmolality and low ECV.**
  - For the collecting duct to excrete water, ADH must be suppressed and solute must be delivered to the tubules.
- **Important terminology:**
  - **Tonicity** is a measure of only **effective** osmoles (mostly sodium salts). Effective osmoles cannot cross the semipermeable membrane and thus pull water via solute drag.
  - **Osmolality** measures both **effective** and **ineffective** osmoles (i.e., alcohols, urea that can cross the membrane freely).
  - Most hyponatremia is hypo-osmolar AND hypotonic. If osmolality is normal or high in a hyponatremia patient, look for additional osmoles.

CONQUER THE BOARDS!

Remember that tonicity is a measure of only effective osmoles (cannot cross semipermeable membrane and thus pull water via solute drag), whereas osmolality measures both effective and ineffective osmoles (i.e., alcohols, urea that can cross the membrane freely). Most hyponatremia is hypo-osmolar AND hypotonic. If osmolality is normal or high in a hyponatremia patient, look for additional osmoles!

Etiology and Classification

Hypo-Osmolar Hyponatremia (*measured* P_{osm} is low [<280])

Most hyponatremia cases seen are hypo-osmolar because *calculated* serum osmolality = (2 × [Na^+]) + (glucose/18) + (BUN/2.8), as seen in the equation, is primarily determined by the sodium concentration and its accompanying anions. Sodium and glucose are effective osmoles, whereas blood urea nitrogen (BUN) is an ineffective osmole.

There are 3 types of hypo-osmolar hyponatremia:

- Hypovolemic hyponatremia.
- Euvolemic hyponatremia.
- Hypervolemic hyponatremia.

Iso-Osmolar Hyponatremia (*measured* **P_{osm}** *is* normal [280 to 295])

- Often referred to as **pseudohyponatremia** and due to:
  - Paraproteinemia (i.e., multiple myeloma—increased light chains or proteins is the additional osmole).
  - Hyperlipidemia—increased lipids are the additional osmole.
- **Pseudohyponatremia:** It is called pseudohyponatremia because it is essentially a product of how sodium is measured and not a true hyponatremia. Plasma consists of a water component, which is 93% water, and a solid component, which is 7%, composed of plasma protein and lipid. Sodium ions are dissolved in the plasma water, so increasing the solid component artifactually decreases the Na^+ concentration. The sodium concentration in the plasma is actually normal.

Hyper-Osmolar Hyponatremia (*measured* **P_{osm} is high**[>295])

- Look for an **additional solute** that is contributing to the osmolality.
  - Is this solute an "effective" or "ineffective" osmole? "Effective osmoles" cannot cross semipermeable membranes and thus pull water, where as "ineffective osmoles" can.
  - Remember that **tonicity is a measure of only effective osmoles**, whereas **osmolality measures both effective and ineffective osmoles.**

CONQUER THE WARDS!

For each 100 mg/dL increase in plasma glucose above normal, there is a decrease in plasma sodium concentration by 1.6 mEq/L.

Corrected Na^+ = [(plasma glucose −100)/100] × 1.6.

CONQUER THE WARDS!

When approaching a hyponatremia patient, the **urine osmolality** tells you about the activity of ADH, while the **urine sodium** can tell you about the patient's effective circulating volume. If the urine sodium is <20, think **low** ECV (i.e., hypovolemia, congestive heart failure, nephrotic syndrome). If the urine osmolality is high (>50 to 100 mOsm/kg), ADH is active.

CONQUER THE WARDS!

Very high urine osmolality and high urine sodium in a euvolemic patient suggest a diagnosis of SIADH.

CONQUER THE BOARDS!

The urine sodium concentration tells you about the effective arteriolar volume, while the urine osmolality tells you about the action of ADH. Use these to narrow down your differential diagnosis. A high urine Na and markedly elevated urine osmolality (higher than the plasma osmolality) indicates euvolemia and high ADH levels, suggesting a diagnosis of SIADH.

- Clinically when there is an additional **"effective osmole," or a substance that will pull water from the intracellular space via solute drag**, this pulled water will dilute and lower plasma sodium concentration.
  - Possible causes are:
    - High glucose (most common).
    - Mannitol.
    - IV immunoglobulins (IVIGs).
    - Glycines or sorbitol used in bladder or prostate irrigations.
  - Always check glucose level.

Diagnostic Workup

In patients with hyponatremia, following are the usual diagnostic workup:

- **Measured plasma osmolality** will help differentiate between hypo-osmolar hyponatremia, iso-osmolar hyponatremia, and hyper-osmolar hyponatremia.
- **Urine osmolality**: This gives you a sense of how well the kidney is diluting urine and the activity of ADH. In hyponatremia, ADH should be very low, as the kidney should be maximally diluting the urine to excrete free water (urine osmolality <100 osm/kg). If urine osmolality is high, then either ADH is inappropriately high (e.g., SIADH) or appropriately high (e.g., dehydration). Remember ADH is turned on by decreases in effective arterial volume.
- **Urine sodium**: Urine Na concentration can reflect effective arteriolar volume (EAV) or intravascular volume (use of diuretics may confound, as the urine Na will be falsely elevated) and also help differentiate causes of hypo-osmolar hyponatremia.

Further workup will depend on what the etiology of hyponatremia is. The causes of hyper-osmolar hyponatremia and iso-osmolar hyponatremia are explained earlier. We will now focus on the differential of hypo-osmolar hyponatremia (Figure 14-6).

HYPO-OSMOLAR HYPONATREMIA

The differential of hypo-osmolar hyponatremia is categorized based on the clinical evaluation of a patient's volume status: hypovolemic, euvolemic, and hypervolemic (see figure 14-5).

HYPOVOLEMIC HYPONATREMIA

- Clinical features of hypovolemia:
  - Low blood pressure (BP), orthostatic hypotension, tachycardia.
  - Dry mucous membranes, poor skin turgor.
  - No pulmonary or peripheral edema, no jugular venous distension (JVD).
- **Urine Na <20 mEq/L** if cause is GI losses (diarrhea, vomiting).
- **Urine Na >20 mEq/L** if cause is due to kidney losses (i.e., diuretics or renal salt wasting, can be seen with cisplatin use).
- **Urine osmolality** can be high or low. Initially in pure volume depletion the urine osmolality will be high because the body will choose volume over osmolality. ADH will be **appropriately high** causing water retention and leading to high urine osmolality but low serum osmolality through low sodium. But once you have corrected the volume the ADH will shut off and

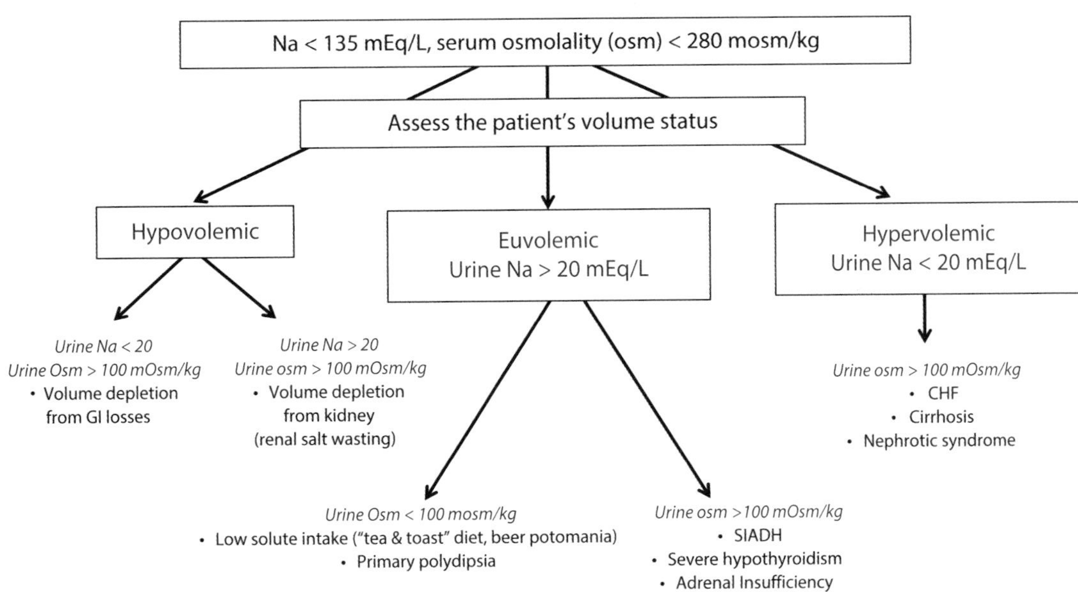

FIGURE 14-6. Hyponatremia Diagnosis Algorithm

the urine osmolality will become low as the body tries to excrete free water to correct the sodium.

EUVOLEMIC HYPONATREMIA

- Clinical features of euvolemia (normal volume status):
  - Normal BP.
  - Normal heart rate.
  - Moist mucous membranes.
  - No pulmonary or peripheral edema, no JVD.
  - Normal skin turgor.
- **Urine Na^+> 20**, indicating normal EAV (may not be accurate in a patient on diuretics).
- **Urine osmolality will help further narrow the differential: LOW urine osmolality <100 mOsm/kg** is usually due to **low solute intake** caused by:
  - "Tea and toast" diet and beer potomania.
  - Patients have adequate liquid intake and appear euvolemic.
  - Their ADH is **appropriately** turned off and trying to excrete maximally dilute water but can't because of low dietary solute intake.
  - Primary polydipsia is due to a patient drinking more water than the kidney can excrete. It usually requires a patient to drink more than 15 L a day. Their ADH is **appropriately** turned off.
- **HIGH urine osmolality >100 mOsm/kg** is caused by the following. Workup usually includes a thyroid-stimulating hormone (TSH) and morning cortisol measurements:
  - **Hypothyroidism** (usually severe and in myxedema coma).
  - **Adrenal insufficiency.**
  - **SIADH** – Remember SIADH is a syndrome and it is important to look for a cause in order to guide treatment. The most common causes of SIADH are listed in Table 14-14.

CONQUER THE WARDS!

A patient with poorly controlled diabetes presents with hyponatremia and an elevated plasma osmolality. Check the glucose level and correct the sodium level for the elevation in glucose. Correction of hyperglycemia should lead to correction of the sodium level.

Table 14-14. Common Causes of SIADH

CNS	Pulmonary	Medications	Malignancy	Other
Stroke Meningitis Trauma Cerebral Hemorrhage	All types of pneumonia Asthma Pneumothorax Tuberculosis Acute respiratory distress syndrome	**Pain medications:** Opiates General anesthesia NSAIDs **Psychiatric medications:** Selective serotonin reuptake inhibitors MAOI Tricyclics **Antiseizure medications:** Carbamazepine Valproate Lamotrigine **Chemotherapy:** Platinum compounds Cyclophosphamide Methotrexate Ifosfamide **Other:** Methylenedioxymethamphetamine (MDMA, ecstasy) Amiodarone Proton pump inhibitors Nicotine	Small cell lung cancer Head and neck cancer Olfactory neuroblastomas	Nausea Pain

CNS, central nervous system; *MAOI*, monoamine oxidase inhibitor; *NSAID*, nonsteroidal antiinflammatory drug.

HYPERVOLEMIC HYPONATREMIA

- Clinical features of hypervolemia with LOW EAV.
  - Pulmonary or peripheral edema, JVD.
  - Ascites.
- **Urine Na is <20**, because patient has low EAV, ***though clinically hypervolemic***.
- **Urine osmolality** is higher than appropriate in the setting of hyponatremia (>100 mOsm/kg) as the body is perceiving a low-volume state. So ADH is **appropriately** turned on.
- Cause is usually CHF, cirrhosis, or nephrotic syndrome.

Treatment

General Rules

- Treatment approach is 2-fold:
  1. Correction of the plasma sodium.
  2. Treatment of the underlying disorder.
- **Symptomatic hyponatremia:** If the patient presents with symptomatic hyponatremia (i.e., seizure, vomiting), hypertonic saline (3% or 2%) may be used to rapidly correct the sodium until symptoms improve. **This is true for all causes of hyponatremia.** But once symptoms improve, the sodium should not be corrected by more than 8 mEq/L overall in a 24-hour period.
- **Maximum correction** should not exceed 6 to 8 mEq/L over 24 hours unless you know for sure that it is acute hyponatremia (<48 hours), but this is often impossible to know, so it is better to assume the hyponatremia is chronic. **Overcorrection of Na^+ can lead to central pontine myelinolysis (CPM)** (see later).

- Treat the underlying disorder if one is present:
  - **Hypovolemic hyponatremia:** Replete volume with isotonic fluid if volume depleted.
  - **Tea and toast diet** or **beer potomania:** Increase solute intake.
  - **SIADH:** Treat underlying cause and treat with water restriction, usually less than 1 L (this value can be estimated by calculating the patient's free water clearance = Urine volume * 1 [(Urine Na + Urine K)/(Serum Na)]. If the volume of free water restriction exceeds the patient's free water clearance, hyponatremia will not improve. If free water restriction alone is ineffective, try increasing free water excretion by using loop diuretics that will disrupt the loop of Henle and prevent ADH from maximally reabsorbing free water. Another strategy is to increase solute intake (e.g., urea or sodium tablets), thus increasing the solute delivered to the kidney and increasing free water excretion. Administration of isotonic or hypertonic fluids may worsen hyponatremia in these cases given the fixed, high urine osmolality—solute will be excreted and water will be reabsorbed.
  - **Hypervolemic hyponatremia:** Restrict water to less than 1 L intake if hypervolemic hyponatremia, diuretics for hypotonic urine excretion.

CONQUER THE WARDS!

During correction of hyponatremia, it is critically important to frequently monitor the urine output, plasma Na^+, urine Na^+, and urine osmolality to avoid rapid correction and devastating neurologic complications, including cerebral pontine myelinolysis, cerebral herniation, and brain death.

Feared Complication: CPM

- Sometimes termed osmotic demyelination syndrome.
- Occurs 2 to 6 days after rapid or overcorrection of hyponatremia.
- A symmetric zone of demyelination occurs in the basis pontis (and extrapontine areas) and is diagnosed by magnetic resonance imaging (MRI).
- Symptoms of CPM include mental status change (confusion, lethargy, obtundation), paralysis, coma, and "locked-in syndrome" (awake but cannot communicate or move). These symptoms are devastating and often irreversible or only partly reversible.

HYPERNATREMIA

General Facts

- **Definition**: Plasma sodium >146 mEq/L.
- In almost all cases except in diabetes insipidus, hypernatremia occurs when there is inadequate intake of free water due to:
  - Defect in thirst mechanism.
  - Lack of access to water.
- Factors implicated in generating hypernatremia:
  - Lack of ADH.
    - Central diabetes insipidus (DI): Lack of ADH production from posterior pituitary.
    - Nephrogenic diabetes insipidus: Tubular resistance to ADH activity
  - Lack of thirst.

Major Causes

Increased water loss, not replaced due to defect in thirst mechanism or lack of access to water.

- Insensible losses:
  - Fever (sweat).
  - Respiratory losses.
- Urinary losses:

- Central or nephrogenic DI.
- Osmotic diuresis (diuresis of free water).
  - Hyperglycemia.
  - Mannitol.

Symptoms

- Chronic hypernatremia (more common hypernatremia present for more than 48 hours).
  - Lethargy.
  - Mental status changes.
- **Central pontine myelinolysis:** Similar to hyponatremia (see earlier). The most dreaded complication of acute hypernatremia is shrinking of the brain quickly, causing shearing of cerebral vessels and intracranial hemorrhage.
- Acute hypernatremia is uncommon but can occur in the setting of IV administration of fluids with high sodium concentrations (i.e., 3% NaCl solution).

Treatment

- Estimate free water deficit (FWD) using the following formula; can be used as a guide for rate of free water replacement:
  - If hypernatremia is chronic (>48 hours), maximum correction should not exceed 8 mEq/L over 24 hours.
  - Give IV fluid that is hypotonic to patient's plasma osmolality (most commonly 5% dextrose in water [D5W] or 0.45% NaCl [1/2 NS]).
  - **Sodium must be checked often, as overcorrection can lead to cerebral edema.**

CONQUER THE **WARDS!**

Calculate the FWD (in liters) to estimate how much water needs to be replaced to reach the target sodium. For a 70-kg man with a sodium of 150 mEq/L and a target sodium of 140 mEq/L:

FWD = TBW × **(Measured Na/Normal Na) – 1)= 42 L× [(Measured Na/Target Na) – 1]**

= 42 L × (150/140 – 1) = 3L

3 L of free water should be replaced over 24 hours to improve the sodium from 150 mEq/L to 140 mEq/L over 24 hours.

OTHER ELECTROLYTE DISORDERS

The following reviews the different types of electrolyte disorders other than hyponatremia and hypernatremia. However, a few general principles of electrolyte disorder management are in order:

- Always check the other electrolytes: Isolated electrolyte abnormalities are uncommon.
- Redraw labs if it appears there was hemolysis in the lab tube.
- If severe, place patient on continuous ECG monitoring.

HYPOKALEMIA

General Facts

Definition: Plasma potassium <3.3 mEq/L. Potassium is mostly stored intracellularly.

Etiology

Hypokalemia is caused by decreased dietary intake (anorexia nervosa), increased shift of cells from extracellular to intracellular, or increased excretion.

- **Net potassium shift from extracellular to intracellular**: This is most commonly caused by the following:

CONQUER THE **WARDS!**

Patients taking digitalis must have their potassium checked regularly because hypokalemia increases the risk and severity of digitalis toxicity.

- Insulin (drives K^+ into cells).
- Beta-adrenergics.
- Catecholamine excess (e.g., acute stress, myocardial infarction).
- Metabolic alkalosis

- **Increased excretion** can occur from kidney or GI causes.
  - Increased kidney potassium excretion:
    - Medications: **Diuretics** (furosemide and thiazides) are the most common causes. Other common medications causing hypokalemia are amphotericin B, cisplatin, and aminoglycosides.
    - Hypomagnesemia: This is an important reason in the hospital, so it is important to always check a magnesium level when someone is hypokalemic. Magnesium must be repleted before potassium to optimally restore potassium levels.
    - RTA type I (distal) or type II (proximal).
    - Osmotic diuresis due to use of mannitol or hyperglycemia.
    - Increased mineralocorticoid activity.
      - Primary hyperaldosteronism due to an adrenal adenoma.
      - Secondary hyperaldosteronism from CHF, cirrhosis, dehydration, or Cushing syndrome.
    - Rare genetic disorders:
      - Bartter syndrome: Juxtaglomerular cell hyperplasia causing increase in renin/aldosterone, which leads to metabolic alkalosis, hypokalemia, hypercalciuria, muscle weakness, and tetany (seen in young adults).
      - Gitelman syndrome: Defective distal tubule thiazide-sensitive Na^+ Cl^- transporter leads to metabolic alkalosis, hypokalemia, hypomagnesemia, and hypocalciuria. Less severe in presentation compared to Bartter syndrome.
- **Increased GI losses**
  1. Vomiting: Hypokalemia is caused by secondary hyperaldosteronism from dehydration.
  2. Diarrhea.

Signs and Symptoms

- Impaired gastric motility, nausea, and vomiting.
- Mild muscle weakness to overt paralysis depending on severity.
- Rhabdomyolysis.
- Atrial and ventricular dysrhythmias.

Treatment

Replace potassium (PO or IV, depending on severity). IV infusion of K^+ should not exceed 20 mEq/L/hr, but may be combined with simultaneous oral administration.

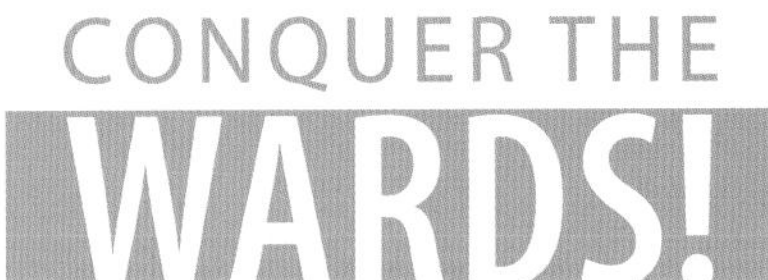

A 10-mEq infusion will raise the serum K by approximately 0.1 mEq/L.

CONQUER THE WARDS!

Chronic, slowly developing hyperkalemia is better tolerated than acute changes (i.e., less likely to have cardiac changes).

HYPERKALEMIA

General Facts

Definition: Serum K >5.5 mEq/L.

CONQUER THE WARDS!

Perform an ECG on patients with new onset of hyperkalemia (>5.5 mEq/L).

Etiology

- Always consider **pseudohyperkalemia** (falsely elevated measurement due to hemolysis of specimen and leakage of potassium from lysed cells in the tube). Need to repeat test.
- **Intracellular to extracellular potassium** shifting occurs in metabolic acidosis, insulin deficiency, beta-blockers, and digitalis toxicity.
- **Increased** potassium load occurs with IV potassium supplementation, potassium-containing medications, and increased cellular breakdown.
- **Decreased** potassium excretion occurs with oliguric kidney injury, potassium-sparing diuretics, ACE inhibitors, and aldosterone deficiency.

Signs and Symptoms

- Neurologic: Muscle cramps, weakness, paresthesias, paralysis, areflexia, tetany.
- Respiratory insufficiency.
- Cardiac: Arrhythmias, arrest.

Diagnosis

ECG changes:

- Initial changes are **tall, peaked T waves in ALL ECG leads** (see Figure 14-7) and then QRS widening, flattened P wave, and ultimately the QRS degrade into a "sine-wave" pattern.
- Eventually these changes can lead to ventricular fibrillation, complete heart block, or asystole.

CONQUER THE BOARDS!

Treatments for hyperkalemia:
Controlling ***K*** ***I***mmediately **D**iverts **B**ad **A**rrhythmias.

Calcium
Kayexalate, Diuretics
Insulin and glucose
Dialysis
Bicarbonate
Albuterol

Treatment

- **Immediate**: The following therapies are only temporizing measures of lowering potassium until definitive therapy for potassium removal is initiated. *Remember: Your job is not done until definitive potassium-lowering therapy is given.*

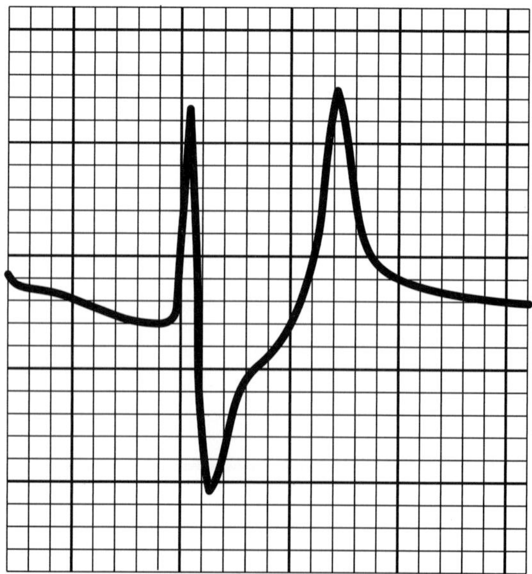

FIGURE 14-7. Peaked T waves in Hyperkalemia

- **IV calcium gluconate**: Goal is immediate cardiac membrane stabilization; acts in minutes.
- **Insulin** has a potent effect on driving potassium into cells and acts in minutes.
  - Shifts K^+ from extracellular fluid to intracellular fluid.
  - Must give glucose to prevent hypoglycemia in the form of D50 IV push.
- **Albuterol** (beta-adrenergic agonist) **nebulizer** also shifts K^+ into cells.

■ **Definitive therapy**: The following therapies provide removal of total body potassium:
- **Cation exchange resin** that causes bowel movements such as polystyrene sulfonate. Can take hours to remove K^+.
- **Diuretics** (e.g., furosemide) and normal saline increase kidney K^+ excretion and may be given together if patient is euvolemic.
- **Hemodialysis** is the most effective therapy to lower total body potassium but is reserved for refractory hyperkalemia, or hyperkalemia with life-threatening arrhythmias, because it requires the placement of a central line.

CONQUER THE WARDS!

Kayexalate, diuretics, cationexchangers (e.g., Kayexalate), normal saline, and dialysis are needed to remove potassium from the body.

HYPOPHOSPHATEMIA

General Facts

Definition: Serum phosphate <2.5 mg/dL.

Etiology

Usually alcoholism or malnutrition is the cause. Also seen with diabetic ketoacidosis (DKA) and hyperparathyroidism.

Symptoms

- Neurologic (mental status change, agitation) and muscle weakness.
- Severe hypophosphatemia (<1 mg/dL) can result in rhabdomyolysis or seizures.

Treatment is with phosphate supplementation orally, or if phosphate <1 mg/dL, intravenously.

HYPERPHOSPHATEMIA

General Facts

Definition: Plasma phosphate >5 mg/dL.

Etiology

- Kidney injury.
- Tumor lysis syndrome (rapid necrosis of tumor after chemotherapy).
- Iatrogenic (excessive amounts given IV or PO).

Treatment

- Phosphorus binders: These bind phosphate in the gut and decrease absorption. (calcium-containing binders: calcium carbonate and calcium acetate, and non-calcium-containing binder: sevelamer).
- Low-phosphorus diet

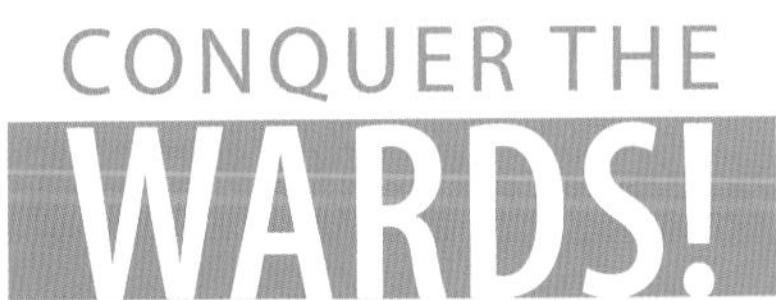

A common cause of high phosphate serum values is in vitro hemolysis. Most labs will report that the specimen was hemolyzed, however.

HYPOMAGNESEMIA

General Facts

Definition: Serum magnesium <1.8 mg/dL.

Etiology

- **Medications:** Loop diuretics, antibiotics (amphotericin, gentamicin), PPIs, and insulin.
- Hungry bone syndrome: Occurs in patients with prolonged high PTH after parathyroidectomy.

Treatment

Oral and/or IV magnesium supplementation.

CONQUER THE WARDS!

When supplementing calcium or potassium, always check for hypomagnesemia.
The calcium and potassium levels will not correct if magnesium is low.

HYPERMAGNESEMIA

General Facts

Definition: Serum magnesium >2.3 mg/dL.

Etiology

- Iatrogenic (during treatment of eclampsia/preeclampsia).
- Magnesium-containing drugs (some laxatives, antacids) if given to a patient with kidney injury.

Treatment

- IV fluids.
- Calcium if there are ECG changes.
- Hemodialysis if it is refractory.

CHAPTER 15 RHEUMATOLOGY

OVERVIEW OF HIGH-YIELD TOPICS IN RHEUMATOLOGY

VASCULITIS

General Facts

The primary vasculitides are a heterogenous group of disorders characterized by inflammation within the blood vessel wall. This inflammation leads to downstream ischemia and tissue damage. These diseases are typically categorized by the size of the blood vessel involved, from large vessels (aorta and major branches) to medium vessels to small vessels (capillaries and venules) (see Figure 15-1). Additionally, some vasculitides can affect both the arteriole and venous circulation. The clinical presentation and epidemiology are very different among these diseases (see Table 15-1). However, all have the potential for significant organ damage.

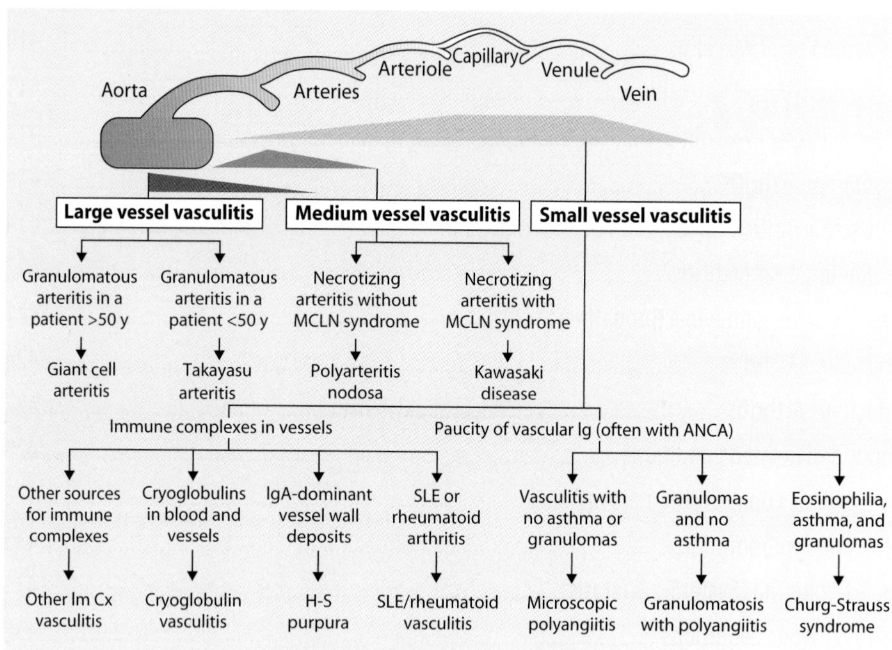

FIGURE 15-1. Diagram illustrating the vascular distribution of major types of vasculitis. ANCA, antineutrophil cytoplasmic antibody; H-S purpura, Henoch-Schönlein purpura; Im Cx, immune complex; MCLN, mucocutaneous lymph node syndrome; SLE, systemic lupus erythematosus. (Modified, with permission, from Jennette JC, Falk RJ. Nosology of primary vasculitis. *Curr Opin Rheumatol.* 2007;19:10.)

LARGE VESSEL VASCULITIS

- Affects the aorta and major branches (e.g., subclavian arteries).
- There are 2 types:
  - **Giant cell arteritis** (GCA; also called temporal arteritis):
    - It is by far the **most common primary vasculitis** and typically involves **the extracranial branches of the carotid artery**.
    - GCA exclusively affects patients >50 with the peak incidence at age 75.
    - It is most common in patients of northern European descent.
  - **Takayasu arteritis**:
    - Typically affects patients <40 with a female predominance.
    - It has a predilection for the **intrathoracic large arteries**.

MEDIUM VESSEL VASCULITIS

- Affects vessels that are smaller than the major aortic branches but still contain **an intima, internal elastic lamina, muscular medial, and adventitia**. Typically these vessels are large enough to be visualized on imaging studies (not just histopathology).
- There are 2 types:
  - **Polyarteritis nodosa**:
    - Affects **adults** and has a **strong association with hepatitis**.
    - Predilection for mesenteric arteries.
  - **Kawasaki disease**:
    - Affects **children** and is associated with fevers and mucocutaneous inflammation (conjunctivitis, tongue redness, cervical lymphadenopathy).
    - Usually self-limited, lasting for 12 days.
    - Can be complicated by vascular inflammation leading to coronary artery aneurysms, heart failure, and peripheral artery occlusions.

CONQUER THE **BOARDS!**

Cryoglobulinemia is often seen in association with hepatitis C, autoimmune disease (e.g., lupus or Sjögren disease), or hematologic malignancies.

CONQUER THE **WARDS!**

Giant cell arteritis is associated with polymyalgia rheumatic (PMR; a disease of intense inflammation of the periarticular shoulder and hip girdle) about 50% of the time. Only about 15% of patients with PMR will have GCA.

SMALL VESSEL VASCULITIS

General Facts

- Affects **arterioles, capillaries, and venules**. The diagnosis is typically made histologically.
- These diseases are typically categorized as follows:
  - **Immune complex vasculitis:** Significant immune complex deposition is seen on biopsy.
    - Cryoglobulinemia.
    - IgA vasculitis (formally Henoch-Schöenlein purpura).
    - Anti-GBM disease (Goodpasture syndrome).
  - **ANCA-associated vasculitis:** These diseases are associated with a **positive blood test called antineutrophil cytoplasmic antibodies (ANCA)**.
    - Eosinophilic granulomatous with polyangiitis (EGPA; formally Churg–Strauss).
    - Granulomatous with polyangiitis (GPA; formally Wegener granulomatosis).
    - Microscopic polyangiitis (MPA).

CONQUER THE **BOARDS!**

gA vasculitis is a different disease from IgA nephropathy (see Chapter 14- Section Nephritic syndrome).

Clinical Features

The typical signs and symptoms of vasculitis depend on the size of the blood vessel involved. In general, low-grade fevers, fatigue, unintentional weight loss, myalgias, and arthralgias are common in all types (see Table 15-1).

Table 15-1. Common symptoms of Vasculitis

Large Vessel	Headache, visual changes, and jaw claudication (especially GCA) Limb claudication (especially Takayasu) Hypertension due to involvement of the renal artery (especially Takayasu)
Medium Vessel	Abdominal pain due to involvement of the visceral arteries Cutaneous ulcers Neuropathy (especially intense pain and foot drop) Hypertension due to involvement of the renal arterioles
Small Vessel	Pulmonary hemorrhage Glomerulonephritis Palpable purpura Neuropathy (especially intense pain and foot drop); "mononeuritis multiplex" is the term for sequential development of acute painful peripheral neuropathies in distinct distributions

Some vasculitides have additional important features see table 15-2:

- **Giant cell arteritis:** Visual loss or double vision in GCA is an emergency requiring immediate high-dose corticosteroid treatment (this should be started even before confirmation of the diagnosis).
- **Takayasu disease** is also called "pulseless disease" because chronic inflammation of the subclavian arteries can lead to subclavian stenosis and loss of radial pulses.
- **Polyarteritis nodosa** rarely affects the lungs.
- **GPA,** in addition to pulmonary and renal involvement, typically affects the upper airway, including the paranasal sinus, nasopharynx, and larynx (subglottic stenosis).
- **EGPA** typically presents with a prodrome of difficult-to-control asthma and allergic rhinitis with eosinophilia prior to the vasculitic phase of the disease.
- **IgA vasculitis and cryoglobulinemia** usually present with prominent palpable purpura (see figure 15-2).
- **Anti-GBM disease** typically presents with acute pulmonary hemorrhage and renal failure from glomerulonephritis.

Table 15-2. Physical Exam Findings

Large Vessel	**GCA:** ■ Nodular, tender temporal artery but not specific or sensitive ■ Loss of temporal artery pulse **Takayasu disease:** ■ Loss of radial pulses
Medium Vessel	**Polyarteritis nodosa:** ■ Abdominal tenderness ■ Foot drop–associated sensory loss in the distribution of the peroneal nerve ■ Lower extremity ulcerations **Kawasaki disease** ■ Conjunctivitis – bilateral and nonexudative ■ Erythema of lips and oral mucosa ■ Cervical LAD
Small Vessel	Palpable purpura is common in small vessel vasculitis Lower extremity swelling if renal involvement Foot drop due to peroneal nerve infarction Bilateral crackles if lungs involved Eye redness due to scleritis in ANCA-associated vasculitis

Diagnostic Workup

If vasculitis is suspected, the basic workup includes a complete blood count, basic metabolic panel, urinalysis, and nonspecific markers of inflammation such as erythrocyte sedimentation rate (ESR) and C-reactive protein (CRP). Depending on which vasculitis you are suspecting, more specialized tests can be ordered (see table 15-3).

- Anemia due to chronic inflammation can be seen.
- Urinalysis can show an active urinary sediment (positive red blood cells [RBCs] that are dysmorphic, RBC casts, positive white blood cells [WBCs]).
- If small vessel vasculitis is suspected, **ANCA** should be sent, which is usually positive in GPA and MPA and about 50% of the time in EGPA. **Complement levels** can help differentiate between immune-complex vasculitis (low levels) and ANCA-associated vasculitis (normal levels).

The diagnosis of vasculitis is typically made histologically, with some exceptions (see table 15-3).

CONQUER THE **BOARDS!**

Cocaine use can give a false-positive ANCA test (and can also present with skin findings that mimic vasculitis). False-positive ANCA tests can also be seen in endocarditis, inflammatory bowel disease, and cystic fibrosis.

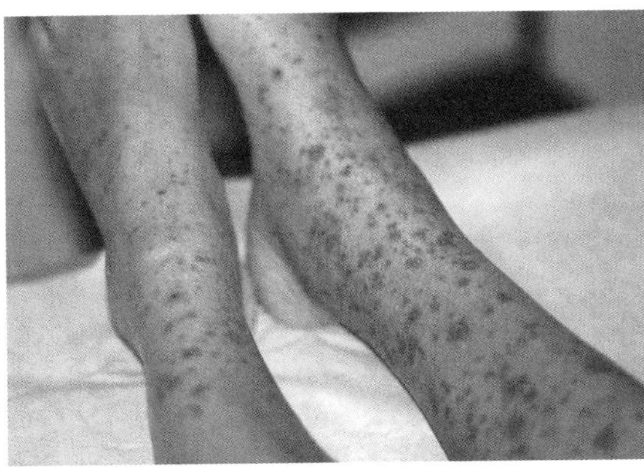

FIGURE 15-2. Palpable purpura with some superficial ulcerations in a patient with Henoch-Schönlein purpura. Note also the presence of right ankle swelling due to arthritis. (Reproduced, with permission, from Imboden JB, Hellmann DB, Stone JH, eds: *Current Diagnosis & Treatment: Rheumatology*, 3rd ed. www.accessmedicine.com. Copyright © McGraw-Hill Education. All rights reserved.)

CONQUER THE WARDS!

"Leukocytoclastic vasculitis" (LCV) is a histologic term referring to vascular inflammation of the small blood vessels of the skin. In addition to the small vessel vasculitides listed here, this finding can be caused by infections or medications (most commonly antibiotics), or it can be idiopathic.

Table 15-3. Workup for Vasculitis

Large Vessel	**GCA: Temporal artery biopsy** is the gold standard for GCA. Some institutions will also use temporal artery ultrasound (looking for the "halo sign" of inflammation surrounding the temporal artery) as an adjunctive modality. **Takayasu arteritis**: Diagnosis made via **CT angiography or MRA of the chest** to look for vessel wall edema, stenosis, and aneurysm formation (see figure 15-3).
Medium Vessel	**Biopsy:** Can be confirmed histologically with nerve biopsy (if nerve involvement) or skin biopsy of a cutaneous ulcer. **Mesenteric angiography** shows typical saccular microaneurysms in polyarteritis nodosa.
Small Vessel	**Skin or renal biopsy** is typically performed. Antineutrophil cytoplasmic antibody tests are helpful, as noted earlier. Anti-GBM antibodies are positive in Goodpasture disease.

CONQUER THE BOARDS!

Plasma exchange is used for anti-GBM disease (Goodpasture syndrome), since these antibodies are pathogenic.

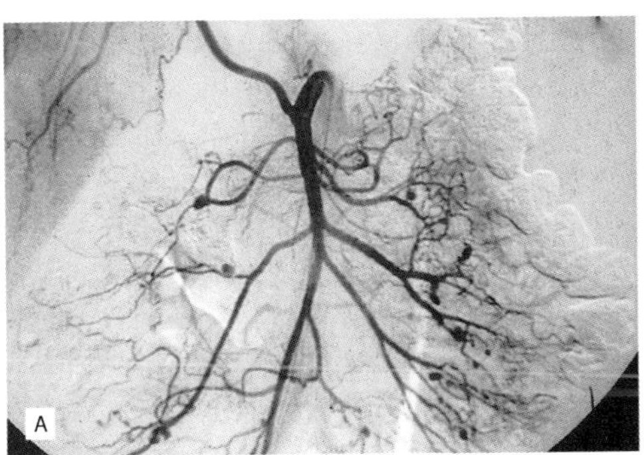

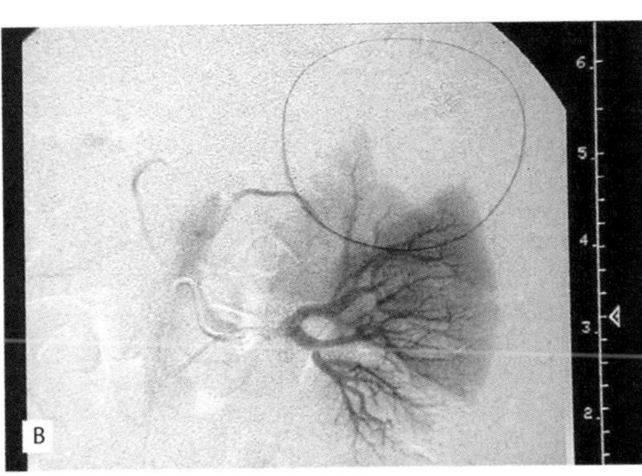

CONQUER THE BOARDS!

If there is a suspicion for GCA, start steroids immediately, as once visual loss occurs, it is typically permanent. You have at least a week on steroids to do the TA biopsy for confirmation of the diagnosis.

FIGURE 15-3. Angiographic features of polyarteritis nodosa. A: Mesenteric angiogram showing multiple microaneurysms. B: A wedge-shaped renal infarction. (Reproduced, with permission, from Stone JH. Vasculitis: a collection of pearls and myths. *Rheum Dis Clin North Am*. 2007;33(4):691–739.)

CONQUER THE WARDS!

Infections are a major cause of death in these patients, especially in the first 6 months after diagnosis.

Table 15-4. Treatment for Vasculitis

Large Vessel	**Tocilizumab** for giant cell arteritis
Medium Vessel	**Cyclophosphamide** for severe disease (e.g., neurologic deficit or gastrointestinal ischemia)
Small Vessel	**Rituximab or cyclophosphamide** especially if there is pulmonary or renal involvement

Management

Corticosteroids are the cornerstone for acute control of inflammation in all vasculitides. "Pulse-dose" therapy (IV solumedrol 1000 mg for 3 to 5 days) is given if there is acute organ-threatening involvement, for example, if there is pulmonary hemorrhage or rapidly rising creatinine. After this patients are typically transitioned to prednisone 1 mg/kg with a slow taper, depending on response. Additional medications include rituximab and cyclophosmamide (see Table 15-4).

HIGH-YIELD LITERATURE

RAVE trial:

Stone JH, et al. Rituximab versus cyclophosphamide for ANCA-associated vasculitis. *N Engl J Med.* 2010;363(3):221-232.

PROMINENT ARTHRITIS

OSTEOARTHRITIS

General Facts

Osteoarthritis (OA) is by far the most common type of arthritis and the most common cause of disability in the elderly.

- It is considered a noninflammatory, slowly progressive arthritis associated with both cartilage loss and bony productive changes (osteophytes, aka bone spurs).
- There is a predilection for the following joints:
  - Hips.
  - Knees.
  - First metatarsophalangeal (MTP).
  - Carpometacarpal (CMC) joint.
  - Proximal interphalangeal joints.
  - Distal interphalangeal joints.
  - Lumbar spine.
- It uncommonly affects the elbows, wrist, or ankles unless there is a history of trauma.

Clinical Features

Patients typically endorse slowly progressive, achy pain in the affected joint, typically triggered by exertion and relieved with rest. Some morning stiffness may be present, but it is less long and debilitating as opposed to inflammatory arthritis.

Risk Factors

- Age is the strongest nonmodifiable risk factor, but there is a large genetic contribution as well.
- Obesity is by far the most common modifiable risk factor.
- Previous trauma to the joint (e.g., meniscal injuries).
- Congenital abnormalities (e.g., hip dysplasia).
- Metabolic abnormalities (e.g., hemochromatosis—will present with OA in atypical sites, such as second and third MCP joints).

Physical Exam Findings

- Unlike with inflammatory arthritis, affected joints are not red and warm (see Figure 15-4).
- Small joint effusions may be present, especially in the knee, but they are cool and slowly developing.
- Crepitus (crunching sound with movement) can be present.
- Range of motion of the joint can be decreased (e.g., knee flexion or internal rotation of hips).
- Heberden nodes and Bouchard nodes are a manifestation of bony productive changes and can be seen in the distal interphalangeal (DIP) and proximal interphalangeal (PIP) joints, respectively (see Figures 15-5 and 15-6).
- Disuse atrophy of the periarticular muscles can be present if the patient has been using the joint less due to pain.

Diagnostic Workup

Radiographs (should be weight bearing for lower joints) show joint-space narrowing, subchondral sclerosis, subchondral cysts, and osteophytes (see

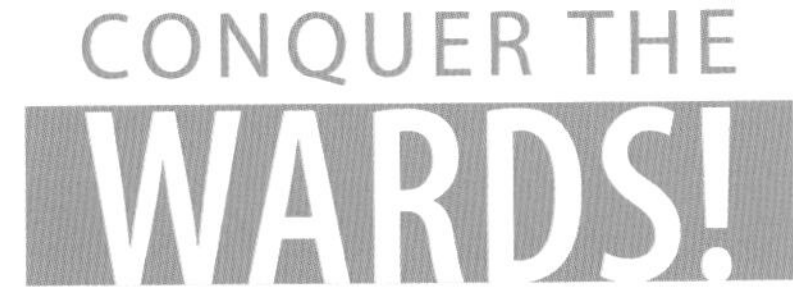

ESR and CRP rise naturally with age. A good rule of thumb is normal ESR = age / 2 in men, age + 10 / 2 in women.

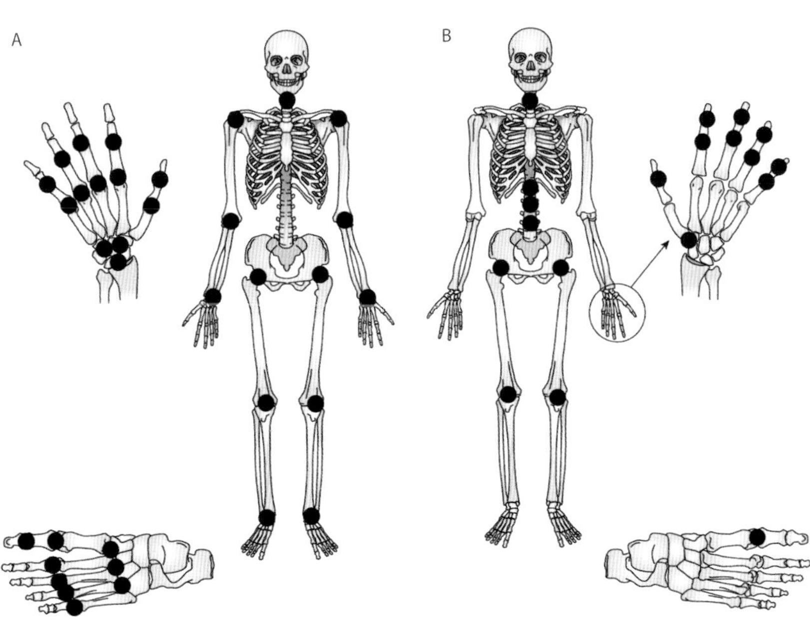

FIGURE 15-4. The joint distribution of the two most common types of arthritis are compared: rheumatoid arthritis (A) and osteoarthritis (B). Rheumatoid arthritis involves almost all synovial joints in the body. Osteoarthritis has a much more limited distribution. Importantly, rheumatoid arthritis rarely, if ever, involves the distal interphalangeal joints, but osteoarthritis commonly does. (Reproduced, with permission, from Imboden JB, Hellmann DB, Stone JH, eds: *Current Diagnosis & Treatment: Rheumatology*, 3rd ed. www.accessmedicine.com. Copyright © McGraw-Hill Education. All rights reserved.)

Figures 15-5 and 15-7). Unlike with rheumatoid arthritis (RA), erosions of the bone are usually absent.

- Systemic markers of inflammation (ESR, CRP) should be normal, and aspiration of the joint shows noninflammatory joint fluid (<2000 WBC).

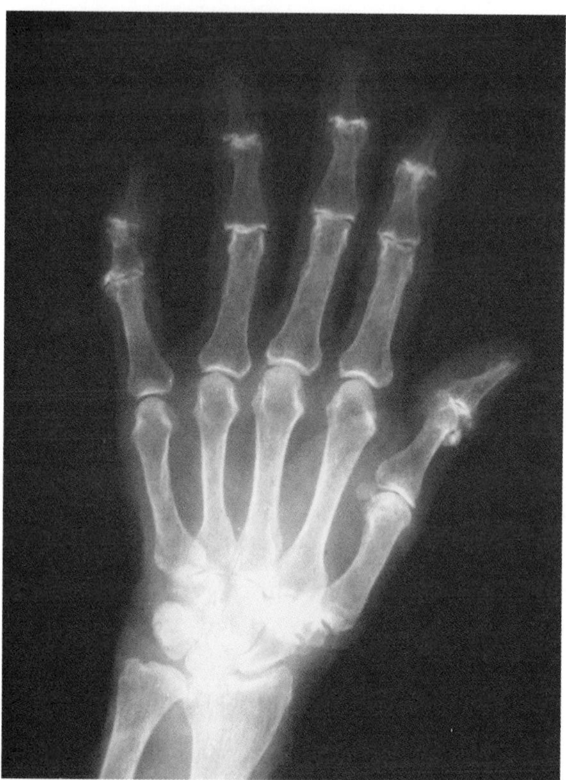

FIGURE 15-5. Radiograph of a hand showing osteoarthritis of the distal interphalangeal (DIP), proximal interphalangeal (PIP), and first carpometacarpal (CMC) joints. Note the joint-space narrowing of the DIP and PIP joints compared to the metacarpophalangeal joints, as well as the bony sclerosis (eburnation) of all joints involved by the osteoarthritis process. (Reproduced, with permission, from Imboden JB, Hellmann DB, Stone JH, eds: *Current Diagnosis & Treatment: Rheumatology*, 3rd ed. www.accessmedicine.com. Copyright © McGraw-Hill Education. All rights reserved.)

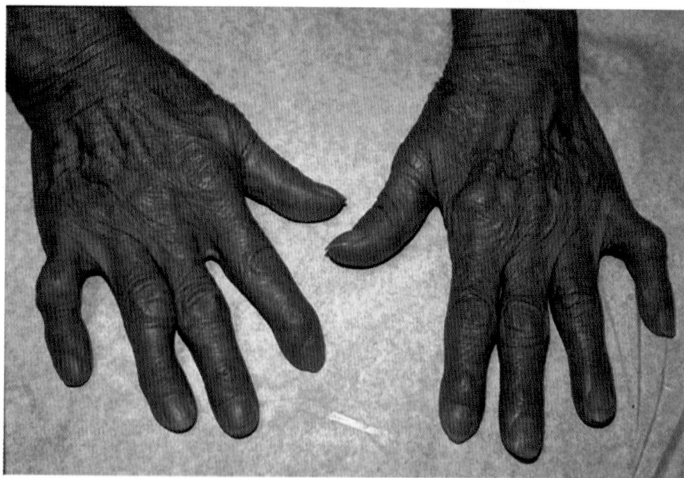

FIGURE 15-6. Bony enlargement of some distal interphalangeal (DIP) and proximal interphalangeal (PIP) joints consistent with Heberden (DIP) and Bouchard (PIP) nodes. (From Usatine RP, Smith MA, Mayeaux EJ Jr, Chumley HS. *The Color Atlas and Synopsis of Family Medicine*, 3rd ed. New York: McGraw-Hill, 2019. Reproduced with permission from Richard P. Usatine, MD.)

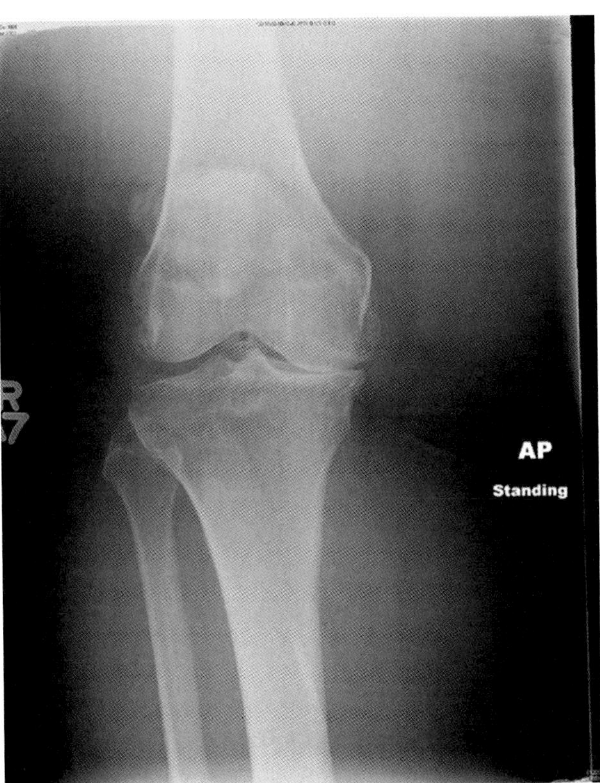

FIGURE 15-7. Osteoarthritis of the knee causing joint space narrowing, sclerosis, and bony spurring in all three compartments of the right knee, most pronounced in the medial compartment. (From Usatine RP, Smith MA, Mayeaux EJ Jr, Chumley HS. *The Color Atlas and Synopsis of Family Medicine*, 3rd ed. New York: McGraw-Hill, 2019. Reproduced with permission from Heidi Chumley, MD.)

Management

Unfortunately, currently there are no disease-modifying medications (unlike with RA or other inflammatory arthritis, see later).

- Acetaminophen and nonsteroidal antiinflammatory drugs (NSAIDs) can be used for pain.
- Intraarticular injections of corticosteroids and hyaluronic acid are common, but the effectiveness of these compared to placebo injection is controversial.

Nonpharmacologic therapy is crucial:

- Weight loss has been shown to improve pain.
- Physical therapy to strengthen the muscles around the joint.
- Orthotic devices and mobility assistance.
- Joint replacement surgery provides definitive treatment. Indications for surgery include pain that significantly interferes with a patient's quality of life. Notably, joint replacement surgery is much more effective if patients diligently participate in postsurgical rehab therapy; thus, it is not a good option for patients who are too frail.

RHEUMATOID ARTHRITIS

General Facts

RA is the most common inflammatory arthritis in America, affecting about 1% of the population. Untreated, it leads to chronic bone destruction and chronic joint deformities. However, the last 20 years have seen an incredible improve-

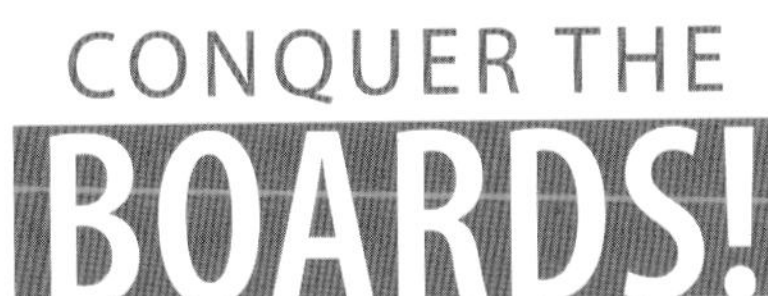

Smoking not only increases one's risk for rheumatoid arthritis, but also decreases response to therapy.

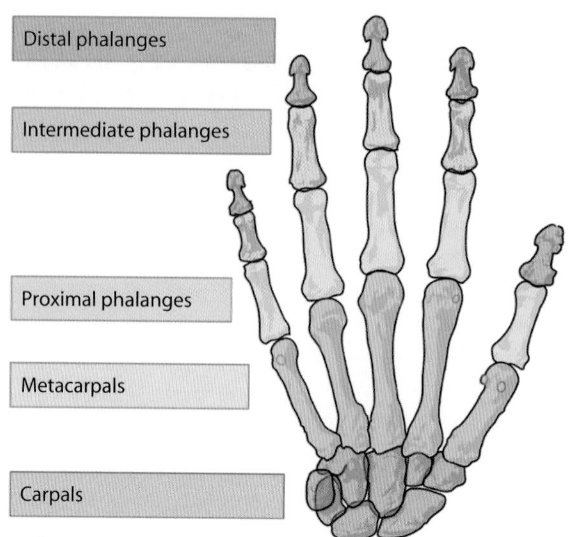

FIGURE 15-8. Hand and Finger Bones

ment in the management of this condition due to a plethora of new therapies. Smoking is the strongest environmental risk factor. The "shared epitope," which is a common amino acid sequence found in some HLA-DR4, -DR14, and -DR1 beta chains, is the most common genetic risk factor.

Clinical Features

- Patients typically present with subacute, bilateral achy pain of **peripheral joints** (see Figure 15-8)**:**
  - Hands.
    - MCP joint.
    - PIP joint.
  - Feet (MTPs).
    - MTP joints.
    - Ankles.
  - Elbows (loss of extension).
  - Knees.
- Joints not affected:
  - DIP joints.
  - Spine (exception is the atlantoaxial [C1/C2] joint).
- Joints affected later on in the disease:
  - Hips.
  - Shoulders.
- Pain is typically worse in the morning, associated with significant joint swelling, and >1 hour of morning stiffness. Often patients will endorse functional limitations (e.g., difficulty putting on their clothes or brushing their teeth).
- **Extraarticular complications** can occur with more severe disease, including inflammation of the eye (scleritis), interstitial lung disease, and rheumatoid vasculitis (typically in a medium/small vessel distribution, presenting with LE ulcerations and neuropathy). Importantly, all RA patients are at a 2-fold risk of developing cardiovascular disease due to their chronic inflammatory state.

Physical Exam Findings

- Initially, exam findings can be subtle and consist of boggy swelling of the joints. Patients might have trouble closing their hands.

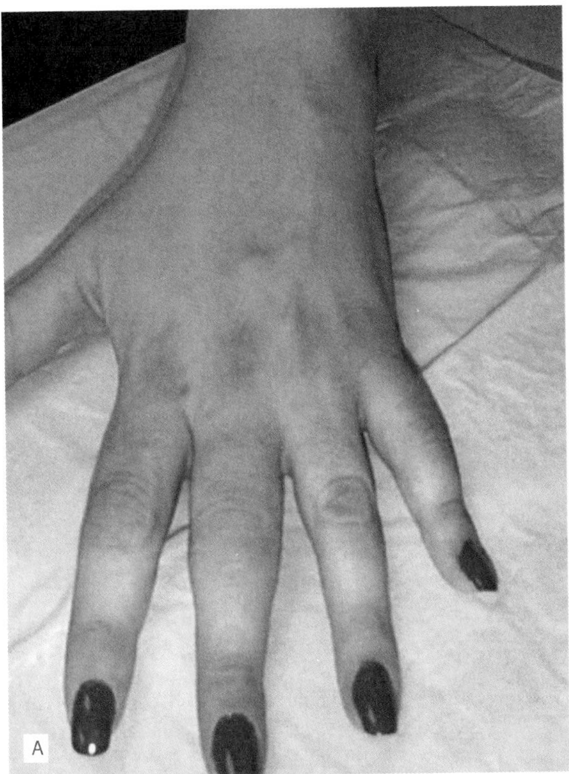

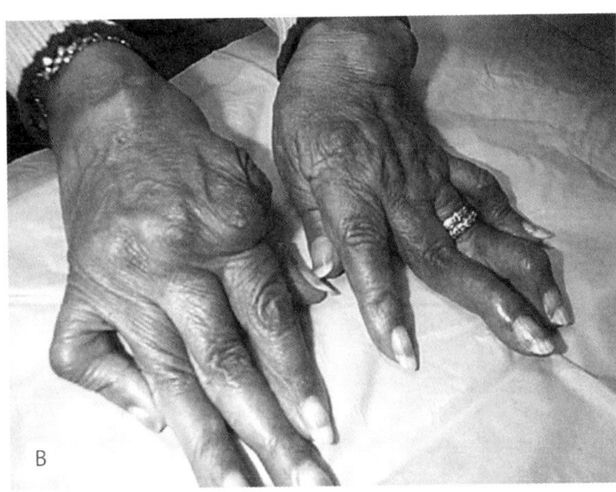

FIGURE 15-9. A: A patient with early rheumatoid arthritis. There are no joint deformities, but the soft tissue synovial swelling around the third and fifth proximal interphalangeal (PIP) joints is easily seen. B: A patient with advanced rheumatoid arthritis with severe joint deformities including subluxation at the metacarpophalangeal joints and swan-neck deformities (hyperextension at the PIP joints). (Reproduced, with permission, from Imboden JB, Hellmann DB, Stone JH, eds: *Current Diagnosis & Treatment: Rheumatology*, 3rd ed. www.accessmedicine.com. Copyright © McGraw-Hill Education. All rights reserved.)

- Over time with untreated disease, more chronic deformities can occur, such as ulnar deviation of the fingers, swan neck/boutonniere deformities, subluxation at the MCPs, or ulnar prominence (see Figures 15-9 and 15-10).

Diagnostic Workup

- **Elevated inflammatory markers** (ESR/CRP) are common.
- **Rheumatoid factor** (RF) is an immunoglobulin M (IgM) molecule that binds to the Fc portion of immunoglobulin G (IgG). It is about 75% sensitive but is less specific; it can be seen in the setting of chronic infections such as hepatitis C, or even in normal aging.

CONQUER THE BOARDS!

TNF is important in granuloma formation. Thus, patients on TNF-alpha inhibitors have a uniquely elevated risk for tuberculosis (TB). All patients must be screened for latent TB before starting these medications.

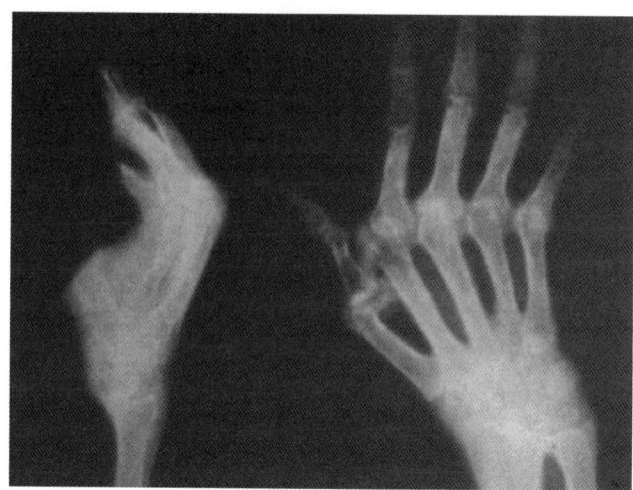

FIGURE 15-10. Radialward displacement of the metacarpals in rheumatoid arthritis. (Reproduced, with permission, from Chapter 9. Hand surgery. In: Skinner HB, McMahon PJ. *Current Diagnosis & Treatment in Orthopedics*, 5th ed. New York: McGraw-Hill, 2014.)

- **Citrullinated peptide (CCP) antibodies** are more specific (95%).
- It is important to note that about 20% to 25% of patients with RA are "seronegative"; thus, a negative RF/CCP does not rule out the diagnosis.
- X-rays can be normal early in the disease. Periarticular erosions and joint-space narrowing can occur with inadequately treated disease.

Management

- **Window of treatment:** Patients with RA have a window of treatment for the initiation of disease-modifying therapy (medications that interfere with the pathogenesis of the disease and prevent long-term complications), typically considered **3 to 6 months** after the onset of symptoms. Patients treated within this window have a lower rate of long-term complications. Anyone suspected of having RA needs an early referral to rheumatology.
- **Acute treatment: NSAIDs and systemic corticosteroids** are used for acute pain relief, but they do not seem to interfere with the chronic destructive process. Additionally, they have significant long-term adverse effects.
- **Chronic treatment: Methotrexate** is typically the first-line disease-modifying antirheumatic drug (DMARD) and is usually the backbone of therapy. Typically, if the patient still has active disease after 3 months, additional therapy (either "triple therapy," see later, or a biologic agent) is added. Patients are subsequently seen at regular intervals, and therapies are adjusted based on patient response ("treat to target" strategy). Most therapies are given 3 to 6 months to demonstrate effectiveness (see Table 15-5).

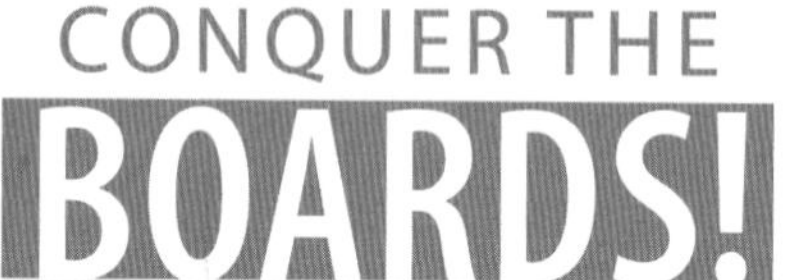

NSAIDs and steroids are NOT adequate as monotherapy for rheumatoid arthritis.

Table 15-5. Conventional DMARDs

Medication	Side Effects	Note
Methotrexate	GI; cytopenia; oral ulcers; liver toxicity; mild infections. (Note: Liver toxicity and cytopenia risks can be decreased with concurrent folic acid use.)	"Anchor drug" for RA. Most responsible for improved outcomes compared to pre-DMARD therapy. Cleared renally, so cannot be used if significant renal dysfunction.
Hydroxychloroquine (Plaquenil)	GI (mild); rash Retinal toxicity (rare)	Mildest therapy, not immunosuppressive.
Sulfasalazine	GI; rash; leukopenia	Often used in combination with methotrexate and hydroxychloroquine as "triple therapy."
Leflunomide	GI; infections	Often used if methotrexate cannot be tolerated.

- **Biologics and small-molecule inhibitors** are typically used if patients still have active disease despite methotrexate. Although the mechanisms of action are different, in general, these medications have the same level of efficacy and risk. Infectious complications are the most clinically relevant and are most related to patient age, comorbidities (e.g., chronic obstructive pulmonary disease [COPD] or diabetes), and concurrent prednisone use (see Table 15-6).

CONQUER THE BOARDS!

Combining biologic DMARDs significantly increases infection risk and has not been shown to improve efficacy.

Table 15-6. Biologics and Small Molecule Inhibitors for RA Treatment

Medication Class	Drugs	Comment
TNF inhibitors	Infliximab (Remicade) Etanercept (Enbrel) Adalimumab (Humira) Certolizumab (Cimzia) Golimumab (Simponi)	Oldest and still most commonly prescribed biologics.
B-cell inhibitors	Rituximab (Rituxan)	Only used for seropositive patients.
Co-stimulation blockage	Abatacept (Orencia)	Possibly lowest infection risk among biologics.
IL-6 inhibitors	Tocilizumab (Actemra) Sarilumab (Kevzara)	Risk (low) of GI perforation.
JAK inhibitors	Tofacitinib (Xeljanz) Baricitinib (Olumiant) Upadacitinib	Oral medications. Can cause elevated LDL but do not increase CAD risk.

CONQUER THE WARDS!

Randomized controlled trials have shown similar efficacy for "triple therapy" vs. the MTX/TNF combination.

SERONEGATIVE SPONDYLOARTHROPATHIES

General Facts

- **Definition:** A group of diseases associated with inflammatory arthritis that are negative for rheumatoid factor/CCP and share common clinical features: inflammatory back pain, asymmetric oligoarthritis, enthesitis (inflammation at attachment sites of ligaments and tendons to bone), dactylitis (sausage digits), and uveitis.
- Historically, these diseases have been categorized into psoriatic arthritis, ankylosing spondylitis, reactive arthritis, and inflammatory bowel disease (IBD)–associated arthritis; clinically these names are still commonly used. However, because of overlapping clinical features, they are now more broadly grouped into **peripheral spondyloarthropathies** and **axial spondyloarthropathies** based on the dominant location of their joint involvement.

Clinical Features

- **Inflammatory back pain:** Unlike RA, spinal involvement is common, especially in the sacroiliac joints (sacroiliitis). Inflammatory back pain has the following features:
  - Onset <40 years of age.
  - Prolonged (usually >1 hour) morning stiffness.
  - Insidious onset.
  - Improvement with exercise.
  - No improvement with rest.
  - Awakens patient at night.

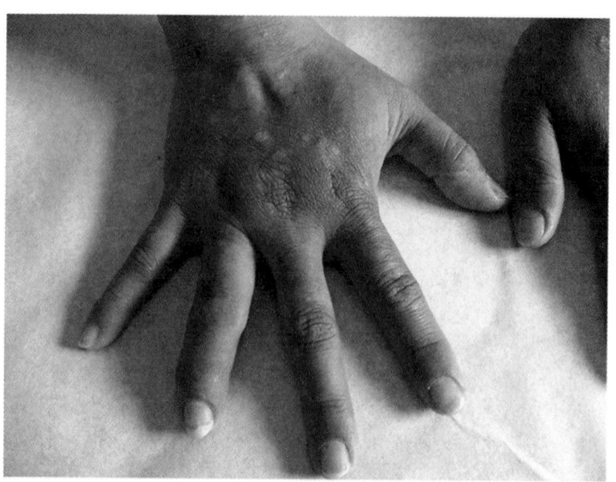

FIGURE 15-11. Dactylitis of the ring finger of a patient with psoriatic arthritis. (From Imboden JB, Hellmann DB, Stone JH, eds: *Current Diagnosis & Treatment: Rheumatology*, 3rd ed. www.accessmedicine.com. Copyright © McGraw-Hill Education. All rights reserved. Used with permission from Dr. J. Graf, University of California, San Francisco.)

- **Asymmetric oligoarthritis:** Joint involvement is typically asymmetric and oligoarticular. Involved joints will be swollen with stiffness (like RA).
- **Enthesitis** (inflammation of where the tendons insert into bones) is a prominent clinical feature, especially in the Achilles tendon, plantar fascia, patellar tendon, pelvis, chest wall, elbows, and shoulders.
- **Dactylitis:** Unlike synovitis, swelling involves the entire digit, including the flexor tendon, tendon sheath, soft tissue, bone, and joints.
- **Extraarticular:** A number of extraarticular features can be seen: psoriasiform rashes, uveitis, oral ulcers, and gastrointestinal inflammation.

CONQUER THE WARDS!

Chlamydia causes reactive arthritis; gonorrhea does not. Gonorrhea can, however, cause disseminated gonococcal infections, which have prominent articular involvement (see Infectious Arthritis section).

Other Clinical Features of Specific Spondyloarthropathies

Reactive Arthritis

- **Classic clinical triad of arthritis, urethritis, and conjunctivitis** ("can't see, can't pee, can't climb a tree"). However, only a subset of patients have all 3 features. Aseptic urethritis can be seen whether the triggering infection was gastrourinary (GU) or gastrointestinal (GI).
- Reactive arthritis is considered an immune response to certain bacterial infections. It is typically triggered by:
  - *Chlamydia trachomatis* (most common in United States).
  - *Yersinia, Salmonella, Shigella,* or *Campylobacter.*
  - *Rarely, it can be also triggered by Escherichia coli, Clostridium difficile,* or *Chlamydia pneumonia.*
- The articular manifestations occur usually 1 to 4 weeks after the inciting infection. As it is an immune response to infection and not a direct joint infection, bacteria cannot be cultured from the inflamed joint.

CONQUER THE WARDS!

Skin manifestations of psoriasis can be subtle in patients with psoriatic arthritis. In a patient with an undiagnosed inflammatory arthritis, it is important to carefully examine places where psoriasis can hide, including the scalp, behind the ears, gluteal cleft, intertriginous areas (inverse psoriasis), and especially the nails.

Psoriatic Arthritis

- About 25% of patients with psoriasis have psoriatic arthritis (PsA).
- Psoriasis usually precedes the arthritis by years, but in about 15% of cases, the joint and skin disease present simultaneously, or the arthritis develops first.

Diagnostic Workup

- **HLA-B27** is positive in the vast majority of patients with ankylosing spondylitis. It is a useful screening test in younger white patients with inflammatory low back pain; however, further advanced imaging (see later) should be done if diagnostic uncertainty remains. HLA-B27 is positive in about 50% of patients with reactive arthritis and 25% of PsA. In general, patients who are HLA-B27 positive have more axial and ophthalmic involvement.
- **Imaging:**
  - **X-rays of sacroiliac region and affected joints**: In patients with spondyloarthropathies, x-rays typically show evidence of not just bone and cartilage destruction (as in RA) but also new bone formation, including periostitis and enthesophytes (bony growth at tendon attachment). Extensive new bone formation leads to "ankylosis" (loss of joint space due to new bone formation) (see Figure 15-12).
  - **Magnetic resonance imaging (MRI) of the sacroiliac (SI) joint** is more sensitive and shows subchondral bone marrow edema before structural changes (e.g., erosions) are evident. However, this finding can also be seen in patients with mechanical low back pain, patients with a history of pregnancy, athletes, and even normal subjects. Thus, the entire clinical picture must be considered when considering the diagnosis.
- Stool cultures for pathogens known to cause reactive arthritis, or urine testing for *Chlamydia*. However, by the time the arthritis appears, the active infection has usually resolved and thus these tests are often negative.

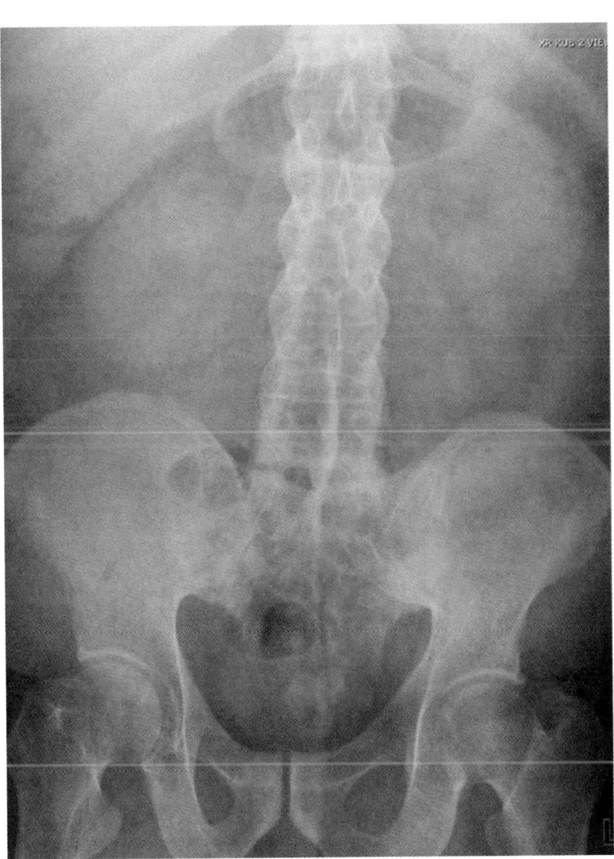

FIGURE 15-12. Kidney, ureter, bladder (KUB) view showing bamboo spine and fusion of both sacroiliac joints. (From Usatine RP, Smith MA, Mayeaux EJ Jr, Chumley HS: *The Color Atlas and Synopsis of Family Medicine*, 3rd ed. Reproduced with permission from Richard P. Usatine, MD.)

CONQUER THE **WARDS!**

Only about 5% of HLA-B27 carriers have a spondyloarthropathy, so a positive HLA-B27 test, while increasing risk for these diseases, in itself is not diagnostic.

CONQUER THE **WARDS!**

In ankylosing spondylitis, typical x-ray findings include bilateral sacroiliac (SI) joint erosions, sclerosis, and ankylosis (note that these changes are usually unilateral in reactive arthritis and psoriatic arthritis). However, it takes 5 to 10 years of symptoms before radiographic changes occur.

Serologic testing can be performed as well, but these do not differentiate between recent and remote infection.

Management

- NSAIDs and corticosteroids can help control acute inflammation but have significant long-term side effects.
- Conventional DMARDs like sulfasalazine, leflunomide, and methotrexate can be used for peripheral involvement but are minimally effective for axial involvement.
- **Biologic DMARDs are very effective.** In addition to anti–tumor necrosis factor (TNF) therapies, biologic DMARDs that target the IL-17/23 pathway such as secukinumab, ixekizumab, and ustekinumab can be used. These newer agents are similar in efficacy for articular disease to the anti-TNF therapies but are more effective for cutaneous disease (e.g., psoriatic skin rashes).
- **Prognosis:** About 50% of patients with reactive arthritis have symptoms that resolve in 6 months. PsA patients have similar long-term disability to RA patients.

CONQUER THE **BOARDS!**

Biologic DMARDS that target the IL-17/23 pathway do not appear to have the same risk of TB reactivation as the anti-TNF medications.

CRYSTALLINE ARTHRITIS

General Facts

There are two main types of crystalline arthritides:

- **Gout** is the most common inflammatory arthritis in the United States, affecting ~4% of the population. It results from the deposition of uric acid (monosodium urate) crystals in the joints and tendons. Notably, high levels of uric acid are seen in 20% to 25% of the population. Thus, high uric acid levels are NOT diagnostic of gout (hyperuricemia appears to be necessary but not sufficient to develop gout).
- **CPPD** disease is arthritis caused by calcium pyrophosphate crystals. It can present as acute CPPD arthropathy (formally known as "pseudogout") or as chronic CPPD arthropathy with various clinical manifestations (see below).

CONQUER THE **WARDS!**

Most animals do not get gout because they have the enzyme uricase, which degrades uric acid within the body. Humans have lost this enzyme in our evolution.

Clinical Features

Both gout and acute CPPD arthropathy (pseudogout) present with acute, red, swollen joints and are usually exquisitely painful.

- **Gout:** A patient's first attack of gout is almost always in the first MTP (see Figure 15-13), midfoot, or ankle. Gout can affect other joints (e.g., knee, wrist) but usually only after previous attacks in the distal lower extremities.
- **Acute CPPD arthropathy**: In contrast to gout, the first attack often affects the wrist or knee.
- Chronic CPPD arthropathy can present with low-grade joint swelling in the small joints of the hands ("pseudo-RA" pattern). It can also be associated with osteoarthritis in atypical sites, for example, the metacarpophalangeal joints or wrists.

CONQUER THE **BOARDS!**

Crystalline and septic arthritis present similarly, with an acute inflamed and painful joint. There is no vital sign, physical exam maneuver, or blood test that can differentiate the two; only an aspiration can give definitive diagnosis.

Physical Exam Findings

Affected joints of acute gout and CPPD are red, warm, swollen, and very tender to palpation. Chronic uric acid crystal deposition leads to nodular lesions called tophi, which often occur on the MTP, extensor surfaces (e.g., olecranon bursa), fingers, or ears.

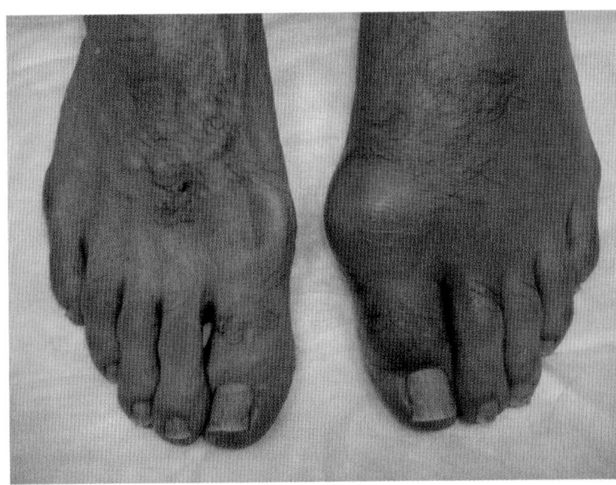

FIGURE 15-13. Podagra: Gout. The left first MTP joint is swollen and exquisitely tender; the entire forefoot is erythematous and warm. Note also the bunions (L > R). (Reproduced, with permission, from LeBlond RF, Brown DD, Suneja M, Szot JF. *DeGowin's Diagnostic Examination*, 10th ed. New York: McGraw-Hill, 2015.)

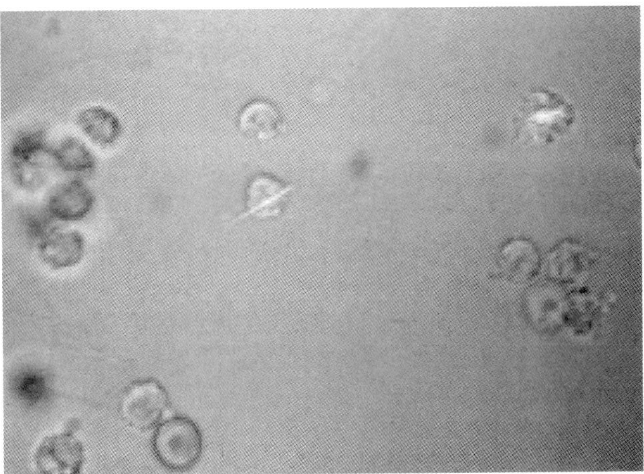

FIGURE 15-14. Urate crystal ingested by a polymorphonuclear leukocyte in synovial fluid. This finding is pathognomonic for acute gouty arthritis. (Reproduced, with permission, from Imboden JB, Hellmann DB, Stone JH, eds: *Current Diagnosis & Treatment: Rheumatology*, 3rd ed. www.accessmedicine.com. Copyright © McGraw-Hill Education. All rights reserved.)

Diagnostic Workup

- Joint aspiration is essential, both to identify the responsible crystals and to rule out infection. **Gout** joint fluid has **monosodium urate crystals** that appear as needle-shaped and **negatively birefringent** (see Figure 15-14). **CPPD arthropathy** joint fluid **has calcium pyrophosphate crystals** that are typically rhomboid shaped and can be **positively birefringent**.
- Imaging is unnecessary to diagnose acute gout or CPPD. Imaging modalities are only used when a patient presents with a history compatible with gout or CPPD arthritis, but no active inflammatory joint fluid that can be aspirated.
  - X-rays in chronic gout can show "rat-bite" erosions (juxta-articular, "punched out" erosions with overhanging edges).
  - X-rays in CPPD arthropathy can show calcification of the knee meniscus or triangular fibrocartilage of the wrist ("chondrocalcinosis") (see Figure 15-15). However, most patients with this finding never develop clinical CPPD arthropathy (either acute or chronic).
  - Ultrasound in chronic gout can show a "double contour sign" of urate deposition deposited on cartilage, as well as directly visual tophaceous deposits. Dual-energy computed tomography (CT) scan shows urate deposits directly as well.

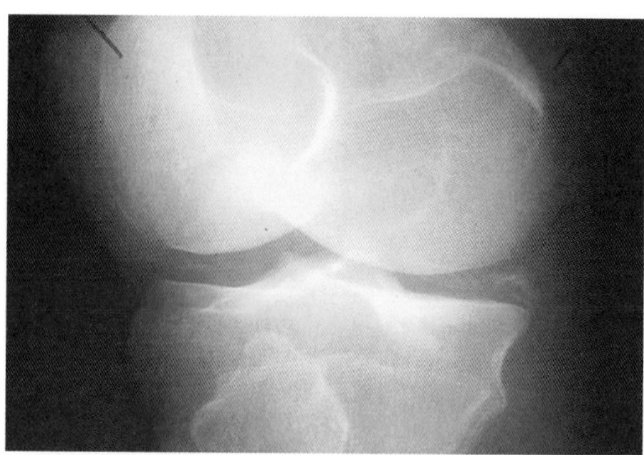

FIGURE 15-15. Chondrocalcinosis of the knees. (Reproduced, with permission, from Imboden JB, Hellmann DB, Stone JH, eds: *Current Diagnosis & Treatment: Rheumatology*, 3rd ed. www.accessmedicine.com. Copyright © McGraw-Hill Education. All rights reserved.)

Table 15-7. Acute Management of Crystalline Arthritis

Drug	Comment
Colchicine	Decrease dose if renal disease. Less effective if given >48 hours after symptom onset. GI upset common with high dosing.
NSAIDs	Avoid in renal disease and should be avoided if patient has multiple risk factors for GI bleeding.
Intraarticular corticosteroid injection	Excellent option if 1–2 joints involved. Can still raise blood sugar in diabetics.
Systemic corticosteroids	Most commonly used if severe polyarticular disease. Can raise blood sugar and increase infection risk. Too rapid taper can lead to rebound flare.
Anakinra	IL-1 beta antagonist. Effective but very expensive and carries infection risk. Painful daily subcutaneous injection.

CONQUER THE WARDS!

Allopurinol is frequently underdosed in clinical practice and can be safely increased to up to 800 mg if done slowly, even in patients with chronic kidney disease.

Management

In the acute setting, NSAIDs, colchicine, corticosteroids (either intraarticular or systemic), and anti-IL-1 agents are used for acute pain relief in both acute gout and acute CPPD arthropathy. There is no single best agent. All 3 have their advantages and side effects, so the choice of agent is dependent on patient risk factors (Table 15-7). Icing the affected joints can also be helpful.

CONQUER THE WARDS!

A lower-dose colchicine regimen (2 tabs followed by 1 tab an hour later) is as effective as a higher-dose regimen (hourly dosing until diarrhea) for treatment of acute gout.

Chronic Therapy

If a patient with gout has multiple attacks (>2/year), risk factors for recurrence (e.g., chronic kidney disease), evidence of tophi on exam, or radiographic erosions, long-term therapy to lower serum urate levels ("urate-lowering therapy") is recommended. The goal is usually a serum uric acid <5. Therapeutic options are listed in Table 15-8.

There is no "urate-lowering therapy" equivalent for CPPD arthropathy. If a patient has frequent, recurrent attacks of acute pseudogout, then daily colchicine can be used as prophylaxis.

Table 15-8. Chronic Management of Crystalline Arthritis

Drug	Mechanism of Action	Comment
Allopurinol	Xanthine oxidase inhibitor (enzyme involved in the production of uric acid)	Most commonly prescribed drug for chronic gout. Rare severe cutaneous hypersensitivity reaction associated with HLA B*5801.
Febuxostat	Xanthine oxidase inhibitor	Used if allopurinol ineffective or not tolerated. May have increased cardiovascular (CV) risk compared to allopurinol.
Probenecid	Blocks renal reabsorption of uric acid	Can be combined with allopurinol. Multiple doses/day. Cannot be used if chronic kidney disease (CKD) or history of nephrolithiasis.
Pegloticase	Uricase enzyme that converts uric acid to soluble allantoin	IV infusion every 2 weeks. Extremely effective in lowering uric acid levels. High rate of infusion reactions and extremely expensive. Used only if massive tophaceous deposits.

INFECTIOUS ARTHRITIS

General Facts

- The osteoarticular system can be infected by many types of bacteria, as well as viruses, fungi, and protozoa.
- "Septic arthritis" typically refers to an acute suppurative bacterial arthritis, mostly commonly *Staphylococcus aureus* or *Streptococcus*. Immunocompromised patients are also at risk for gram-negative infections.
- Bacteria typically reach the joint hematogenously, though spread from an adjacent bone or soft tissue infection, or via penetrating trauma, can also occur.

Clinical Features

Patients with septic arthritis present with an acute, red, hot, exquisitely painful and tender joint.

The knee is the most commonly affected joint, although almost any joint can be involved. About 10% of patients can have a polyarticular infection. It should be noted that up to 50% of patients will not have a fever.

Risk Factors for Septic Arthritis

- Very young or very old.
- Underlying joint damage (rheumatoid arthritis, prosthetic joints, recent joint surgery).
- Intravenous drug use (IVDU).
- Alcoholism.
- Diabetes mellitus.

Other Noteworthy Specific Causes of Bacterial Arthritis

- **Gonorrhea** is the most common cause of septic arthritis in a young, sexually active person. Patients can present either with a single swollen joint or with tenosynovitis (inflammation around tendon sheaths), fever, and purpuric pustular skin rashes (disseminated gonococcal infection [DGI]).
- ***Borrelia burgdorferi*** can cause joint symptoms at any stage, though it only causes a true inflammatory arthritis in the tertiary stage (weeks/months

CONQUER THE BOARDS!

Parvovirus should always be considered in a patient who presents with <6 weeks of symmetric small joint polyarthritis, especially if there is any exposure to children.

after initial infection). Usually 1 to 2 joints are involved. Though effusions are large, the pain is typically less than a suppurative bacterial infection. Diagnosed serologically; typically 10/10 IgG bands are seen on Western blot in true infectious arthritis.

- A number of viruses can cause infectious arthritis, most notably **parvovirus, chikungunya, and dengue.**
- Immunocompromised patients are at risk for chronic fungal infections or tuberculosis. These usually present insidiously and affect the joint and surrounding bone.

Diagnostic Workup

- **Aspiration** should be done immediately when an infectious arthritis is suspected.
- The higher the synovial fluid WBC count, the more likely the cause is septic arthritis; however, diagnosis is only confirmed when the organism is cultured.
- Peripheral WBC count and inflammatory markers will not distinguish septic arthritis from mimickers (e.g., acute gout).
- Peripheral blood cultures are positive in about half of patients with septic (bacterial) arthritis.

Management

- Untreated suppurative bacterial infections progress rapidly and can destroy joints within hours/days, so antibiotic therapy should be initiated immediately after aspiration, before cultures have returned.
- Empiric coverage should begin with covering methicillin-resistant *S. aureus* (MRSA) (vancomycin is a good first choice). Gram-negative coverage should also be added (e.g., ceftriaxone or cefepime) if the patient is immunocompromised.
- If septic arthritis is confirmed by the growth of bacteria from the initial aspiration, the joint should be drained, typically with arthroscopic surgical drainage. Usually a single surgical procedure is enough, but the patient should be monitored closely for recurrent swelling so that additional drainage can be performed. Antibiotics are tailored based on the organism identified and continued for 2 to 6 weeks.
- Some bacteria-specific treatment regiments:
  - *B. burgdorferi* arthritis is treated with 1 month of doxycycline.
  - Gonococcal arthritis is treated with 1 week of ceftriaxone.
  - Viral arthritides are treated with supportive care (e.g., NSAIDs, fluids).
  - Fungal or *Mycobacteria* infections are treated with prolonged courses of therapy.

LUPUS AND RELATED CONDITIONS

SYSTEMIC LUPUS ERYTHEMATOSUS

General Facts

Systemic lupus erythematosus (SLE) is the prototypical autoimmune disease.

- Typically affects women of childbearing age, though children and older adults can be affected as well.
- Clinically more severe in African Americans, Asians, and Hispanics, as compared to whites.

- Certain medications (e.g., hydralazine, procainamide) can also cause drug-induced lupus.
- **The nomenclature of lupus and lupus-like disease can be confusing.**
  - **Undifferentiated connective tissue disease (aka "incomplete lupus")** refers to patients with a few features of lupus but not enough to meet classification criteria.
  - **Overlap syndrome** refers to patients who meet **criteria for 2 different rheumatic diseases**.
  - **Mixed connective tissue disease** refers to a specific disease that has features of **lupus** and **scleroderma** and is characterized by **a positive RNP antibody**.

Clinical Features

- Lupus can affect virtually any organ system in the body.
- Lupus is a heterogenous disease. Some patients can present with a mild rash and joint pain, while others present fulminantly with severe neurologic or renal involvement.
- Table 15-9 lists the common clinical features by system. The **most common manifestations** are:
  - Rashes (e.g., malar rash).
  - Arthralgias: One of the earliest manifestations and occur in over 90% of patients. Tends to be mildly painful, polyarticular, and symmetrical. Rarely destructive, unlike RA.
  - Serositis (pleural or pericardial inflammation/effusions).
  - Hematologic involvement.
  - Renal involvement. **Lupus nephritis** is the most common cause of morbidity in patients with lupus.

Table 15-9. Clinical Manifestations of SLE

General	Fatigue, fever, unintentional weight loss
Skin	Photosensitive rashes especially the malar rash Hair loss Raynaud disease
Eyes	Dry eyes
ENT	Oral or nasal ulcers, usually painless
CV	Pericardial effusion Increased risk of coronary artery disease
Pulm	Pleural effusion
Heme	Leukopenia, thrombocytopenia, hemolytic anemia Lymphadenopathy DVT/PE
Neuro	Neuropsychiatric lupus Acute confusional state Seizures Transverse myelitis Acute psychosis Peripheral neuropathy
MSK	Joint pains
GU	Renal failure and proteinuria
GYN	Preeclampsia, pregnancy loss

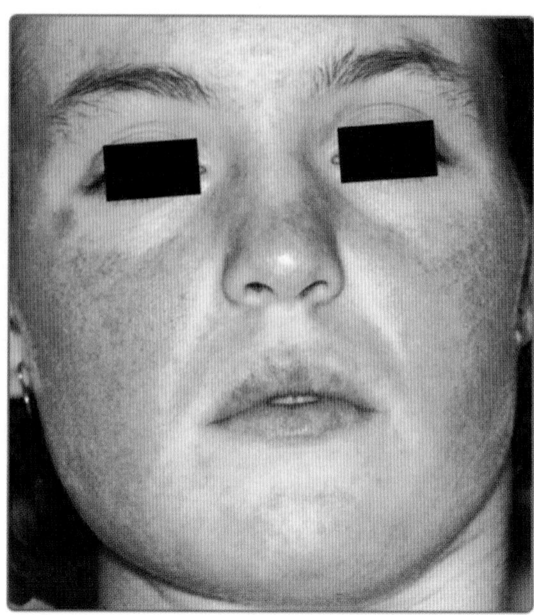

FIGURE 15-16. Localized acute cutaneous lupus erythematosus. Erythematous, slightly edematous, sharply demarcated erythema, is seen on the malar areas in a "butterfly" distribution. (Reproduced, with permission, from Kang S, Amagai M, Bruckner AL, et al, eds. *Fitzpatrick's Dermatology,* 9th ed. New York: McGraw-Hill, 2019.)

Physical Exam Findings

Here are some of the typical findings of SLE; note this is not an exhaustive list.

Skin

- **Malar rash (see Figure 15-16)**:
  - Seen in about half of patients with lupus.
  - Typically erythematous, mildly raised, and involves both checks and nasal bridge.
  - Classically **spares the nasolabial fold**.
- **Discoid lupus**:
  - Erythematous papules and plaques that subsequently can evolve into chronic lesions with atrophy and plugging of the hair follicles (see Figure 15-17).
  - The lesions have a **predilection for the head and neck and, importantly, will scar** (thus causing permanent hair loss if located in the scalp).

HEENT

- **Oral ulcers**:
  - Look like typical aphthous ulcers.
  - Affect the cheeks, hard palate, and "wet line" of the inner lip. In contrast to herpetic ulcers, **they are not usually painful** and do not appear on the vermillion border.

MSK

- Joints may show bogginess and tenderness.
- Unlike in RA, irreversible deformities are seldom seen.

CV/Pulm

- Heart or lung sounds can be distant if there is pleural or pericardial effusion.
- Pleural or pericardial rubs can be heard.

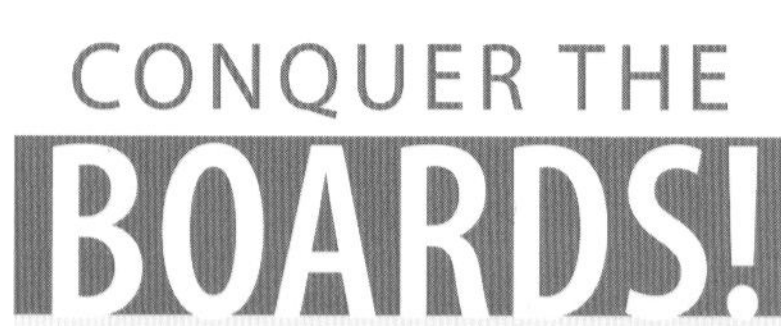

Patients can have isolated cutaneous lupus without having systemic lupus. This is especially common in discoid lupus; only about 5% of patients with discoid lupus limited to the head and neck have systemic lupus.

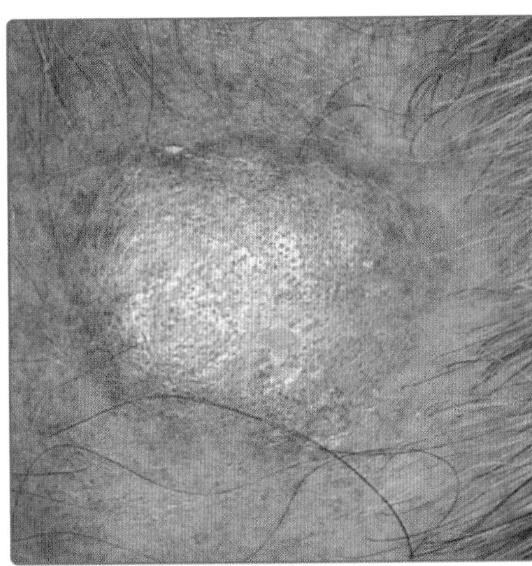

FIGURE 15-17. Classic discoid lupus erythematosus. Typical early erythematous plaque on the forehead demonstrating hyperkeratosis and accentuation of follicle orifices in a 60-year-old man with a 25-year history of cutaneous lupus erythematosus. The lesion had been present for 3 months; no dermal atrophy was present at this stage. (Reproduced, with permission, from Kang S, Amagai M, Bruckner AL, et al, eds. *Fitzpatrick's Dermatology,* 9th ed. New York: McGraw-Hill, 2019.)

Diagnostic Workup

Table 15-10 presents the 2012 SLICC Classification Criteria (need at least 4, with 1 clinical and 1 immunologic criteria).

Virtually ALL patients with lupus have positive antinuclear antibodies (ANA), typically at high titer. However, the vast majority of people with a positive ANA do NOT have lupus. Thus, the ANA is a sensitive, but not specific, test for lupus. Additional lab tests to send in the workup for lupus are listed in Table 15-11.

CONQUER THE **BOARDS!**

An antinuclear antibody test should not be sent for isolated nonspecific symptoms like fatigue and myalgias.

Table 15-10. 2012 SLICC SLE Classification Criteria

Clinical Criteria	Laboratory Criteria
Acute cutaneous lupus (most common below) ■ Malar rash ■ Diffuse maculopapular rash	Antinuclear antibody
Chronic cutaneous lupus (discoid lupus)	Anti-DS DNA antibody
Oral/nasal ulcers	Anti-Smith antibody
Nonscarring alopecia (diffuse thinning without other causes)	Anti-phospholipid antibodies
Arthritis (effusion of at least 2 joints)	Low complement levels
Serositis (pleural/pericardial inflammation)	Direct Coombs test
Renal ■ >500 mg protein per 24 hours ■ Red blood cell casts	
Neurologic	
Hemolytic anemia	
Leukopenia (<4000) or lymphopenia	
Thrombocytopenia (<100,000)	

Table 15-11. SLE Laboratory Workup

Test	Relevance
DS DNA antibodies	Most specific test for lupus. Titer can correlate with disease activity (not seen with other antibodies).
Smith antibodies	Specific antibodies for lupus.
RNP antibodies	Can be seen in lupus but also mixed connective tissue disease.
SSA/B antibodies	Also can be seen in Sjögren syndrome. SSA is associated with neonatal lupus syndrome due to passive transfer of this antibody across the placenta.
Histone antibodies	Positive in drug-induced lupus but often seen in idiopathic lupus as well.
Coombs test	Can be positive even if no active hemolysis.
Antiphospholipid antibodies (anti-cardiolipin, beta 2 glycoprotein, lupus anticoagulant)	Increased risk of blood clots and pregnancy morbidity.
Complement levels (C3, C4)	Low, as deposition of immune complexes leads to consumption of serum complement proteins.
ESR	Elevated due to polyclonal gammopathy.
Urinalysis	Proteinuria and red blood cell casts suggest active lupus nephritis.

CONQUER THE **WARDS!**

There is often an ESR/CRP discrepancy in active lupus, with a very high ESR and only mildly elevated CRP. If a patient with lupus has a very high CRP, infection must be ruled out.

CONQUER THE **WARDS!**

Renal biopsies are crucial in any lupus patient presenting with renal insufficiency or proteinuria and typically show a proliferative glomerulonephritis. Immunofluorescence shows "full house" staining (e.g., positive for IgG, IgA, IgM, C3, and C1q).

HIGH-YIELD LITERATURE

ANA and Lupus

Abeles AM, Abeles M. The clinical utility of a positive antinuclear antibody test result. *Am J Med*. 2013;126(4):342-348.

CONQUER THE **WARDS!**

Classification criteria can be used as a guide but should not be used solely for diagnosis at the bedside.

Management

In general, the management of patients with lupus is tailored to the severity of their disease (more severe involvement requires more aggressive medication; Table 15-12). The exception is that essentially all patients should be on **hydroxychloroquine (Plaquenil)**. This is a nonimmunosuppressant antimalarial medication that has been shown to prevent flares, lessen chronic damage, and improve mortality in patients with lupus.

CONQUER THE **WARDS!**

If a patient with lupus is admitted for fever, it is essential to rule out infection prior to attributing the fevers to lupus, especially if they are already on immunosuppressive medications.

Table 15-12. Management of Severe SLE

Corticosteroids	Mainstay of treatment for acute control of inflammation. However, many long-term side effects even at relatively low doses.
Hydroxychloroquine	In addition to above, often very effective for skin and arthritic involvement.
Methotrexate	Often for joint disease; never renal involvement.
Belimumab (Benlysta)	Biologic against the cytokine B-cell activating factor. Used for mild/moderate involvement, especially to decrease corticosteroid burden. Not used for severe disease such as renal or neurologic.
Mycophenolate mofetil (Cellcept) or cyclophosphamide	Used for severe disease, including renal and neurologic. Mycophenolate mofetil is more typically used due to a better side effect profile.

Other Treatment Considerations

- **Photoprotection:** All lupus patients need to be vigilant about photoprotection, as ultraviolet (UV) light can flare not just skin but systemic lupus.
- **Cardiovascular disease:** This is the major cause of death in patients with SLE. Smoking cessation and exercise should be stressed for all patients with this condition.
- **Pregnancy:**
  - Most patients with lupus can have a normal healthy pregnancy.
  - However, patients with lupus are at higher risk of adverse pregnancy outcomes such as fetal loss and preeclampsia, especially if they have anti-phospholipid antibodies.
  - **Neonatal lupus syndrome**: Characterized by rash and (most feared) cardiac conduction abnormalities, including irreversible heart block. Caused by passive transfer of SSA antibody.
  - Pregnancy can also flare the mother's lupus.
  - **Importantly, outcomes for both the mother and baby are improved if the mother's SLE is in remission prior to conception.**

CONQUER THE WARDS!

Hydroxychloroquine is typically very well tolerated. With long-term use there is a low risk of retinal toxicity. Patients need yearly eye exam screenings while on this medication.

SJÖGREN'S SYNDROME

General Facts

- Sjögren syndrome (SS) is a chronic autoimmune inflammatory disorder that always affects lacrimal and salivary gland function. However, it can also have extraglandular complications.
- SS can either be primary (idiopathic) or secondary (seen in the context of another autoimmune disease, most notably rheumatoid arthritis or lupus).
- It is almost exclusively seen in women, with most diagnosed in the forties and fifties.

Clinical Features

- **Severe dry eyes and mouth** without an underlying cause are seen in virtually all patients. Patients complain of a dry, gritty sensation in their eyes; sometimes they feel a foreign body. They often use artificial tears with minimal improvement.
- **Fatigue** is quite common in patients with SS and is multifactorial in etiology.
- **Extraglandular disease:** About one-third of patients with SS will have clinically significant extraglandular disease, including
  - Interstitial lung disease.
  - Joint pain – typically symmetric and nonerosive, affecting the hands, wrists, and knees.
  - Peripheral neuropathy.
  - Rashes – annular plaques as well as dry skin.
  - Tubulointerstitial nephritis, but also glomerulonephritis.
  - Cutaneous vasculitis due to cryoglobulinemia.
  - Lymphoma: increased risk of lymphoma in patients with SS.

Physical Exam Findings

- A variety of oral lesions reflecting poor salivary gland production can be seen, including dry mucous membranes, tongue fissuring and hypolobulation, and dental caries in atypical locations. Parotid swelling is often seen (see Figure 15-18).

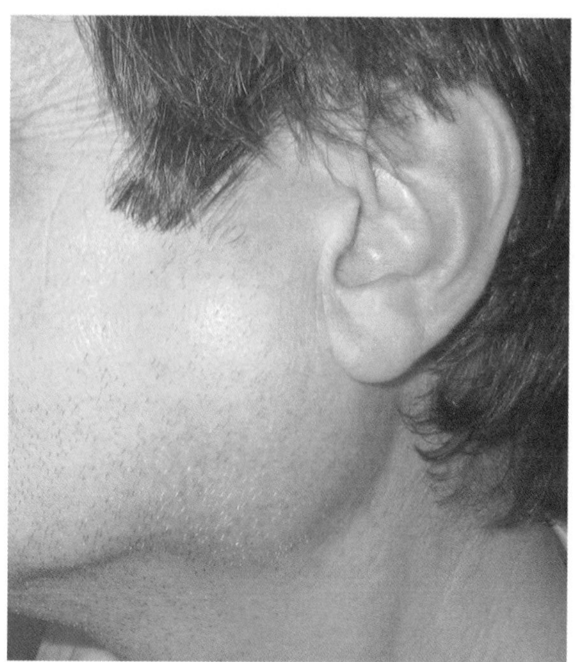

FIGURE 15-18. Parotid enlargement. (Reproduced, with permission, from Imboden JB, Hellmann DB, Stone JH, eds: *Current Diagnosis & Treatment: Rheumatology*, 3rd ed. www.accessmedicine.com. Copyright © McGraw-Hill Education. All rights reserved.)

- The ophthalmologist can see areas of devitalized tissue in the corneas with special stains.

Diagnostic Workup

The diagnosis is made with a combination of:

- Subjective symptoms of dry eyes and dry mouth.
- Objective findings of abnormal lacrimal or salivary glands.
  - **Positive Schirmer test**: Filter paper is placed on the eyelid and the tear production is measured over time.
  - **Abnormal eye exam** showing devitalized tissue in the cornea,
  - **Abnormal parotid gland ultrasound**.
  - **Positive serologies (SSA/B antibody)**:
    - About 25% of patients with SS are "seronegative," meaning they test negative for the SSA/B antibody. In these patients a biopsy of the inner lip can be helpful, since the inner lip contains minor salivary gland tissue. The characteristic finding in SS is focal lymphocytic sialadenitis (collections of 50 lymphoid cells around normal acinar tissue).

Management

- Unfortunately, immunosuppression for the treatment of dry eyes and dry mouth in SS has not been found to be effective.
- **Treatment of dry eyes:**
  - Avoid dry or windy environments.
  - **Preservative-free artificial tears** should be frequently used, and nighttime lubricating ointment can be added.
  - **Topical cyclosporine** is used if more aggressive measures are needed.
- **Treatment of dry mouth** requires a multifactorial approach that includes:
  - Drinking water frequently.
  - Artificial saliva.
  - Salivary stimulation with sugar-free gum or lozenges.

- Frequent dental cleanings at least every 3 months.
- If these measures are ineffective, then:
  - **Sialogogues** (muscarinic agonists) like pilocarpine or cevimeline are used.
  - These medications must be taken multiple times per day.
  - Associated with frequent side effects due to their mechanism of action of cholinergic stimulation (sweating, flushing, increased urinary frequency, nausea, diarrhea).

- **Treatment of extraglandular manifestations:** Rituximab has been most frequently used.
- **Increased risk for lymphoma**.
  - Typically non-Hodgkin lymphoma. MALT lymphomas (often arising from the parotid gland) or diffuse large B-cell lymphoma are the most common subtypes.
  - Patients have the highest risk for lymphoma among rheumatic diseases (approximately 5- to 10-fold).
  - Lymphoma usually develops 5 to 10 years after the initial diagnosis.
  - Risk factors for lymphoma include persistent salivary gland enlargement, cutaneous vasculitis, cryoglobulinemia, glomerulonephritis, hypocomplementemia, and monoclonal gammopathy.
  - How and when to screen for the development of this complication is unknown, but should be strongly considered if a patient with SS develops constitutional symptoms (fever, weight loss, night sweats), persistent salivary gland enlargement (especially parotid), or persistent lymphadenopathy.

SCLERODERMA (SYSTEMIC SCLEROSIS)

General Facts

- Scleroderma (systemic sclerosis) is characterized by fibrosis of skin and internal organs, vasculopathy, and the production of autoantibodies.
- It is rare, with ~20 new cases per million per year in the United States.
- The disease has traditionally been categorized into "limited" and "diffuse" based on the extent of skin involvement, with "limited" involvement being distal to the elbows and knees. However, importantly, BOTH limited and diffuse skin disease can be characterized by severe internal organ involvement.

More recently, there is a trend to move toward a serologic classification (see later) of disease.

CONQUER THE **WARDS!**

The pneumonic "CREST" (calcinosis, Raynaud disease, esophageal dysmotility, sclerodactyly, telangiectasias) was previously used to describe a subset of patients with limited SS. However, this has fallen out of favor, as all these features can be seen in any form of scleroderma.

Clinical Features

- **Raynaud disease:** Almost all patients with scleroderma have severe Raynaud disease (fingers/toes turn white, then blue, then red in response to cold or stress), often leading to digital ischemia without treatment. Skin thickening starts in the fingers ("sclerodactyly") and progresses proximally; it can make affected digits difficult to use.
- **GI:** Esophageal dysmotility and gastroparesis cause dysphagia with postprandial abdominal pain and bloating. Symptoms of gastroesophageal reflux disease (GERD) are quite common. Some degree of GI involvement is seen in almost all patients and can be the most problematic manifestation, causing severe symptoms and nutritional deficiencies.
- **Pulmonary:**
  - **Interstitial lung disease.**
  - **Pulmonary hypertension** causes shortness of breath. If there is subsequent right-sided heart dysfunction, lower extremity edema can be seen.

- **Renal**: **Scleroderma renal crisis** is characterized by the rapid onset of high blood pressure and acute renal failure, often leading to pulmonary edema. It is usually seen soon after diagnosis in the setting of worsening skin disease and is associated with particular autoantibodies (see Table 15-15).
- **Other**: Cardiac involvement (frequently with decreased ejection fracture, pericardial effusion, and conduction defects due to cardiac fibrosis), myositis, and inflammatory arthritis.
- Scleroderma physical exam findings are summarized in Table 15-13.

CONQUER THE WARDS!

Telangiectasias are dilated post-capillary venules that **blanch** with pressure

Table 15-13. Physical Exam Findings

Skin (Figure 15-19)	• Diffuse; "puffy fingers" may be first sign of the disease. • Skin feels thick and hardened. • Telangiectasias especially on palms, lips, face, and chest. • Fingertip ulcerations. • Nailfold capillaries are dilated and disorganized. • "Scleroderma facies" with purse-string lips, decreased oral aperture, and loss of wrinkles.
Lung	Velcro-like crackles if interstitial lung disease (ILD).
CV	Loud P2 if pulmonary arterial hypertension (PAH).
Articular	Tendon friction rubs, especially wrist/ankle.

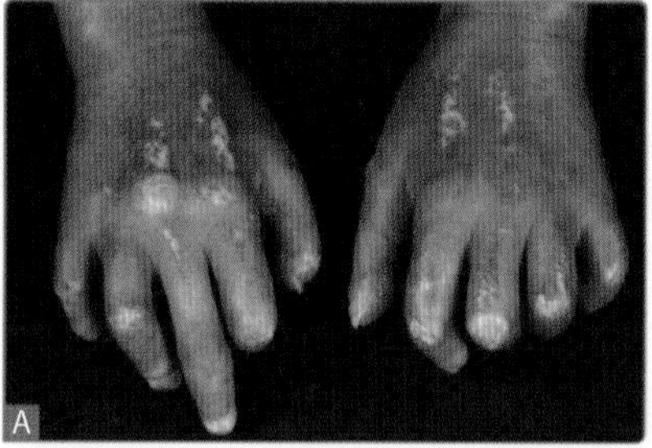
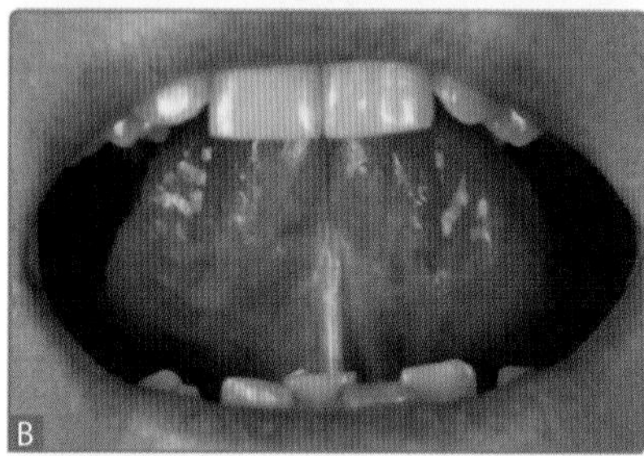
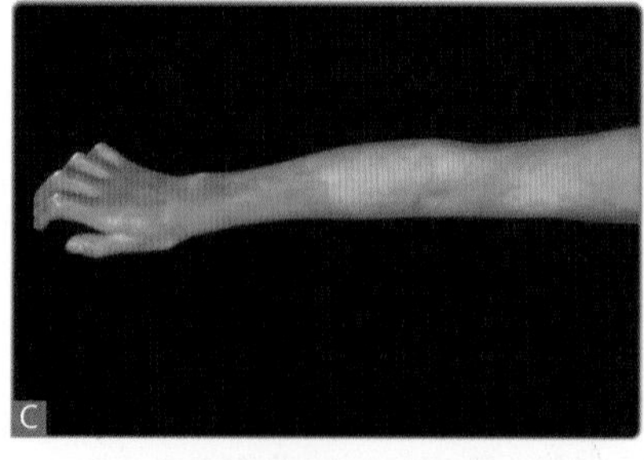
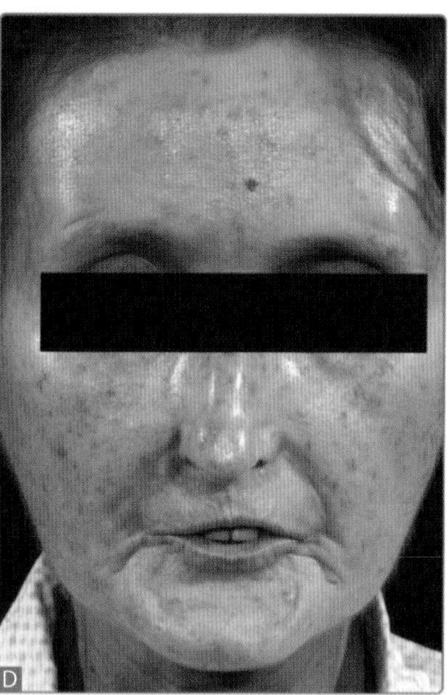

FIGURE 15-19. Extensive skin involvement in patients with diffuse cutaneous systemic sclerosis. A: Sclerodactyly with dermatogenous contractures (restricted mobility of digital joints) and salt-and-pepper hyperpigmentations and hypopigmentations. B: Microstomia (radial furrowing around the mouth) with frenulum sclerosis. C: Skin thickening proximal of the metacarpophalangeal joints. D: Typical scleroderma facial physiognomy with hypermimia, microstomia, telangiectasias, and a beaked nose. (Reproduced, with permission, from Kang S, Amagai M, Bruckner AL, et al, eds. *Fitzpatrick's Dermatology,* 9th ed. New York: McGraw-Hill, 2019.)

Table 15-14. ACR/EULAR Criteria for Classification of Scleroderma

Item	Subitem	Weight/Score
Skin thickening of the fingers of both hands extending proximal to the metacarpophalangeal joints *(sufficient criterion)*		9
Skin thickening of the finger (only count the higher score)	Puffy fingers Sclerodactyly of the fingers (distal to the metacarpophalangeal joints but proximal to the proximal interphalangeal joints)	2 4
Fingertip lesions *(only count the higher score)*	Digital tip ulcers Fingertip pitting scars	2 3
Telangiectasia		2
Abnormal nailfold capillaries		2
Pulmonary arterial hypertension (HTN) and/or interstitial lung disease (ILD) *(maximum score is 2)*	Pulmonary artery HTN ILD	2 2
Raynaud phenomenon		3
SSc-related autoantibodies (anticentromere, anti-topoisomerase I [anti-Scl-70], anti-RNA polymerase III) *(maximum score is 3)*	Anticentromere Anti-topoisomerase I Anti-RNA polymerase III	3

ACR, American College of Rheumatology; *EULAR,* European League Against Rheumatism.

CONQUER THE WARDS!

Pulmonary hypertension will cause a low DLCO out of proportion to the FVC. Interstitial lung disease causes a similar decrease in both these parameters.

Table 15-15. Scleroderma Subserologies

Antibody	Clinical Features
Centromere	Limited skin disease. Increased risk of pulmonary hypertension, less of interstitial lung disease.
SCL -70 (topoisomerase I)	Diffuse skin disease. Increased risk of interstitial lung disease.
RNA polymerase III	Diffuse skin disease. Associated with malignancy. Increased risk of scleroderma renal crisis and gastric antral vascular ectasias.

Diagnostic Workup

- Scleroderma is a clinical diagnosis, though classification criteria have been published. Patients with a total score of ≥9 are classified as definitely having scleroderma (see Table 15-14).
- If scleroderma is suspected, ANA immunofluorescence and subserologies (see Table 15-15) should be sent. ANA is almost always positive.
- Skin biopsy would show excessive collagen, but is rarely necessary for diagnosis.

Management

Unlike most rheumatic diseases, corticosteroids are not routinely used for scleroderma, especially as high doses (>10 mg) increase the risk for scleroderma renal crisis. Instead, a multimodal approach is taken, depending on the symptoms the patient displays. The major cause of death is lung involvement (ILD or PAH).

CONQUER THE BOARDS!

In PAH alone, PFTs show low DLCO with normal FVC. If there is ILD, both of these parameters will be low.

- **Calcium channel blockers** that work peripherally (amlodipine, nifedipine) and PDE-5 agents (sildenafil up to 20 mg TID) are used for Raynaud disease, especially if there is concurrent ulceration or digital ischemia.
- **Methotrexate and mycophenolate mofetil** are used for skin disease.
- **Proton pump inhibitors** help with GERD. Promotility agents can be used for GI tract involvement.
- **Cyclophosphamide or mycophenolate** are used for ILD.
- Pulmonary hypertension is not treated with immunosuppression, but rather with vasodilatory agents like any other cause of pulmonary arteriole hypertension.
- **Angiotensin-converting enzyme (ACE) inhibitors:** In the past, scleroderma renal crisis (SRC) was a common cause of death, but this can now be effectively treated with ACE inhibitors. Typically captopril is started at a dose of 12.5 mg q6h but is rapidly uptitrated to the dose needed to control the blood pressure. Of note, ACE inhibitors do not prevent SRC and are not recommended as prophylaxis.

HIGH-YIELD LITERATURE

Tashkin DP, et al. Mycophenolate mofetil versus oral cyclophosphamide in scleroderma-related interstitial lung disease (SLS II): A randomised controlled, double-blind, parallel group trial. *Lancet Respir Med*. 2016;4(9):708-719.

MISCELLANEOUS CONDITIONS

INFLAMMATORY MYOPATHIES

General Facts

- Inflammatory myopathies are idiopathic diseases characterized by autoimmune muscle inflammation and (typically) proximal muscle weakness.
- Historically these diseases have been categorized based on their muscle biopsy findings, as either polymyositis (PM), dermatomyositis (DM), immune-mediated necrotizing myopathy (IMNM), or inclusion body myositis (IBM). However, the discovery of different autoantibodies ("myositis-specific antibodies") has identified unique subsets of patients with characteristic clinical features, response to treatment, and prognosis (see later). About 70% of patients with DM can have a detectable autoantibody with current testing, depending on the lab technique.
- IBM deserves special mention: It is the most common inflammatory myopathy of patients >50, has a particular pattern of muscle involvement (see later), and importantly, does NOT respond to immunosuppressive agents, since the primary pathology is thought to be neurodegenerative, with the inflammatory infiltrates as a secondary phenomenon.

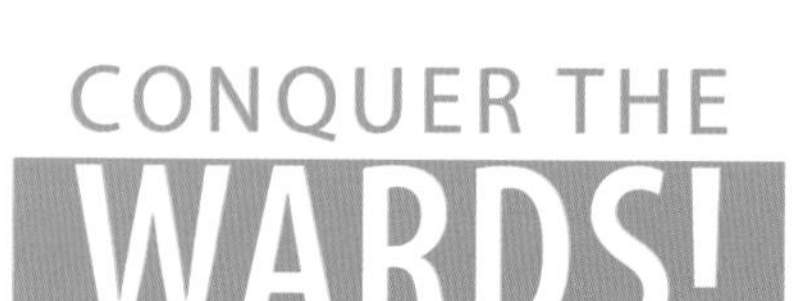

If an elderly patient has "treatment-refractory" polymyositis, the diagnosis is probably inclusion body myositis.

Clinical Features

- Most patients present with subacute (weeks to a few months) proximal muscle weakness. They describe difficulty rising from a chair, walking upstairs, reaching to grab items from cabinets, or brushing hair.
- Muscle pain is atypical, but can be seen especially in patients with immune-mediated necrotizing myopathy.
- A number of extramuscular features can be seen, including rashes (often with prominent itching), ILD, and joint inflammation.

- A subset of patients will have extramuscular (especially cutaneous) features alone ("amyopathic dermatomyositis").
- **Anti-synthetase syndrome** occurs in 30% of myositis patients and is a constellation of the following symptoms (not all have to be present):
  - Constitutional symptoms (e.g., weight loss and fever).
  - Myositis.
  - Raynaud phenomenon.
  - Mechanic's hands (fissures on the radial fingers).
  - Nonerosive arthritis.
  - ILD.
  - Positive antibody to aminoacyl-transfer ribonucleic acid synthetase enzymes (mostly commonly Jo-1 antibody).

Physical Exam Findings

- **HEENT:** Look for eyelid edema and **heliotrope** rash on eyelids (purplish discoloration) (see Figure 15-20).
- **Neuro:** Muscle weakness, typically of the proximal muscles, including arm abduction and thigh flexion. Sensory function is generally preserved, and muscle atrophy is a late finding.
- **Skin**: Many signs can be seen. The most common are:
  - **V sign** (violaceous erythema in a V distribution on chest).
  - **Shawl sign** (violaceous erythema on upper back).
  - **Gottron papules** (erythematous papules overlying the MCPs, PIPs) (see Figure 15-21).
  - Ischemic ulcers on hands and extensor surfaces (MDA-5 antibody).
  - Cutaneous calcinosis.
- **MSK**: Pain and swelling in small joints of hands.

Diagnostic Workup

- If a myositis is suspected, initial tests should include **muscle enzymes (CPK, aldolase)**, which are usually elevated. An **MRI** of the affected muscles will show edema within the muscles. However, both of these features are nonspecific and can be seen in other diseases affecting the neuromuscular

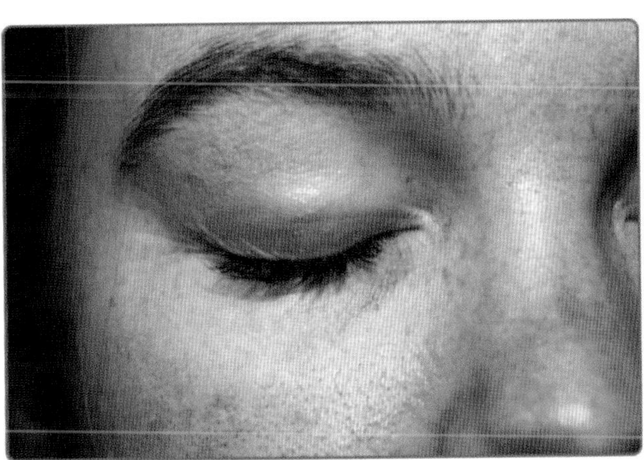

FIGURE 15-20. Heliotrope sign. Violaceous to pink erythema and edema on the upper eyelid. (Reproduced, with permission, from Kang S, Amagai M, Bruckner AL, et al, eds. *Fitzpatrick's Dermatology*, 9th ed. New York: McGraw-Hill, 2019.)

CONQUER THE WARDS!

Statin medications can cause muscle pain in a number of ways. Most commonly, patients may endorse mild myalgias without true muscle weakness. Statins can also cause a direct toxic effect on muscles, leading to muscle weakness and elevated CPK. This syndrome improves a few weeks after withdrawal of the medication. Lastly, and much more rarely, statins can trigger the development of an immune-mediated necrotizing myopathy, with very high CPK values, intense muscle pain, and weakness. Importantly, in these patients withdrawal of the medication is not sufficient and immunosuppressive medication is necessary.

CONQUER THE BOARDS!

Inclusion body myositis presents with a characteristic pattern of muscle weakness, with prominent weakness of the finger flexors and quadriceps.

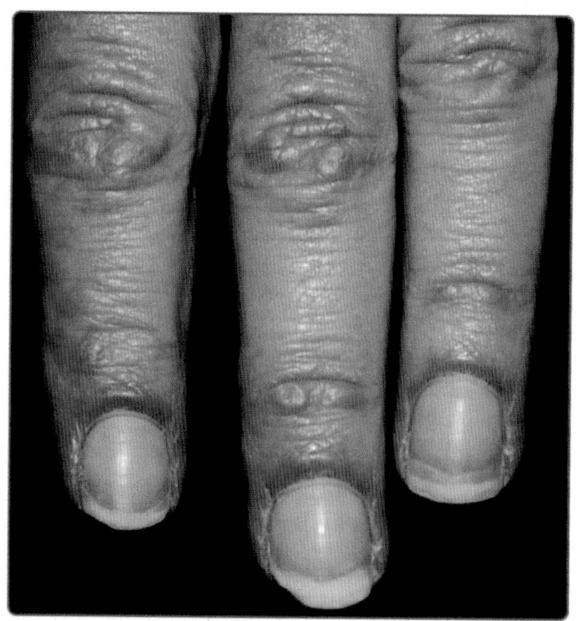

FIGURE 15-21. Gottron papules. Light pink, ill-defined papules over the proximal and distal interphalangeal joints, few with central umbilication. Deep red erythema, edema of the proximal nailfolds, and dilated nailfold capillaries are evident. (Reproduced, with permission, from Kang S, Amagai M, Bruckner AL, et al, eds. *Fitzpatrick's Dermatology,* 9th ed. New York: McGraw-Hill, 2019.)

system. The following tests should then be run to confirm the diagnosis (Table 15-16).

- **Myositis-specific antibodies:** This is a crucial step in the diagnostic workup (see Table 15-16).
- **Muscle biopsy** remains an important tool, both to identify an inflammatory myopathy and rule out mimickers (e.g., drug-induced myopathy, muscular dystrophy) (See Table 15-17).

Table 15-16. Myositis-Specific Antibodies

Autoantibody	Histopathology	Characteristics
Mi-2	DM	Classic DM skin rashes and muscle weakness; good response to steroids.
TIF-gamma	DM	Strong malignancy association.
NXP-2	DM	Cutaneous calcinosis, muscle pain, and edema.
MDA-5	DM	Rapidly progressive pulmonary involvement, minimal muscle disease, ischemic cutaneous ulcerations.
Anti-synthetase (Jo-1 most common, but also PL-7, PL-12, EJ, OJ)	DM or PM	Anti-synthetase syndrome (see the previous page).
SRP	IMNM	Myalgias and very elevated creatinine phosphokinase (CPK).
HMCOa-reductase	IMNM	Myalgias and very elevated CPK. Often seen in the setting of statin use, but can be idiopathic as well.

DM, dermatomyositis; *IMNM,* immune-mediated necrotizing myopathy; *PM,* polymyositis.

Table 15-17. Inflammatory Myopathy Biopsy Findings

Polymyositis	Endomysial inflammation with CD8+ T cells, with invasion of nonnecrotic muscle fibers
Dermatomyositis	Perimysial inflammation with CD4+ T cells and perifascicular atrophy
Inclusion body myositis	Endomysial inflammation with CD8+ T cells, with invasion of nonnecrotic muscle fibers, rimmed vacuoles, cytoplasmic inclusion bodies on EM
Immune-mediated necrotizing myopathy	Muscle cell necrosis and macrophage infiltration

Management

- **Corticosteroids** are first-line and are typically started at 1 mg/kg.
- **IV immunoglobulin** is often used in combination with steroids for acute control of disease, especially if there is severe dysphagia.
- A variety of **steroid-sparing agents** are used, including azathioprine, methotrexate, mycophenolate mofetil, and rituximab. These do not work in the acute setting.
- **IBM** is not treated with immunosuppression. Unfortunately, there are no disease-modifying therapies for IBM at the current time, and treatment is based on physical therapy and assistive devices.
- **Association with cancer:**
  - DM is a common paraneoplastic syndrome.
  - Risk of cancer among patients with DM is increased approximately 5-fold overall compared to the general population in the years surrounding the diagnosis.
  - A wide variety of cancers, both liquid and solid, have been reported in association with DM.
  - Anyone diagnosed with DM should be screened for age-appropriate cancers.
  - The risk of malignancy is strikingly high with certain autoantibodies, most notably TIF-1 gamma. In patients carrying this antibody, additional imaging, including a positron-emitting tomography (PET) scan, should be strongly considered.

As mentioned above, inclusion body myositis does not respond to immunosuppression.

HIGH-YIELD LITERATURE

Fiorentino DF, et al. Most patients with cancer-associated dermatomyositis have antibodies to nuclear matrix protein NXP-2 or transcription intermediary factor 1γ. *Arthritis Rheum*. 2013;65(11):2954-2962.

IGG4-RELATED DISEASE

General Facts

- IgG4-related disease (IgG4-RD) is a relatively newly described clinical entity of tumefactive (tumor-like) lesions that have the potential to affect multiple organ symptoms, with the biopsy findings consistent across organ symptoms.
- Many of its clinical manifestations were previously described as idiopathic single-organ diseases, such as Mikulicz disease and Riedel thyroiditis.

Clinical Features

- Patients are not typically systemically ill with fevers and major constitutional symptoms.
- IgG4-RD can affect almost any organ system; single or multiple organ systems can be affected either simultaneously or sequentially, and thus the diagnosis can be challenging. The most commonly affected organs are:
  - GI tract:
    - Autoimmune pancreatitis.
    - Sclerosing cholangitis.

- Sialadenitis (salivary gland): Typically parotid and (more common) submandibular gland swelling.
- Dacryoadenitis: Lacrimal gland enlargement.
- Renal: Tubulointerstitial nephritis.
- Retroperitoneal fibrosis and periaortitis.

Physical Exam Findings

- Dacryoadenitis (lacrimal gland enlargement) and submandibular gland enlargement are commonly seen.
- Lymphadenopathy is common.
- Nonspecific papules, plaques, or nodules can be seen on the skin.

Diagnostic Workup

- **ESR** is often elevated due to polyclonal hypergammaglobulinemia.
- **Eosinophilia or elevated IgE levels** may be helpful, as they are uncommonly elevated in other rheumatic diseases.
- **Serum IgG4 levels** are frequently measured, but they are not sensitive or specific for the diagnosis.
- **Imaging:**
  - **Magnetic resonance cholangiography (MRCP)** will show bile duct abnormalities similar to primary sclerosing cholangitis.
  - **CT of the abdomen** will show fusiform swelling of the pancreas, often with a surrounding capsule-like rim. IgG4-RD can also present as a pancreatic mass that can be confused with pancreatic cancer.
  - **CT of the lungs** can show numerous findings, including bronchovascular thickening, pulmonary nodules/masses ("pseudotumor of the lung") that can be mistaken for lung cancer, and ILD.
- **Biopsy is the gold standard.**
  - **IgG4-RD is considered a histologic diagnosis.** Careful review with the pathologist is essential.
  - The characteristic biopsy features are typically seen across organ symptoms (just as noncaseating granulomas are seen across organ systems in sarcoidosis): lymphocytoplasmic infiltrate (with at least 40% IgG plasma cells of IgG4), storiform (whirled pattern) fibrosis, obliterative phlebitis, and eosinophilic infiltration.

Management

- Corticosteroids are the mainstay of therapy (usually started at 1 mg/kg) and typically provide rapid improvement in clinical features.
- Rituximab has been successfully used in cases where steroids are unable to be tapered.

SARCOIDOSIS

General Facts

- Chronic granulomatous disease that can affect any organ system, though most commonly the lungs, skin, and eyes.
- The biopsy of noncaseating granulomas is consistent across organ systems.
- African Americans and patients with northern European heritage are at highest risk for sarcoidosis. Typically sarcoidosis presents in the third or fourth decade of life.

Clinical Features

- Like many rheumatic diseases, sarcoidosis is a heterogenous disease.
- Can be found **incidentally**, with a chest x-ray done for other reasons, demonstrating the classic bilateral hilar adenopathy.
- Can also present **acutely**, with Lofgren syndrome (erythema nodosum and polyarthritis).
- Chronic manifestations are listed in Table 15-18.

Diagnostic Workup

- Overall, **sarcoidosis is a histologic diagnosis**, with the findings of epithelioid noncaseating granulomas in the setting of a compatible clinical presentation and the exclusion of alternative diagnoses.
- **Chest x-ray (CXR)** to identify typical intrathoracic findings is usually the first step and often scored according to the Scadding staging system (these stages are not chronologic) (see Table 15-19 and Figure 15-22).
- **Cardiac MRI** is frequently used to identify sarcoid infiltration of the myocardium. Typical findings are patchy and multifocal late gadolinium enhancement.
- Granulomas can lead to low 25-vitamin D but elevated 1–25 (activated) vitamin D, and consequently elevated serum calcium levels.

Table 15-18. Chronic Manifestations of Sarcoidosis

Organ System	Manifestation	Comment
Pulmonary	Hilar adenopathy, upper lobe opacities	>90% of patients have some form of lung involvement
Ocular	Uveitis (can be anterior, posterior, or panuveitis) Lacrimal gland enlargement	~25%
Skin	Erythema nodosum Maculopapular or plaque lesions	~25%; considered "great mimicker" of other skin diseases
Hepatic	Alkaline phosphatase elevation	Common but rarely clinically significant
Cardiac	Heart block, arrhythmias, heart failure	5%–10% clinically significant, but overall underrecognized cause of death
Neurologic	Bell palsy (most common) Pituitary disease Leptomeningeal enhancement on MRI Peripheral neuropathy	5%–10% clinically significant
Musculoskeletal	Lofgren syndrome Chronic arthritis	Chronic arthritis very uncommon

Table 15-19. Scadding Chest X-Ray Staging in Sarcoidosis

Stage	CXR Findings
0	Normal
1	Bilateral hilar adenopathy
2	Bilateral hilar adenopathy with pulmonary infiltrates
3	Parenchymal infiltrates alone
4	Pulmonary fibrosis

CONQUER THE WARDS!

Sarcoidosis is one of the few systemic autoimmune diseases that has a predilection for the upper lung fields (most involve lower lobes).

CONQUER THE WARDS!

"Lupus pernio" refers to a sarcoid skin lesions characterized by violaceous plaques on the central face. It is commonly seen with concurrent respiratory tract involvement. If untreated, it can cause destruction and disfigurement. It is not related to systemic lupus erythematosus.

CONQUER THE WARDS!

Serum ACE levels are often sent but have poor sensitivity and specificity for the diagnosis of sarcoidosis.

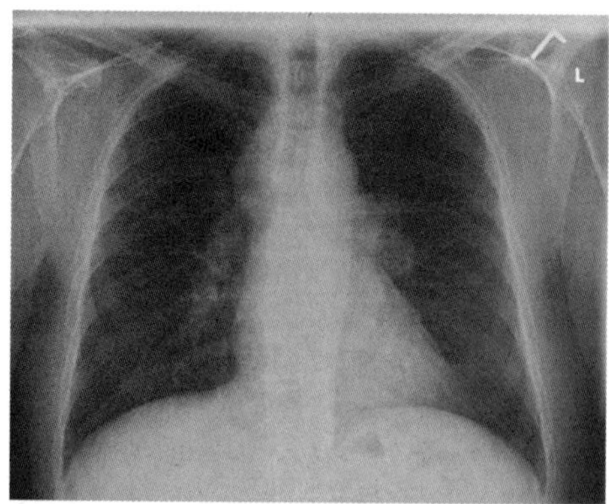

FIGURE 15-22. Posterior-anterior chest roentgenogram demonstrating bilateral hilar adenopathy, stage 1 disease. (Reproduced, with permission, from Jameson JL, Fauci AF, Kasper DL, et al, eds: *Harrison's Principles of Internal Medicine*, 20th ed. www.accessmedicine.com. Copyright © McGraw-Hill Education. All rights reserved.)

Management

- Corticosteroids are the mainstay for acute treatment, though it should be noted that sarcoidosis often can go into spontaneous remission (especially Scadding stage 1).
- A variety of steroid-sparing agents have been used, but none are Food and Drug Administration (FDA) approved. Methotrexate is probably the most common. Anti-TNF therapy is increasingly used, especially for neurologic, ocular, or cardiac involvement.

BEHÇET SYNDROME

General Facts

- Behçet disease is an inflammatory disease of unknown cause characterized by recurrent oral aphthae and various systemic manifestations.
- It typically presents in the second through fourth decade of life and is more severe in men.
- It is most common in patients from east Asia to the Mediterranean, especially Turkey.

Clinical Features

- **Severe, painful oral ulcers:** All patients with Behçet disease have oral ulcers. They resemble aphthous stomatitis, but the episodes of oral ulceration are more frequent and often involve multiple ulcers at once (see Figure 15-23). Other manifestations are listed in Table 15-20.

CONQUER THE WARDS!

The presence of pathergy can be tested by inserting a small needle into the subcutaneous tissue of the forearm; if pathergy is present, a small pustule will appear in the area after 1 to 2 days. It is seen in about half of Turkish patients with Behçet disease, but only about 10% of patients in the United States.

Diagnostic Workup

- Behçet disease is a clinical diagnosis and there is no diagnostic test.
- The 1990 International Study Group for Behçet's Disease criteria are the most frequently used classification criteria which include:
  - Recurrent oral ulcers (at least 3 in a 12-month period).

  AND
  - At least 2 of the following:
    - Recurrent genital ulcers.
    - Uveitis.
    - Skin lesions (as described earlier).
    - Pathergy phenomenon.

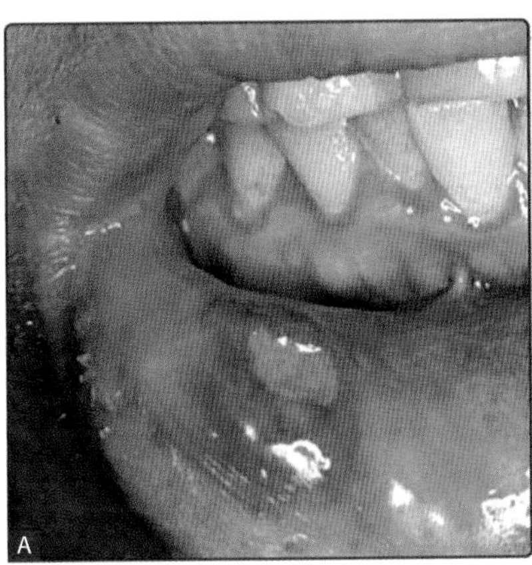

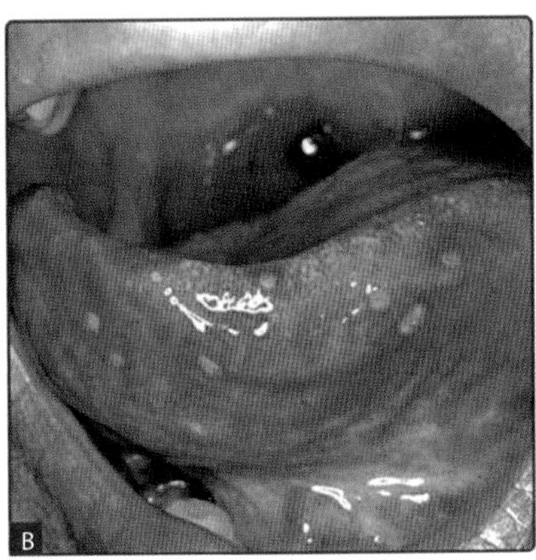

FIGURE 15-23. (A) Single and (B) multiple oral aphthous ulcers. (Part A from Altenburg A, et al. Epidemiology and clinical manifestations of Adamantiades-Behçet disease in Germany—current pathogenetic concepts and therapeutic possibilities. *J Dtsch Dermatol Ges*. 2006;4:49, with permission. Copyright © 2006 John Wiley & Sons. Part B reproduced, with permission, from Kang S, Amagai M, Bruckner AL, et al, eds. *Fitzpatrick's Dermatology,* 9th ed. New York: McGraw-Hill, 2019.)

Table 15-20. Additional Manifestations of Behçet Disease

System	Manifestation	Frequency
Genital	■ Painful genital ulcers resembling oral aphthae. On scrotum of men, vulva of women. Scarring is common.	75%
Cutaneous	■ Erythema nodosum–like lesions ■ Papulopustule/pseudofolliculitis ■ Acneiform lesions ■ Pathergy phenomenon (sterile pustules develop after minor trauma)	75%
Vascular	■ Deep venous thrombosis (DVT) ■ Pulmonary artery aneurysms (major cause of mortality) ■ Superficial thrombophlebitis ■ Cutaneous ulcerations	15%
Eye	■ Uveitis: often posterior or panuveitis, and bilateral. Major cause of morbidity; blindness if untreated	50%
Musculoskeletal	■ Nonerosive arthritis of medium to large joints, occurring intermittently	50%
Neurologic	■ Parenchymal disease (with predilection for diencephalon) ■ Venous sinus thrombosis	10%
GI tract	■ Ulcerations that can occasionally be difficult to differentiate from inflammatory bowel disease. More common in Far Eastern populations	10%–50%

Management

- The management is tailored to the severity of the disease.
- **Oral and genital ulcers** can be treated with topical corticosteroids and **colchicine** for prevention of recurrence.
- More severe disease (e.g., neurologic manifestations) is often treated with either azathioprine and/or TNF-alpha inhibitor therapy.
- It is controversial as to whether the thrombotic manifestations (e.g., DVT) should be treated with anticoagulation or immunosuppression.

CONQUER THE WARDS!

Saddle nose deformity can be seen in relapsing polychondritis, granulomatosis with polyangiitis, and syphilis. However, cocaine abuse is probably the most common cause.

CONQUER THE BOARDS!

In contrast to a cellulitis of the ear, in RLP the noncartilaginous portion of the ear (the lobule) is spared.

RELAPSING POLYCHONDRITIS

General Facts

- Rare inflammatory disease characterized by inflammation of cartilaginous structures.
- The cause is unknown.
- In about 10% to 20% of patients, usually older men, it is seen in the setting of myelodysplastic syndrome.

Clinical Features

- Inflammation of the auricular, nasal, laryngotracheal, and costal cartilages is characteristic.
- Inflammatory eye disease, usually scleritis, is often seen.
- There is an association with large vessel vasculitis, usually aortitis, in about 10% of cases.

Physical Exam Findings

- Swelling, erythema, and tenderness of the pinna of the ear or the nasal septum (see Figure 15-24).
- Tenderness on the costal cartilage of the chest wall.
- If there is laryngotracheal involvement, wheezing or stridor can be heard.
- With long-standing disease, saddle nose deformity due to destruction of the nasal cartilage can occur.

Diagnostic Workup

- Diagnosis is typically made clinically.
- There are no serologic markers.
- Biopsy showing cartilage inflammation can be done, but is typically not necessary.

Management

- Corticosteroids are used for acute inflammatory control.

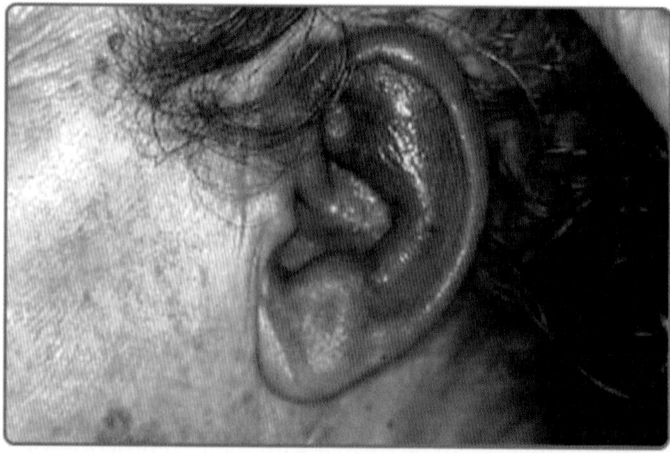

FIGURE 15-24. Relapsing polychondritis. Painful inflammation of the cartilaginous portion of ear. (Reproduced, with permission, from Kang S, Amagai M, Bruckner AL, et al, eds. *Fitzpatrick's Dermatology,* 9th ed. New York: McGraw-Hill, 2019.)

SOFT TISSUE RHEUMATISM

TENDINOSIS/BURSITIS

General Facts

Tendinosis

- All tendons in the body can develop tendinosis, and it becomes more common with age.
- Diabetes is a major risk factor for tendinosis.
- The most common sites of tendinosis are:
  - Rotator cuff tendons of the shoulders (especially the supraspinatus).
  - Extensor tendons of the forearm that insert into the lateral elbow (tennis elbow).
  - First compartment tendons of the wrist (de Quervain tenosynovitis).
  - Achilles tendon of the ankle.
  - Plantar fascia (not technically a tendon but presents similarly).

Bursa

- Bursa are fluid-filled sacs that make it easier for tissues to glide over each other.
- Often bursitis is secondary to local trauma (though bursitis due to a bacterial infection—aka "septic bursitis"—or gout can also occur).
- There are >100 bursa in the body, but only a few can become inflamed, including the:
  - Subacromial bursa of the shoulder.
  - Olecranon bursa of the elbow.
  - Trochanteric bursa of the hip.
  - Pes anserine bursa of the knee.
  - Prepatellar bursa of the knee.

Clinical Features

Tendinosis

- The pain is typically gradually increasing.
- Typically affected tendons feel stiff, improve with initial activity, but can worsen with prolonged activity.
- Often the patient gives a history of new/increased activity (e.g., new workout routine or new activity).

Bursitis presents with relatively acute sharp pain in the area of the affected bursa.

Physical Exam Findings

Tendinosis

- Usually, no obvious physical findings.
- Typically has pain when the tendon is stressed (either active or passive range of motion [ROM]).

Bursitis

- Focal tenderness.
- Bursa can be swollen and appear concerning, for example, the olecranon bursa of the elbow or the prepatellar bursa of the knee (see Figure 15-25).

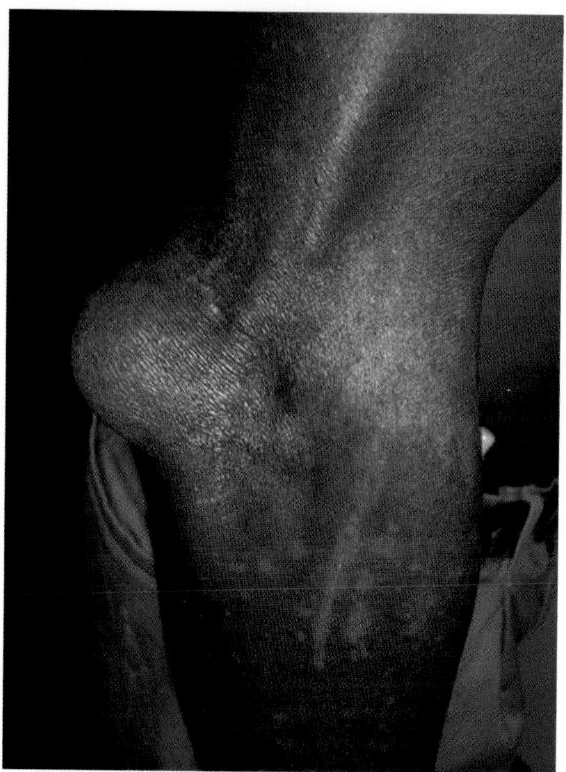

FIGURE 15-25. Chronic aseptic olecranon bursitis without erythema or tenderness. (Used, with permission, from Richard P. Usatine, MD, in Usatine RP, Smith MA, Mayeaux EJ Jr, Chumley H. *The Color Atlas of Family Medicine*, 2nd ed. New York: McGraw-Hill, 2013.)

- Bursas are generally not contiguous with the joint, and thus the joint should have full ROM.

Diagnostic Workup

- Diagnosis can typically be made clinically.
- MRI or ultrasound can be used if there is confusion.

Management

- Stopping the activity that is bringing on the pain is most important.
- NSAIDs and ice can be effective.
- Local corticosteroid injection can help the bursitis. This is typically not recommended for tendinosis due to risk of tendon rupture.

NERVE COMPRESSION

General Facts

- The most common nerve compression syndrome is **carpal tunnel**, in which the median nerve becomes compressed at the level of the wrist.
- Other common locations include:
  - **Cubital tunnel:** Ulnar nerve compression at the elbow.
  - **Tarsal tunnel:** Posterior tibial nerve compression in the medial ankle.

Clinical Features

- Paresthesias distal to the site of entrapment are most common (e.g., volar first 3 fingers in carpal tunnel syndrome).
- With time, sensory loss and weakness of the supplied musculature may occur.

Physical Exam Findings

- Stressing the nerve at the site of compression can sometimes bring on paresthesias.
- **Tinnel sign** at the wrist is done by tapping over the medical nerve on the volar wrist. If there is subsequent tingling in the thumb, index, middle finger, and radial half of the fourth digit, this suggests carpal tunnel.
- **Phalan sign** is performed by hyperflexing the wrists. If there is tingling similar to Tinnel sign, then this suggests carpal tunnel.
- Both Tinnell and Phalan have relatively low sensitivity and specificity.
- Atrophy of the muscles supplied by the obstructed nerve (e.g., muscles of the thenar eminence of the thumb) is a late finding.

Diagnostic Workup

- Often the diagnosis can be made on clinical grounds.
- A nerve conduction study can be done if there is confusion.
- A bedside ultrasound can show dilation of the nerve proximal to the obstruction; it can also identify cause of the obstruction, for example, nearby tendon inflammation.
- **Electromyography (EMG) and ultrasound are approximately equally sensitive for the diagnosis of carpal tunnel syndrome.**

Management

- Use of splints/braces to prevent positions that exacerbate compression is important.
- Local corticosteroid injections can be helpful.

LOW BACK PAIN

General Facts

- Both acute and chronic low back pain are extremely common symptoms in the general population.
- **Acute low back pain**:
  - Typically due to a muscle strain or ligamentous sprain.
  - Vast majority improve within 6 weeks.
- **Chronic low back pain** (pain >12 weeks):
  - Typically multifactorial and is often categorized as "chronic nonspecific low back pain."
  - There is often a component of central pain sensitization, in which there is amplification of neural signaling within the central nervous system leading to pain hypersensitivity.
- Low back pain can also be a sign of a systemic disease, and thus when a patient presents with this symptom, it is important to review red flags for serious pathology, including fevers, neurologic dysfunction (especially bowel/bladder), pain severe enough to wake up from sleep, history of cancer, or history of trauma.

CONQUER THE WARDS!

"Sciatica" refers to pain that radiates from the buttocks to the leg in the distribution of the sciatic nerve. The most common cause is compression of a lumbar nerve root by disk material that has ruptured through the surrounding annulus fibrosus.

Clinical Features

Acute Low Back Pain

- Typically due to a muscle or ligamentous strain. Patients will endorse achy, nonradiating pain, often in the paraspinal musculature.

CONQUER THE WARDS!

A history of cancer is the strongest risk factor for back pain caused by bone metastasis. Breast, prostate, lung, and multiple myeloma are the most common causes of skeletal metastasis.

CONQUER THE BOARDS!

Most radiculopathies involve the L5 and S1 nerve roots.

CONQUER THE WARDS!

Cauda equina syndrome describes an acute compression of nerves in the cauda equina. Patients endorse new problems with bowel/bladder control, anesthesia in a saddle distribution, and weakness. This can occur due to a herniated disc, infection, inflammation, cancer, or spinal stenosis. It is a neurosurgical emergency.

- But can be due to more serious conditions, such as:
  - Bony metastasis characteristically has nighttime pain.
  - Epidural abscesses have severe pain and fevers.
  - Herniated discs:
    - Pain is sudden in onset.
    - Pain that radiates down one leg, especially if associated with numbness or weakness in that distribution, suggests nerve compression.

Chronic Low Back Pain

- Patients with chronic, nonspecific low back pain have poorly localized, achy pain that typically worsens with activity and prolonged sitting.
- If a young patient has chronic low back pain with associated prolonged morning stiffness, think spondyloarthropathy (see seronegative spondyloarthropathy section).
- Less common, but specific, chronic low back pain conditions include:
  - **Spinal stenosis**: Patients have pain that radiates into the lower extremity triggered by walking or prolonged standing and relieved by rest or lumbar flexion (shopping cart sign).
  - **Chronic radiculopathy** (often due to facet hypertrophy causing foraminal stenosis, or spondylolisthesis): Patients endorse pain, sensory loss, and weakness in the area supplied by the involved nerve root.
  - **Vertebral compression fracture:** In patients with underlying osteoporosis, especially those on chronic steroids. Often there is no trauma history.

Physical Exam Findings

For most cases of low back pain, the exam is nonspecific, but a focused exam should be done in every patient to identify those who need further acute work-up. Palpation over the spine and a neurologic exam targeting the nerve roots supplying the lower extremities (L2–S1) are important. Physical exam findings of the different causes of back pain are summarized below in Table 15-21.

Table 15-21. Characteristics in Common Back Pain Causes

Cause of Back Pain	Physical Exam
Acute muscle strain	Nonspecific, often tenderness of paraspinal muscles
Herniated disk	Positive straight leg raise test (elevating leg with patient supine causes worsening radicular pain) suggests L5 nerve impingement. Associated neurologic findings (weakness, sensory loss) in the affected nerve root.
Compression fracture	Focal tenderness
Bony metastasis	Focal tenderness
Epidural abscess/vertebral osteomyelitis	Severe discomfort, focal tenderness, fever
Chronic nonspecific low back pain	Nonspecific tenderness over spine and musculature
Spinal stenosis	Often normal, can lead to wide-based gait
Radiculopathy	Associated neurologic findings (weakness, sensory loss) in the affected nerve root

Nerve Root	Motor Function	Sensory Function
L2	Hip flexion	Anterior thigh
L3	Knee extension	Anterior Thigh
L4	Ankle dorsiflexion	Knee
L5	Toe dorsiflexion	Dorsal foot
S1	Ankle plantarflexion	Lateral foot

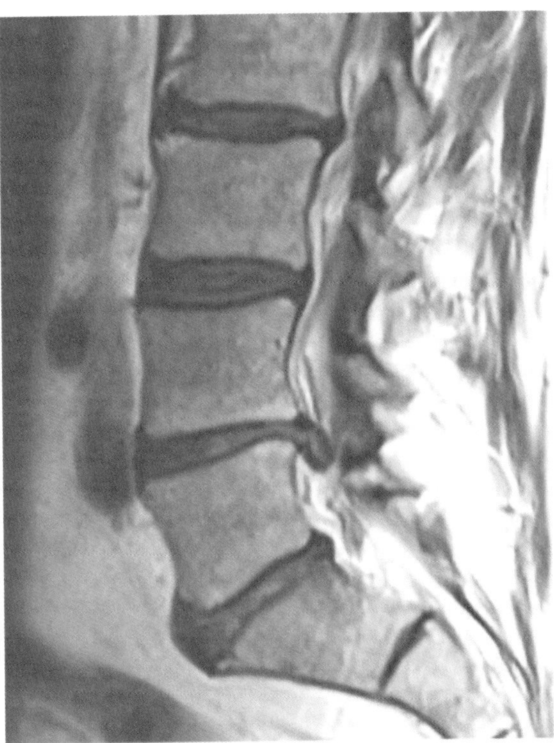

FIGURE 15-26. Sagittal MRI scan of the lumbar spine showing L4–5 disc extrusion. Note the persistence of high signal intensity within the center of the disc and herniation. (Reproduced, with permission, from Maitin IB, Cruz E. *Current Diagnosis & Treatment: Physical Medicine & Rehabilitation*. New York: McGraw-Hill, 2015.)

Diagnostic Workup

The vast majority of patients with either acute or chronic low back pain do not need imaging.

Notably, an MRI is not helpful for chronic, nonspecific low back pain, as most of the findings seen (e.g., facet arthritis, mild herniated disk) are common in the general population and do not change management (see Figure 15-26). There are certain scenarios in which an MRI should be obtained urgently ("red flags"):

- New urinary retention or incontinence.
- Saddle anesthesia.
- Loss of motor function not limited to a single nerve root.
- Signs of acute infection.

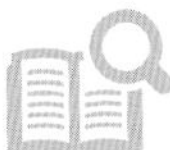

HIGH-YIELD LITERATURE

Chou R, Qaseem A, Owens DK, Shekelle P, Clinical Guidelines Committee of the American College of Physicians. Diagnostic imaging for low back pain: Advice for high-value health care from the American College of Physicians. *Ann Intern Med*. 2011;154(3):181-189.

Management

- Acute low back pain typically resolves spontaneously after a few weeks, but acetaminophen and NSAIDs can be used.
- Chronic nonspecific low back pain is most effectively treated with multimodal therapy, which includes:

- Physical or aquatic therapy.
- Pain control in a stepwise approach:
  - First line: Nonnarcotics – acetaminophen and NSAIDs.
  - Second line: Duloxetine or tramadol or tricyclic antidepressants (e.g., nortriptyline).
  - Third line: Muscle relaxants and/or opioids. However, extreme care must be taken in starting these agents, as opioids have addictive properties and both medication types' side-effect profile is more dangerous. Opioids in randomized trials have not shown long-term benefit for chronic low back pain.
- Cognitive behavioral therapy and mindfulness-based stress reduction.
- Weight loss is crucial.
- Steroid injections (e.g., facet joint injections) are also sometimes used, but the efficacy vs placebo is controversial.

HIGH-YIELD LITERATURE

Qaseem A, Wilt TJ, McLean RM, Forciea MA, Clinical Guidelines Committee of the American College of Physicians. Noninvasive treatments for acute, subacute, and chronic low back pain: A clinical practice guideline from the American College of Physicians. *Ann Intern Med*. 2017 4;166(7):514-530.

CHAPTER 16 NEUROLOGY

OVERVIEW OF HIGH-YIELD TOPICS IN NEUROLOGY

CONQUER THE WARDS!

Familiarity with different groups of anatomic localization will assist you in forming a comprehensive list of differential diagnoses.

LOCALIZATION AND TIME COURSE: THE KEYS TO NEUROLOGIC DIAGNOSIS

In neurology, the determination of localization and time course are critical to making an accurate diagnosis.

"Localization" and "localizing the lesion" are terms frequently used by neurologists and refer to the practice of pinpointing the anatomic structure(s) of the nervous system affected by a disease. Localization is most broadly divided into points in the central nervous system versus the peripheral nervous system, which is then further subdivided (Table 16-1). When approaching a case, one should consider where the most proximal location in the nervous system is that a symptom could potentially originate from and then think about every possible location all the way through the most distal point; this is the so-called "ceiling to floor" approach. Using this method, the clinician will avoid a common diagnostic error of inaccurate localization simply because he or she does not expand his or her assessment enough to include the correct point. It is important to remember that some disease processes do not have a singular localization. Instead, they might result in a multifocal localization (simultaneous optic neuritis and thoracic myelitis in multiple sclerosis [MS]), a systemic presentation (motor neuron dysfunction in amyotrophic lateral sclerosis [ALS]), or global dysfunction (altered mental status due to drug toxicity).

Time course refers to the temporal progression of the symptoms: how rapidly they developed, how quickly they plateaued, how long they lasted, etc. The time course of a disease can be practically divided into 3 major categories: **acute, subacute, and chronic** (Table 16-2). Incorporating the time course into the process allows the clinician to begin to determine the underlying pathophysiology.

Table 16-1. Anatomic Localization of Neurologic Deficits

Anatomic Localization	Examples of Specific Structures	Examples of Neurologic Disease at Localization
Central		
Cortical areas – outermost layers of brain, purely gray matter	Language centers and visual processing centers	Large vessel stroke and seizure
Subcortical brain – inner layers of brain, contains both gray and white matter tracts and deep structures that run from cortex to brainstem/spinal cord	Basal ganglia and thalamus	Small vessel stroke and multiple sclerosis
Brainstem	Cranial nerves and medial longitudinal fasciculus	Brainstem stroke and acoustic schwannoma
Spinal cord	Corticospinal tract and spinothalamic tract	Transverse myelitis and spinal cord compression
Peripheral		
Motor neuron	Anterior horn cell	Amyotrophic lateral sclerosis
Nerve root	C8 nerve root	Cervical radiculopathy and lumbar radiculopathy
Nerve plexus	Posterior cord of brachial plexus	Neuralgic amyotrophy and diabetic amyotrophy
Peripheral nerve	Median nerve and peroneal nerve	Polyneuropathy and focal compression neuropathy
Neuromuscular junction	Acetylcholine receptors	Myasthenia gravis and Lambert–Eaton syndrome
Muscle	Muscle fiber fascicles and type I muscle fibers	Statin-induced myopathy and Duchenne muscular dystrophy

Table 16-2. Time Course of Neurologic Diseases		
Time Course	**Pathophysiologic Process**	**Examples of Neurologic Disease**
Acute (maximal in onset of seconds to minutes)	Vascular event, aberrant electrical discharge, and cortical-spreading depression	Stroke, seizure, and migraine
Subacute (symptom onset over days to weeks)	Evolving inflammation, growth of a space-occupying lesion	Multiple sclerosis, tumor, infection, Guillain–Barré syndrome (GBS)
Chronic (symptom worsening over months to years)	Neurodegeneration and nutritional deficiencies	ALS, Parkinson disease, Alzheimer dementia, and polyneuropathy

Table 16-3. Types of Ischemic Stroke		
	Large Vessel Ischemic Stroke	**Small Vessel Ischemic Stroke**
Etiology	Large vessel atherosclerosis (e.g., carotid artery atherosclerosis), cardioembolism (e.g., atrial fibrillation)	Lipohyalinosis of terminal arterioles secondary to "small vessel disease" (e.g., hypertension, diabetes)
Anatomic regions affected	Cortical and subcortical regions	Subcortical areas and brainstem
Size of infarcted tissue	Large, wedge-shaped	Small and rounded, also known as a "lacune"
Classic distinguishing neurologic deficits	Often includes cortical deficits and multiple tracts	May involve only 1 tract (see Table 16-6 for specific syndromes)
Acute treatment	TPA and mechanical embolectomy	TPA

- **Acute** onset of symptoms denotes a sudden change over seconds or minutes. Examples include a hemorrhage or infarct caused by vessel dysfunction, a seizure caused by electrical discharge, or a migraine aura caused by cortical-spreading depression.
- **Subacute** onset over days and weeks suggests that there is a **growing or evolving process** causing the symptoms. Examples include tumor, demyelinating disease, and infection.
- **Chronic** onset of symptoms over months or years denotes a **degenerative process**. Dementias, Parkinson disease, progressive MS, and ALS would be included in this subgroup.

Determination of localization and time course enables the clinician to form a comprehensive yet focused differential diagnosis. This differential is the basis for further diagnostic testing.

STROKE

General Facts

- Stroke is a sudden onset of a new neurologic deficit caused by a disruption of blood flow. The major types of stroke are **ischemic** and **hemorrhagic**.
- **Ischemic stroke** is divided into **large vessel** and **small vessel** (Table 16-3).
  - **Large vessels** include the middle cerebral artery (MCA), anterior cerebral artery (ACA), posterior cerebral artery (PCA), and basilar artery (BA) (see Figure 16-1). Importantly, patients with large vessel strokes commonly present with one or more **cortical signs** (Table 16-4) in addition to other deficits. See Table 16-5 for common stroke syndromes of large vessel strokes.

Table 16-4. Cortical Signs Commonly Seen in Large Vessel Strokes

Deficit/Signs	Anatomic Localization
Expressive (Broca) aphasia: Difficulty in language production (both writing and speaking). Speech lacks proper rhythm and intonation and is often ungrammatical. Word finding difficulty is prominent. Patient is often frustrated by their deficit	Broca area in language-dominant (usually left) frontal lobe
Receptive (Wernicke) aphasia: Difficulty in language understanding (both reading and listening). Sometimes called "fluent aphasia" or "word salad" because the patient will speak with a normal rhythm and intonation, but the content will be unintelligible	Wernicke area in language-dominant (usually left) temporal lobe
Acalculia: Inability to perform basic calculations	Parietal lobe
Alexia: Inability to read with preservation of writing	Occipital lobe
Agraphia: Inability to write	Frontal or parietal lobe
Apraxia – Inability to perform a previously learned motor task (e.g., brushing teeth)	Frontal or parietal lobes (usually left)
Hemispatial neglect: Lack of awareness and processing of sensory stimuli from one side. Related deficits include alien hand syndrome and extinction to double simultaneous stimulation	Parietal lobes (either side, but more pronounced when on the right hemisphere)
Homonymous hemianopsia: Blindness in one half of the visual field affecting both eyes	Occipital lobes and optic tract radiations
Gaze deviation: Both eyes are forcefully deviated to one side	Frontal eye fields (eyes are deviated toward the side of the lesion)

CONQUER THE **WARDS!**

Gaze deviation can also be secondary to lesions in the paramedian pontine reticular formation, which results in forced deviation of eyes AWAY from the lesion.

- **Small vessel** strokes arise from occlusion of distal terminal branches of these arteries and usually present with a more restricted symptom profile (Table 16-6).

- **Hemorrhagic stroke** is divided into:
  - **Intracerebral hemorrhage (ICH)**
  - **Epidural hemorrhage**
  - **Subdural hemorrhage**
  - **Subarachnoid hemorrhage (SAH)**
- **Other important terms:**
  - **Transient ischemic attack (TIA)** is a sudden new neurologic deficit attributable to ischemia in a cerebral vascular territory that resolves completely within 24 hours (usually within 30 minutes) and results in no identifiable infarcted tissue on magnetic resonance imaging (MRI).
  - **Penumbra** refers to the area of potentially salvageable tissue around the core of the stroke.

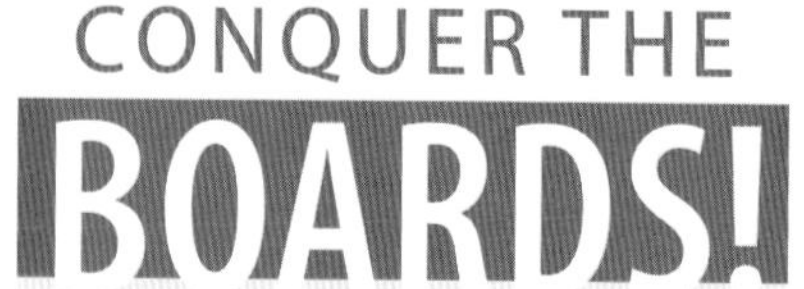

The number-one modifiable risk factor for stroke is hypertension.

- **Risk factors:**
  - Stroke in general–**hypertension**, diabetes, tobacco use, hyperlipidemia, atrial fibrillation, drug use, hypercoagulable states.
  - Specific to hemorrhagic stroke–bleeding diathesis, anticoagulation, trauma.
  - Specific to ICH–amyloid angiopathy, tumors.
  - Specific to SAH–arteriovenous malformations, ruptured aneurysms.

Table 16-5. Important Stroke Syndromes by Vascular Distribution (see Figure 16-1)

Syndrome	Deficits
Middle cerebral artery (MCA)	■ Contralateral hemiparesis (arm and face more than leg) ■ Contralateral hemisensory deficit ■ Homonymous hemianopsia ■ Aphasia (usually dominant/left hemisphere) ■ Contralateral hemispatial neglect (more pronounced on nondominant/right hemisphere)
Anterior cerebral artery (ACA)	■ Contralateral weakness of leg ■ Expressive aphasia ■ Abulia (lack of motivation)
Internal carotid artery (ICA)	■ Combination of middle cerebral and anterior cerebral artery syndromes
Posterior cerebral artery (PCA)	■ Contralateral homonymous hemianospia ■ On language-dominant side, alexia (inability to read) without agraphia (inability to write) can occur
Posterior inferior cerebellar artery (PICA) • Aka lateral medullary syndrome or Wallenberg syndrome	■ Nausea ■ Vertigo ■ Hoarseness ■ Ataxia ■ Ipsilateral Horner syndrome* ■ Ipsilateral palate and tongue weakness ■ Contralateral sensory disturbance ■ Dysphagia and dysarthria
Anterior inferior cerebellar artery (AICA)	■ Ipsilateral facial weakness ■ Gaze palsy ■ Deafness ■ Tinnitus
Lacunar syndromes (small vessel syndromes)	Common presentations include ■ Pure motor – contralateral hemiparesis affecting equally face, arm, and leg without other deficits ■ Pure sensory – contralateral hemisensory loss without other deficits ■ Ataxic hemiparesis – contralateral hemiparesis and appendicular ataxia ■ Clumsy hand dysarthria – contralateral appendicular ataxia and weakness of hand with associated dysarthria and dysphagia

- **Epidemiology:**
  - Stroke is a #1 cause of preventable disability worldwide.
  - Stroke is the fifth leading cause of death in the United States.
  - One in four patients with stroke have had a previous stroke.

Clinical Features

- Sudden onset; the peak of symptom severity will generally be within minutes.
- **Ischemic stroke**–caused by an embolic (e.g., heart) or thrombotic clot. Neurologic symptoms and signs are confined to a region of the brain supplied by a common vascular distribution (e.g., MCA).
- **Hemorrhagic stroke:**
  - Clinical syndromes are less well defined because the expansion of blood does not "respect" vascular territories and causes deficits attributable to multiple territories.

CONQUER THE **WARDS!**

It is important to distinguish between aphasia and dysarthria, as the 2 have different potential localizations and clinical implications.

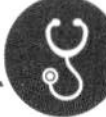

***Horner's Syndrome**

HORNE

H – hemianhidrosis (loss of sweating)

O – one eye (usually unilateral)

R – relaxed eyelid (ptosis)

N – narrow pupil (miosis)

E – enophthalmos (sunken eye)

Table 16-6. Subcortical or Brainstem Signs Commonly Seen in Small Vessel Strokes

Deficit/Signs	Anatomic Localization
Hemiparesis: Motor weakness on one side of the body	Precentral gyrus, basal ganglia, corticospinal tract
Hemisensory deficit: Loss of sensation on one side of the body	Postcentral gyrus, thalamus, spinothalamic tract
Facial droop	Precentral gyrus, basal ganglia, cranial nerve VII
Dysarthria: Difficulty in speech production	Precentral gyrus, basal ganglia, cranial nerves (IX, X, XII)
Dysphagia: Difficulty in swallowing	Precentral gyrus, basal ganglia, cranial nerves (IX, X, XII)
Appendicular ataxia: Dyscoordination of limbs	Cerebellum, cerebellar tracts in brainstem, basal ganglia

- **Epidural hemorrhage** is most often associated with trauma to the temporal bone with associated injury to the **middle meningeal artery.**
- **Subarachnoid hemorrhage** is associated with **"thunderclap" headache**, which is a headache that reaches peak intensity within seconds and is often described by patients as the worst headache of their life.
- **Subdural hemorrhage** may have a subacute onset over days to weeks, as it is typically the result of a venous bleed.
- Can be associated with early signs and symptoms of increased intracranial pressure (see the next section) (e.g., nausea and vomiting).

- **Hypoperfusion (i.e., "watershed") stroke:**
  - Caused by sudden and profound drops in cerebral perfusion.
  - Affects vulnerable regions that are in between the major cerebral artery territories.
  - Classic presentation includes deficits in occipital region (blindness, field cut) with weakness in shoulder and thighs and sparing the face, hands, and feet ("man-in-a-barrel").
- **Venous stroke:**
  - Uncommon type of stroke secondary to cerebral venous sinus thrombosis.
  - Often has components of both ischemic and hemorrhagic stroke.
  - As it is not arterial, associated deficits do not respect vascular territories.
  - Seizure is a common sequela.

Diagnostic Workup

- Imaging for acute management and diagnosis:
  - Noncontrast computed tomography (CT) scan of head: Most useful to assess for bleeds and subacute or chronic stroke. This is the most important test in acute strokes eligible for tissue plasminogen activator (TPA).
  - Computed tomography angiography (CTA) or magnetic resonance angiography (MRA) of head and neck: Identifies occlusion of large vessels, including carotid stenosis, and vascular malformations (e.g., aneurysms, arteriovenous malformations). Either one of these tests must be performed to assess patients who are potential candidates for thrombectomy (see management).
  - Patients presenting between 6 and 24 hours of last known well (LKW) should have perfusion imaging (e.g., CT perfusion, MR perfusion) to

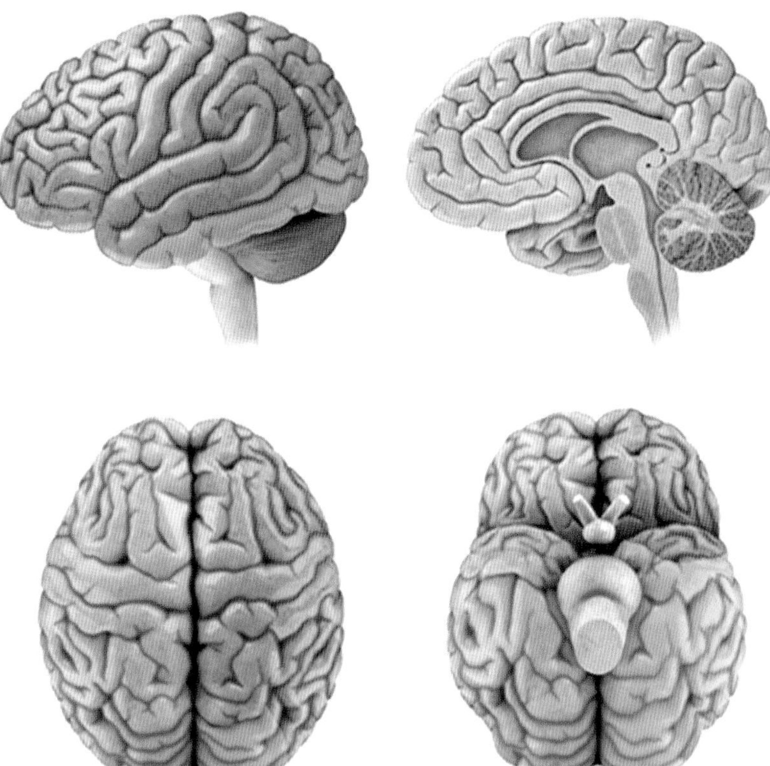

FIGURE 16-1. Vascular territories of major (large) vessels of brain. The anterior cerebral artery region (blue) includes the motor and sensory cortices for the leg and face. The middle cerebral artery region (pink) includes the motor and sensory cortices for the arm and the language centers (on dominant hemisphere). The posterior cerebral artery region (green) includes the primary visual cortex, the thalamus, and the midbrain. (Used, with permission, from Elsayes KM, Oldham SAA: *Introduction to Diagnostic Radiology*. www.accessmedicine.com. Copyright © McGraw-Hill Education. All rights reserved.)

assess for salvageable ischemic brain tissue to determine if they are a good candidate for thrombectomy.
- MRI of brain: Most sensitive imaging modality for acutely infarcted tissue. This is the best test in strokes not requiring acute intervention with TPA or thrombectomy (see management).

- Workup for secondary prevention of stroke:
  - Electrocardiogram (ECG)/telemetry: Assesses for cardiac disease, including atrial fibrillation. Should be performed in all acute stroke patients after imaging.
  - Carotid ultrasound: A more cost-friendly way to assess for carotid atherosclerosis. Performed in nonacute management to assess patients for stroke risk factors.
  - Cardiac echocardiography: Looks for cardioembolic sources, including ventricular thrombus and patent foramen ovale (PFO). Transesophageal echocardiography (TEE) is more invasive but more sensitive than transthoracic echocardiography (TTE).
  - Bloodwork to assess for stroke risk factors: Hemoglobin A1C, lipid panel, complete blood count, basic metabolic panel.

CONQUER THE WARDS!

LKW ≠ symptom onset. If a patient wakes up with symptoms, his or her LKW is when he or she went to bed.

CONQUER THE WARDS!

A negative CT head during the acute phase does NOT rule out an ischemic stroke.

Management

- Acute ischemic stroke (aka stroke code management):
  - Initial stroke code management is focused on 3 things:
    - Determination of **last known well (LKW)**: That is, when was the patient last seen or confirmed to have been normal?
    - Brief neurologic exam via the **National Institutes of Health Stroke Scale (NIHSS)**, which is an ordinal grading system for stroke severity based on neurologic exam findings, including mental status, visual fields, eye movement, facial strength, limb strength, sensation, coordination, language, and speech. A higher score suggests a worse stroke severity (see).
    - **Acute stroke imaging:** Noncontrast CT scan of head is always obtained to assess the patient for hemorrhagic stroke (to see if the patient is a candidate for TPA) and to assess for other potential pathology, including early ischemic changes. CTA of the head and neck and CT perfusions are used to assess for large vessel occlusion strokes that are intervenable by mechanical thrombectomy.
  - Intravenous tissue plasminogen activator (IV tPA):
    - Indications:
      - Patients must be within 4.5 hours of LKW.
      - Patients must have clinical evidence of possible stroke.
    - Contraindications:
      - Hemorrhagic stroke identified on CT head.
      - Blood pressure >185/110.
      - Predisposition to hemorrhage (e.g., anticoagulants, thrombocytopenia, elevated international normalized ratio [INR]).
    - Most serious adverse effect is cerebral hemorrhage.
  - Mechanical thrombectomy (aka mechanical embolectomy, thrombus retrieval):
    - Typically requires resources of a comprehensive stroke center.
    - Available to patients within 24 hours of LKW, as thrombectomy beyond this time frame has not been shown to have benefit.
    - Patients must have vascular imaging (CTA or MRA) with evidence of large vessel occlusion (e.g., MCA, ACA, basilar).
    - If not contraindicated, patients with large vessel occlusions that present in the appropriate time period should also receive IV TPA.
  - Postacute ischemic stroke:
    - Start aspirin (if TPA was given, first wait 24 hours and confirm lack of hemorrhagic conversion on repeat CT head).
    - If atrial fibrillation is discovered, start oral anticoagulation instead of aspirin (see cardiology section).
    - Start high-intensity statin.
    - Blood pressure should be "permissive" in first 24 to 48 hours poststroke (i.e., allowed to rise to up to 220/110 without pharmacologic intervention in order to allow for perfusion).
    - Cardiac telemetry to monitor for atrial fibrillation.
    - Speech therapy, physical therapy, and occupational therapy should assess stroke patients.

- Transient ischemic attack (TIA):
  - Patients with TIA are at higher risk for stroke, especially in the first 48 hours.
  - TIA severity can be rated by the ABCD2 score (**A**ge, **B**P [blood pressure], **C**linical, **D**uration, **D**iabetes).
    - Age ≥40 (1 point).
    - Systolic blood pressure (SBP) ≥140 or diastolic blood pressure (DBP) ≥90.
    - Symptoms of weakness +/– speech (2 points).
    - Symptoms of speech only (1 point).
    - Other symptoms (1 point).
    - Duration <10 minutes (0 points).
    - Duration 10 to 59 minutes (1 point).
    - Diabetes (1 point).
  - Patients with higher-risk TIAs (ABCD2 ≥4) should be considered for hospital admission for neurologic monitoring (q4h) and workup to identify potential etiologies of future stroke (Refer to Risk factors under stroke).
- Hemorrhagic stroke:
  - Maintain SBP <180 to prevent further bleeding. IV antihypertensives such as labetalol and nicardipine are typically used.
  - Monitor and treat increased intracranial pressure when appropriate (see the next section).
  - Vascular imaging (e.g., CTA head and neck or MRA head and neck) should be performed to assess for potential underlying vascular malformations. These include aneurysms, arteriovenous malformations, and tumors. If discovered, neurosurgical consultation should be considered.
  - ECG and cardiac telemetry.
  - Speech, physical, and occupational therapy.

HIGH-YIELD LITERATURE

Overview of the NIHSS:

Lyden P. Using the National Institutes of Health Stroke Scale. *Stroke*. 2017;48(2):513-519.

One of the landmark trials that pioneered mechanical thrombectomy for acute stroke intervention:

Berkhemer OA, Fransen PSS, Beumer D, et al. A randomized trial of intraarterial treatment for acute ischemic stroke. *N Engl J Med*. 2015;372(1):11-20.

INCREASED INTRACRANIAL PRESSURE AND BRAIN HERNIATION

General Facts

- **Brain herniation** is the movement of brain tissue into a space that it normally does not occupy as a result of abnormally increased intracranial pressure.
- Brain herniation relates to the **Monro–Kellie hypothesis,** which states the cranial compartment is incompressible and the volume inside the cranium

is fixed, and thus any increase in intracranial contents (blood, cerebrospinal fluid [CSF], brain tissue) will lead to a decrease in volume of other contents.

- Especially when sudden, it may be irreversible and frequently leads to coma and death.
- Involvement of the medulla can disrupt the respiratory center and lead to central respiratory failure.
- Etiologies include stroke, hemorrhage, tumors, and infection.

Clinical Features and Physical Exam Findings

- **Increased intracranial pressure (ICP):**
  - Alteration of mental status: Drowsiness, confusion, lack of response to physical stimuli.
  - Nausea and vomiting.
  - Headache.
  - Papilledema.
- **Uncal herniation:** Uncal gyrus herniates **downward** through the tentorium.
  - Third nerve palsy on ipsilateral side ("down and out," blown pupil).
  - Either contralateral or ipsilateral hemiparesis due to involvement of motor tracts in brainstem.
- **Subfalcine herniation**: Cingulate gyrus herniates **sideways across** the midline under the falx (see Figure 16-2).
  - Can compromise blood flow through ACA and present with unilateral or bilateral leg weakness.
- **Central herniation**: The entire cerebral hemisphere herniates across the tentorium (see Figure 16-2).
- **Ascending (upward) transtentorial herniation**: As a result of increased ICP in the posterior fossa, the cerebellum and brainstem herniate **upward** through the tentorium (see Figure 16-2).
- **Tonsillar herniation:** As a result of increased ICP in the posterior fossa, the cerebellar tonsils and brainstem herniate **downward** through the foramen magnum (see Figure 16-2).
- **Transdural/transcranial herniation:** Herniation of brain tissue **outward**. Seen in posttrauma or postcraniotomy patients with increased ICP (see Figure 16-2).

Diagnostic Workup

- Monitoring of respiratory and cardiac function.
- Noncontrast CT scan of head: Allows for assessment for bleeds, mass lesions, and radiographic evidence of increased ICP and herniation.

Management

- Temporizing measures to reduce ICP.
  - Raise head of bed 30 degrees.
  - Hyperventilation to reduce pCO_2, which reduces cerebral blood flow.
  - Mannitol and hypertonic saline: Hyperosmotic agents that reduce intraparenchymal water content.
  - Hypothermia.
  - Neuromuscular blockage.
- Decompression:
  - Almost invariably required in cases of pending brain herniation.
  - Generally begins with placement of extraventricular drain (EVD) for both ICP monitoring and drainage of CSF to relieve increased ICP.
  - Surgical decompression via craniotomy, if necessary.

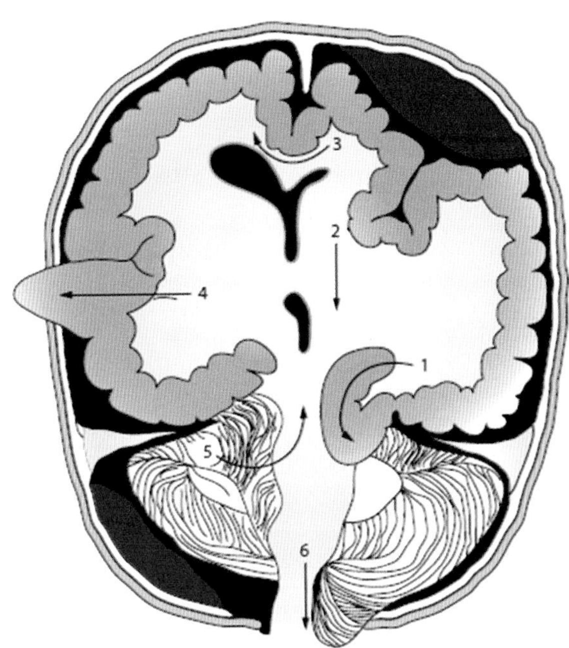

FIGURE 16-2. Examples of herniation pathways. Supratentorial masses can cause (1) uncal, (2) central, (3) subfalcine, and (4) transdural/transcranial herniation, whereas infratentorial masses can lead to (5) ascending transtentorial and (6) tonsillar herniation. (Used, with permission, from Hall JB, Schmidt GA, Kress JP. *Principles of Critical Care*, 4th edition. www.accessmedicine.com. Copyright © McGraw-Hill Education. All rights reserved.)

Common Questions Asked on Rounds

- What are the first signs of increased ICP?
  - Alteration of mental status, headache, nausea, vomiting.
- What are the common etiologies of increased ICP?
  - Tumor, stroke, hemorrhage, infection.

HIGH-YIELD LITERATURE

Review on Management of Intracranial Pressure

Freeman WD. Management of intracranial pressure. *Contin Lifelong Learn Neurol*. 2015;21(5 Neurocritical Care):1299-1323.

SEIZURE DISORDERS

General Facts

- **Seizures** are abnormal and excessive neuronal discharges causing transient disturbance of cerebral function.
- Seizures can be "provoked," meaning that there is a transient abnormality that increased a patient's likelihood for seizure.
  - Provoking factors include central nervous system (CNS) infections, fever, metabolic disturbances, and acute head injuries.
- **Epilepsy** is the enduring predisposition to have seizures.
- A patient has epilepsy if he or she has 2 unprovoked seizures occurring more than 24 hours apart. The most recent definition of epilepsy, however, also includes patients who have 1 unprovoked seizure and other risk factors for recurrent seizures.
  - These risk factors for recurrence include identification of a focal brain lesion, electroencephalogram (EEG) abnormalities, and diagnosis of genetic epilepsy syndromes.

Clinical Features

- Seizures vary widely in their presentations. Patients and bystanders may report:
  - Sudden onset of symptoms.
  - Uncontrollable shaking of limbs.
  - Inability to respond during events.
  - Urinary incontinence during events (note: this is nonspecific and can be seen in other cases of loss of consciousness, including syncope).
- Seizures are classified by 2 attributes:
  - **Site of onset**: Can be partial (one side of brain) or generalized (bilateral onset).
  - **Level of awareness:** ANY alteration in consciousness qualifies as impaired awareness. This includes a patient who appears slightly distracted to one who is obtunded.
- Examples of classifications:
  - **Focal-aware motor seizure** (aka "simple partial motor seizure"): Movement associated with seizure in one specific part of a brain with complete retention of consciousness (e.g., epilepsy partialis continua).
  - **Focal-impaired awareness seizure** (aka "complex partial seizure"): Impairment of consciousness with seizure onset in a specific part of the brain (classically the temporal lobe) +/− motor features.
  - **Focal to bilateral seizure**: Begins on one side of the brain and then spreads to both sides.
  - **Generalized impaired awareness nonmotor seizure** (aka "absence seizure" and "petit mal"): Change in awareness, classically manifesting as "staring spell" +/− automatic or repetitive movements (i.e., automatisms) such as lip smacking secondary to seizure with generalized onset. Classic seizure for **childhood absence epilepsy** with EEG pattern of generalized 3 Hz spike and wave pattern.
  - **Generalized impaired awareness motor seizure** (aka "generalized tonic-clonic" or "grand mal" seizure): Generalized onset manifesting as loss of awareness with limb stiffening (tonic) phase and limb jerking (clonic) phase.
- **Status epilepticus** is an emergency situation where a seizure lasts longer than 5 minutes or when multiple seizures occur in close succession without recovery.
- **Nonepileptic seizure** (aka psychogenic seizures, nonepileptic events): An event that has features of seizure, including uncontrollable limb movement and alteration of consciousness, but is not related to abnormal and excessive neuronal discharge.
  - Considered a form of conversion disorder and associated with a history of abuse.
  - EEG during these events is normal.
  - Certain clinical features may be suggestive of nonepileptic seizures, including hip thrusting and hip gyration movements, lack of stereotypical consistency in events, lack of postictal confusion, and bilateral limb movements without alteration of consciousness.
  - A portion of epilepsy patients also experience nonepileptic seizures. Even skilled epilepsy doctors may not be able to discern between true seizures and nonepileptic seizures in each case. Therefore, proper workup should be done to confirm seizure type in these patients.

CONQUER THE BOARDS!

Absence seizure = generalized 3 Hz spike-and-wave on EEG.

CONQUER THE WARDS!

When describing seizure events, focus on precise descriptions of time course and movements. This is more useful than simply describing events as "grand mal" or "petit mal."

Physical Exam Findings

- During events:
  - Lack of awareness and responsiveness.
  - Stereotypical movements that are reproduced in multiple events.
  - Inability of examiner to distract or suppress movements.
- Acutely after events:
  - Tongue bite on lateral side of tongue.
  - **Postictal confusion** (i.e., postseizure confusion): Generally lasts a few hours.
  - **Postictal paralysis** (aka **Todd paralysis**): Motor weakness in limbs affected by seizure (e.g., patient with left hemisphere focal motor seizure with residual and transient right limb weakness after the seizure stops). Typically lasts for hours to a few days.
- It is common for patients with seizures to have a baseline normal neurologic examination.

Diagnostic Workup

- Brain imaging:
  - CT head scan should be prioritized if there is concern for an acute intracranial process that is responsible for the seizure (e.g., hemorrhage).
  - MRI of the brain has higher resolution and much more sensitivity for small and subtle findings and should be performed to either clarify findings on the CT scan or to further evaluate a normal-appearing CT of the head.
- Routine blood tests and toxicology screen to assess for metabolic or drug-induced seizures.
- EEG to assess for ongoing seizures and/or findings associated with increased seizure risk (i.e., epileptiform activity, epileptogenic potentials).
- Antiepileptic drug (AED) levels: Useful in patients with epilepsy to assess for medication noncompliance, insufficient medication dosing, and medication toxicity.

CONQUER THE WARDS!

A normal EEG does not rule out a diagnosis of epilepsy, as it may be abnormal only during a seizure. This highlights the fact that epilepsy is a clinical diagnosis.

Management

- Address underlying etiology of seizure if possible (most common etiologies to consider include hyponatremia, hypocalcemia, fever, sepsis, CNS infections, acute head injuries, stroke).
- Address ABCs if necessary: Prolonged seizures can lead to airway failure and cardiovascular collapse.
- Most seizures self-resolve in less than 1 minute and do not require acute intervention. Prolonged seizures require acute therapies with IV benzodiazepines, loading doses of AEDs, and in severe cases IV sedatives such as barbiturates, as the risk of neurologic injury or death from status epilepticus is significant.
- Prescription of AEDs for daily use should only be given to patients with epilepsy (i.e., at high risk for recurrent seizures). Patients with seizures without high risk of recurrence (e.g., provoked seizures) do not require AEDs.
- Numerous AEDs have similar efficacy in preventing seizures. Therefore, selection of AEDs is largely based on their side effect profile (see Table 16-7).

- Newer AEDs include **levetiracetam**, **lamotrigine**, and **lacosamide**. Older AEDs include **valproic acid**, **carbamazepine**, **phenytoin**, and **phenobarbital**.
- Newer medications generally have a better tolerable side effect profile. Older medications generally have a worse side effect profile but are cheaper and available in nonoral formulations.

Table 16-7. Antiepileptic Medications, Route of Metabolism, and Adverse Effects

AED	Metabolism	Adverse Effects
Phenobarbital	Liver	Sedation, osteoporosis, decreased IQ
Phenytoin	Liver	Sedation, arrhythmia, hypotension, dizziness, rash, gingival hyperplasia, cerebellar degeneration, osteoporosis
Carbamazepine	Liver	Sedation, dizziness, rash, Stevens–Johnson syndrome, osteoporosis, hyponatremia, mild transient leukopenia, agranulocytosis, hair loss, weight gain
Oxcarbazepine	Liver	Sedation, dizziness, hyponatremia, weight gain, rash
Valproic acid	Liver	Sedation, liver effects, hemorrhagic pancreatitis, aplastic anemia, rash, hyperammonemia, thrombocytopenia
Lamotrigine	Liver	Rash, Stevens–Johnson syndrome, dizziness, insomnia, GI distress
Clobazam	Liver	Sedation, dry mouth, constipation
Zonisamide	Liver	Sedation, renal stones, acute angle glaucoma
Topiramate	Renal	Sedation, productive aphasia, renal stones, weight loss, paresthesias, acute angle glaucoma
Levetiracetam	Renal	Sedation, behavioral agitation, depression
Lacosamide	Renal	Sedation, ataxia
Vigabatrin	Renal	Sedation, retinal toxicity, diplopia

Common Questions Asked on Rounds

- What type of seizure did the patient have?
- What AED would you prescribe and why?

HIGH-YIELD LITERATURE

Antiepileptic drugs

Abou-Khalil BW. Antiepileptic drugs. *Contin Lifelong Learn Neurol.* 2016;22(1, Epilepsy):132-156.

BRAIN TUMORS

General Facts

- Many different types that vary widely in prognosis and management see table 16-8.
- Clinical presentation is generally nonspecific. Diagnosis is dependent on imaging and biopsy.

- In adults, the most common brain tumors are due to metastases from other primary cancers. Primary cancers most commonly responsible for brain metastases are carcinomas (lung, breast, kidney, colorectal) and melanoma.

Clinical Features

- Cognitive impairment.
- Headache, nausea/vomiting caused by increased ICP.
- Headache is often worse at night due to transient increases in CO_2 leading to vasodilation. Headache sometimes worsened with rise in intrathoracic pressure such as coughing or sneezing.
- Seizures.
- Weight loss.

CONQUER THE WARDS!

Metastatic tumors from renal cell carcinoma, breast cancer, lung cancer, papillary thyroid carcinoma, and melanoma are the most likely to hemorrhage.

Table 16-8. Brain Tumors

Astrocytoma	■ Most common primary intracranial tumor ■ Categorized in stages I–IV based on rate of tumor cell growth ■ Those occurring in adults are usually high grade and have a poor prognosis ■ **Glioblastoma multiforme (GBM)** is a stage IV astrocytoma • Mean survival 12–15 months • Classic imaging finding of "butterfly" shape from crossing the midline (Figure 16-3)
CNS lymphomas	■ Commonly also affects spinal cord, eyes, leptomeninges ■ Can be diagnosed with identification of malignant lymphocytes on biopsy or CSF sample
Oligodendrogliomas	■ Associated with calcification on imaging studies ■ Particularly epileptogenic ■ Can either be high or low grade
Ependymoma	■ In adults, more commonly found in spinal canal ■ In children, more commonly found in fourth ventricle and posterior fossa ■ Associated with "drop metastases," which is the spread of disease more caudally in spinal canal
Medulloblastoma	■ **Most common malignant primary brain tumor of childhood** ■ Posterior fossa tumors commonly found in cerebellum and frequently cause compression of brainstem ■ Associated with "drop metastases"
Meningioma	■ **Most common benign primary intracranial tumor** ■ Commonly asymptomatic ■ Associated with imaging finding of "dural tail" (Figure 16-4) ■ Less commonly can be high grade
Vestibular schwannoma	■ Formerly known as "acoustic neuroma" ■ **Most common benign tumor involving cranial nerves** ■ Associated with unilateral deafness ■ Mass effect may cause an ipsilateral CN VII palsy (i.e., Bell palsy) ■ Associated with neurofibromatosis type 2 > type 1
Metastatic tumors to CNS	■ **Most common type of brain tumor in adults** ■ Associated with carcinomas (lung, breast, kidney, colorectal) and melanoma ■ Particularly associated with edema out of proportion to size of tumor (Figure 16-5)

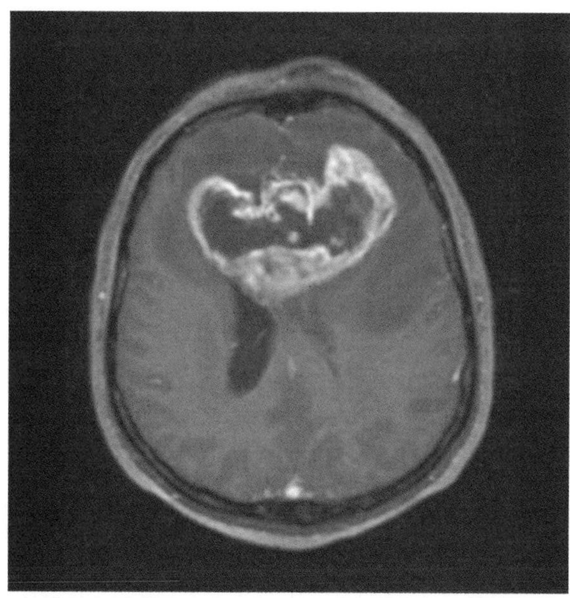

FIGURE 16-3. Brain MRI (T1 contrast sequence, axial view) showing an infiltrating glioblastoma multiforme that has crossed the corpus collosum, aka "butterfly glioma." (Used, with permission, from Reisner HM. *Pathology: A Modern Case Study.* New York, NY: McGraw-Hill; 2015.)

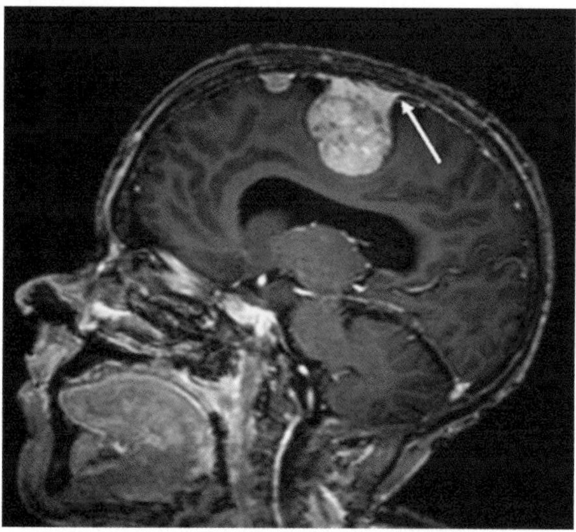

FIGURE 16-4. Brain MRI (T1 contrast sequence, sagittal view) of a meningioma. Note the classic appearance of a contrast-enhancing lesion with a dural base, aka dural tail (arrow).

Physical Exam Findings

- As with clinical findings, physical exam findings are nonspecific and depend on tumor burden and location.
- Findings of increased ICP, including papilledema, cranial nerve (CN) VI deficit, and lethargy.

Diagnostic Workup

- Brain imaging with CT head and MRI brain with contrast. See figures 16-3 and 16-4.
- CT chest/abdomen/pelvis or positron emission tomography (PET) scan to assess for potential primary tumor elsewhere in the body.
- Brain biopsy for pathologic diagnosis.

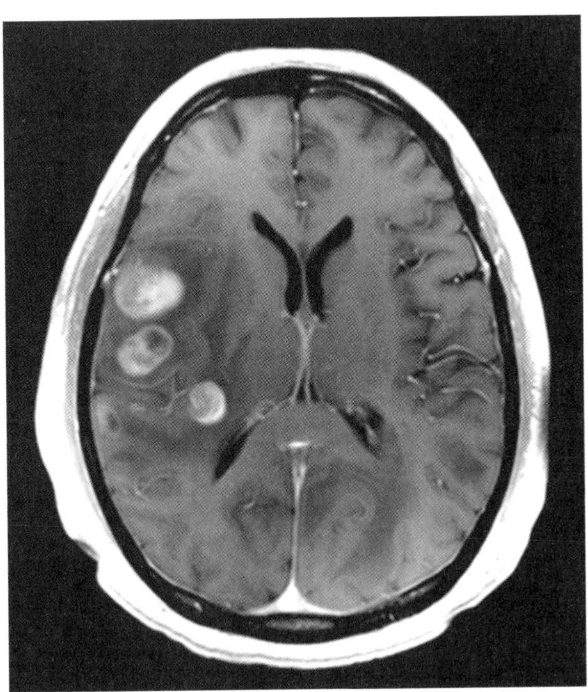

FIGURE 16-5. Brain MRI (T1 contrast sequence, axial view) of metastatic tumors from renal cell carcinoma. Multiple lesions are seen in the right hemisphere. There is surrounding edema that respects the gyral margins, which is classic for vasogenic edema.

- EEG if seizures are suspected.
- CSF studies for cytology if leptomeningeal involvement is suspected (e.g., CNS lymphoma).

Management

- Acutely, patients may require management of **increased ICP.**
- Treatment of tumors themselves can involve a mix of:
  - Surgical resection.
  - Chemotherapy.
  - Radiation therapy.
- Management of common neurologic sequalae include:
  - AEDs.
  - Corticosteroids for edema (dexamethasone 4 mg q6h is most common dose).

Common Questions Asked on Rounds

- What are common primary tumors that cause CNS metastasis?
  - Lung, breast, colorectal, kidney, melanoma.
- What tests are necessary to reach a diagnosis for a brain tumor?
  - Initial diagnosis is made with brain imaging (generally MRI brain). Definitive diagnosis and subtyping require tissue biopsy.

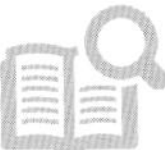

HIGH-YIELD LITERATURE

Pruitt AA. Medical management of patients with brain tumors. *Contin Lifelong learn Neurol.* 2015;21 (2, Neuro-oncology):314-331.

OVERVIEW OF HEADACHE

General Facts

- Most patients with headache will have **primary headache disorders**. Most primary headaches are caused by tension-type and migraine headaches, which are discussed later. These are headache disorders where there is no structural abnormality in the brain (i.e., there is no imaging or lab abnormality to explain the headache).
- The more serious and potentially life-threatening causes of headache, however, are **secondary headache disorders**, or headaches that are secondary to abnormalities in the brain and often are associated with abnormalities on imaging, serum labs, and CSF labs. Examples include headache secondary to subdural hematoma, idiopathic intracranial hypertension (IIH, pseudotumor cerebrii), meningitis, and temporal arteritis.
- When assessing a patient with a headache, it is paramount to recognize if he or she has any features of secondary headache disorders.
- After ruling out secondary headache, the assessment should focus on characterizing the headache features to determine which primary headache disorder is most likely the diagnosis.
  - It is important to note that the headaches associated with secondary headache disorders often have nonspecific features and can appear similar to primary headache disorders.

Clinical Features

- The following findings on history are **red flags** for potential secondary headache disorders:
  - Older age of onset (>45 years), as primary headaches uncommonly begin after this age.
  - Fever (meningitis).
  - Confusion and loss of consciousness (meningitis, mass lesion, bleed, increased ICP).
  - Headaches that are worse with supine position (increased ICP).
  - Weight loss and night sweats (malignancy).
  - Severe nausea and vomiting (increased ICP).
  - Visual loss (mass lesion, IIH).
- Headaches in general should be characterized by the following features:
  - **Length**: When did the headaches start?
  - **Frequency**: How many headache days do you have in a month?
    - Note that it is important to ask about number of "headache days" as opposed to number of headaches, as a single headache can last an entire month.
  - **Duration of episodes**: How long does a headache typically last?
  - **Location of pain**: Part of head and face, unilateral vs bilateral.
  - **Quality of pain:**
    - Pulsating and bandlike pain are classically associated with migraine.
    - Dull and pressure-like pain are classically associated with tension headache.
  - **Preceding symptoms** before the pain (aka aura), namely visual and sensory symptoms.
  - **Associated symptoms**: Nausea, vomiting, dizziness, fatigue.

Physical Exam Findings

- The following physical exam findings are **red flags** for potential secondary headache disorders:
  - Abnormal mental status exam, confusion (increased ICP, meningitis).
  - Neck stiffness (meningitis).
  - Papilledema (increased ICP, IIH).
  - Abnormalities on neurologic exam suggestive of a focal lesion (e.g., hemiparesis, ataxia).
- In patients with primary headache disorders, the neurologic exam is typically normal between attacks.

Diagnostic Workup

- Primary headache disorders are generally diagnosed clinically and do not require further testing.
- The presence of red flags for secondary headache disorder in the history or exam should prompt further workup, which can include:
  - Imaging: Either CT head or MRI brain. CT head is often sufficient to screen for causes of secondary headache disorders, but MRI brain will offer better resolution and diagnostic value.
  - Lumbar puncture (LP): Obtained in cases of suspected infection or idiopathic intracranial hypertension. LP should not be performed in patients with increased ICP secondary to identifiable structural lesion.
  - Laboratory workup if warranted: For example erythrocyte sedimentation rate and C-reactive protein in suspected cases of temporal arteritis.
- In patients with a new diagnosis of primary headache disorder without red flag findings, it is reasonable to obtain one-time brain imaging to solidify the diagnosis and rule out secondary headache disorder.

MIGRAINE HEADACHE

General Facts

- Second most common form of primary headache (behind tension headache).
- A leading cause of lost job productivity.
- Females more commonly affected than males.

Clinical Features

- Headache lasting at least 4 hours (but can last days to weeks).
- Pain with unilateral location and pulsating quality.
- Aggravation by physical exertion.
- Photophobia and/or phonophobia.
- Nausea and/or vomiting.
- **Aura**: Some patients experience focal transient neurologic deficits associated with their headaches lasting between 5 and 60 minutes. Common auras include visual (e.g., scintillating scotoma) and sensory (e.g., limb paresthesias and numbness).

Physical Exam Findings

- Neurologic exam generally should be normal between attacks. During an attack, however, subtle physical findings include:
  - Allodynia: Abnormal sensitivity or painful response to a nonpainful stimulus.

CONQUER THE WARDS!

"Primary" headache refers to headaches without associated structural disease. "Secondary" headache refers to headaches due to structural disease.

CONQUER THE WARDS!

When asking a patient about headache frequency, ask about how many "headache days" in a month instead of how many headaches. A single headache can last weeks!

- Tenderness near nerves that innervate sensory function of face and head (e.g., the trigeminal nerve as it exits the supraorbital notch, the greater occipital nerve as it exits the occipital ridge).
- Photophobia.

Diagnostic Workup

- Primarily a clinical diagnosis.
- MRI brain for previously undiagnosed patients to assess for secondary cause of headache.
- Obtaining imaging with MRI brain is particularly important for patients with red flag symptoms of secondary headache (see the previous section).

Management

- Lifestyle modification for minimizing headaches including regular sleep, regular meals, and identifying triggers (e.g., specific foods, smells).
- Acute therapies for headache include nonsteroidal antiinflammatory drugs (**NSAIDs**) and **triptans** (e.g., sumatriptan).
- IV therapies for acute headache include dopamine antagonists (e.g., **metoclopramide**), IV NSAIDs (e.g., **ketorolac**), and **IV valproic acid**.
- Chronic preventive medications for patients with frequent headaches (more than 7 days a month) include tricyclic antidepressants (e.g., **amitriptyline and nortriptyline**), antiepileptic medication (e.g., **topiramate** and **valproic acid**), and beta-blockers (e.g., **metoprolol, propranolol**).
- **Botulinum toxin** injection may be useful as a chronic preventive treatment in patients with "chronic migraine" (more than 14 headache days a month).
- Patients are instructed to keep a "headache diary" to track their migraine frequency and severity to assess for disease progression and efficacy of treatments.

HIGH-YIELD LITERATURE

Dodick DW. Migraine. *Lancet*. 2018;391(10127):1315-1330.

CLUSTER HEADACHES

General Facts

- Considered one of the most painful headache syndromes, with patients often reporting attacks as worse than anything else ever experienced.
- Predominantly affects men.
- Attacks come in "clusters" and last weeks to months, which are punctuated by periods of remission lasting between months and years.
- Part of a larger group of disorders known as **trigeminal autonomic cephalgias**, which are a group of headache disorders characterized by unilateral head pain with associated ipsilateral cranial autonomic features (conjunctival injection, lacrimation, nasal congestion, rhinorrhea).

Clinical Features

- Severe unilateral orbital, supraorbital, or temporal pain lasting between 15 and 180 minutes.
- A sense of restlessness and agitation.
- Associated nasal congestion, rhinorrhea.

Physical Exam Findings

- During attacks, there are autonomic features ipsilateral to the side of headache, including conjunctival injection, lacrimation, miosis, and ptosis.
- In between attacks, the neurologic exam is normal.

Diagnostic Workup

- Primarily a clinical diagnosis.
- MRI brain for previously undiagnosed patients to assess for secondary cause of headache.

Management

- **100% oxygen therapy** and **triptans** are used for acute attacks.
- **Verapamil** is the standard for preventive treatment.

Common Questions Asked on Rounds

- What differentiates migraine from cluster headache?
  - Cluster headaches are "activating," and patients are normally anxious and agitated during attacks. During migraines, patients are "low," preferring silence and isolation.
  - Cluster headaches have a high male predominance, whereas migraine affects more females than males.
  - Cluster headaches are associated with orbital or supraorbital pain. Migraine is more associated with head pain.
- Cluster headaches are associated with trigeminal autonomic symptoms. Migraines are associated with nausea, dizziness, and aura.

HIGH-YIELD LITERATURE

Goadsby PJ. Trigeminal autonomic cephalalgias. *Contin Lifelong Learn Neurol.* 2012;18(4):883-895.

TENSION-TYPE HEADACHES

General Facts

- The most common type of headache.
- Aggravated by mental and physical stress.
- Generally mild to moderate in intensity.

Clinical Features

- Bilateral mild- to moderate-intensity pain.
- Nonpulsating, tightening, and constricting quality of pain.
- Not associated with vomiting and nausea.
- Not associated with aura or transient focal neurologic deficits.

Physical Exam Findings

- During attacks patients may have tenderness in pericranial and cervical muscles.
- Physical exam is otherwise normal.

Diagnostic Workup

- Primarily a clinical diagnosis.
- Diagnosis relies on excluding other headache disorders with more specific features (e.g., migraine) and looking for **red flag** signs of secondary headache.
- MRI brain for previously undiagnosed patients to assess for secondary cause of headache.

Management

- **Acetaminophen** and **NSAIDs** for acute treatment.
- **Tricyclic antidepressants** for preventive therapy if headache frequency ≥15 headache days a month.

Common Question Asked on Rounds

- What differentiates tension-type headaches from migraines?
  - Tension-type headaches do not have aura and typically are not debilitating like migraines.

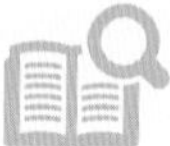

HIGH-YIELD LITERATURE

Kaniecki RG. Tension-type headache. *Contin Lifelong Learn Neurol.* 2012;18(4):823-834.

IDIOPATHIC INTRACRANIAL HYPERTENSION

General Facts

- **IIH** (i.e., **pseudotumor cerebrii**) is a disorder of increased ICP without evidence of an associated brain mass lesion.
- Delayed diagnosis and treatment can lead to permanent blindness.
- The pathophysiology of the disease is poorly understood.
- IIH is predominantly found in women and has a strong association with obesity.
- Other risk factors include vitamin A toxicity, steroid use, contraceptives, and anemia.

Clinical Features

- Headache.
- Visual complaints ranging from transient visual obscurations to sustained loss of acuity.

- Pulsatile tinnitus.
- Symptoms worse with activities that increase ICP, including Valsalva maneuver.

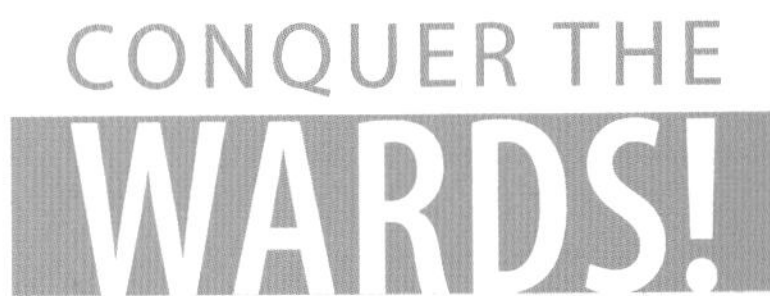

It is important to check a fundoscopic exam in all patients with headache to assess for IIH, as it is commonly missed!

Physical Exam Findings

- **Papilledema** on fundoscopic exam.
- Reduced visual acuity.
- Reduced visual fields.
- Patients can have CN deficits secondary to ICP increases (most commonly CN VI palsies).

Diagnostic Workup

- MRI brain to assess for structural etiology of increased pressure.
- MR venogram to assess for venous sinus thrombosis, a common mimic.
- LP to assess for opening pressure, which is necessary for diagnosis.
- Formal visual field testing, which is helpful for tracking disease progression and treatment efficacy.

Management

- Carbonic anhydrase inhibitors (e.g., **acetazolamide** and **topiramate**).
- **Furosemide**.
- Serial LPs.
- Surgical treatments in select patients, which include optic nerve sheath fenestrations and CSF shunt procedures.
- Weight loss.

Common Questions Asked on Rounds

- What workup is necessary in a patient suspected of having IIH?
  - Brain imaging to rule out mass lesion.
  - LP to assess for CSF opening pressure.
- What are the potential risks of not treating a patient with IIH?
  - Blindness, which may occur insidiously and is largely irreversible.

HIGH-YIELD LITERATURE

Mollan SP, Davies B, Silver NC, et al. Idiopathic intracranial hypertension: Consensus guidelines on management. *J Neurol Neurosurg Psychiatry*. 2018;89(10):1088-1100.

MULTIPLE SCLEROSIS AND INFLAMMATORY DEMYELINATING CENTRAL NERVOUS SYSTEM DISEASES

General Facts

- **MS** is the most common inflammatory demyelinating CNS disease.
- Most common cause of disability in young people, excluding trauma.
- Diagnosis usually between twenties and fifties, with mean age of onset of 27.
- Women are more commonly affected than men with a ratio of 2 to 3:1.

Clinical Features

- Two ways to accumulate disability in MS:
  - **Relapse**: New symptom that is localizable and manifests over days and weeks in the absence of fever or infection, caused by subacute formation of demyelinating lesion.
  - **Progressive disease**: Gradual worsening of symptoms over months and years, caused by chronic degeneration of neurons and axons.
- Symptoms of MS may vary depending on part of the CNS involved. Common presenting symptoms include:
  - Fatigue.
  - Blurry vision: May be caused by optic neuritis.
  - Double vision: Indicative of brainstem relapse.
  - Numbness and tingling in limbs: Caused by spinal cord or brain lesions.
  - Loss of coordination with limbs: May be suggestive of cerebellar lesions.
  - Weakness: Caused lesion in corticospinal tract in brain or spinal cord.
- MS can be classified by the various types of disease courses.
  - **Relapsing and remitting MS (RRMS):**
    - Eighty-five percent of patients are diagnosed with RRMS at onset.
    - Clearly defined relapses and new lesion formation. **In between relapses patient is clinically stable** (though the patient may have a residual symptom from previous attack).
  - **Primary progressive MS**: Disease progression from onset without definite relapse, worsening typically occurs over years with occasional plateaus and only minimal improvements.
  - **Secondary progressive multiple sclerosis**: Initially RRMS that later develops consistent disease progression over a period of years.

Physical Exam Findings

Various neurologic syndromes are associated with MS and present with characteristic examination findings.

- **Optic neuritis:**
  - Inflammation of the optic nerve (CN II).
  - Decreased visual acuity or blindness.
  - Pain with eye movement.
  - Afferent pupillary defect (APD) on exam.
    - When shining a light in affected eye, the pupil will not constrict (loss of direct pupillary constriction). When shining a light in the nonaffected eye, the affected eye will constrict (maintained consensual pupillary constriction).
  - Acutely the fundoscopic exam is normal. Chronically, the optic disc can appear pale.
- **Internuclear ophthalmoplegia (INO):**
  - Due to lesion in medial longitudinal fasciculus in the brainstem, which is a pathway that maintains conjugate eye movement.
  - On lateral gaze, there is failure in adduction with normal abduction (Figure 16-6).
  - The abducting eye will also demonstrate fast beating nystagmus toward the midline.
- **Myelitis** (aka transverse myelitis) (Figure 16-7).
  - Inflammation of spinal cord, typically patchy and eccentric (near outer edge of spinal cord, as opposed being centrally located).
  - May result in **motor symptoms**: Hemiparesis or paraparesis.

A

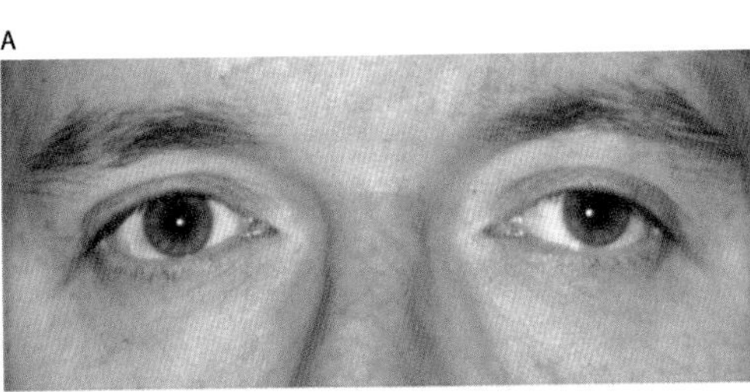

B

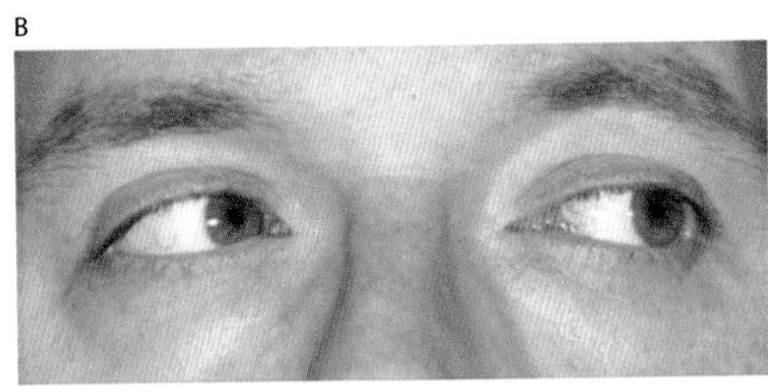

C

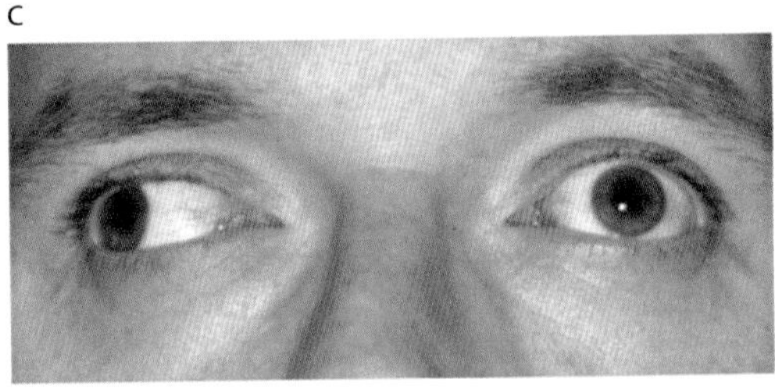

FIGURE 16-6. Left internuclear ophthalmoplegia presenting with (A) normal primary gaze, (B) normal left horizontal gaze, and (C) failure of adduction of left eye on rightward horizontal gaze. Reproduced, with permission, from Jameson JL, Fauci AF, Kasper DL, et al, eds: *Harrison's Principles of Internal Medicine*, 20th ed. www.accessmedicine.com. Copyright © McGraw-Hill Education. All rights reserved.)

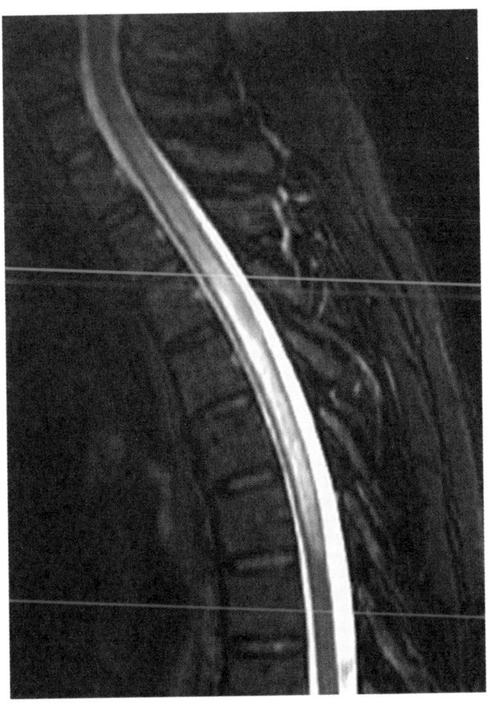

FIGURE 16-7. Spine MRI (sagittal view of T2 sequence), in which water is bright [e.g., CSF] and fat is dark (e.g., axon myelin sheath), of transverse myelitis demonstrated by T2 hyperintensity (increased white in spinal cord) in the cervicothoracic spinal cord. This patient has neuromyelitis optica, which is associated with longitudinally extensive transverse myelitis.

- **Sensory level**: Sensory deficits from toes up to a circumferential level of their body, generally in the torso.
- May include **bowel and bladder incontinence**.
- For more details regarding potential clinical findings, see section on spinal cord injury and radiculopathy.

Diagnostic Workup

- **MRI of brain, cervical spine, and thoracic spine with and without contrast**: MRI is required for identification of lesions associated with MS, as CT scans are insufficient for identifying demyelinating lesions. Given that lesions are frequently asymptomatic, scanning of the entire CNS (brain and spinal cord, which ends in the thoracic spine) is warranted at the time of diagnosis to understand the complete picture.
  - **Contrast-enhancing lesions** are subacute (30 to 60 days), whereas **non-enhancing lesions** are chronic (older than 60 days).
- **Lumbar puncture** for CSF analysis:
  - The presence of **oligoclonal bands** supports a diagnosis of MS and is present in 90% of MS cases.
  - Pleocytosis of greater than 50 white blood cells is inconsistent with MS and suggests another cause.
- A diagnosis of MS is made when a patient has experienced 2 or more attacks in 2 or more areas of the CNS. This is otherwise known as **"dissemination in time" (DIT)** and **"dissemination in space" (DIS)**.
- Clinical evidence alone can be enough for a diagnosis of MS, but evidence of both DIT and DIS can be found using MRI. Similarly, the presence of CSF oligoclonal bands substitutes for evidence of DIT in the most recent criteria.

> CONQUER THE **WARDS!**
>
> Patients with potential MS relapse may instead be having a pseudo-relapse. It is important to obtain a urinalysis to assess for UTI, even in asymptomatic patients.

Management

- Acute attacks and relapses:
  - If the patient is symptomatic, start IV methylprednisolone 1 gram q24h for 3 to 5 days.
  - If a contrast-enhancing lesion is not seen, especially if the symptoms are similar to previous, a diagnosis of "pseudo-relapse" should be considered.
    - A pseudo-relapse may be precipitated by infections (e.g., urinary tract infections), stress, electrolyte imbalance, and exposure to high heat.
- Preventive management
  - Disease-modifying therapies (DMTs) (Table 16-9), which can be administered orally, subcutaneously, or IV. Choice of DMT depends on disease severity, compliance, and side effect profile.
  - Goal of DMTs is to stop new lesion formation, new relapse, and any clinical progression.

> CONQUER THE **WARDS!**
>
> Teriflunomide is also found in sperm, and men also need to undergo drug elimination as a part of family planning.

Notes on Other Related Diseases Included in Differential Diagnosis of MS

Neuromyelitis Optica Spectrum Disorder

- Originally thought to be an extremely severe variant of MS, but now identified as its own disease entity.
- Associated with **aquaporin-4 antibody.**
- Classic presentation with bilateral optic neuritis and longitudinally extensive transverse myelitis (lesions extending over 3 or more vertebrae) (see Figure 16-8).
- Prognosis is generally worse, though patients may do very well with treatment.
- Usually treated with IV glucocorticoids and plasma exchange.

> CONQUER THE **BOARDS!**
>
> All patients considered for natalizumab should be initially screened for JC virus antibody and subsequently screened every 6 months.

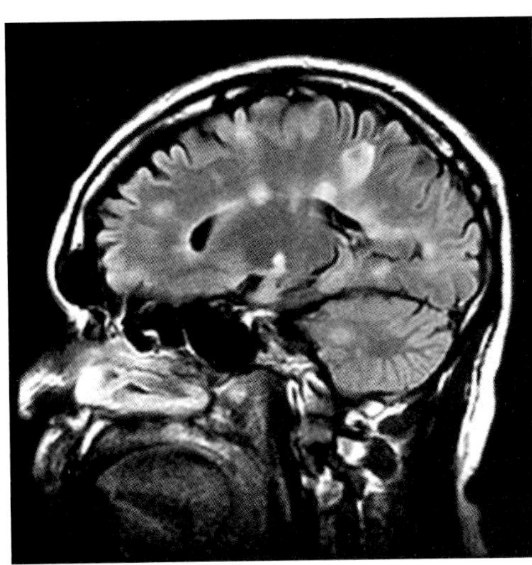

FIGURE 16-8. MRI brain (sagittal FLAIR view) of a patient with multiple sclerosis demonstrating classic finding of pericallosal ovoid lesions that are perpendicular to the ventricles (aka Dawson fingers).

Table 16-9. Disease-Modifying Therapies for Multiple Sclerosis

Medication	Route and Frequency of Administration	Risk/Adverse Effects	Other Notes
Interferon	SubQ or IV	■ Flulike symptoms ■ Fever ■ Elevated liver enzymes	■ Oldest DMT; rarely used as first-line therapy today
Glatiramer acetate	SubQ daily or 3× weekly	■ Injection site reaction	■ Minimal side effect profile ■ Likely less efficacious than newer drugs
Fingolimod	PO daily	■ Bradycardia on first day of dosing ■ Macular edema ■ Infection, including PML rarely	■ Risk of rebound of activity if drug is discontinued
Siponimod	PO daily	■ Bradycardia risk for some ■ Infection	■ Indicated for SPMS as well as RRMS ■ Requires genetic testing to determine correct dose
Cladribine	PO daily × 5 days, repeated in 1 month and then entire cycle repeated in 1 year	■ Infection ■ Lymphopenia ■ May increase risk for malignancy	■ Dosing based on weight
Dimethyl fumarate	PO, twice daily	■ Flushing and GI side effects initially ■ Lymphopenia ■ PML rarely	
Teriflunomide	PO, daily	■ Temporary hair thinning ■ Elevated liver enzymes ■ Teratogenicity	
Natalizumab	IV, every 4 weeks	■ Many associated cases of **progressive multifocal leukoencephalopathy (PML)**, which is associated with latent **JC virus**; can lead to permanent disability and death	■ Monitoring of twice annual serum JC antibody, safest use in those that are JC antibody negative
Alemtuzumab	IV, once yearly for 2 successive years; not dosed again unless there is new lesion or relapse	■ Autoimmune disease (thyroid, lung, liver) ■ Infection (due to temporary depletion of both B and T cells)	
Ocrelizumab	IV, twice yearly	■ Infection	■ Indications for both RRMS and PPMS ■ First drug approved for MS that specifically targets B cells, high level of efficacy

Acute Disseminated Encephalomyelitis (ADEM)

- More common in children.
- Associated with recent infection, concomitant fever, and encephalopathy.
- Patients with ADEM often have a fulminant, multifocal presentation, which may include encephalopathy.
- Radiographically, ADEM classically presents with uniformly enhancing white matter lesions in contrast to MS, where there is a mixture of nonenhancing and enhancing lesions.
- Unlike MS, ADEM is self-limited without future relapse.

HIGH-YIELD LITERATURE

Thompson AJ, Banwell BL, Barkhof F, et al. Diagnosis of multiple sclerosis: 2017 revisions of the McDonald criteria. *Lancet Neurol.* 2018;17(2):162-173.

MENINGITIS

General Facts

- Acute infection of the subarachnoid space and leptomeninges.
- Can be caused by bacteria, viruses, and fungi.
- Increased risk in those with sinusitis, otitis, and head trauma.

Clinical Features

- Bacterial meningitis:
  - Classic triad of headache, fever, and stiff neck.
  - Mental status changes (e.g., confusion, lethargy, coma).
  - Seizures.
  - Nausea, vomiting, photophobia.
- Most common causative bacteria (in descending order of incidence):
  - *Streptococcus pneumoniae.*
  - *Neisseria meningitidis* (aka meningococcemia) (young adults).
  - *Listeria monocytogenes* (immunocompromised hosts, very young and very old).
  - *Haemophilus influenzae* (unimmunized adults).
  - Group B *Streptococcus* (neonates).
- Viral meningitis (aka aseptic meningitis):
  - Most commonly caused by enterovirus.
  - Similar features to bacterial but can be less pronounced.
  - Treatment is supportive (except in cases of herpes simplex or varicella).
- Herpes meningoencephalitis:
  - Acute to subacute course of confusion and psychiatric symptoms may be the predominant finding, more so than meningismus.
  - +/− Seizure.
  - History of non-CNS herpes simplex infection.
  - MRI brain may show abnormalities in **temporal lobes.**
- Tuberculosis meningitis:
  - Associated with "basilar meningitis" and manifests with multiple **cranial nerve deficits** and increased ICP.
  - Suspect in immunocompromised patients.

- Fungal meningitis:
  - Can have a subacute or chronic course.
  - May also cause cranial neuropathies.
  - Associated with increased ICP, especially with *Cryptococcus.*
  - Rare in immunocompetent patients. Suspect in immunocompromised patients.

Physical Exam Findings

- Meningismus: Inability to flex the neck *forward* either actively or passively.
- **Kernig sign**: Extending the knee with the hip flexed causes pain in back and hamstring.
- **Brudzinski sign**: Forced neck flexion results in flexion at knee and hip.
  - Both Kernig and Brudzinski signs are specific but not sensitive in identifying meningitis.
- *Neisseria meningitidis* is associated with a maculopapular rash that occurs on days 1 to 3 of illness and is prominent in areas of skin subject to pressure.

Diagnostic Workup

- Blood culture.
- CT scan before LP to assess for abscess and to rule out mass effect.
  - Performing an LP in the presence of increased ICP can lead to brain herniation.
- LP for CSF analysis, including cell count, protein, glucose, opening pressure, herpes simplex virus (HSV), and varicella-zoster virus (VZV) polymerase chain reaction (PCR), and antibody titers (Table 16-10).

Management

Bacterial Meningitis

- *Streptococcus pneumoniae:* Vancomycin + cefotaxime or ceftriaxone.
- *N. meningitidis:* Ceftriaxone.
- If patient is at risk for *Listeria*, add ampicillin.
- In patients with suspected bacterial meningitis, dexamethasone should be started and continued only if *Streptococcus pneumoniae* is confirmed as the causative pathogen.

Viral Meningitis

- Treatment is supportive except in cases of suspected herpes simplex or varicella infections where antiviral therapy with acyclovir is warranted until PCR results are known.

Table 16-10. CSF Findings in Meningitis and Abscess

	WBCs (cells/μL)	Differential	Protein (mg/dL)	Glucose (mg/dL)	Opening Pressure (normal <20 mm Hg)
Bacterial meningitis	>100 (can be in 1000s)	Neutrophils	100–500	<10–40	Elevated
Viral meningitis	5–1000	Lymphs/monos	50–300	>40	Normal or elevated
TB/fungal meningitis	5–1000	Lymphs/monos	50–300	<10–40	Elevated
Brain abscess	5–100	Neutrophils	50–300	<10–40	Elevated

Choosing Empiric Antibody Therapy

- Treatment should be started before CSF test results.
- If there is suspicion for a bacterial meningitis, cover broadly with vancomycin and ceftriaxone/cefotaxime. In elderly patients, cover for *Listeria* with ampicillin.
- If there is suspicion for herpes simplex based on clinical findings, then start acyclovir.

Common Questions Asked on Rounds

- What do you expect to see on the CSF analysis in this patient with bacterial meningitis?
  - The answer should be high WBC, and protein and low glucose.
- Why should one obtain a CT head before attempting an LP?
  - To rule out a mass lesion causing increased ICP, which is a contraindication for LP, as it may lead to brain herniation.

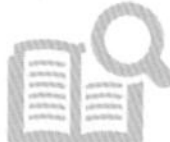

HIGH-YIELD LITERATURE

Steroids in Acute bacterial Meningitis

van de Beek D, de Gans J, McIntyre P, Prasad K. Steroids in adults with acute bacterial meningitis: A systematic review. *Lancet Infect Dis*. 2004;4(3):139-143.

AUTOIMMUNE AND PARANEOPLASTIC ENCEPHALITIS

General Facts

- The **autoimmune and paraneoplastic encephalitides** are a heterogeneous group of severe inflammatory disorders of the brain associated with antibodies against neuronal proteins.
- Frequently, but not necessarily, associated with a malignancy.
- **Anti-NMDA encephalitis** is the most commonly and best characterized form, which classically affects young women and is associated with **ovarian teratoma**. (NMDA receptors are proteins that control electrical impulses in the brain especially critical for judgment, human interaction, memory formation, and autonomic functions such as breathing).
- An important differential in a patient with unexplained encephalopathy, psychiatric symptoms, and seizures.

Clinical Features

- Acute to subacute time course: **Rapidly progressive usually in less than 2 months**.
- Somnolence.
- Personality changes.
- Psychiatric symptoms, including depression, mania, psychosis, and insomnia.
- Abnormal movements.
- Seizures.

Physical Exam Findings

- Decreased level of consciousness.
- Memory deficits.

- Movement disorders (e.g., **oral-buccal dyskinesias,** tremor, chorea, dystonias).
- **Autonomic instability** (e.g., hyperthermia, fluctuant blood pressure and heart rate).
- Language dysfunction (e.g., mutism, echolalia).

Diagnostic Workup

Because this is a challenging diagnosis, most of the following tests are done if you suspect an autoimmune or paraneoplastic encephalitis.

- EEG: May show epileptiform activity. Some patients have characteristic EEG finding of **delta brush.** This should be prioritized to treat for seizure with AEDs.
- MRI brain: May show characteristic findings of T2 hyperintensities in hippocampus and limbic regions.
- CSF analysis may show lymphocytic pleocytosis, but the CSF may also have no white cells. Therefore CSF fluid should be sent for autoimmune and paraneoplastic antibodies.
- Serum testing for autoimmune and paraneoplastic antibodies, which includes antibodies for NMDA receptor, voltage-gated potassium channel (VGKC), LGI-1, CASPR2, AMPA receptor, antineuronal nuclear antibodies (ANNAs), Purkinje cell cytoplasmic antibodies (PCA), amphiphysin (AMPH), and CRMP-5.

Management

- Treatment of underlying malignancy if present.
- Seizure control with antiepileptic medications.
- Aggressive treatment with IV methylprednisolone, intravenous immunoglobulin (IVIG), and/or plasma exchange (PLEX).
- If initial therapies are ineffective, add secondary immunosuppressive therapies such as rituximab or cyclophosphamide.

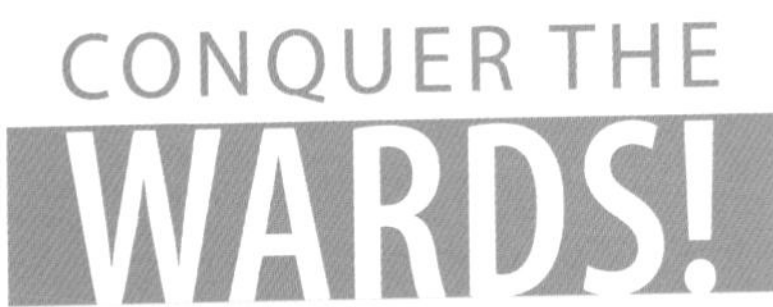

Removal of ovarian teratoma in patients with anti-NMDA encephalitis can be curative.

Common Questions Asked on Rounds

- What malignancy is commonly associated with anti-NMDA encephalitis?
  - Ovarian teratoma.
- How do you differentiate autoimmune encephalitis from infectious encephalitis?
  - Infectious encephalitis: CSF with bacterial growth or viral antibodies, fever, more acute.
  - Autoimmune encephalitis: More subacute course, autoimmune encephalitis/paraneoplastic antibody identified on serum or CSF.

HIGH-YIELD LITERATURE

Graus F, Titulaer MJ, Balu R, et al. A clinical approach to diagnosis of autoimmune encephalitis. *Lancet Neurol.* 2016;15(4):391-404.

PARKINSON DISEASE

General Facts

- Complex progressive neurodegenerative disease involving motor and cognitive function.
- Mean age of diagnosis 70 years.
- Associated with degeneration of dopamine-producing neurons in **substantia nigra**.

Clinical Features

- Classic triad of **tremor, bradykinesia, and rigidity**.
- **Tremor:** Patients typically complain of tremulousness. Sometimes tremor may not be bothersome to the patient and noticed mainly by others.
- **Bradykinesia**: Typically starts in manual dexterity such as buttoning clothes and with difficulty standing from a chair and dragging legs.
- **Rigidity:** Stiffness that usually starts unilaterally on same side as tremor progressing to the contralateral side.
- **Sleep disorders**: Affect majority of patients and consist of insomnia, daytime sleepiness, and restless leg syndrome.
- **Cognitive decline** is a late feature.
- **Nonmotor features** such as decreased sense of smell, constipation, urinary retention, and cognitive dysfunction may also occur.

Physical Exam Findings

- **Masked facies** (aka hypomimia): Lack of emotional facial expression, decreased eye blink rate, and hypophonia (decreased volume of speech).
- Resting tremor:
  - Oscillating movement generally in distal arm or leg that occurs while at rest and extinguishes with movement of limb.
  - Classically described as a "**pill-rolling tremor**."
  - Generally begins unilaterally and spreads to the contralateral limb after several years.
- Bradykinesia: Slowness of movement that can be witnessed in various parts of neurologic exam.
  - Slow speed in finger-to-nose testing.
  - Slowness and "getting stuck" during fine motor testing such as finger tapping.
  - Decreased arm swing during gait exam.
- Rigidity: Increased tone in limb that is not dependent on the velocity of limb movement (contrast with spasticity, which is increased tone predominantly with high-velocity limb movements).
  - "**Cogwheel rigidity**" refers to the ratchet pattern of resistance and relaxation when testing for tone.
  - Like tremor, begins unilaterally and eventually spreads contralaterally.
- Postural instability:
  - Generally a later sign.
  - Assessed with "**pull test**" where the examiner stands behind the patient and tugs backwards on the shoulders. Normally a patient will be able to catch his or her balance in one step. In a patient with Parkinson disease, it may take several steps (or they may not regain balance at all).
- Autonomic dysfunction: Generally a later sign.

> **CONQUER THE WARDS!**
>
> Resting tremor is classically found in Parkinson disease. Postural or action tremor is classically found in essential tremor.

Diagnostic Workup

- Primarily a clinical diagnosis based on history and examination.
- Dopamine transporter single-photon emission computed tomography (SPECT) imaging (DaTscan) may be helpful in cases of unclear diagnosis, but is not required for diagnosis.

Management

- **Carbidopa-levodopa**: First-line therapy. Other therapies added if symptoms persist.
  - Levodopa is converted to dopamine in the CNS.
  - Carbidopa inhibits conversion of levodopa to dopamine in peripheral tissue.
- Anticholinergics (e.g., **trihexyphenidyl, benztropine**) – block cholinergic inhibition of dopaminergic neurons.
- Dopamine receptor agonists (e.g., **bromocriptine, pergolide**): Can be used as adjunctive or secondary therapy. Higher risk of dopamine-toxicity mood symptoms, including hyperimpulsivity and hypersexuality.
- Monoamine oxidase inhibitors (e.g., **selegiline**): Used as adjunctive therapy. Blocks central metabolism of dopamine. Must be wary of serotonin syndrome in patients also on other serotonergic medications (e.g., antidepressants).
- In select cases **deep brain stimulation (DBS)** has proven very effective at decreasing symptom burden and medication requirements.

Note on Potential Differentials

- Parkinson disease is the most common disease that causes "**parkinsonism**," which are the symptoms and signs described earlier. However, other conditions must be included in the differential diagnosis.
- **Drug-induced parkinsonism:**
  - Secondary to chronic antidopaminergic use (e.g., antipsychotics) and other drugs with antidopaminergic effects such as metoclopramide and prochlorperazine.
  - More likely to affect gait earlier in course.
  - More likely to be symmetric in onset.
  - May or may not be reversible with discontinuation of offending medication.
- Other neurodegenerative diseases can cause parkinsonism and must be on the differential. These are collectively known as the "**Parkinson-plus syndromes**."
- **Progressive supranuclear palsy:**
  - Patients have early postural instability and cognitive impairment.
  - Classically associated with vertical gaze is better ophthalmoparesis.
  - Parkinsonism features are generally symmetric at onset.
  - Poorly responsive to levodopa.
- **Multiple systems atrophy:**
  - Patients have early involvement of autonomic and cerebellar dysfunction.
  - Postural instability occurs early in the disease.
  - Parkinsonism features are generally symmetric at onset.
- **Dementia with Lewy body:**
  - Dementia generally precedes parkinsonism or occurs early in disease course.
  - Associated with visual hallucinations and fluctuating levels of consciousness.
- **Corticobasal degeneration:**
  - Progressive asymmetric movement disorder commonly first affecting one limb with combinations of rigidity, dystonia, tremor, chorea, and myoclonus.
  - Cortical dysfunction may manifest as aphasia, apraxia, and alien limb phenomenon.

Common Questions Asked on Rounds

- What is the classic triad of Parkinson disease?
  - Bradykinesia, rigidity, and tremor.

HIGH-YIELD LITERATURE

Hess CW, Okun MS. Diagnosing Parkinson disease. *Contin Lifelong Learn Neurol.* 2016;22(4 Movement Disorders):1047-1063.

CHANGE IN MENTAL STATUS

General Facts

- **Terminology:** Change in mental status is often categorized into 3 levels of consciousness:
  - **Coma:** Lack of response to external stimuli.
  - **Delirium:** Acute or subacute presentation with fluctuating symptoms, which is different from dementia, where the symptoms occur over a longer period and do not fluctuate.
  - **Dementia:** See later in this section.
- For the purposes of this section, we will focus on **delirium**, as this is the most commonly seen neurologic diagnosis on medical wards. You may also hear other terms such as acute confusional states or encephalopathy. For the most part, these terms are describing a change in mental status, which for practical purposes encompasses delirium.
- **Delirium** in nearly 30% of older hospitalized patients.

Clinical Features

- **Delirium is characterized by 5 key features in the DSM-V:**
  - Disturbance in attention and awareness.
  - **Acute or subacute (over hours to days) AND fluctuating symptoms.**
  - Cognitive disturbance (memory deficit, disorientation, perceptual changes).
  - Not explained by preexisting neurocognitive disorder.
  - Evidence from history, physical exam, or labs that delirium is due to an underlying medical issue.
- **Risk factors for delirium:**
  - **Increase in baseline vulnerability:**
    - Underlying brain diseases, most commonly dementia, stroke, and Parkinson disease.
    - Advanced age.
    - Sensory impairment.
  - **Precipitating factors** are extensive, but the most common are:
    - Medications: Polypharmacy, antihistamines.
    - Infection (e.g., urinary tract infection [UTI], pneumonia, cellulitis, abdominal pain, meningitis, viral upper respiratory infection [URI], sinusitis).
    - Electrolyte disturbances (hyponatremia, hypocalcemia, hyperglycemia).
    - Low perfusion states (dehydration, heart failure, shock).
    - Immobility (especially use of restraints).

- Foley catheters, central lines.
- Endocrine disturbances: Thyroid, parathyroid, pituitary, adrenal.
- Pulmonary issues: Hypoxemia, hypercarbia.
- Pain.
- Constipation.

Diagnostic Workup

- **Step 1: High index of suspicion.** Some studies show a failure to recognize delirium in 70% of cases. A change in the level of consciousness is the first observable clue and can be as subtle as a patient's inability to focus during history taking.
- **Step 2:** Perform a **mini mental status exam** or even a brief test of attention such as serial-sevens or spelling "world" backwards to assess attention. A more formalized tool is the **Confusion Assessment Method (CAM)** which can be used to diagnose delirium. It has a sensitivity of up to 100% and specificity of 95%.
- **Step 3: Focused history and physical exam looking for underlying causes.** Due to delirium, getting a history or a physical is challenging. It is important to speak with family members or caretakers to find out history. It is especially important to obtain a thorough medication history, focusing on any new medications and any alcohol or illicit drug use. Focus your physical exam on the common causes outlined earlier under precipitating factors.
- **Step 4: Laboratory tests.** Basic workup includes complete metabolic panel, complete blood count, toxic screen for illicit drug use, and an arterial blood gas if signs of respiratory issues. Imaging, like a head CT, is not routinely recommended unless there are focal neurologic exam findings or a history suggesting head trauma. Other tests such as EEG, LP, and MRI are also not done routinely unless history and physical suggest a need for these tests.

Management

- Treatment of underlying cause of the delirium whether that is antibiotics, fluids, or correction of electrolyte or endocrine disturbances.
- **Severe agitation:** Sometimes patients with delirium can become severely agitated. **Antipsychotics** such as Haldol 0.5 mg or 1 mg can be used as needed only. Continuous or prophylactic use of antipsychotics is not recommended due to limited evidence showing their efficacy. Benzodiazepines should be avoided because they may worsen delirium.
- **Prognosis:**
  - **Mortality** can be twice that of patients without delirium.
  - **Cognitive dysfunction:** Symptoms may persist for 12 months or longer, especially in patients with dementia.
- **Prevention:** Because there is no proven treatment for delirium and it has an overall poor prognosis, prevention is key. These also can be used when patients have delirium to help with recovery.
  - Orientation protocols: Having clocks, calendars, and windows with outside views. Frequent verbal reorientation. Having family and friends visit.
  - Sleep protocols: Avoiding nursing, medical procedures during usual sleeping hours, and decreasing nighttime noise (e.g., ear plugs).
  - Early mobilization.
  - Avoiding physical restraints that limit mobility and removing tethers when they are no longer medically necessary. Tethers include Foley catheters, continuous IV fluids, serial leg compression devices, or telemetry.

DEMENTIA

General Facts

- Cognitive disorders are characterized by their effect on the different cognitive domains, which include:
  - Memory.
  - Attention.
  - Orientation.
  - Executive function (decision-making).
  - Visuospatial.
  - Language.
  - Calculation.
- **Mild cognitive impairment (MCI)** is the presence of decreased cognitive function in at least one domain.
- **Dementia** is the loss of cognitive function in 2 domains AND loss of ability to independently maintain activities of daily living.
- Differential diagnosis includes:
  - Neurodegenerative disease (Alzheimer disease, Lewy body dementia, frontotemporal dementia).
  - Stroke (aka vascular dementia).
  - Infection (syphilis, HIV, Creutzfeldt–Jakob disease).
  - Vitamin deficiency (B_{12}, thiamine, niacin).
  - Normal-pressure hydrocephalus.
  - Trauma.
  - Tumors.
  - Depression (aka pseudodementia).

CONQUER THE WARDS!

Reversible causes of dementia include hypothyroidism, syphilis, and vitamin B_{12} deficiency and must always be checked in the dementia workup.

Diagnostic Workup

The main focus of the workup is to rule out reversible or modifiable causes of the cognitive decline. Also see delirium section.

- Complete blood count (CBC).
- Chemistry panel.
- Vitamin B_{12}.
- Thyroid-stimulating hormone (TSH).
- Rapid plasma reagin (RPR).
- Brain imaging (CT or MRI)
- EEG if seizures are suspected.

Management

- Treatment of specific disorder.
- Optimize sensory functions (visual aids, hearing aids).
- Simplify activities of daily living (e.g., simplify floor plans, minimize staircases).
- Modify home life for physical safety (e.g., bed rails, home health aides).
- Encourage social engagement with family and community.
- Minimize polypharmacy and sedating medications when possible.
- Occupational therapy consult.

Common Questions Asked on Rounds

- What is the initial blood workup for a patient suspected to have dementia?
  - CBC, chemistry panel, vitamin B_{12}, TSH, RPR.

- What measures can family members take at home to minimize the complications of dementia?
  - Modify home for physical safety and encourage social engagement.

ALZHEIMER DEMENTIA

General Facts

- Most common cause of dementia.
- Generally occurs in older individuals (>65 years).
- Neurodegenerative disorder of unclear etiology but associated with accumulation of **beta-amyloid and tau protein deposition** in the brain.
- Higher incidence in **Down syndrome.**

Clinical Features

- Chronic progressive and insidious course.
- Memory is commonly affected.
  - Declarative memory (memory of specific events) is usually profoundly affected.
  - Procedural and motor learning memory spared until late disease.
  - Semantic memory (vocabulary, facts) spared until late disease.
- Executive function dysfunction: Less organized, less motivated, difficulty with abstract reasoning.
- Neuropsychiatric dysfunction: Depression, apathy, agitation, aggression, psychosis.

Physical Exam Findings

- Aside from cognitive findings, physical exam is generally normal.
- Other neurologic exam findings, especially early in the disease, should prompt consideration for a different diagnosis.

Diagnostic Workup

- Primarily a clinical diagnosis.
- General dementia workup to assess for other and potentially reversible causes (see Dementia section).

Management

- **Donepezil**, **memantine**, and **galantamine** may slow cognitive decline.
- Exercise, mental activity, and social engagement may be protective.
- Treatment of behavioral symptoms with antipsychotics and antidepressants.

Common Questions Asked on Rounds

- What type of memory is most commonly affected in early Alzheimer disease?
  - Declarative memory.
- What types of medications are available for the treatment of Alzheimer disease?
  - Donepezil, memantine, and galantamine.

NORMAL-PRESSURE HYDROCEPHALUS

General Facts

- Clinical syndrome associated with pathologically enlarged ventricles with normal ICP.
- There is an absence of an "obstructive" cause of hydrocephalus (e.g., tumor).

CONQUER THE BOARDS!

Normal Pressure Hydrocephalus (NPH) has the classic triad of "wet, wild, and wobbly."

Clinical Features and Physical Exam Findings

- Classic triad of **dementia, incontinence, and gait dysfunction**.
- Gait dysfunction:
  - **"Magnetic" gait**, which is thought to be due to apraxia. It appears the patient's feet are glued to the floor.
  - Small steps, often with a wide base; difficulty in turning.
  - Postural instability often demonstrated by pull test.
  - Often responsive to treatment.
- Dementia:
  - Executive dysfunction: Difficulty with complex planning and decision-making.
  - Memory deficits with poor retrieval.
  - Poor concentration and attention.
- Pertinent negatives:
  - Lack of headaches, nausea, and vomiting.
  - Patient is classically unconcerned about urinary incontinence.
  - Lack of papilledema.

CONQUER THE WARDS!

Testing of gait before and after lumbar puncture and drain is used to determine if a patient is likely to respond to placement of a VP shunt.

Diagnostic Workup

- Brain imaging to evaluate for enlarged ventricles (CT or MRI) (see Figure 16-9).

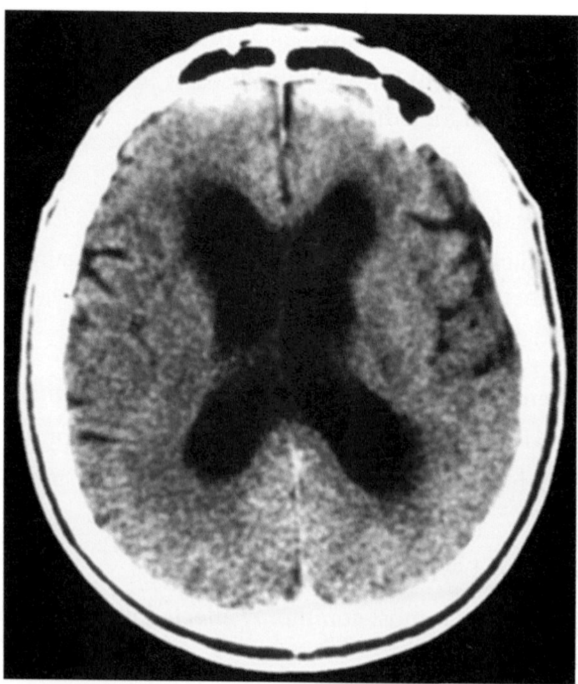

FIGURE 16-9. CT head of patient with normal-pressure hydrocephalus. Note the enlarged lateral ventricles without evidence of enlarged sulci (the presence of which may be more suggestive of enlarged ventricles secondary to brain atrophy). (Used, with permission, from Simon RP, Aminoff MJ, Greenberg DA: *Clinical Neurology*, 10th ed. Copyright © McGraw-Hill Education. All rights reserved.)

- Lumbar puncture and/or lumbar drain to assess for normal opening pressure and for improvement in symptoms after drainage of CSF.

Management

- **Ventriculoperitoneal shunt (VP shunt)**: Device that diverts CSF from ventricles to peritoneal space, with goal of relieving hydrocephalus and associated symptoms.
- Patients with moderate to severe dementia are unlikely to improve after placement of shunt.

Common Questions Asked on Rounds

- What is the classic triad of normal-pressure hydrocephalus?
  - "Wet, wobbly, and wacky": Incontinence, shuffling gait, dementia.
- Which patients are most likely to respond to placement of a VP shunt?
  - Patients who have not yet developed dementia.

HIGH-YIELD LITERATURE

Halperin JJ, Kurlan R, Schwalb JM, Cusimano MD, Gronseth G, Gloss D. Practice guideline: Idiopathic normal pressure hydrocephalus: Response to shunting and predictors of response: Report of the Guideline Development, Dissemination, and Implementation Subcommittee of the American Academy of Neurology. *Neurology*. 2015;85(23):2063-2071.

APPROACH TO DIZZINESS

General Facts

- Dizziness is one of the most common reasons for neurologic referral and consultation.
- Three main groups of disorders must be differentiated in dizziness:
  - CNS causes.
  - Peripheral nervous system causes.
  - Non-neurologic causes.
- The distinction between these types of dizziness is important, as central neurologic dizziness can be associated with stroke and tumor.

Terminology

- Dizziness is a nonspecific complaint and may be suggestive of one of the following more specific disorders.
  - **Vertigo:** Sensation of self-motion in the absence of motion (e.g., room spinning sensation). Classically associated with vestibular dysfunction. Can be present in both central and peripheral neurologic disorders.
  - **Presyncope:** Sensation of lightheadedness ("feeling faint"). Associated with cardiovascular diseases (e.g., orthostatic hypotension).
  - **Unsteadiness:** Feeling of being unstable while seated, standing, or walking without a directional preference. Nonspecific complaint that can be associated with both vestibular and cerebellar disorders.
  - **Oscillopsia:** The false sensation that the visual surrounding is oscillating or vibrating. Associated with nystagmus.

Clinical Features

- Details on timing and physical findings are key in distinguishing between different etiologies of dizziness.
- **Central neurologic dizziness:**

- Dizziness is frequently persistent.
- Accompanied by cranial nerve, motor, sensory, or cerebellar abnormal exam findings.
- Nystagmus that changes direction or is multidirectional.
- Skew deviation of eyes: Eyes will deviate from their normal conjugate positions (generally vertically) after eye opening or after eye movements.

- **Peripheral neurologic dizziness:**
  - Dizziness is frequently episodic.
  - Nystagmus that is unidirectional.
  - Sensorineural hearing loss.
  - Tinnitus.
  - Lack of other neurologic abnormalities on exam.
- **Non-neurologic dizziness:**
  - Orthostatic worsening of dizziness.
  - Loss of consciousness.

Diagnostic Workup and Management

- Central neurologic etiologies of dizziness can almost universally be evaluated with an MRI brain.
- Peripheral neurologic etiologies of dizziness are frequently clinical diagnoses.
- See Table 16-10 for further details.

Table 16-10. Neurologic Disorders of Dizziness

Disease	Central or Peripheral	Distinguishing Features	Management
Posterior circulation stroke	Central	■ Acute onset ■ Cerebellar and cranial nerve deficits ■ Dizziness is persistent ■ **"HINTS exam"** for clinical assessment of dizziness-related stroke vs peripheral etiology (see high-yield literature)	■ See the section Stroke
Brainstem encephalitis	Central	■ Altered mental status ■ Fever	■ CSF analysis of infectious and paraneoplastic markers and subsequent treatment of underlying cause
Vestibular schwannoma	Peripheral	■ Subacute to chronic onset ■ May be associated with increased intracranial pressure ■ Occasionally associated with ipsilateral seventh nerve palsy	■ Surgical resection
Vestibular neuronitis	Peripheral	■ Subacute to chronic onset ■ Dizziness is persistent ■ Associated with recent infection	■ Short course of steroids
Ménière syndrome	Peripheral	■ Episodic vertigo lasting minutes to several hours ■ Associated with episodic sensorineural hearing loss and ear fullness (endolymphatic hydrops)	■ Initial treatment with diet modification (salt and caffeine reduction) and diuretics ■ Secondary treatment involves surgical and "destructive" therapies such as intratympanic gentamicin injections
Benign paroxysmal positional vertigo (BPPV)	Peripheral	■ Episodic vertigo lasting seconds to minutes ■ Associated with specific head movement or positioning ■ Can be diagnosed at bedside with **Dix–Hallpike maneuver** (See High-Yield Literature)	■ Can be treated with bedside maneuver – **Epley maneuver**

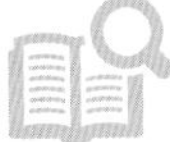

HIGH-YIELD LITERATURE

Fife TD. Positional dizziness. *Contin Lifelong Learn Neurol*. 2012;18(5 Neuro-otology):1060-1085.

Kattah JC, Talkad AV, Wang DZ, Hsieh Y-H, Newman-Toker DE. HINTS to diagnose stroke in the acute vestibular syndrome. *Stroke*. 2009;40(11):3504-3510.

BELL PALSY

General Facts

- **Bell palsy** is an idiopathic acute paresis of the peripheral facial nerve (aka CN VII).
- Commonly mistaken for stroke.
- Must consider other causes of CN VII palsy associated with another neurologic disorder including Guillain–Barré syndrome and vestibular schwannomas.

Clinical Features

- Acute onset of unilateral facial weakness. Can continue to progress over days to weeks.
- Difficulty eating and drinking.
- Eye irritation.
- Change in taste.
- Change in hearing.
- Although CN VII is largely a nonsensory nerve, patients will frequently complain of an abnormal sensation in their face (see Figure 16-10).
- Absence of neurologic symptoms elsewhere in the body.

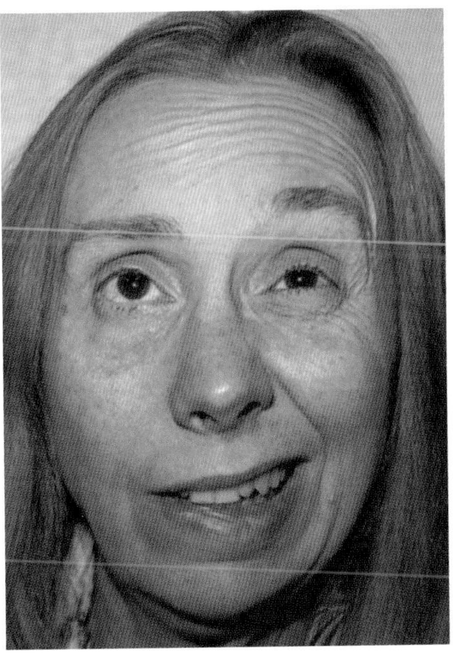

FIGURE 16-10. Bell palsy of right face. In addition to the right facial droop, there is an inability to elevate the right forehead and a widened right palpebral fissure. (Used, with permission, from Knoop KJ, Stack LB, Storrow AB, Thurman RJ, eds: *The Atlas of Emergency Medicine*, 4th ed. www.accessmedicine.com. Copyright © McGraw-Hill Education. All rights reserved. Photo contributor: Lawrence B. Stack, MD.)

CONQUER THE **WARDS!**

Understanding the difference between peripheral and central facial paresis is key to successfully differentiating Bell palsy from a stroke.

Physical Exam Findings

- Findings specific to **peripheral facial paresis** include (see Figure 16-10):
  - Weakness in forehead movement, sometimes appreciated by loss of wrinkles on side of the forehead (frontalis muscle).
  - Weakness in eye closure (orbicularis oculi muscle).
  - Loss of taste on anterior two-thirds of tongue.
  - Hyperacusis.
- Lower facial weakness (asymmetric smile, nasolabial fold flattening) is found in both central and peripheral facial paresis.
- Absence of neurologic deficits in other cranial nerves and in the limbs.

Diagnostic Workup

- MRI brain can be ordered to exclude stroke in unclear cases.
- **Lyme disease** serology if there is clinical suspicion, especially with a bilateral presentation (a common infectious cause of facial palsy).
- Electromyography (EMG) of face can be considered for prognostication in cases that do not resolve in several weeks.

Management

- Corticosteroids (e.g., **prednisone**) for 1 week.
- Eye care to prevent corneal abrasions (e.g., wearing eye patch, lubricating eye drops).

Common Question Asked on Rounds

- What findings differentiate a central and peripheral facial droop?
  - Peripheral facial droop involves eye closure and forehead elevation, whereas central does not.

HIGH-YIELD LITERATURE

Management of Bells Palsythis

Zandian A, Osiro S, Hudson R, et al. The neurologist's dilemma: A comprehensive clinical review of Bell's palsy, with emphasis on current management trends. *Med Sci Monit*. 2014;20:83

SPINAL CORD INJURY AND RADICULOPATHY

General Facts

- **Spinal cord injury** (i.e., spinal cord compression) is an important entity to recognize clinically, as it may be a neurologic and/or neurosurgical emergency due to the potential for quadriplegia (cervical cord injury) and paraplegia (cervical or thoracic cord injury).
- **Radiculopathy** is often associated with similar disease processes as spinal cord compression. Unlike spinal cord compression, it is not an emergency. Distinguishing the 2 clinically is important for triaging patients.
- **Degenerative disc disease** of the spine is the most common cause of both spinal cord compression and radiculopathy. The cervical and lumbar spine are most commonly affected. Involvement of the thoracic spine is rare.
- Other etiologies of spinal cord injury:
  - Tumors and mass lesions.
  - Trauma.

- Vascular (e.g., anterior spinal artery stroke).
- Infection (e.g., HTLV-1, HIV).
- Inflammatory (e.g., transverse myelitis in multiple sclerosis, systemic lupus erythematöus, Sjögren syndrome).
- Nutritional (e.g., deficiencies in vitamin B_{12}, vitamin E, copper).

- Other etiologies of radiculopathy:
  - Infection (e.g., HIV, cytomegalovirus [CMV]).
  - Leptomeningeal carcinomatosis.
  - Inflammatory (e.g., Guillain–Barré syndrome).
  - Tumors and mass lesions.
  - Trauma.

Clinical Features

- Neck and back pain is present in both spinal cord compression and radiculopathy.
- Spinal cord injury:
  - Weakness and sensory symptoms are typically bilateral.
  - Bowel and bladder symptoms.
  - Saddle paresthesia.
  - **Spinal cord compression is a neurologic emergency, especially when symptoms are severe or rapidly progressing.**
- Radiculopathy:
  - Shooting pain from neck down the arm (cervical radiculopathy) or from low back down the leg (lumbar radiculopathy).
  - Weakness and sensory symptoms are typically unilateral.

Physical Exam Findings

- Spinal cord injury:
  - Hyperreflexia below the level of the lesion.
  - Weakness below a myotomal level (e.g., spinal cord compression at C5 can cause weakness in muscles innervated by C5 roots and below).
  - Sensory deficits distal to an entire dermatomal level (e.g., spinal cord compression at T1 can cause sensory loss in dermatomes in the T1 roots and below).
  - Increased tone and spasticity.
  - Brown–Sequard syndrome (aka hemicord injury). Characterized by unilateral weakness and loss of vibration and position sense below the level (due to involvement of corticospinal tract and posterior columns) and contralateral pain and temperature loss below the level (due to involvement of the spinothalamic tract).
- Radiculopathy:
  - Weakness and atrophy of muscles in affected myotome.
  - Sensory deficits in affected dermatome.
  - Hyporeflexia at level of lesion.

Diagnostic Workup

- MRI of spine (specific areas of spine depending on symptoms) (see Figure 16-11).
- Lumbar puncture for CSF analysis if there is suspicion for infectious, inflammatory, or neoplastic etiologies.

CONQUER THE WARDS!

A good way to determine if your patient has saddle paresthesia is to ask if he or she has numbness when he or she wipes after using the toilet.

CONQUER THE WARDS!

While neuropathic pain medications are good for symptoms of tingling and shooting pain, they are ineffective in the treatment of numbness.

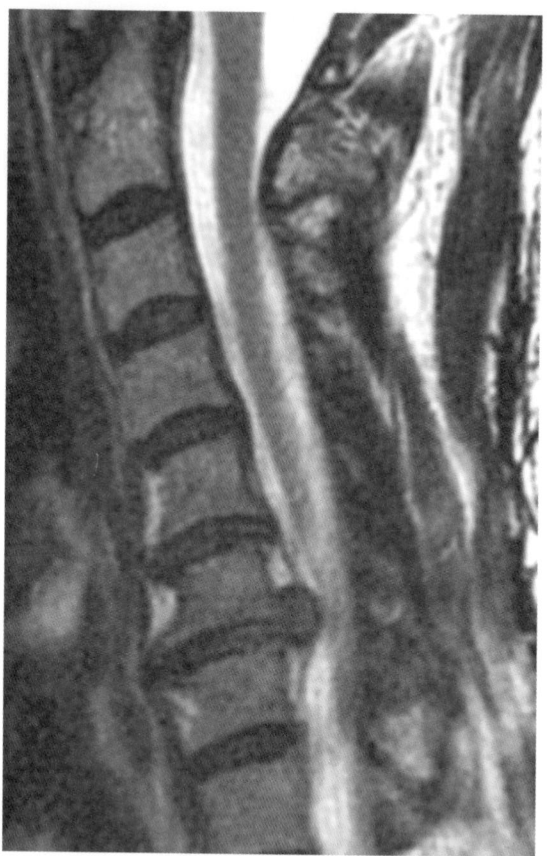

FIGURE 16-11. Cervical spine MRI (T2 sequence, sagittal view) of cervical disc herniation at C6–C7. Smaller disc bulges are seen at C4–C5 and C5–C6. (Reproduced with permission from Chapter 11. Pain in the Back, Neck, and Extremities. In: Ropper AH, Samuels MA, Klein JP, eds. *Adams & Victor's Principles of Neurology*, 10e. New York, NY: McGraw-Hill; 2014.)

Management

- Neuropathic pain medications (e.g., **gabapentin, pregabalin, duloxetine**).
- Physical and occupational therapy.
- Surgery in select cases.
- Treatment of underlying etiology.

HIGH-YIELD LITERATURE

Diagnosis and management of Cervical Radiculopathy

Iyer S, Kim HJ. Cervical radiculopathy. *Curr Rev Musculoskelet Med*. 2016;9(3):272-280.

AMYOTROPHIC LATERAL SCLEROSIS

General Facts

- **Amyotrophic lateral sclerosis (ALS)** is a progressive disorder that affects motor neurons in the cerebral cortex, brainstem, and spinal cord.
- Part of a larger spectrum of "motor neuron disease." ALS is differentiated by involvement of both upper and lower motor neuron degeneration. Other motor neuron diseases include **primary lateral sclerosis** (upper motor neuron only) and **progressive muscular atrophy** (lower motor neuron only).

Clinical Features

- Early features include loss of exercise tolerance, cramps, and fatigue.
- Weakness without sensory symptoms or pain.
- Bulbar and respiratory involvement generally occurs later but can be a presenting feature.

Physical Exam Findings

- Upper motor neuron (UMN) signs: Hyperreflexia, pathologic reflexes.
- Lower motor neuron signs: Muscle atrophy, fasciculations in tongue as well as in limbs.

Diagnostic Workup

Diagnosis is dependent on a combination of **clinical** and **electrodiagnostic** test findings.

- **Nerve conduction and needle electromyography** (collectively shortened to EMG): Findings of denervation in multiple myotome distributions are required for diagnosis of ALS. Furthermore, EMG is useful for assessing for other differentials, including demyelinating neuropathies (e.g., multifocal motor neuropathy).
- **MRI of brain and spinal cord**: Assesses for alternative causes of UMN findings (e.g., degenerative spine disease, demyelinating brain disease).
- **Serum laboratory studies** to exclude other mimics: HIV, HTLV, heavy metal, TSH.
- **Cancer screening**: ALS can be a paraneoplastic phenomenon.

Management

- **Riluzole**: Oral therapy that modestly slows down disease progression and improves survival.
- **Edaravone**: Infusion therapy that modestly slows down functional decline.
- Multidisciplinary care: Ideally patients with ALS should be cared for at a comprehensive ALS center where they can receive unified care from multiple subspecialties, including:
  - Speech and swallow therapy.
  - Respiratory therapy.
  - Physical and occupational therapy.
  - Nutrition.
- Positive-pressure ventilation in patients with reduced vital capacity.
- Tracheostomy in patients requiring mechanical ventilation.
- Gastrostomy tube in patients with dysphagia refractory to diet modification.

HIGH-YIELD LITERATURE

Costa J, Swash M, de Carvalho M. Awaji criteria for the diagnosis of amyotrophic lateral sclerosis: A systematic review. *Arch Neurol*. 2012;69(11):1410-1416.

GUILLAIN–BARRÉ SYNDROME

General Facts

- Guillain–Barré syndrome (GBS) is also known as acute inflammatory demyelinating polyradiculoneuropathy (AIDP).
- Classically follows a viral infection (classically *Campylobacter jejuni*).
- Can be a **neurologic emergency**.

Clinical Features

- Earliest symptom is typically paresthesias in fingertips and toes.
- Over several days, ascending paralysis begins, starting with lower extremities.
- Eventually quadriparesis and ventilatory failure can occur.
- Deep aching pain is a common feature.
- Nadir of symptoms occurs **before 4 weeks** (compare to CIDP in next section).
- Generally, a monophasic disease, but residual deficit is common, and rarely some patients may even experience relapses.
- There are various atypical presentations (e.g., **Miller Fisher syndrome**).

CONQUER THE BOARDS!

The most frequently associated viral infection is *Campylobacter jejuni*, which causes a diarrheal illness.

CONQUER THE BOARDS!

Miller Fisher syndrome's classic triad is areflexia, ataxia, and opthalmoparesis.

Physical wExam Findings

- Cranial nerve deficits (e.g., CN VII palsies).
- **Ascending weakness** in legs > arms.
- **Areflexia**.
- Sensory deficits affecting distal > proximal limb.
- Autonomic dysfunction: Tachyarrhythmias, hypotension.

Diagnostic Workup

- Diagnosis is frequently clinical, as CSF and EMG testing are frequently normal early in the disease.
- CSF demonstrates increased protein with normal WBC count (aka **cytoalbuminologic dissociation**): Occurs 1 week after disease onset.
- EMG shows signs of acquired demyelinating neuropathy (e.g., conduction block; may not manifest for 1 week).
- MRI of brain and spine should overall be unremarkable but may occasionally demonstrate increased T2 signal in CN and nerve roots.
- Pulmonary function tests (PFTs) to assess for ventilatory stability.

CONQUER THE WARDS!

PFTs, specifically negative inspiratory force (NIF) and vital capacity (VC), are most useful for assessing respiratory stability in patients with neuromuscular causes of ventilatory failure (e.g., MG, GBS).

Management

- Most patients require hospitalization for cardiac and respiratory monitoring.
- Mechanical ventilation for patients with respiratory muscle paralysis may be necessary.
- Plasma Exchange (PLEX) and/or Intravenous immunoglobulin (IVIG) should be used early and has been shown to hasten recovery.
- Corticosteroids are ineffective.

Common Questions Asked on Rounds

- What are the expected CSF findings for GBS?
  - Normal WBC count and cytoalbuminologic dissociation.
- What are the serious complications of GBS?
  - Respiratory failure and cardiac arrhythmia.

HIGH-YIELD LITERATURE

Dimachkie MM, Barohn RJ. Guillain-Barré syndrome and variants. *Neurol Clin*. 2013;31(2):491-510.

CHRONIC INFLAMMATORY DEMYELINATING POLYRADICULONEUROPATHY

General Facts

- **Chronic inflammatory demyelinating polyradiculoneuropathy (CIDP)** is a progressive and relapsing neuropathy.
- Often simplified to "chronic GBS" due to similar clinical and EMG findings, but it is likely an entirely different disease.
- Generally presents in adults (peak incidence at 30 to 60 years).

Clinical Features

- Subacute to chronic in time course.
- Lower extremity weakness and sensory symptoms are frequent presenting symptoms.
- Nadir of symptoms occurs >**8 weeks** after symptom onset (compare to GBS).
- Atypical presentations include pure sensory and pure motor forms.

Physical Exam Findings

- Symmetric and frequently non-length-dependent pattern of weakness.
- Cranial nerve deficits (e.g., CN VII palsy).
- **Areflexia**.
- Sensory deficits in distal leg and hands.

Diagnostic Workup

- EMG: Required for diagnosis. Expect findings of acquired demyelination (e.g., conduction block).
- CSF demonstrating albuminocytologic dissociation.
- MRI of brain and spine should overall be unremarkable but may occasionally demonstrate increased T2 signal in CN and nerve roots.
- Immunofixation and serum electrophoresis to assess for monoclonal protein, which is associated with 30% of cases of CIDP and should prompt further hematologic workup.
- Other serum laboratory studies for other causes of neuropathy (see next section): CBC, chemistry (kidney function testing), LFT, hemoglobin A_{1c}, hepatitis B and C, antinuclear antibodies, vitamin B_{12}, TSH.

Management

- **Corticosteroids** are first-line therapy (compare to GBS, where corticosteroids are ineffective).
- Immunosuppressants (e.g., **mycophenolate**).
- **Chronic IVIG and/or PLEX** at variable intervals depending on patient response.

CONQUER THE WARDS!

"Length dependent" is a term used to describe neuropathies that affect muscles innervated by the longest nerves (e.g., distal leg) before shorter nerves (e.g., proximal muscles, face).

Common Questions Asked on Rounds

- What differentiates GBS from CIDP?
    - GBS is an acute to subacute illness, generally reaches its nadir within 4 weeks, and is generally monophasic.
    - CIDP is a chronic illness and generally reaches its nadir after 8 weeks of symptom onset.
- What differentiates CIDP from more common chronic polyneuropathies?
    - CIDP is a demyelinating neuropathy.
    - Common chronic polyneuropathies (e.g., diabetic polyneuropathy) are axonal neuropathies.

HIGH-YIELD LITERATURE

Management of Chronic Inflammatory Demyelinating Polyradiculoneuropathy

Van den Bergh PYK, Hadden RDM, Bouche P, et al. European Federation of Neurological Societies/Peripheral Nerve Society guideline on management of chronic inflammatory demyelinating polyradiculoneuropathy: Report of a joint task force of the European Federation of Neurological Societies and the Peripher. *Eur J Neurol.* 2010;17(3):356-363.

CHRONIC POLYNEUROPATHY

General Facts

- **Chronic polyneuropathies (aka peripheral neuropathies, axonal sensorimotor polyneuropathies)** are a heterogeneous collection of disorders that systemically affect peripheral nerves.
- Often secondary to another systemic disease, which are numerous (metabolic, endocrine, infection, autoimmune, hematologic, toxic). Polyneuropathy is often the **heralding finding of many undiagnosed systemic diseases.**
- **Diabetic polyneuropathy** is the most common chronic polyneuropathy.
- Generally affects older individuals, as it is frequently the product of chronic diseases.

CONQUER THE **WARDS!**

Diabetic polyneuropathy is the most common chronic polyneuropathy, and as a result is responsible for many symptoms in terms of difficulty walking and foot pain.

Clinical Features

- More commonly "length-dependent" and affects legs before arms, distal portions of limbs before proximal. Less common "non-length-dependent" forms can affect limbs in a patchier distribution.
- Sensory symptoms are frequently more prominent than motor symptoms.
- Common sensory symptoms include numbness, tingling, shooting, and electrical pain.
- Most common motor symptom is difficulty walking.

Physical Exam Findings

- Weakness in distal leg muscles (e.g., ankle dorsiflexion).
- Atrophy of distal leg muscles.
- Loss of vibration, pin, and joint position sense in feet.
- Hyporeflexia or areflexia.
- Presence of Romberg sign (from loss of proprioception).
- Abnormal gait.

Diagnostic Workup

- EMG to assess for systemic and length-dependent **axonal changes** of peripheral nerves. Also helpful in assessing for differentials, including **mononeuropathy multiplex** (associated with vasculitis) and **demyelinating neuropathies**.
- Serum laboratory workup to assess for secondary cause of neuropathy: CBC, chemistry (kidney function testing), LFT, hemoglobin A_{1c}, hepatitis B and C, antinuclear antibodies, vitamin B_{12}, TSH, immunofixation, SPEP.
- MRI imaging of spine in select patients to assess for degenerative spine disease.

Management

- Treatment of underlying disease.
- Neuropathic pain medications (e.g., **gabapentin, pregabalin, duloxetine**).

Common Questions Asked on Rounds

- What is the most common cause of chronic polyneuropathy?
  - Diabetes.
- What are important differential diagnoses for chronic polyneuropathy?
  - Mononeuritis multiplex and demyelinating neuropathies (e.g., CIDP).

HIGH-YIELD LITERATURE

Peripheral nerve and motor disorders

Li Y. Axonal sensorimotor polyneuropathies. *Continuum (Minneap Minn)*. 2017;23(5, Peripheral Nerve and Motor Neuron Disorders):1378-1393. Federation of Neurological Societies and the Peripher. Eur J Neurol. 2010;17(3):356-363.

NEUROCUTANEOUS SYNDROMES

General Facts

- Also known as phacomatoses, a group of genetic disorders that present with a combination of neurologic and cutaneous features.
- Management involves treatment of associated neurologic disorders and screening for associated systemic disorders.

HIGH-YIELD LITERATURE

Neurocutaneous disorders

Rosser T. Neurocutaneous disorders. *Contin Lifelong Learn Neurol.* 2018;24(1):96-129.

PRESYNAPTIC NEUROLOGIC DISORDERS

MYASTHENIA GRAVIS

General Facts

- **Myasthenia gravis (MG)** is an autoimmune disease affecting the acetylcholine receptors in the neuromuscular junction.
- Most common disease that affects the neuromuscular junction.
- Bimodal age of onset with female predominance.

Table 16-11. Neurocutaneous Syndromes

Disease	Genetics	Cutaneous Disorders	Neurologic Disorders	Other Disorders
Neurofibromatosis type 1	Autosomal dominant, 17q, *NF1* gene	■ Café au lait spots ■ Axillary freckling	■ Peripheral neuropathy due to neurofibromas ■ Plexiform neurofibromas, which can undergo malignant transformation ■ Optic gliomas	■ Lisch nodules
Neurofibromatosis type 2	Autosomal dominant, 22q, *NF2* gene	■ Plaque-like hyperpigmented areas of skin ■ Café au lait spots (less common than NF1)	■ Vestibular schwannomas (frequently bilateral) ■ Meningiomas of brain and spine ■ Neurofibromas	■ Cataract
Tuberous sclerosis complex	Autosomal dominant, 9q and 16p, *TSC1* and *TSC2* genes	■ Hypomelanotic macules ■ Facial angiofibromas ■ Shagreen patches (orange-peel lesions)	■ Epilepsy ■ Cerebral hamartomas (tubers) ■ Subependymal nodules ■ Subependymal giant cell astrocytomas	■ Retinal hamartomas ■ Cardiac rhabdomyomas ■ Renal angiomyolipoma
Sturge–Weber syndrome	Sporadic, 9q, *GNAQ* gene	■ Facial port-wine birthmark	■ Cerebral vascular malformations ■ Epilepsy ■ Migraines ■ Strokelike episodes	■ Glaucoma

Clinical Features

- Fluctuating symptoms with "**fatiguability**" (e.g., worse at the end of the day or after exertion).
- Ocular symptoms—namely ptosis and diplopia—are frequent.
- Dysarthria, dysphagia.
- Proximal weakness more common than distal weakness.
- **Myasthenic crisis** refers to exacerbations of MG that require hospitalization for respiratory monitoring and/or intubation.

Physical Exam Findings

- Fatiguability is often demonstrable on exam with various maneuvers, including sustained effort on strength testing and sustained upward gaze.
- Extraocular movements may be abnormal and dysconjugate with a predilection to affect the **medial rectus muscles**.
- **Ptosis**, which is often bilateral.
- Weakness in neck flexion or extension.
- Absence of sensory symptoms.
- Reflexes are generally normal despite weakness.

Diagnostic Workup

- **Acetylcholine receptor antibody testing**.
- **MUSK antibody testing** (a more severe, bulbar predominant form of MG).
- **Edrophonium test**: A small dose of a fast-acting acetylcholinesterase inhibitor is administered, and the patient is observed for resolution of a deficit (e.g., ptosis).

CONQUER THE **BOARDS!**

Single-fiber EMG looking for the presence of jitter has the highest sensitivity for a diagnosis of a neuromuscular junction disorder. However, it is not performed routinely because it is time intensive.

- **EMG**: Assesses for health of neuromuscular junction with repetitive nerve stimulation testing. Also useful for assessing for other differentials, including neuropathies and myopathies.
- **CT chest**: Assesses for thymic hyperplasia or thymoma, which can be associated with MG.

Management

- **Pyridostigmine**: Acetylcholinesterase inhibitor.
- DMTs:
  - Corticosteroids (e.g., prednisone).
  - Immunosuppressants (e.g., **mycophenolate, azathioprine**).
  - IV monoclonal antibodies (e.g., **rituximab**).
- **Thymectomy** for patients with thymic hyperplasia or select young patients (see Myasthenia Gravis).
- Myasthenic crisis management:
  - **IVIG and/or PLEX.**
  - Respiratory support (e.g., intubation, noninvasive positive-pressure ventilation).

Common Questions Asked on Rounds

- What EMG finding is associated with MG?
  - Decrement on repetitive nerve stimulation.
- What is a bedside test that is diagnostic for neuromuscular junction disorder?.
  - Edrophonium test.

HIGH-YIELD LITERATURE

Myasthenia Gravis

Silvestri N, Wolfe G. Myasthenia gravis. *Semin Neurol*. 2012;32(03):215-226.

Wolfe GI, Kaminski HJ, Aban IB, et al. Randomized trial of thymectomy in myasthenia gravis. *N Engl J Med*. 2016;375(6):511-522.

LAMBERT–EATON MYASTHENIC SYNDROME

General Facts

- **Lambert–Eaton myasthenic syndrome (LEMS)** is an acquired presynaptic neuromuscular junction disorder secondary to autoantibodies directed against VGKCs.
- Most frequently a paraneoplastic disorder but can be a primary autoimmune disorder.

Clinical Features

- Subacute onset.
- Lower extremity more common than upper extremity weakness.
- Fatigue.
- Muscle aching and stiffness during or after exertion.
- History of malignancy.

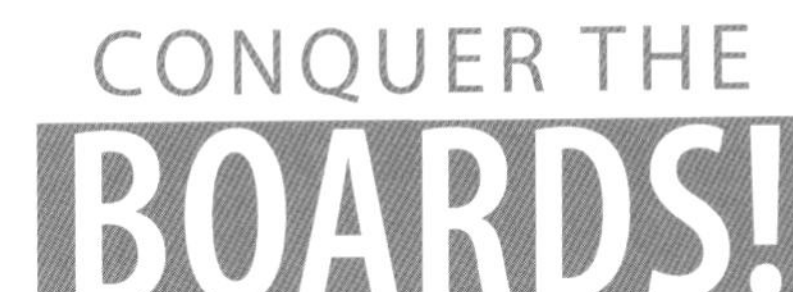

The most common malignancy associated with LEMS is non-small-cell lung cancer.

Physical Exam Findings

- Most common pattern of weakness is proximal leg weakness.
- Brief exercise may temporarily improve strength (a common feature to all disorders affecting the presynaptic neuromuscular junction).

- Ptosis and ophthalmoparesis (generally milder than MG).
- Ventilatory failure is rare.

Diagnostic Workup

- EMG.
- VGKC antibody testing.
- Cancer screening.
- Serum CK.
- Acetylcholine receptor antibody.

Management

- Treatment of underlying malignancy.
- Acetylcholinesterase inhibitor (e.g., pyridostigmine).
- **3,4 diaminopyridine (3,4 DAP):**
  - Blocks voltage-dependent potassium channel conductance.
  - Risk of seizures and cardiac conduction defects.
- **IVIG and/or PLEX.**

Common Questions Asked on Rounds

- What clinical feature differentiates presynaptic and postsynaptic neuromuscular junction disorders?
  - In presynaptic disorders, brief exercise may temporarily improve strength.
- What are examples of presynaptic and postsynaptic neuromuscular junction disorders?
  - Presynaptic: LEMS, botulism.
  - Postsynaptic: MG.

HIGH-YIELD LITERATURE

Lambert_Eaton Syndrome

Sanders DB. Lambert-Eaton myasthenic syndrome: Diagnosis and treatment. *Ann N Y Acad Sci.* 2003;998:500-508.

BOTULISM

General Facts

- **Botulism** is a paralytic disease caused by *Clostridium botulinum*, resulting in blockage of acetylcholine release at the presynaptic neuromuscular junction.
- Associated with wound contamination and ingestion of improperly home canned foods.
- In infants, associated with ingestion of honey.

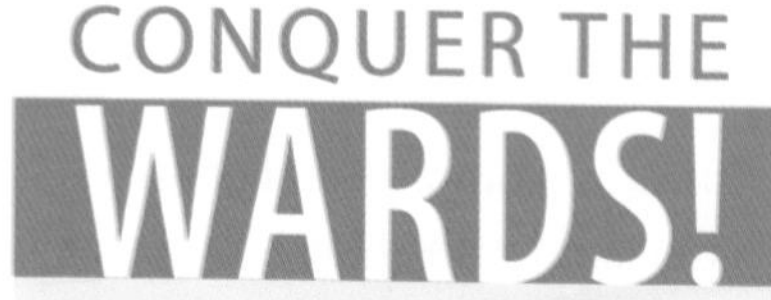

The 5 Ds of botulism: Diplopia, dysarthria, dysphagia, dyspnea, and descending weakness.

Clinical Features

- Acute onset. Incubation period of 18 to 36 hours.
- Diplopia.
- Dysphagia.
- Dysarthria.
- Dyspnea.
- Nausea, vomiting, dry mouth, dry eyes (from anticholinergic effects).

Physical Exam Findings

- Ptosis.
- Ophthalmoparesis.
- Facial paresis.
- Descending weakness with limb involvement later in disease course.

Diagnostic Workup

- **Serum testing for neurotoxin**, which is only available at specialized labs.
- Primarily a clinical diagnosis, and treatment should begin before laboratory confirmation.

Management

- **Botulism antitoxin**.
- Respiratory support with mechanical ventilation if needed.

Common Questions Asked on Rounds

- What is the classic presentation of botulism?
  - **Ascending paralysis without sensory symptoms.**
- What are associated risk factors for botulism?
  - Ingestion of improperly canned foods and ingestion of honey in infants.

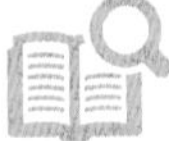

HIGH-YIELD LITERATURE

Botulism

Sobel J. Botulism. *Clin Infect Dis.* 2005;41(8):1167-1173.

MYOPATHY

General Facts

- **Myopathy** is a large collection of heterogeneous disorders that affect muscles and can be secondary to genetic, toxic, autoimmune, metabolic, and endocrine etiologies.
- Identifying underlying cause is critical to management, as different diseases can have conflicting treatment plans.
- A diagnosis is often considered with an elevated serum creatine kinase.

Clinical Features

- Complaints of weakness in proximal muscles (e.g., difficulty ascending stairs, difficulty lifting objects).
- Muscle cramp, ache, and fatigue with or without exertion.
- **Lack of neuropathic sensory symptoms** including numbness, tingling, and electrical and shooting pains.
- Common causes include
  - Statin- and steroid-induced myopathy.
  - Thyroid disease.
  - Dermatomyositis and polymyositis.
  - Muscular dystrophies.

Physical Exam Findings

- Proximal > distal weakness.
- Muscle atrophy.
- Reflexes are preserved except in cases of severe weakness.
- Lack of sensory exam deficits.

Diagnostic Workup

- Serum labs for evidence of muscle breakdown: **Creatine kinase, serum aldolase, liver function tests.**
- MRI testing of affected limbs to assess for evidence of myopathy and area to biopsy.
- **Muscle biopsy** is often required for diagnosis.
- **Genetic testing** can be diagnostic for inherited myopathies.
- EMG findings for myopathy are often nonspecific, but help to exclude other conditions on the differential.

Management

- Varies between disease types.
- Treatment of rhabdomyolysis with IV fluids.

Common Questions Asked On Rounds

- What medications are associated with myopathy?
  - Statins and steroids.
- What test is generally needed for specific diagnosis of myopathy?
  - Muscle biopsy and/or genetic testing.

HIGH-YIELD LITERATURE

Venance SL. Approach to the patient with hypercalcemia. *Contin Lifelong Learn Neurol*. 2016;22(6):1803-1814.

CHAPTER 17 AMBULATORY MEDICINE

OVERVIEW OF HIGH-YIELD TOPICS IN AMBULATORY MEDICINE

INTRODUCTION TO AMBULATORY CARE

AMBULATORY CARE TRAINING TIPS

There is a wide variety of ambulatory care training experiences across U.S. medical schools, but the following advice is broadly applicable:

- **Know Expectations:** Make sure you get clear guidance from your clerkship director and clinic preceptors on what is expected of you. What is the expected level of autonomy? How are you being evaluated? What is the clinic flow?
- **Efficiency Is Key:** Unlike in the hospital where time may not be as much of an issue, the providers you will be working with will have between 15 and 20 minutes per patient, so you will need to have an efficient strategy for gathering information.
- **Agenda Setting**: Since you need to be efficient, make sure to set the agenda with the patient. Make sure to elicit all complaints/concerns up-front so you can prioritize. You should ask patients what brings them in and any other concerns they have. You may have to help them prioritize—you won't necessarily be able to talk about everything during one visit! Be sure to review the agenda you set with the patient at the end of the visit when you summarize your plan!
- **Ask About Health Prevention**: In addition to your symptom-driven questions, be sure to ask about health maintenance (nutrition, exercise, weight changes), accident prevention (seat belt use, firearm safety), toxic habits (alcohol, tobacco, drug use), and sexuality (sexually transmitted infection [STI] prevention, contraception).
- **Keep Disease Prevalence in Mind**: Common things are common. Be sure to include common etiologies of outpatient complaints first in your differential. In this section, we have included the most common causes of death and most common causes of emergency department (ED) and urgent care visits in the United States for this purpose. These lists can also inform your studying during your ambulatory rotation.
- **But Still Keep Differentials Broad**: In the hospital, patients on medicine have generally been triaged there from the emergency room or clinic, and thus have "medicine problems." In the clinic, the patients are the ones doing the triaging, so your differential needs to be broader for acute complaints (e.g., while you will likely not see appendicitis on the medicine floor, these patients can certainly present to a general medicine clinic with a complaint of abdominal pain).
- **Ask Your Preceptors How to Structure Presentations**: Presentations may be trickier in the clinic, as there is often not a "chief" complaint, but rather multiple issues (acute and chronic) to address. Most typically, your presentation will have the following structure:
  1. **Reason(s) for visit:** "Mr. X is here for follow-up on diabetes and a new complaint of abdominal pain" or "Mr. X is here for his yearly visit."
  2. **History for each individual element** you discussed with the patient.
  3. **General and focused exam.**
  4. **Plan by problem**: Generally it is easier to follow if you make it clear about the transition from problem to problem ("For his diabetes, I want to recheck his A_{1c} and check a urine microalbumin/creatinine ratio to screen for nephropathy. I expect his A_{1c} to be stable, so no medication changes should be indicated. For his abdominal pain, I think it most likely GERD because of X, Y, Z....")

- **Pre-Chart (When You Can)**: Figure out how to see who is scheduled for your preceptor the following day so you can do some preparation and reading on the issues likely to come up in clinic tomorrow.

SCREENING AND PREVENTION INTRODUCTION

Primary vs. Secondary vs. Tertiary Prevention

- **Primary prevention:** Prevent disease or injury before it occurs. Examples include nutritional counseling for heart disease prevention or vaccinations to prevent infectious diseases (see Table 17-1).
- **Secondary prevention**: Aims to reduce the impact of disease or injury that has already occurred by enabling early detection and treatment. Examples include all cancer screenings, as well as screening for diabetes and hypertension (see Tables 17-2 and 17-3).
- **Tertiary prevention**: Aims to reduce the impact of ongoing chronic diseases or injuries. Examples include rehabilitation programs after strokes or any number of treatments for diabetes and hypertension.

CONQUER THE WARDS!

Most clinicians combine/conflate secondary and tertiary prevention into one thing. The key distinguishing factor is that primary prevention means preventing the disease from ever happening (not just catching it early).

U.S. Preventive Service Task Force Guidelines

- The U.S. Preventive Service Task Force (USPSTF) is an independent panel of national experts who make evidence-based recommendations about prevention services.
- Grading:
  - **Grade A**: **Recommends service.** High certainty that net benefit is **substantial**.
  - **Grade B**: **Recommends service.** High certainty that net benefit is **moderate** or there is moderate certainty that the net benefit is moderate to substantial.
  - **Grade C**: **Patient-specific decision**. There is at least moderate certainty that the net benefit is small.
  - **Grade D: Recommends against**. There is moderate or high certainty that the service has no net benefit or that harms outweigh benefits.
  - **Grade I**: **Current evidence is insufficient**.

CONQUER THE BOARDS!

The USPSTF Guidelines form a huge chunk of the ambulatory/prevention questions on the shelf exam. Find the list of their A and B level recommendations online and read them!

DISEASE EPIDEMIOLOGY IN THE UNITED STATES

Most Common Causes of Death in the United States (2016)

- Heart disease (23%).
- Cancer (22%).
- Injuries (6%).
- Chronic respiratory disease (6%).
- Cerebrovascular disease (5%).
- Alzheimer dementia (4%).
- Diabetes mellitus (3%).
- Influenza and pneumonia (2%).
- Kidney disease (2%).
- Suicide (2%).

CONQUER THE WARDS!

Sixty percent of Americans have at least one chronic medical condition.

Most Common Chronic Conditions in the United States

- Hypertension (27%) (see Cardiology).
- Hyperlipidemia (21%) (see Cardiology).
- Mood disorders (12%) (see Ambulatory Medicine).

CONQUER THE WARDS!

If there are things on this list of common acute complaints and chronic diseases you don't feel comfortable evaluating, read the accompanying sections in this book!

TABLE 17-1. Adult Vaccinations

Vaccination	Who to Vaccinate	When and Vaccination Options	Comments
Influenza	All adults	Annually: Two types of vaccines: 1. Inactivated Influenza vaccine for most. Can consider high dose inactivated for adults >65 years old. 2. The live-attenuated intranasal vaccine has lower efficacy and has been recommended against by the CDC in multiple recent influenza seasons.	Make sure to ask about egg allergy before giving inactivated influenza vaccine. The traditional inactivated influenza vaccine should be your choice for most patients. Give the high-dose flu shot to older patients if available, but the added benefit of the higher dose is small (0.5% absolute risk reduction for lab-confirmed influenza in the main study published in *NEJM*).
Tetanus, Diphtheria, and Pertussis (TDAP)	All adults.	Should get TD booster every 10 years. Substitute TDaP vaccination if they have never received pertussis vaccination.	
Herpes Zoster	Adults 50 years or older.	Two-dose series given at least 2–6 months apart. Recombinant vaccine (Shingrix) is preferred.	Insurance coverage can be variable and vaccines are expensive, so double-check before giving!
Human Papilloma Virus (HPV)	Age 9–26 years old.	Three-dose series at 0, 2, and 6 months.	Recently FDA approved for use in adults 27–45 years old, but no clear guidelines about use in this population as of early 2019.
Measles, Mumps, and Rubella (MMR)	All adults.	Give one dose of MMR vaccine to adults with no evidence of immunity to measles, mumps, or rubella.	In practice, many clinicians will only assess MMR immunity in pregnancy, immunosuppression, or potential for workplace exposure (health care, school).
13-Valent Pneumococcal (PCV13)	Immunocompetent adults 65 and older, or adults with risk factors (immunodeficiency disorders, HIV, asplenia, or CKD).	Give a maximum of one dose before age 65 and one dose after age 65.	Whenever PCV13 and PPSV23 are indicated, give PCV13 first and will generally wait 1 year between pneumonia vaccines.
23-Valent Pneumococcal (PPSV23)	Immunocompetent adults 65 and older, or adults with risk factors (immunosuppression, or chronic heart disease, lung disease, liver disease, alcoholism, diabetes, or tobacco use).	Give a maximum of one dose before age 65 and one dose after age 65.	Should wait at least 5 years between doses of PPSV23 (e.g., if patient gets a dose at age 63 for CHF, their post-65 dose should be given at age 68).
Hepatitis A	Nonimmune adults at risk (travel to high-risk country, men who have sex with men, illicit drug use, chronic liver disease, occupational risk).	Two doses, 6–12 months apart. First dose takes 4 weeks to work.	
Hepatitis B	Nonimmune adults at risk (chronic liver disease, HIV, risk of exposure to blood, diabetics who monitor glucose regularly, sexual risk factors).	Three-dose series at 0, 1, and 6 months.	
Meningitis (Meningococcal)	Adolescents at risk, and adults with risk factors (asplenia, complement deficiencies, or occupational exposure).	Two- or 3-dose series depending on vaccine.	

TABLE 17-2. Cancer Screening

Cancer Screening	When/How to Screen	Screening Options	USPSTF Guidance*	Commentary and Key Points
Breast Cancer	**1. Women 50–74 yo** (universally accepted) **2. Women 40–50 yo** (controversial with divergent recommendations from guideline writing bodies)	**Mammography** - Every 1–2 years depending on the guidelines.	**Grade C:** 40–49 yo **Grade B:** 50–74 yo Recommends screening every 2 years with mammography	**Conquer the Wards!** Given the conflicting recommendations, a patient-centered approach to decision-making is always best!
Cervical Cancer	**Women 21–65 yo.** Ends at age 65 if 3 consecutive normal Pap smear	1. **Pap smear with cytology** every **3 years** from **age 21 until age 30.** 2. Pap smear with cytology **and HPV co-testing** every **5 years** from **age 30 until 65.**	**Grade A**	**Conquer the Boards!** NEVER test for HPV in women younger than 30. It is very common to have transient HPV positivity, and screening does not improve outcomes in this group.
Colon Cancer	**All adults >50 yo** until life expectancy <10 years	1. **Colonoscopy** - **Every 10 years** - Most common option 2. **Stool-based testing** - Annual FOBT** - Annual FIT*** - FIT-DNA**** every 3 years 3. **CT colonography** every 5 years 4. **Flexible sigmoidoscopy** every 5 years	**Grade A:** 50–75 yo **Grade C:** 76–85 yo No stated preference between tests.	**Conquer the Wards!** The best colon cancer screening approach is the one your patient will accept!
Lung Cancer	1. **Adults 55–80 yo and the following:** - 30 pack-year smoking history + - Currently smoker or have quit within the past 15 years 2. Stop screening once the patient has not smoked for 15 years or develops health problems that substantially limit life expectancy	**Annual low-dose CT**	**Grade B**	Lung cancer screening is the most effective cancer screening test currently recommended, with proven reductions in all-cause mortality in this high-risk cohort.
Prostate Cancer	1. CONTROVERSIAL consider **men 55–69 yo** Incredibly controversial with conflicting and problematic data. Previously recommended for by most guidelines, then against, and now quite unclear.	Digital rectal exam (DRE) and PSA annually	**Grade C**	Do not recommend universal screening. Will need to make decisions on a patient-by-patient basis, given the limitations of our current evidence and guidelines.

* USPSTF, United States Preventive Services Task Force: Funded, and appointed by U.S. Department of Health and Human Services and made up of primary care physicians and epidemiologists.

** FOBT, Fecal occult blood testing usually requires three separate samples; compliance is poor with this test.

*** FIT, Fecal immunochemical test, which tests for hidden blood in the stool.

**** FIT-DNA, FIT test + detection of altered DNA (cancer cells) in the stool.

TABLE 17-3. Other Screening Measures (USPSTF Recommended)

Screening Intervention	Who/When to Screen	How to Screen
Abdominal Aortic Aneurysm (AAA)	One-time screening of adult males aged 65–75 who have ever smoked (>100 cigarettes total)	Ultrasound
Chlamydia/Gonorrhea	Screen in all sexually active women younger than age 24 and in all older adults at risk for STIs: new sexual partners, multiple partners, partners with STIs, previous STIs, and those exchanging sex for money or drugs	Urine GC/*Chlamydia* (or endocervical swab if doing at same time as exam/Pap smear)
Syphilis	All adults at risk for syphilis: men who have sex with men, persons with HIV, history of incarceration, and living in areas of high incidence	RPR or VDRL testing
HIV	All adults aged 15–65 should be screened at least once. Can consider regular intervals (annually) in those at risk, but evidence unclear about optimal screening interval	Fourth-generation antigen/antibody HIV-1/2 assay
Hepatitis B	Adults at high risk (birth in endemic country, lack of childhood vaccination, CKD or ESRD, immunosuppression)	Hepatitis B surface antigen and antibody, hepatitis B core antibody (confirm with HBV DNA)
Hepatitis C	One-time screening for adults born between 1945 and 1965. Screen others who are at high risk (blood transfusion before 1992, injection drug use history, intranasal drug use, unregulated tattoos, history of incarceration)	Hepatitis C antibody (confirm with HCV RNA)
Depression	All adults	PHQ-2 (annually)
Falls	Community-dwelling adults 65 years or older	Ask about history of recent falls or patient concern for future falls
Obesity	All adults	Check BMI at each visit
Osteoporosis	Women 65 years and older	DEXA (axial skeleton)
Tuberculosis	All adults at increased risk (birth in endemic country and known or potential exposures)	PPD or interferon-gamma release assay (IGRA)

- Diabetes mellitus (10%) (see Endocrine).
- Osteoarthritis (6%) (see Rheumatology).
- Asthma (6%) (see Pulmonary).
- Coronary artery disease (5%) (see Cardiology).

Most Common Reasons for Urgent Clinic and ED Visits in the United States

- Superficial injuries.
- Musculoskeletal complaints (see Rheumatology).
- Dermatologic issues and infections (see Dermatology).
- Abdominal pain (see Gastroenterology).
- Headaches (see Neurology).
- Chest pain (see Cardiology).
- Urinary tract infections (see Infectious Disease).
- Upper respiratory infections (see Infectious Disease).
- Complications of chronic diseases.

ROUTINE BLOOD TESTING IN CLINIC

There is a wide variety across practices in terms of what blood work is done "routinely" as part of disease screening and health maintenance. You will likely see significant variability between providers even within one practice. Following are the guideline-driven recommendations for common tests ordered in clinic, though going beyond these is not necessarily wrong (though many professional societies through the Choosing Wisely campaign of the ABIM have included elements recommending against routine screening blood work):

- Complete blood count (CBC): Not recommended in the absence of symptoms.
- Basic metabolic panel (BMP): Annual screening in those with hypertension on antihypertensives or in diabetic patients. No routine screening otherwise.
- Hepatic panel: Not recommended in the absence of symptoms.
- Thyroid-stimulating hormone (TSH): Not recommended in the absence of symptoms.
- Vitamin D (25-OH vitamin D): There are no recommendations or evidence for universal vitamin D screening, though it is often done.
- Hemoglobin A_{1c}: The USPSTF recommends screening adults 40 to 70 years old who are overweight or obese, with a rescreening interval of every 3 years. The American Diabetes Association (ADA) recommends screening any adult with a body mass index (BMI) >25 and any other risk factor for diabetes, with a rescreening interval of every 3 years.
- Lipid panel: Variable guidance, with USPSTF most recently recommending screening starting at age 40, with 5-year rescreening intervals. Previous guidance recommended starting screening at 35 years in men and 45 years in women, with consideration of initiation of screening 10 years prior to that in the presence of risk factors.

ADULT SAFETY SCREENING MEASURES

INTIMATE PARTNER VIOLENCE

- **Definition and epidemiology:**
  - "Intimate partner violence" describes actual or threatened psychological, physical, or sexual harm by a current or former partner or spouse.
  - Lifetime prevalence ranges from 20% to 40% depending on the study and population.
- **When to suspect:**
  - Inconsistent explanation of injuries.
  - Delays in seeking treatment from injuries.
  - Frequent emergency department (ED) or urgent visits for injuries/accidents.
  - Late initiation of prenatal care in pregnancy.
  - Overly attentive or verbally abusive partner.
  - Bruises of different ages.
  - Bruises or wounds on forearms, head, or neck.
- **Screening:**
  - USPSTF **Grade B Recommendation** to screen **women of child-bearing age**.
  - No universally recommended screening tools exist, but important to screen for both potential psychological (yelling/screaming, repeated criticism, financial punishments) and physical components of abuse.

- Most important steps are to show concern and interest in the patient and to begin with open-ended questions.
- **Interventions:**
  - Specific interventions will depend on local resources, but important for you to express empathy, validate the patient's feelings, and assess for safety.
  - Provide information about local resources and shelters; utilize social worker support if available.
  - Can work with patient to create safety plan (where will they go if they feel unsafe, what do they need to bring).

CONQUER THE WARDS!

You only need prophylaxis for procedures that involve the face and mouth, with GI endoscopies being an exception.

PRIMARY PROPHYLAXIS AND VACCINATIONS

ENDOCARDITIS PROPHYLAXIS

When assessing for the need for endocarditis prophylaxis, you need to 1) assess the patient's risk of infective endocarditis and 2) assess the risk of the procedure. Only patients who have risk factors AND are undergoing certain high-risk procedures need to receive endocarditis prophylaxis.

- **Who Needs Endocarditis Prophylaxis?** Consider prophylaxis in patients with one of the following:
  - Prosthetic or mechanical cardiac valve.
  - Previous episodes of infective endocarditis.
  - Congenital heart disease, including unrepaired cyanotic disease, completely repaired congenital heart defect with prosthetic material, or repaired congenital heart disease with residual defects.
  - Valvulopathy following cardiac transplantation.
- **When Is It Needed?** Only give to high-risk patients prior to the following procedures:
  - Dental procedures that involve manipulation of gingival tissue.
  - Procedures that involve biopsy of respiratory tract mucosa.
- **What Should Be Given?**
  - Amoxicillin 2 g ONCE prior to procedure.
  - If penicillin-allergic, can consider clindamycin 600 mg ONCE or azithromycin 500 mg ONCE or cefazolin/ceftriaxone 1 g ONCE prior to procedure.

CONQUER THE BOARDS!

Small ASDs or VSDs that have not undergone repair and do not cause cyanosis are not an indication for prophylaxis.

CONQUER THE WARDS!

Download the AHRQ ePSS app for your phone—you can see all the USPSTF recommended interventions for your patients in just a few steps!

ASPIRIN PRIMARY PROPHYLAXIS

- Controversial and complicated, with shifting guidelines over last several years and considerable variability in use.
- USPSTF Grade B Recommendation: Consider low-dose aspirin for primary prevention of cardiovascular disease in adults aged 50 to 59 who 1) have >10% 10-year cardiovascular disease risk (ASCVD Risk Calculation), 2) are not an increased risk of bleeding, 3) have a life expectancy >10 years, and 4) are willing to take low-dose aspirin daily for at least 10 years.

CONQUER THE WARDS!

Based on the guideline recommendations, you can probably guess that the magnitude of the benefit is small and takes at least 10 years to be realized. As such, the decision to prescribe aspirin is often individualized, taking into account the patient's preferences and risk factors.

HIGH-YIELD LITERATURE

Zoster vaccination – The ZOE-50 trial:

Lal H, Cunningham AL, Godeaux O, et al. Efficacy of an adjuvanted herpes zoster subunit vaccine in older adults. *N Engl J Med.* 2015;372:2087-2096.

NUTRITION

OBESITY

In the United States, more than 70% of adults are overweight, and more than 35% of adults are obese. There have been parallel increases in rates of hypertension, diabetes, and cardiovascular disease and death. There are hundreds of health co-morbidities associated with obesity, the most important of which are listed here.

- **Overview and definition:**
  - Obesity is defined as a body mass index (BMI) >30 kg/m^2.
  - Patients are classified as overweight if their BMI falls between 25 and 30 kg/m^2.
  - Weight is all about energy balance: Resting energy expenditure (organ and muscle function) + additional expenditure from physical activity cannot be significantly outweighed by caloric intake in the long term without weight gain.
- **Complications:**
  - Metabolic: Hyperlipidemia, metabolic syndrome, type 2 diabetes.
  - Cardiovascular: Premature atherosclerosis, hypertension, coronary artery disease, stroke.
  - Pulmonary: Deconditioning, obstructive sleep apnea.
  - Musculoskeletal: Osteoarthritis, gout.
  - Gastrointestinal: Biliary disease.
  - Genitourinary: Nephrolithiasis, chronic kidney disease (CKD), incontinence.
  - Malignancy: Endometrial cancer, breast cancer, ovarian cancer, colon cancer, rectal cancer.
- **Dietary and lifestyle interventions:**
  - Patient counseling and individualization of dietary planning are essential. Ask patients what they think they can accomplish. Your goal for them should be to lose around 1 pound per week, which correlates with an energy deficit of around 3500 calories/week.
  - Recommend increasing aerobic exercise, with 150 minutes of moderate aerobic activity (brisk walking, swimming) per week.
  - Overall goal is ~10% weight loss over a 6-month period.
  - Muscle is highly metabolically active (so muscle mass can hasten weight loss), so encourage strength training as patients are able.

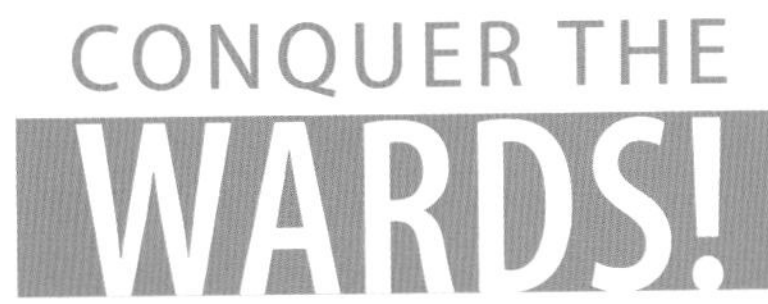

Download the CDC Vaccine Schedule App for real-time reference in the clinic.

HIGH-YIELD LITERATURE

Bariatric surgery and mortality: A cohort study from Israel, finding decreases in all-cause mortality at 4.5 years out from bariatric surgery as compared to usual medical care alone:

Reges O, Greenland P, Dicker D, et al. Association of bariatric surgery using laparoscopic banding, Roux-en-Y gastric bypass, or laparoscopic sleeve gastrectomy vs usual care obesity management with all-cause mortality. *JAMA.* 2018;319:279-290.

TABLE 17-4. Vitamin disorders

Vitamin	Deficiency	Excess
Vitamin B_6 (pyridoxine)	Stomatitis, glossitis, peripheral neuropathy. Other than as a side effect of isoniazid (INH) therapy this is rarely seen.	None (water-soluble).
Vitamin B_{12} (cobalamin)	Anemia, macrocytosis, hypersegmented neutrophils, neurologic abnormalities. Can be seen in strict vegans, malabsorptive syndromes affecting the ileum, pernicious anemia, or those on metformin therapy.	None (water-soluble).
Vitamin D (25-OH vitamin D)	Most with mild deficiency are asymptomatic. Those with low vitamin D and accompany elevated PTH can have accelerated bone loss (osteopenia, osteoporosis). With severe deficiency, can see muscle weakness and gait abnormalities.	Rare, but can see hypercalcemia and its accompanying symptoms (polyuria, vomiting, muscle weakness, confusion), nephrocalcinosis, and nephrolithiasis.
Folic Acid	Anemia, macrocytosis, hypersegmented neutrophils, weight loss. Very rare due to cereal fortification, but could be concerned in those with long history of alcohol abuse.	None (water-soluble).

- **Other interventions:**
  - Pharmacologic therapies do exist for weight loss, but a combination of limited efficacy, lack of insurance coverage, and serious side effects significantly limit their use. Medications that are currently approved for weight loss include liraglutide (GLP-1 agonist), lorcaserin (serotonin agonist), orlistat (pancreatic lipase inhibitor), phentermine-topiramate (phentermine is a sympathomimetic; topiramate is an anticonvulsant), and bupropion-naltrexone (bupropion is an antidepressant; naltrexone is an opioid receptor antagonist). Can consider these therapies in those with a BMI >30 and complications from obesity.
  - Bariatric surgery: For those with a BMI >40 or a BMI >35 with complications of obesity. Excellent data support bariatric surgery, though it is an invasive surgery with risks. Prospective randomized controlled trials (RCTs) have shown significant improvements in complications of obesity (diabetes, hypertension, etc.), and a recent cohort study suggested a mortality benefit to bariatric surgery vs. medical care alone.

VITAMIN DEFICIENCY AND EXCESS

Most vitamin derangements are rarely seen in clinic, but several of the more commonly evaluated vitamins and the syndromes associated with deficiency and excess are listed in Table 17-4. Other vitamin abnormalities (A, B_1, B_2, B_3, B_5, biotin, C, E, and K) are rarely considered in clinical practice outside of severe malnutrition or malabsorptive syndromes.

MENTAL HEALTH

With national limitations in access to psychiatry services (due to insufficient numbers of practicing psychiatrists), the role of screening, diagnosis, and first-line treatment often falls to primary care physicians in the clinic. Patients with severe depression or anxiety, refractory depression or anxiety, or mental health conditions such as schizophrenia and bipolar disorder should be referred for psychiatric evaluation.

DEPRESSION

Epidemiology and Screening

- Lifetime prevalence of major depression in the United States has been found to be as high as 17%, and the annual prevalence rate is nearly 7%.
- Rates of depression are higher in patients with chronic medical illness (~25% lifetime risk).
- Risk factors include prior episodes, family history, female gender, poor social support, life stressors, childhood traumas, chronic medical illnesses, and a history of substance use.
- Screening recommendation from USPSTF is to screen all patients during routine visits.
- Use the PHQ-2 to screen, with a positive answer to either question indicating possible depression and the need to follow up. The 2 questions are: "During the last month, have you often been bothered by feeling down, depressed, or hopeless?" and "During the last month, have you often been bothered by having little interest or pleasure in doing things?"
- After an initial positive PHQ-2 screen, proceed to a full PHQ-9 to evaluate for the presence of depression and assess severity.

CONQUER THE WARDS!

For the precise diagnostic criteria, see the DSM-5. The PHQ-9 is based on these 9 symptoms and is the tool most providers use in clinic to diagnose and assess disease severity.

Diagnostic Criteria

The DSM-5 diagnostic criteria for depression are as follows: A) 5 or more of the following symptoms must be present during the same 2-week period, with one of the symptoms being either depressed mood or loss of interest or pleasure; B) the symptoms cause significant distress; C) the episode is not attributable to medical conditions or substance use; D) there is no other psychiatric disorder present that better explains the symptoms; and E) there has never been a manic or hypomanic episode.

- Depressed mood.
- Anhedonia (markedly diminished interest or pleasure in activities).
- Weight changes (gain or loss).
- Sleep changes (insomnia or hypersomnia).
- Psychomotor agitation or retardation.
- Low energy.
- Feelings of worthlessness or guilt.
- Poor concentration.
- Recurrent thoughts of death or suicidal ideation.

CONQUER THE WARDS!

Though we should screen all patients, you should especially consider screening patients with fatigue, chronic pain, insomnia, or otherwise unexplained symptoms.

Principles of Initial Treatment

- Goal of therapy is to restore baseline functionality.
- Screen ALL patients for suicidality (passive or active).
- Options include psychotherapy and pharmacotherapy, with the evidence suggestion that combination therapy (both psychotherapy and pharmacotherapy) is superior to either option alone.
- For pharmacotherapy, selective serotonin reuptake inhibitors (SSRIs) are generally the first-line therapy with no evidence to support one particular

CONQUER THE WARDS!

Though there is no specific data indicating these must be the first-line choices, the most commonly prescribed first-line SSRIs in the United States are sertraline, citalopram, and escitalopram.

agent (recent meta-analyses have found conflicting results). There is no evidence that initial therapy with multiple agents achieves superior outcomes.

- The choice of initial therapy should be individualized, considering potential drug–drug interactions, patient preference, cost/availability, and side effect profiles.

GENERALIZED ANXIETY DISORDER

General Facts

- **Definition:** Generalized anxiety disorder: Excessive anxiety and worry that is difficult to control and causes distress or impairment, occurring more days than not for at least 6 months, about a number of events or activities.

Differential Diagnosis

- Depression with anxiety.
- Panic disorder.
- Adjustment disorder.
- Substance use disorder.

Principles of Initial Treatment

- The first step is to assess the degree of disability or impairment to determine the need for medical treatment.
- Options include psychotherapy (cognitive-behavioral therapy [CBT]) or pharmacotherapy, or a combination of the 2.
- The decision to start CBT is largely based on patient preference and resource availability.
- SSRIs or serotonin-norepinephrine reuptake inhibitors (SNRIs) are first-line, with the decision between agents made on the drug's side effect profile, drug–drug interactions, and patient preference.
- For patients on medical therapy with only a partial response to SSRI or SNRI therapy, buspirone can be added as an adjunct (but is generally not used as monotherapy given its limited efficacy).
- Benzodiazepines can be a potentially useful adjunct, but have numerous potential side effects that limit their long-term use, including risk of dependence or abuse, rebound after discontinuation, and worsening of any depressive symptoms. As such, they are generally reserved for more refractory cases.

CONQUER THE BOARDS!

When choosing medical therapy for generalized anxiety disorder and panic disorder, antidepressants (SSRIs or SNRIs) are always first-line therapy, not benzodiazepines or buspirone.

PANIC DISORDER

Clinical Manifestations and Diagnosis

- Panic attacks generally present with acute-onset, intense episodes that can last minutes to an hour. In a panic disorder, the patient experiences recurrent episodes.
- Diagnostic criteria for a panic attack include an abrupt surge of intense fear or discomfort peaking within a minute, during which time at least 4 of the following occur: Palpitations, sweating, shaking, shortness of breath, choking/gagging sensations, chest pain, nausea or abdominal pain, dizziness or lightheadedness, chills or hot flashes, paresthesias, depersonalization (being detached from oneself), fear of losing control or "going crazy," or fear of dying.
- A diagnosis of panic disorder implies a history of recurrent panic attacks, with attacks followed by a month or more of persistent concern or worry

about future attacks and with attacks not attributable to other psychiatric disorders, substance use, or chronic medical conditions.

Differential Diagnosis

The differential diagnosis can be quite wide, depending on the predominant symptom that the patient is describing, but considerations should include:

- Substance use disorders.
- Other anxiety disorders (generalized anxiety disorders, phobia, social anxiety).
- Cardiac conditions (angina, arrhythmias).
- Pulmonary conditions (pulmonary embolism, chronic obstructive pulmonary disease [COPD], asthma).
- Hyperthyroidism.
- Pheochromocytoma.

Principles of Initial Treatment

- First-line therapy generally consists of SSRI or SNRI therapy, generally at lower doses than used in management of depression. Tricyclic antidepressants (TCAs) are also a possible option, though have more side effects, which can prove limiting. The decision about what agent to prescribe should be individualized based on patient preference, drug–drug interactions, and side effect profiles.
- Benzodiazepines can be a useful adjunct, as they are effective and quick acting, though there is potential for abuse. They are often prescribed along with an antidepressant early in treatment to hasten response, but can be used long-term in selected patients.

CONQUER THE WARDS!

Generally speaking, patients who have typical and recurrent panic attacks can be diagnosed with having panic disorder without an extensive workup, but brief consideration should be given to the potential disease mimics.

SUBSTANCE USE DISORDERS

TOBACCO USE

Epidemiology

- About 1 in 6 adult Americans use tobacco products.
- Smoking is the leading preventable cause of mortality.
- On surveys, nearly two-thirds of smokers say they want to quit, and nearly half of all smokers report a quit attempt in the last year. However, only ~5% of smokers who make an unaided attempt to quit are still abstinent at 1 year.

Complications of Tobacco Use

- Increases risk of death (cardiac, pulmonary, cancer).
- Malignancy: Increases risk of numerous types of cancer, including lung cancer, head and neck cancer, bladder cancer, esophageal/gastric/colon cancer, and pancreatic cancer.
- Cardiovascular: Premature atherosclerosis, coronary artery disease, stroke, peripheral vascular disease.
- Pulmonary: Chronic cough, COPD, increased risk of pulmonary infections.

Barriers to Quitting

- One of the main barriers to quitting is the addictiveness of nicotine and the withdrawal symptoms. Symptoms peak in the first 3 days of cessation and subside over several weeks, and can include appetite changes, weight gain, mood changes, irritability, insomnia, difficulty concentrating, and restlessness.
- Another barrier to quitting are social triggers—patients need to identify their triggers and reshape their habits.

Smoking Cessation Counseling (The 5 A's)

- **ASK**: Ask all patients about tobacco use (in all forms, including secondhand smoke).
- **ADVISE**: Advise all tobacco users of harms of smoking and benefits to quitting in clear and brief language. There is high-quality evidence that interventions <5 minutes have effectiveness in improving quit rates.
- **ASSESS**: Assess readiness to change.
  - Precontemplation: Not ready to quit.
  - Contemplation: Considering a quit attempt.
  - Preparation: Actively planning a quit attempt.
  - Action: Actively involved in a quit attempt.
  - Maintenance: Achieved smoking cessation.
- **ASSIST**: If the patient is contemplative (or stages beyond), provide assistance to the patient. This may include 1) setting a quit date, 2) addressing barriers to quitting, 3) discussing potential effects of quitting (both withdrawal symptoms and long-term benefits), 4) discussing behavioral interventions to overcome barriers, and 5) discussing pharmacologic agents to increase success rates.
- **ARRANGE**: Arrange follow-up with patient within 1 to 2 weeks of quit date for short-term follow-up.

CONQUER THE **BOARDS!**

For smoking cessation on the shelf exam, choose behavioral therapy PLUS either varenicline OR 2 forms of nicotine replacement therapy (patch and a short-acting agent for PRN use).

Behavioral and Pharmacotherapy for Smoking Cessation

- Therapy for smoking cessation generally consists of behavioral therapy plus either A) 2 forms of nicotine replacement therapy or B) varenicline, with single-agent nicotine replacement therapy or bupropion being other options.
- **Behavioral therapy**: Effective, especially when paired with pharmacologic agents. If no office-based therapy is available, referral to free telephone quitlines (1800-QUIT-NOW in the United States) or online resources can be helpful.
- **Nicotine replacement therapy (NRT)**: Patch is main long-acting option, with short-acting options including lozenge, gum, spray, or tablets. Will generally pair a patch to control baseline nicotine withdrawal symptoms with a short-acting agent to control cravings on an as-needed (PRN) basis.
- **Varenicline**:
  - Mechanism: Partial agonist of the alpha-4 beta-2 nicotinic receptor, which works to partially stimulate the receptor and decrease symptoms from nicotine withdrawal, and blocks nicotine from tobacco smoke from binding to the receptor.
  - Reduces cravings and withdrawal symptoms.
  - Will generally start varenicline and then have patient set tobacco quit date around 1 week later.
  - Side effects: Initial concerns for neuropsychiatric and cardiovascular effects have not been borne out in literature. Does increase risk of headaches, insomnia, and vivid dreams.
- **Bupropion:**
  - Mechanism: Enhances central nervous system (CNS) noradrenergic and dopaminergic release.
  - Contraindicated in patients with seizure disorder, as it reduces seizure threshold.
  - Side effects: Insomnia, agitation, dry mouth, headache.
- Electronic cigarettes (e-cigarettes):
  - Not traditionally recommended by physicians, but many patients use them or may ask you about them! Emerging data (see "high yield literature" later) suggest these may play an important role in smoking cessation.

CONQUER THE **WARDS!**

While the CAGE questionnaire has a long history of being taught to medical students, it has poor data to support its use, relatively poor performance in real-world settings (especially in women), and is less commonly used than other screening tools.

- E-cigarettes contain nicotine, ethylene glycol, and flavorings, so the patient still ingests nicotine but avoids many of the toxic constituents of cigarette smoke.
- The benefits and harms of e-cigarettes are not well-understood, but are widely thought to be significantly less risky than usual cigarettes, so may be an option for patients who will consider them but are not willing to stop using nicotine products.

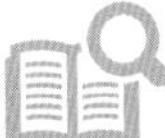

HIGH-YIELD LITERATURE

E-cigarettes vs. nicotine-replacement therapy for smoking cessation:

In this small RCT, e-cigarettes resulted in significantly better smoking cessation outcomes than other forms of nicotine-replacement therapy:

Hajek P, Phillips-Waller A, Przulj D, et al. A randomized trial of e-cigarettes versus nicotine-replacement therapy. *N Engl J Med.* 2019;380:629-637.

ALCOHOL USE DISORDER

Consequences of Alcohol Use

Alcohol use has numerous potentially harmful effects, including:

- CNS: Cerebellar dysfunction, memory issues.
- Cardiovascular: Hypertension, stroke, cardiomyopathy, coronary artery disease.
- Gastrointestinal: Pancreatitis (acute and chronic), chronic liver disease and cirrhosis, gastroesophageal reflux disease (GERD), esophagitis, and peptic ulcer disease (PUD).
- Endocrine: Accelerated bone loss, hypogonadism.
- Malignancy: Oral cancer, head and neck cancers, laryngeal cancer, esophageal/gastric/colon cancer, pancreatic cancer, liver cancers, and breast cancer.

Screening for Alcohol Use Disorder and Diagnosis

- Recommended limits of alcohol use are for men no more than 5 drinks/day and no more than 14 drinks/week on average and for women no more than 3 drinks/day and no more than 7 drinks/week on average.
- Numerous screening and diagnostic tools exist (some are reviewed later; see Table 17-5), but most often will begin with initial question of how often a patient has exceeded the previously noted limits.
- Other tools used in clinical practice include the AUDIT-C (3 items), AUDIT (10 items), or CAGE (4 items).
- The DSM-5 Diagnostic Criteria require presence of 2 of 11 symptoms in the past year. Dependence and tolerance are 2 of these symptoms, and together can clinch the diagnosis but are NOT required to diagnose alcohol use disorder.

Outpatient Management of Alcohol Use Disorder

- The main decision is whether patients should undergo psychosocial counseling, pharmacologic management, or both. For patients with more mild alcohol use disorder, they may only require counseling or support groups such as Alcoholics Anonymous (AA).

TABLE 17-5. AUDIT-C Questionnaire for Detecting Alcohol Use Disorder

Question	Scoring (Points)				
	1	2	3	4	5
How often do you have a drink containing alcohol?	Never	Monthly or less	2–4 times per month	2–3 times per week	4 or more times per week
How many standard drinks containing alcohol do you have on a typical day?	1 or 2	3 or 4	5 or 6	7 to 9	10 or more
How often do you have 6 or more drinks on one occasion?	Never	Less than monthly	Monthly	Weekly	Daily or almost daily

Maximum score of 12. A score ≥4 in men or ≥3 in women is considered positive.

- First-line medication options include naltrexone or acamprosate. Other agents with some evidence supporting their use include disulfiram, topiramate, and gabapentin.
  - Naltrexone: Available in oral and injectable formulations. Blocks the mu-opioid receptor and can reduce cravings. Generally thought to be the most effective option. Can cause transaminitis, so liver function tests (LFTs) should be periodically monitored.
  - Acamprosate: Mechanism not entirely clear, but works to reduce craving. Must be taken 3 times daily, which may limit adherence. Less effective than naltrexone.
  - Disulfiram: Inhibits aldehyde dehydrogenase and prevents alcohol's metabolism, resulting in accumulation of acetaldehyde and accompanying sweating, flushing, nausea, and vomiting. Only to be used in very motivated patients who will take medication daily.

Management of Alcohol Withdrawal

- **General management**: Many patients require hospitalization. Replete thiamine before giving glucose and folate to patient.
- Withdrawal syndromes can vary from mild anxiety and tremor, to alcohol withdrawal seizures, to delirium tremens.
- **Alcohol withdrawal can be life-threatening and should be aggressively treated with benzodiazepine tapers**. Usual onset is 12 to 24 hours after last drink.
- Data are superior for symptom-triggered therapy using a symptom score (such as CIWA; see Figure 17-1), but many hospitals use long-acting benzodiazepines such as chlordiazepoxide with a slow taper.
- **Alcohol withdrawal seizures**: Generally occur 12 to 48 hours after last drink (see Figure 17-2). Should treat with more aggressive use of agents for alcohol withdrawal (benzodiazepines, phenobarbital, and/or propofol) rather than use of antiepileptics.
- **Delirium tremens**: Occurs in about 5% of patients, and if untreated can result in mortality rate of almost 30%. Clinical syndrome of hallucinations, disorientation, tachycardia, diaphoresis, hypertension, and hyperthermia in the setting of alcohol cessation. Requires intensive care unit (ICU) level of care for treatment escalation.
- Refractory alcohol withdrawal (refractory to benzodiazepine therapy) necessitates ICU-level monitoring, airway protection, and potential adjunctive use of medications such as phenobarbital or propofol.

Patient: ______________________ Date: __________ Time: ____:____

Pulse or heart rate, taken for one minute: ________ Blood pressure: ____/____

Nausea and vomiting. Ask 'Do you feel sick to your stomach? Have you vomited?"
Observation:
0—No nausea and no vomiting
1—Mild nausea with no vomiting
2—
3—
4—Intermittent nausea with dry heaves
5—
6—
7—Constant nausea, frequent dry heaves, and vomiting

Tremor. Ask patient to extend arms and spread fingers apart.
Observation:
0—No tremor
1—Tremor not visible but can be felt, fingertip to fingertip
2—
3—
4—Moderate tremor with arms extended
5—
6—
7—Severe tremor, even with arms not extended

Paroxysmal sweats
Observation:
0—No sweat visible
1—Barely perceptible sweating; palms moist
2—
3—
4—Beads of sweat obvious on forehead
5—
6—
7—Drenching sweats

Anxiety. Ask "Do you feel nervous?"
Observation:
0—No anxiety (at ease)
1—Midlity anxious
2—
3—
4—Moderately anxious or guarded, so anxiety is inferred
5—
6—
7—Equivalent to acute panic states as occur in severe delirium or acute schizophrenic reactions

Agitation
Observation:
0—Normal activity
1—Somewhat more than normal activity
2—
3—
4—Moderately fidgety and restless
5—
6—
7—Paces back and forth during most of the interview or constantly thrashes about

Tactile disturbances. Ask 'Do you have you any itching, pins and needles sensations. burning. or numbness, or do you feel like bugs are crawling on or under your skin?"
Observation:
0—None
1—Very mild itching, pins and needles sensation, burning, or numbness
2—Mild itching, pins and needles sensation, burning, or numbness
3—Moderate itching, pins and needles sensation, burning, or numbness
4—Moderately severe hallucinations
5—Severe hallucinations
6—Extremely severe hallucinations
7—Constant nausea, frequent dry heaves, and vomiting

Auditory disturbances. Ask 'Are you more aware of sounds around you? Are they harsh? Do they frighten you? Are you hearing anything that is disturbing to you? Are you hearing things you know are not there?"
Observation:
0—Not present
1—Very mild harshness or ability to frighten
2—Mild harshness or ability to frighten
3—Moderate harshness or ability to frighten
4—Moderately severe hallucinations
5—Severe hallucinations
6—Extremely severe hallucinations
7—Continuous hallucinations

Visual disturbances. Ask "Dose the light appear to be too bright? Is its color different? Dose it hurt your eyes? Are you seeing anything that is disturbing to you? Are you seeing things you know are not there?"
Observation:
0—Not present
1—Very mild sensitivity
2—Mild sensitivity
3—Moderate sensitivity
4—Moderately severe hallucinations
5—Severe hallucinations
6—Extremely severe hallucinations
7—Continuous hallucinations

Headache, fullness in head. Ask "Dose your head feel different/ Does it feel like there is a band around your head?"
Do not rate for dizziness or lightheadness: otherwise, rate severity.
0—Not present
1—Very mild
2—Mild
3—Moderate
4—Moderately severe
5—Severe
6—Very severe
7—Extremely severe

Orientation and clouding of sensorium. Ask "What day is this? Where are you? Who am I?"
Observation:
0—Orientated and can do serial additions
1—Cannot do serial additions or is uncertain about date
2—Date disorientation by no more than two calendar days
3—Date disorientation by more than two calendar days
4—Disorientated for place and/or person

Total score: ________ (maximum - 67) Rater's initials ______

FIGURE 17-1. CIWA Score

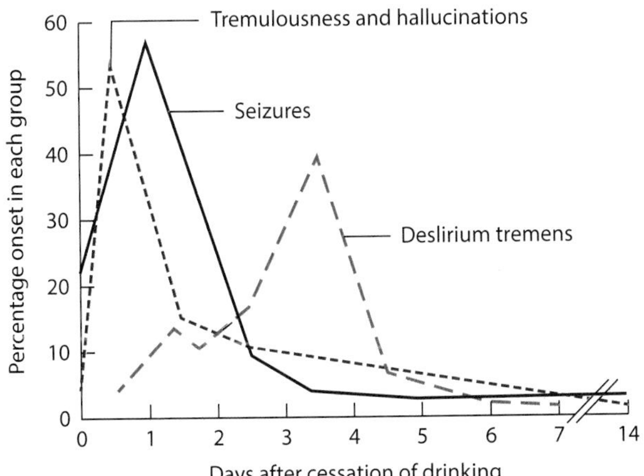

FIGURE 17-2. Timing and Manifestations of Alcohol Withdrawl (From Simon RP, Aminoff MJ, Greenberg DA: *Clinical Neurology*, 10th ed. Copyright © McGraw-Hill Education. All rights reserved. Figure created using data from Victor M, Adams RD. The effect of alcohol on the nervous system. Res Publ Assoc Res Nerv Ment Dis. 1952;32: 526-573.)

HIGH-YIELD LITERATURE

Standing benzodiazepines vs. symptom-triggered benzodiazepine use in alcohol withdrawal:

Saitz R, Mayo-Smith MF, Roberts MS, Redmond HA, Bernard DR, Calkins DR. Individualized treatment for alcohol withdrawal: A randomized, double-blind controlled trial. *JAMA.* 1994; 272(7): 519.

OPIOID USE DISORDER

Epidemiology and Pharmacology

- Over the last decade in the United States, there has been a significant rise in the use of both heroin and illicit prescription medications.
- Opioids are now the most common cause of drug overdose death in the United States.

Clinical Manifestations

- During acute intoxication, you can see significant sedation with associated slurring of speech. On examination, you may see miosis (constricted pupils). For those with chronic use, they may have a normal examination.
- Health consequences of long-term opioid use include risk of overdose (including respiratory depression and death), opioid-induced constipation, opioid-induced hyperalgesia (paradoxical increase in pain and sensitivity), and any consequences of route of administration (e.g., endocarditis or infections such as HIV/hepatitis C virus [HCV]/hepatitis B virus [HBV] if injecting).

CONQUER THE WARDS!

Given that there is no universally recommended screening tool for opioid use disorder, ask your clinic preceptor what the clinic uses. If they don't have a good answer, consider using the Rapid Opioid Dependence Screen.

Screening in the Clinic and Diagnosis of Opioid Use Disorder

- All patients with medical conditions that may have been acquired through opioid use (endocarditis, HIV, HCV, HBV) should be screened.
- Many clinics have adopted universal screening protocols given the significant increase in rates of opioid use throughout the United States.
- There is no single accepted screening technique: Options include the Rapid Opioid Dependence Screen or the DAST-10.

Treatments

Treatment of Acute Intoxication or Overdose

- The main concern is for mental and respiratory status. Need a high index of suspicion in patients without known opioid use disorder.
- Once opioid toxicity is suspected, prompt attention should be paid to the patient's airway and breathing. Naloxone should be given intravenously. If excess naloxone is given, withdrawal may be precipitated, which should be closely monitored (and not empirically treated with opioids). Multiple doses of naloxone may be required depending on the opioid used by the patient.

Treatment of Opioid Withdrawal Syndromes

- Clinical features: Agitation, restlessness, diarrhea, nausea/vomiting, rhinorrhea, myalgias and joint pains, and piloerection.
- Opioid withdrawal can produce significant symptoms and should be treated to prevent relapse, but generally will not result in death even if untreated except in rare circumstances.
- Management may include opioid agonist therapy (methadone, buprenorphine), benzodiazepines, and/or clonidine. Other symptom-driven treatments may also be useful.

Treatment in the Outpatient Setting

- Focus in the clinic should be on harm reduction—aiming for long-term abstinence but ensuring patients are using safely if they are not ready to quit. Harm reduction interventions may include needle exchange programs, never using opioids alone, and developing an overdose plan.
- Prescribe intranasal naloxone for as-needed use on themselves or friends to all patients whether they are currently abstinent or not.
- Refer interested patients for pharmacologic therapy with either methadone (as part of a supervised methadone maintenance program) or buprenorphine-naloxone (prescribed by primary care physicians if they have applied for a waiver).

SYMPATHOMIMETICS

Mechanism and Pharmacology

- Enhances monoamine neurotransmitter (dopamine, norepinephrine, serotonin) activity in the CNS and peripheral nervous system (PNS) by blocking reuptake pumps.
- Cocaine base ("crack" or "freebase") can be smoked but not injected.
- Cocaine salt cannot be smoked, but is readily injected (intravenously or subcutaneously) or insufflated ("snorted") through the nose.
- Intended effects for patients include increased energy, alertness, and sociability, along with feelings of euphoria. However, there are numerous short- and long-term consequences to use.
- Cocaine Intoxication (Acute and Chronic)
- CNS: Increased risk of seizure or stroke.
- Cardiovascular System: Premature atherosclerosis, hypertension, tachycardia, myocardial infarction, cardiomyopathy, myocarditis.
- Pulmonary system: Shortness of breath, wheezing, "crack lung" (acute pulmonary syndrome with fever, hypoxia, diffuse alveolar infiltrates, and respiratory failure).

Management of Acute Cocaine Intoxication

- Initial attention to vital signs (hyperthermia), airway, breathing, and circulation.
- Use benzodiazepines to control excess sympathetic discharge and anxiety.
- Treat organ-specific toxicity. Avoid beta blockade (due to risks of unopposed alpha-adrenergic activity), and consider alpha blockade with agents such as phentolamine for refractory hypertension. Optimal management strategies for "crack lung" are unclear, and efforts should focus on supportive respiratory care.

Cocaine Withdrawal

- Symptoms are bothersome but rarely medically serious.
- Symptoms include depression, anxiety/agitation, cravings, and sleep changes.

Long-Term Management of Cocaine Use Disorders

- Referral to long-term counseling and support groups. Only psychological interventions have shown consistent and long-term improvements in abstinence rates.
- Numerous agents have been examined with varying degrees of data, including dopamine agonists, long-acting amphetamines, and bupropion, but patients should be referred to physicians with experience in addiction medicine.

APPROACH TO COMMON AMBULATORY CHIEF COMPLAINTS

UPPER RESPIRATORY INFECTIONS

Your main role in seeing these patients in clinic is to triage: Differentiating bacterial syndromes (strep pharyngitis, bacterial pneumonia, bacterial sinusitis) vs. influenza vs. "viral URI" (noninfluenza upper respiratory infections).

- **Triage**: Illness scripts for more concerning mimickers of "common cold" include:
  - **Strep pharyngitis**: Fever, pain worst at onset of symptoms, lack of cough.
  - **Bacterial pneumonia**: Fever, productive cough, abnormal pulmonary examination.
  - **Bacterial sinusitis**: Fevers, sinus pain/pressure, purulent nasal discharge.
- **Influenza:**
  - Clinical presentation: Fever, productive cough, prominent myalgia and fatigue.
  - Diagnosis: During the peak of influenza season, patients with suggestive symptoms can be diagnosed clinically. Testing should be obtained in patients who are 1) at high risk for complications from influenza, 2) immunocompromised, or 3) hospitalized.
  - Treatment: Consider supportive therapies for prominent symptoms (e.g., antitussives for cough, pain relief for myalgia, etc.).
    - Low-risk patients can be started on oseltamivir (75 mg BID) if patient is presenting within 48 hours of presentation.
    - High-risk patients can be started on oseltamivir independent of onset (e.g., even if >48 hours from onset).
- **Noninfluenza viral upper respiratory infection:**
  - Umbrella term that encompasses all noninfluenza viral upper respiratory infections including bronchitis and laryngitis. More than 200 viruses can cause URIs.
  - Nearly all therapies for viral URI have limited efficacy and evidence, so goal is to target the most bothersome symptom with 1 to 2 medications:
    - Pain: Acetaminophen or nonsteroidal antiinflammatory drugs (NSAIDs).
    - Runny nose: Antihistamines, nasal saline, intranasal steroids, decongestants (pseudoephedrine or phenylephrine).
    - Cough: Dextromethorphan-guaifenesin, benzonatate.
  - Some evidence for vitamin C in prevention of cold but NOT in treatment. Some evidence for zinc, though must be oral (PO) formulations (intranasal formulations associated with anosmia).

CONQUER THE WARDS!

Older guidelines recommended empiric treatment for strep pharyngitis if all criteria met, but due to improvements in rapid strep sensitivity (fewer missed cases) and more data suggesting that risk of untreated strep pharyngitis is relatively low in adults, we now test everyone and do not empirically treat.

SORE THROAT

Differential Diagnosis/Etiologies

- Most common etiologies are viral etiologies (rhinovirus, adenovirus) and streptococcal infections (group A *Streptococcus*).
- Diagnoses that must be considered (briefly) and cannot be missed include:
  - Primary HIV: Sore throat + fever, rash, adenopathy, fatigue, myalgias
  - Epiglottitis: Sore throat + fever, odynophagia, voice changes, drooling, stridor.
  - Peritonsillar abscess: Sore throat + fever, voice changes, drooling, trismus (spasm of jaw muscles).
  - Submandibular infections (Ludwig angina): Sore throat + fever, chills, mouth pain, stiff neck, dysphagia, drooling.
- Other considerations include non-strep bacteria, including *Mycoplasma*, diphtheria (tightly adherent gray membranes), fusobacterium, and gonorrhea.

Diagnosis

- After excluding rare causes, the main question is whether to test for strep pharyngitis → Modified CENTOR CRITERIA
  - Age (3 to 14 yo = +1, 15 to 44 yo = 0, ≥45 = −1).
  - Fever >38: +1 if present.
  - Tonsillar exudate: +1 if present.
  - Tender anterior cervical lymphadenopathy: +1 if present.
  - Absence of cough: +1 if no cough is present.
- Interpretation of Centor criteria:
  - Score of −1, 0, or 1: No testing, no treatment. Treat for viral pharyngitis.
  - Score of 2 to 5: Rapid strep testing and treatment if positive.

Treatment of Strep Pharyngitis

- Rationale: 1) Reduce severity and duration of symptoms; 2) decrease risk of transmission to others; and 3) reduce risk of complications (rheumatic fever, scarlet fever).
- Therapy:
  - First-line: PO penicillin V 500 mg BID or TID × 10 days.
  - Alternatives: Amoxicillin 500 BID, cephalexin, azithromycin, or clindamycin.
  - No longer contagious after 24 hours of therapy.
  - MUST complete all 10 days to fully reduce risk of complications.

CONQUER THE WARDS!

Rapid strep tests are ~70% to 80% sensitive and ~90% specific, so in most case do not need to obtain cultures. If very high-risk patients (prior episodes of strep pharyngitis, high-risk professionals like medical professionals or school teachers), you may consider also doing a culture to exclude possibility of streptococcal infection.

SINUSITIS

Differentiating Viral from Bacterial Rhinosinusitis

- Bacterial etiologies only account for ~2% of all cases of sinusitis.
- Symptoms of viral sinusitis tend to be less severe, peaking in severity between days 3 and 6 and beginning to resolve after 7 to 10 days.
- Diagnostic criteria for bacterial sinusitis (Infectious Disease Society of America Guidelines): Must meet one of the following:
  - Symptoms more than 10 days without improvement. OR
  - Onset of severe symptoms or signs of high fever and purulent discharge/facial pain for at least 3 consecutive days at the beginning of the illness. OR
  - Symptoms of typical viral illness that slowly improve but then worsen again with more severe symptoms after 5 to 7 days.

Treatment of Viral Sinusitis

- Generally advised to give 1 or 2 agents at a maximum, as efficacy of all therapies is somewhat limited.
- Options include NSAIDs, acetaminophen, nasal saline, intranasal steroids, intranasal decongestants (oxymetazoline), antihistamines, or oral decongestants (such as pseudoephedrine or phenylephrine).
- Some patients like to do nasal irrigation (with a neti pot): Evidence for the efficacy of this therapy is limited, though many patients find it helpful. Incredibly important that patients use sterile water; otherwise, they are putting themselves at risk for iatrogenic infections.

Treatment of Bacterial Sinusitis

- Data for antibiotics is surprisingly mixed, and so can observe patients for additional 7 to 10 days if symptoms are stable and patient is at low risk for complications. Can give same supportive therapies used in viral sinusitis.
- Antibiotics result in a small reduction in symptom burden and duration, but at the cost of increased adverse events (usually minor such as

gastrointestinal [GI] upset). The number needed to treat (NNT) for benefit is around 15, with a number needed to harm (NNH) for adverse effects can be as low as 1.

- If a decision is made to give antibiotics, amoxicillin/clavulanate 875/125 × 5 to 7 days is first-line. Penicillin-allergic patients can use doxycycline or levofloxacin.

CONQUER THE WARDS!

RED FLAG SIGNS for Low Back Pain warrant imaging.

They include:
Incontinence of bowel or bladder
Saddle anesthesia
Lower extremity weakness
Other new neurologic abnormalities
Failure to improve after 4 to 6 weeks

CONQUER THE WARDS!

"Sciatica" refers to pain that radiates from the buttocks to the leg in the distribution of the sciatic nerve. The most common cause is compression of a lumbar nerve root by disk material that has ruptured through the surrounding annulus.

APPROACH TO COMMON MUSCULOSKELETAL COMPLAINTS

Musculoskeletal complaints in clinic are incredibly common, and the workup for each individual joint-related complaint is unique. However, common principles underlie all outpatient/IM musculoskeletal complaints (see Table 17-6):

1. **Rule Out Trauma:** Traumatic evaluation pathways emphasize EARLY imaging. Once you exclude a significantly traumatic etiology to the pain, your history and physical become of paramount importance.
2. **Localize Pain (Exclude Radiation)**: Consider radiation of pain rather than pain from the joint itself (e.g., knee pain that is really radiating from the hip).
3. **Components of Examination**: Your standardized MSK examination will include inspection, palpation, range of motion (passive and active), strength, neurovascular exam, and any special maneuvers for the joint in question. (See Table 17-6.)
4. **Limit Imaging**: Few nontraumatic diagnoses require rapid imaging. Carefully consider how the imaging will change your management of the patient before you order (it often will not).
5. **Choose Medications Carefully**: The evidence for most medications (acetaminophen, NSAIDs) for musculoskeletal complaints is relatively poor, though there is a SIGNIFICANT placebo effect for most of these medications. Carefully consider possible adverse effects of the medications before choosing!

LOW BACK PAIN

General Facts

- Both acute and chronic low back pain are extremely common symptoms in the general population and is the most common musculoskeletal complaint in clinic.
- **Acute low back pain:**
  - Typically due to a muscle strain.
  - Most improve with time.
- **Chronic low back pain** (pain >12 weeks):
  - Typically multifactorial and is often categorized as "chronic nonspecific low back pain."
  - Often a component of central pain sensitization, in which there is amplification of neural signaling within the central nervous system leading to pain hypersensitivity.
- Low back pain can also be a sign of a systemic disease, and thus when a patient presents with this symptom, it is important to review red flags for serious pathology, including fevers, neurologic dysfunction (especially bowel/bladder), pain severe enough to wake up from sleep, history of cancer, or history of trauma.

TABLE 17-6. Brief Descriptions of Selected Musculoskeletal Conditions

Location of Pain	Clinical Syndrome	Typical Presentation	Diagnosis/Imaging	Treatment Notes (in Addition to Acetaminophen vs. NSAIDs and Physical Therapy)
Neck	Neck pain **without** radiculopathy	Localized neck pain without radiation.	No imaging unless symptoms present for more than 8 weeks. X-ray is first-line.	N/A
	Neck pain **with** radiculopathy	Localized neck pain with radiation down one arm.		Steroid injections if persistent pain.
Back	Lower back pain **with** sciatica	Low back pain without radiation. Often see paraspinal muscle tenderness.	No imaging unless more than 6 weeks of symptoms → x-ray.	N/A
	Lower back pain **without** sciatica	Low back pain with radiation all the way down one leg (sciatica).	No imaging unless red flag signs. MRI is first test, after 6 weeks of symptoms without improvement	Can consider gabapentin or pregabalin, steroid injections. Surgery as last recourse.
	Lumbar spinal stenosis	Pseudoclaudication, localized back pain.	MRI as confirmation.	Surgery.
Ankle/ Foot	Ankle sprain	Ankle pain after injury.	Ottawa Ankle Rules help determine if x-ray needed.	Rest, ice, compression, elevation.
	Achilles tendinopathy	Pain on posterior heel, around 4 cm above heel.	Thompson or squeeze test can rule out rupture.	NEVER inject.
	Plantar fasciitis	Foot/heel pain worst in morning getting out of bed ("tearing" sensation).	Pain on palpation when foot is dorsiflexed.	Stretching exercises are essential. Can consider injection vs. surgery if refractory.
Knee	Osteoarthritis +/− Bursitis	Limited morning stiffness, better with rest and worse with exertion.	Areas of bursal inflammation very tender on palpation. See crepitus with OA.	Data for knee replacement surgery is outstanding, so a consideration in severe/ debilitating cases.
	Patellofemoral pain syndrome	Pain worse with sitting, better with moving. Anterior. Often seen in younger women.	N/A	Physical therapy is essential.
	IT band syndrome	Lateral thigh and knee pain, seen in active younger adults.	N/A	Physical therapy
	Ligamentous injury	Knee instability	Positive maneuvers (Lachman, anterior/posterior drawer). Confirm via MRI.	Surgery
	Meniscal Injury	Clicking/locking with knee pain	Positive provocative maneuvers (McMurray, Apley). MRI.	Physical therapy vs. Surgery
Hip	Osteoarthritis	Medial (groin) hip pain, worse with movement.	X-ray	Consider hip replacement if severe.
	Meralgia paresthetica	Anterolateral thigh pain and numbness. Seen in obese patients.	Decreased sensation.	Loose-fitting clothing, weight loss.
	Trochanteric bursitis	Lateral hip pain	Pain on palpation of bursa.	NSAIDs +/− steroid injection.
Hand	Osteoarthritis	PIP and DIP involvement. Worse with use of hands.	Osteophytes, DIP involvement on x-ray.	N/A
	De Quervain tenosynovitis	Thumb/hand pain. Worst at radial aspect of thumb when lifting.	Positive Finkelstein test.	Injections are first-line. Surgery if refractory.
Elbow	Medial epicondylitis	Medial elbow pain.	Pain on wrist flexion.	Bracing. No injections.
	Lateral epicondylitis	Lateral elbow pain.	Pain on wrist extension.	Bracing. No injections.
	Olecranon bursitis	Pain over olecranon bursa. Worse with pressure on elbow.	Must do tap to rule out gout, infection.	Steroid injection vs. NSAIDs.
Shoulder	Rotator cuff tendinopathy	Pain with reaching overhead.	Positive impingement signs. Can confirm on MRI.	Physical therapy.
	Adhesive capsulitis	Pain with moving arm in any plane of direction. Usually a consequence of untreated shoulder pathology.	Clinical diagnosis, confirm via MRI or arthrography.	Physical therapy is very painful. Surgery as last resort.

Clinical Features

Acute Low Back Pain

- Typically due to a muscle or ligamentous strain. Patients will endorse achy, nonradiating pain often in the paraspinal musculature.
- But can be due to more serious conditions such as:
  - Bony metastasis characteristically has nighttime pain.
  - Epidural abscesses have severe pain and fevers.
  - Herniated discs:
    - Pain is sudden in onset.
    - Pain that radiates down one leg, especially if associated with numbness or weakness in that distribution, suggests nerve compression.

Chronic Low Back Pain

- Patients with chronic, nonspecific low back pain have poorly localized achy pain that typically worsens with activity and prolonged sitting.
- Associated with prolonged morning stiffness that improves with activity, suggests a spondyloarthropathy (see Chapter 15- Rheumatology).
- Common causes of chronic low back pain are:
  - **Spinal stenosis**: Patients have pain that radiates into the lower extremity triggered by walking or prolonged standing, and relieved by rest or lumbar flexion (shopping cart sign).
  - **Chronic radiculopathy** (often due to facet hypertrophy causing foraminal stenosis, or spondylolisthesis) endorses pain, sensory loss, weakness in the area supplied by the involved nerve root.

CONQUER THE WARDS!

A history of cancer is the strongest risk factor for back pain due to bone metastasis. Breast, prostate, lung, and multiple myeloma are the most common causes of skeletal metastasis.

CONQUER THE BOARDS!

Most radiculopathies involve the L5 and S1 nerve roots.

Physical Exam Findings

For most cases of low back pain, the exam is nonspecific, but a focused exam should be done in every patient to identify those who need further acute work-up. Palpation over the spine and a neurologic exam targeting the nerve roots supplying the lower extremities (L2–S1) is important.

Cause of Back Pain	Physical Exam
Acute muscle strain	Nonspecific, often tenderness of paraspinal muscles.
Herniated disk	Positive straight leg raise test (elevating leg with patient supine causes worsening radicular pain) suggests at L5 nerve impingement. Associated neurologic findings (weakness, sensory loss) in the affected nerve root.
Compression fracture	Focal tenderness.
Bony metastasis	Focal tenderness.
Epidural abscess/vertebral osteomyelitis	Severe discomfort, focal tenderness, fever.
Chronic nonspecific low back pain	Nonspecific tenderness.
Spinal stenosis	Often normal, can lead to wide-based gait.
Radiculopathy	Associated neurologic findings (weakness, sensory loss) in the affected nerve root.

CONQUER THE WARDS!

The cauda equina syndrome describes an acute compression of nerves in the cauda equine. Patients endorse new problems with bowel/bladder control, anesthesia in a saddle distribution, and weakness. This can occur due to a herniated disc, infection, inflammation, cancer, or spinal stenosis. It is a neurosurgical emergency.

Nerve Root	Motor Function	Sensory Function
L2	Hip flexion	Anterior thigh
L3	Knee extension	Anterior Thigh
L4	Ankle dorsiflexion	Knee
L5	Toe dorsiflexion	Dorsal foot
S1	Ankle plantarflexion	Lateral foot

Diagnostic Workup

The vast majority of patients with either acute or chronic low back pain do not need imaging.

Notably, magnetic resonance imaging (MRI) is not helpful for chronic, nonspecific low back pain, as most of the findings seen (e.g., facet arthritis, mild herniated disk) are common in the general population and do not change management. There are certain scenarios in which an MRI should be obtained urgently (red flag signs) due to concern for spinal cord or cauda equine compression:

- New urinary retention or incontinence.
- Saddle anesthesia.
- Loss of motor function not limited to a single nerve root.
- Signs of acute infection.

HIGH-YIELD LITERATURE

Chou R, Qaseem A, Owen DK, Shekelle P. Clinical Guidelines Committee of the American College of Physicians. Diagnostic imaging for low back pain: Advice for high-value health care from the American College of Physicians. *Ann Intern Med.* 2011;154(3):181-189.

Management

- Acute low back pain typically resolves spontaneously after a few weeks, but acetaminophen and NSAIDs can be used.
- Chronic low back pain is most effectively treated with multimodal therapy, which includes:
  - Pain control in a stepwise approach:
    - First-line: Non-narcotics: Acetaminophen and NSAIDs.
    - Second-line: Duloxetine or tramadol or tricyclic antidepressants (e.g., nortriptyline).
    - Third-line: Muscle relaxants and/or opioids. However, extreme care must be taken in starting these agents, as opioids have addictive properties, and both medication types' side effect profile is more dangerous. Further opioids in randomized trials have shown either no or very small benefits for chronic low back pain.
  - CBT and mindfulness-based stress reduction.
  - Steroid injections are also sometimes used.

HIGH-YIELD LITERATURE

Qaseem A, Wilt TJ, McLean RM, Forceia MA. Clinical Guidelines Committee of the American College of Physicians. Noninvasive treatments for acute, subacute, and chronic low back pain: A clinical practice guideline from the American College of Physicians. *Ann Intern Med.* 2017;166(7):514-530.

APPROACH TO THE RED EYE

History

- Pertinent questions to ask include:
  - Vision changes.
  - Photophobia.

- Trauma to eye or foreign body sensation.
- Does the patient wear contact lenses?
- Discharge.

Physical Examination

- Key steps in the physical exam include:
  - Formal visual acuity testing.
  - Penlight examination: Reactivity of pupils, discharge, pattern of redness on eye.

Selected Differential Diagnosis and Typical Presentations

- The key step for the primary care physician is triage: Is this something I can manage without urgent or emergent consultation from an ophthalmologist? If concerning conditions cannot be excluded, the patient should be urgently referred to an ophthalmologist. **Decreases in visual acuity or significant photophobia raise concern for more serious pathologies and should almost always result in immediate referral to ophthalmology.**
- Benign conditions and their typical presentation:
  - Stye (hordeolum): Bacterial infection of oil gland in eye lid. Results in erythematous bump at edge of eyelid, tender to palpation. No visual changes. Treatment is with warm compresses.
  - Chalazion: Blockage of oil gland in eyelid, may be a result of a stye. Painful, hardened bump at edge of eyelid. Treatment with warm compresses initially. If no response, may need incision by ophthalmology.
  - Viral conjunctivitis: Usually secondary to adenovirus. May see other symptoms of an upper respiratory infection. See conjunctival injection, watery discharge, and a gritty feeling in one eye. The second eye usually becomes involved within 24 to 48 hours. Self-limited process, advise hand hygiene, as highly contagious.
  - Allergic conjunctivitis: Symptomatology similar to viral conjunctivitis, often in patients with known allergies. They may not have more tearing and eye itching.
  - Bacterial conjunctivitis: Redness and mucopurulent discharge in one eye, with affected eye often with prominent symptoms in the morning. See purulent discharge at eyelid margins. Often resolves without treatment unless secondary to chlamydia or gonorrhea (which require prompt treatment). Can treat with antibiotic eye drops if persistent.
  - Episcleritis: Sudden onset of inflammation of the episclera (between the conjunctiva and connective tissue layer). Common, self-limited, either painless or very mild discomfort. Sometimes associated with autoimmune conditions, but most often idiopathic. No vision changes.
  - Corneal abrasion: Scratch to surface of cornea of eye. Patient presents with pain, photophobia, erythema, and a foreign body sensation. Diagnosis via slit lamp examination after fluorescein dye. Treatment is usually with antibiotic ointment to prevent superinfection. May require ophthalmologic consultation if symptoms not improving after 24 to 48 hours.
- Conditions warranting immediate ophthalmologic examination:
  - Angle-closure glaucoma: Presents as acute-onset decrease in vision, severe eye pain, and headache. May be associated with nausea and vomiting, and patients will often describe seeing "halos" around lights. On exam, will see a red eye with increased intraocular pressure.
  - Hyphema: A collection of blood inside the anterior chamber of eye, usually secondary to trauma. Can lead to blindness if untreated.

- Hypopyon: Inflammatory (white blood) cells in the anterior chamber of eye, usually seen with uveitis or iritis.
- Infectious keratitis: Inflammation and infection of the cornea (the clear dome on the front surface of the eye). Patient presents with pain, redness, photophobia, vision changes, and a gritty sensation in the eye.
- Scleritis: Autoimmune condition affecting the sclera (white outer coating of the eye). Often associated with autoimmune diseases, with associated redness, severe eye pain, photophobia, tearing, and decreases in visual acuity.

CHAPTER 18 IN-PATIENT FLOOR EMERGENCIES

OVERVIEW OF HIGH-YIELD TOPICS IN INPATIENT EMERGENCIES

CONQUER THE WARDS!

"Do-Not-Miss" causes of chest pain—MARPE:
Must **A**lways **R**ule out **P**otential **E**mergencies
Myocardial infarction
Aortic dissection
Ruptured esophagus
Pneumothorax
Embolism (pulmonary)

INTRODUCTION

On the inpatient medicine wards, there are 5 common acute complaints that patients will have:

- Chest pain.
- Tachycardia.
- Acute dyspnea.
- Altered mental status.
- Fall.

We will describe here how to initially diagnose the cause and manage these acute complaints. For detailed management of each particular diagnosis, see the appropriate chapter.

Ms. Patel is a 52-year-old female with a known history of hypertension, diabetes, hyperlipidemia, and hypothyroidism who presented with a cough and increased sputum production. Ms. Patel is diagnosed with community-acquired pneumonia and is started on appropriate antimicrobial therapy. On the evening of her first hospital day she complains of the sudden onset of left-sided chest pain.

CHEST PAIN

General Facts

Chest pain is responsible for ~6% of all emergency room visits in the United States, and ~50% of those patients will have noncardiac pain. Chest pain also remains a common complaint of patients already admitted to the hospital for other reasons and may reflect progressive illness, an in-hospital complication, or a clinical response to acute stress. When evaluating a patient with chest pain in the hospital setting, it will be crucial to eliminate the 5 most common life-threatening conditions: including **1) myocardial infarction, 2) aortic dissection, 3) pulmonary embolism, 4) esophageal rupture, and 5) pneumothorax (see Table 18-1).**

Common Clinical Scenario

In 5 Minutes or Less

Before you walk in the room, you should have a differential diagnosis in your head. (See Table 18-1.) Your focused history and exam should be directed toward that differential diagnosis.

TABLE 18-1. Differential Diagnosis for Chest Pain

1. Could the chest discomfort be due to an acute, potentially life-threatening condition that warrants urgent evaluation and management?			
Unstable ischemic heart disease	Aortic dissection	Pneumothorax	Pulmonary embolism
2. If not, could the discomfort be due to a chronic condition likely to lead to serious complications?			
Stable angina	Aortic stenosis	Pulmonary hypertension	
3. If not, could the discomfort be due to an acute condition that warrants specific treatment?			
Pericarditis	Pneumonia/pleuritis	Herpes zoster	
4. If not, could the discomfort be due to another treatable chronic condition?			
Esophageal reflux		Cervical disk disease	
Esophageal spasm		Arthritis of the shoulder or spine	
Peptic ulcer disease		Costochondritis	
Gallbladder disease		Other musculoskeletal disorders	
Other gastrointestinal conditions		Anxiety state	

- **Assess for clinical stability:**
  - Check patient's vitals (blood pressure, pulse, fever, O_2 sat).
  - Assess mental status.
- **Focused history:**
  - Focus on the nature, location, duration, radiation, severity, and any accompanying symptoms. These will be crucial in establishing a cohesive differential diagnosis.
- **Focused physical exam:**
  - Conduct a full cardiopulmonary exam. Remember to target your examination to rule out the most dangerous causes of chest pain (see the Conquer the Wards box on the previous page).
  - Do not forget to assess for murmurs, pulse deficits, and any stigmata of acute heart failure such as jugular venous distention (JVD) or an S3 gallop.
- **Call your resident if** vitals are newly unstable (make sure you know what vitals have been taken):
  - Mean arterial pressure (MAP) <60, heart rate (HR) >110, respiratory rate (RR) >25, O_2 sat <90%, mental status acutely different.
- **If vitals are stable:**
  - Get an electrocardiogram (ECG) (or ask the nurse to).
  - Consider oxygen if O_2 saturation is less than 92%.
  - Stay with the patient until your resident arrives.
  - Be prepared to succinctly tell your resident what you obtained from your focused history, the latest vitals, and your focused exam and what you think the diagnosis is.

Patients who have a more immediate life-threatening etiology for their chest pain tend to appear anxious and in acute distress with possible associated diaphoresis and/or dyspnea.

Laboratory Testing

Based on your findings on history and exam, here are some potential labs to consider getting:

- Troponins: The preferred cardiac biomarker for the diagnosis of an acute myocardial infarction (see Figure 18-1).
- D-Dimer: Among patients with a low pretest probability for a pulmonary embolism. Please remember that D-dimers may be elevated in patients with known malignancy, recent surgeries, and in the setting of sepsis.
- Complete blood count: An elevated white blood cell (WBC) count may be seen in inflammatory states such as myocarditis, pericarditis, and primary pulmonary infections.
- B-type natriuretic peptide (BNP) and NT-ProBNP: Highly sensitive for acute heart failure when levels are greater than 100 pg/mL and/or when the patient has a known baseline value.
- Arterial blood gas: May be used as an adjunct test to diagnose or exclude pulmonary embolism.

Imaging Studies

Based on your findings on history and exam, here are some potential imaging studies to consider getting:

- ECG: A 12-lead ECG should be undertaken within 10 minutes of your encounter.

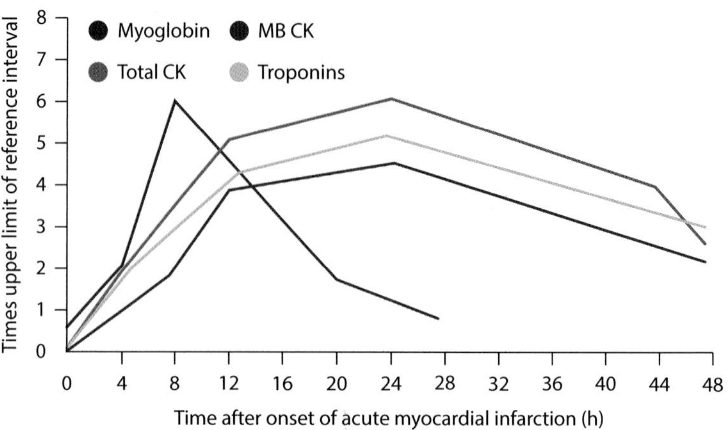

FIGURE 18-1. Time Course of Cardiac Enzyme Markers after Acute Myocardial Infarction (Reproduced, with permission, from Kumar N, Law A: Teaching Rounds: *A Visual Aid to Teaching Internal Medicine Pearls on the Wards.* www.accessmedicine.com. Copyright © McGraw-Hill Education. All rights reserved.)

- Chest x-ray (CXR): Should be obtained in any patient with hemodynamic instability, in which case a portable (STAT) order should be placed.

  Computed tomography (CT) pulmonary angiogram: To rule out pulmonary embolism we can see if there are any issues with the aorta or lung parenchyma.

Mr. Thomas is a 62-year-old male with a known history of hypertension, diabetes, and hyperlipidemia who was admitted for the management and evaluation of a urinary tract infection. On day 2 of his hospitalization Mr. Thomas complains of mild palpitations, and nursing staff report a heart rate of 130 bpm. You are asked to evaluate the patient while your resident is rounding on a new admission.

ACUTE TACHYCARDIA

General Facts

Tachyarrhythmias, by definition, are abnormal heart rhythms with a ventricular rate of 100 or more beats per minute (bpm). It is important to recognize that the clinical presentation of tachycardia may range from mildly symptomatic to fulminant hemodynamic compromise, and the initial minutes of evaluation are critical in preserving clinical stability.

CONQUER THE WARDS!

Signs of unstable tachycardia include **CASH**:
Chest pain (ischemic)
Alteration in mental status
Shortness of breath
Hypotension

Common Clinical Scenario
In 5 Minutes or Less

- **Hemodynamic stability:** Assess rapidly for hemodynamic stability using the pneumonic CASH. If the patient is unstable with hemodynamic compromise, this is a medical emergency, and you need to call a code to activate advanced cardiac life support (ACLS) or a rapid response team. Your hospital may have different terms for each of these, and it is good to know what they are when you start.
- **Targeted history and physical** should focus on:
  - **History:**
    - Cardiac history, especially coronary artery disease or heart failure.
    - Most common causes of tachycardia:
      - Pain.
      - Hypoxia.
      - Infection (fever, cough, dysuria, abdominal pain, skin infections).
      - Medications.
  - **Cardiac exam:** Looking for irregular heartbeats, murmurs, or signs of heart failure (JVD, lower extremity edema, S3 or S4).
- **Twelve-lead ECG** should be obtained while you are doing your history and physical.

- **Rapid review of ECG**, which leads to your differential.
  - Is the QRS narrow or wide (Figures 18-2 and 18-3)?
  - Is the QRS regular or irregular (Figures 18-2 and 18-3)?
  - Are there P waves (Figure 18-2)?

Treatment

In the cardiology section you will find a more detailed discussion about treatment for the various causes of tachycardia. A few general rules:

- **Regular wide complex tachycardia (WCT) and irregular WCT**: You should assume it is ventricular tachycardia or ventricular fibrillation, respectively, unless proven otherwise; if the patient is hemodynamically unstable, treatment should be DC cardioversion.
- **Narrow complex tachycardia**: This often presents with heart rates greater than 150, and it is extremely difficult to discern what type of rhythm it is on an ECG. Here is how this is managed:
  - First: Attach **ECG** leads.
  - Second: Run the **rhythm strip**, which will continuously print (leads V1, II, and V5 only).
  - Third: **Inject 6 mg adenosine** quickly with a quick saline flush as close to the heart as possible. Go to 12 mg if this doesn't work.

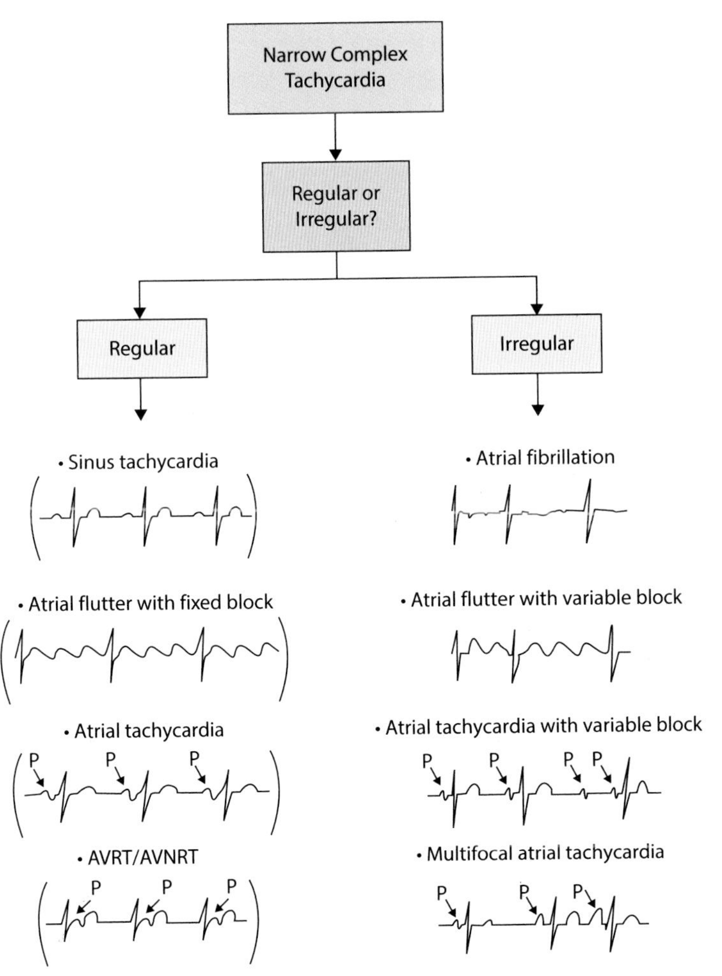

FIGURE 18-2. Narrow Complex Tachycardia Diagnostic Algorithm (Reproduced, with permission, from Kumar N, Law A: *Teaching Rounds: A Visual Aid to Teaching Internal Medicine Pearls on the Wards*. www.accessmedicine.com. Copyright © McGraw-Hill Education. All rights reserved.)

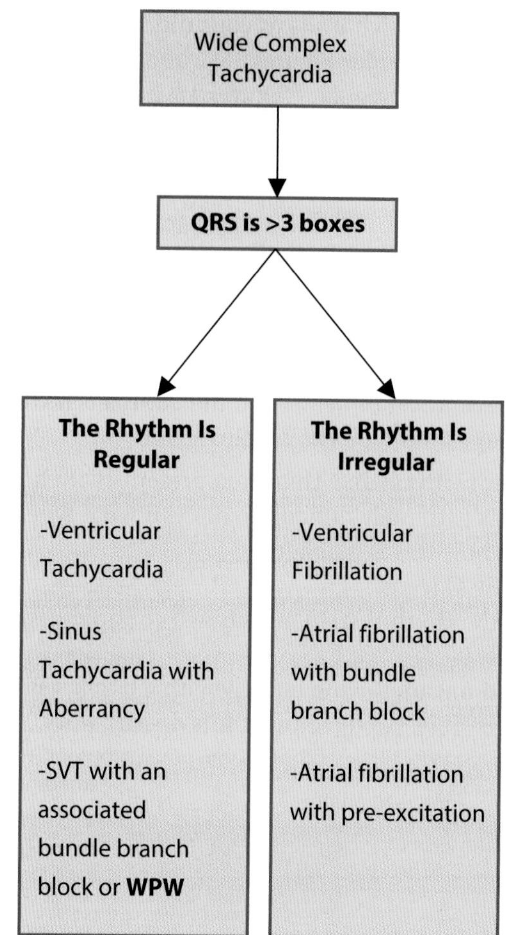

FIGURE 18-3. Wide Complex Tachycardia Diagnostic Algorithm

- Adenosine is extremely short acting (only a few seconds), so it may not work if it is injected from a hand intravenously (IV).
- It is important to warn the patient that he or she may feel his or her heart stop.
- It is important for you to know that the strip may flat-line and that is expected.

• Fourth: Look at the rhythm strip as you inject the adenosine; the underlying rhythm will be revealed and may even stop an AV reentrant tachycardia (AVRT) or AV-nodal reentrant tachycardia (AVNRT) if that is the underlying rhythm.

■ **Beta-blockers** and **calcium channel blockers** are the mainstay of treatment for narrow complex tachycardia. In general, beta-blockers are used first, such as metoprolol, since it can be given IV. But if you give IV (usually 5 mg or 10 mg), remember to think about adding oral (25 or 50 mg initial dose) as well, since it is more long acting. Diltiazem is also commonly used.

CONQUER THE WARDS!

General approach to acute respiratory failure:
Rapid assessment of severity
Action
Cause
Efficacy of treatment

ACUTE RESPIRATORY FAILURE

General Facts

Acute respiratory failure is a common inpatient emergency that requires a time-sensitive and targeted response to prevent further clinical decompensation. It is critical to have an algorithmic initial approach that includes a rapid assessment of severity, early targeted clinical action, ongoing assessment of the underlying cause, and evaluation of the efficacy of your initial treatment interventions.

Common Clinical Scenario
In 5 Minutes or Less

- **Rapid assessment of severity and stability:** Conduct a rapid and focused examination, noting 4 core elements:
  - Level of consciousness.
  - Severity of tachypnea.
  - Use of accessory muscles.
  - Degree of adrenergic stimulation (diaphoresis, tachycardia, hypertension, and agitation).

  If the patient is exhibiting these elements or they are apneic with a pulse, a hospital code should be called with initiation of the appropriate ACLS protocol.
- **Initial diagnostic evaluation for the stable patient should include** (see Figure 18-4):
  - **Oxygen saturation** with continuous monitoring.
  - **Full physical exam.**
  - **Arterial blood gas** to measure pH, O_2, and CO_2 in the blood.
  - **CXR** (portable).
  - Additional laboratory studies, including a complete blood count and basic metabolic panel.
- **Maintain adequate oxygenation:** Oxygen should be administered to patients who have noted hypoxia with an oxygen saturation of <90%. While nasal cannula remains the mode of initial oxygen delivery, it is important to familiarize yourself with the various forms of oxygen delivery available in the hospital setting (see Table 18-2).
- **Establish a targeted differential** based on physical exam findings, biochemical testing, and radiographic studies. The most common diagnoses we see in the hospital are:
  - **Flash pulmonary edema:**
    History: Possible if receiving intravenous fluids (IVF) or recent blood transfusion and/or history of diastolic or systolic heart failure.
    Physical exam: Crackles on exam, sometimes with wheezing.
    Treatment: Furosemide IV 80 mg. Furosemide helps with diuresis but also dilates the pulmonary venous vasculature. Patients will usually improve rapidly over the first hour.
  - **Bronchospasm**:
    History: History of asthma or COPD.
    Physical exam: Diffuse wheezing.
    Treatment: Albuterol nebulizer, repeated until symptoms improve.
  - **Pulmonary embolism:**
    History: Recent surgery or bedbound or hypercoagulable state.
    Physical exam: Normal lung exam or unilateral leg swelling.
    Treatment: Heparin drip and STAT CT pulmonary angiogram.
    Note: If this is suspected, always empirically treat with heparin before getting the angiogram unless the patient is at a high bleeding risk.
  - **Acute respiratory distress syndrome:**
    History: Being treated for a severe infection, or pancreatitis, or history of immunosuppression.
    Physical exam: Diffuse crackles and/or wheezing.
    Treatment: Furosemide, albuterol nebulizers, and possible transfer to the intensive care unit (ICU).

You are called emergently by nursing staff to evaluate Mr. Phillips, who is a 60-year-old male with a history of chronic obstructive pulmonary disease (COPD) who has become more confused in the recent several minutes with a worsening oxygen saturation of 80%.

CONQUER THE **WARDS!**

A patient who is awake, conversant, and responsive to verbal stimulation and is able to manage secretions is protecting their airway.

TABLE 18-2. Different Types of Oxygen Delivery

Type of O_2 Delivery	Flow Rates	FiO_2	How to Titrate	Notes
Low-flow nasal cannula	1–6 L/min	Each L/min adds ~4% FiO_2 above room air[a] 1 L/min = 20% 2 L/min = 24% 3 L/min = 28% 4 L/min = 32% 5 L/min = 36% 6 L/min = 40%	Titrate flow rate only	Best for patients with normal respiratory rates and tidal volumes
Simple face mask	~6–12 L/min	35–60%[a]	Titrate flow rate only	Minimum of 6 L/min flow is required to prevent re-breathing CO_2
Venturi mask	Fixed flow based on adapter chosen	Adapters are usually available in 24%, 28%, 31%, 35%, and 40%	Titrate FiO_2 only	Adapter entrains a set amount of ambient air to deliver a fixed FiO_2
Non-rebreather mask	10–15 L/min	100%	Nontitratable	Short-term bridge therapy only
High-flow nasal cannula	Up to 60 L/min	30–100%	Titrate flow rate and FiO_2	Administers PEEP with high flow rate

[a] Varies based on respiratory rate and minute ventilation.

Source: Kumar N, Law A: Teaching Rounds: A Cisual Aid to Teaching Internal Medicine Pearls on the Wards. www.accessmedicine.com

- As you can see, the common diagnoses can be difficult to differentiate, so it is okay to give furosemide and the albuterol nebulizer together if you are unsure of the diagnosis.
- After you have initiated targeted clinical action, it is critical to re-evaluate and assess the efficacy of your treatment.

Mr. Adams is an 82-year-old male who was admitted to the hospital with lower extremity pain with associated erythema and swelling. He is initiated on appropriate antimicrobial therapy for cellulitis. On the second day of his hospitalization, while doing your morning rounds, you find Mr. Adams to be more confused with increasing bouts of agitation, including attempting to pull out his IV access.

ACUTE ALTERED MENTAL STATUS

General Facts

Alteration in mental status in the hospitalized patient is a common problem that requires both a targeted and timely response in order to initiate appropriate therapeutic interventions. While the etiologies of altered mental status are broad, they can be divided into 4 categories:

- Primary neurologic process.
- Systemic or metabolic disorders affecting the nervous system.
- Exogenous toxins.
- Drug withdrawal.

CONQUER THE WARDS!

Focused history elements for AMS:
- Collateral from family/nursing staff
- In-hospital fall or trauma
- Recent medication administration/modification
- Overt neurologic signs (i.e., seizure activity/slurred speech)

Common Clinical Scenario
In 5 Minutes or Less

- **Focused history** with a focus on differential diagnosis listed in Figure 18-4. MOVE STUPID mnemonic.
- **General physical exam** should include vital signs, assessment of airway stability, and evaluation for acute trauma; look for skin infections, including decubitus ulcers.
- **Neurologic examination** should be undertaken for all patients with an acute change in mental status.

Altered Mental Status Differential Diagnosis

MOVE STUPID

Metabolic: B12 or thiamine deficiency, serotonin syndrome

Oxygen: Hypoxemia (pulmonary, cardiac, anemia)

Vascular: Hypertensive emergency, ischemic/hemorrhagic CVA, Vasculitis, Myocardial Infarction

Electrolyte and **E**ndocrine

Seizure: Status epilepticus, postictal state

Tumor, **T**rauma, **T**emperature, **T**oxins

Uremia: Renal or hepatic dysfunction with hepatic encephalopathy

Psychiatric

Infection

Drugs: Including withdrawal
- (Anticholinergic, TCA's, SSRI's, BZD's, barbituates, alcohol)

FIGURE 18-4. Altered Mental Status Differential Mnemonic. Source: Access Medicine >Principles and Practice of Hospital Medicine, 2e > Acute Respiratory Failure Sylvia C. McKean, John J. Ross, Daniel D. Dressler, Danielle B. Scheurer

- Initial diagnostic workup should include:
  - Complete blood count (CBC), basic electrolytes.
  - Point-of-care glucose.
  - If indicated, an infectious workup based on your exam and history. If you need to search broadly, generally the workup is a urinalysis, CXR, and blood cultures.
- **Imaging studies** should be ordered based on clinical presentation. CT of the head is often warranted as an initial workup for acute stroke or intracranial hematoma.
- Targeted treatment modalities should be initiated based on the differential diagnosis (see Figure 18-4).

FALLS

General Facts

Falls are the most commonly noted adverse events that occur in the hospital environment, with an estimated 700,000 to 1 million falls occurring in hospitals every year. Of these falls approximately 30% result in injury. It is estimated that falls result in $13,000 in operational cost and an increased length of stay of approximately 6 days. Most importantly, it is estimated that 30% of all falls can be prevented.

Ms. Miller is a 59-year-old female who presented to the hospital 2 days ago with intractable back pain for which she is undergoing evaluation. On the second night of her hospitalization, while attempting to ambulate to the bathroom, she falls onto the floor. When you arrive at the bedside, the patient is lying on the floor crying out in pain at her ankle.

Common Clinical Scenario
In 5 Minutes or Less

- **Vitals:** Attain a full set of vitals.
- **Physical exam:** Complete a focused physical examination, targeting evaluation for any injury to the head, spine, or musculoskeletal system.
- **History:** Attain collateral historical elements related to the fall from the patient and/or any bystanders. Pay special attention to whether she lost consciousness or hit her head. Table 18-3 lists other symptoms that would be concerning.

- Provide more immediate supportive care, including analgesia and the application of ice if appropriate.
- **Contact your resident** to review the immediate events and determine the need for further targeted imaging.
- **Incident report:** In coordination with your resident, an incident report will need to be documented, as a fall in the hospital is an important patient safety issue. All falls are reviewed by hospitals because it is deemed a never event by the Centers of Medicare and Medicaid Services.

TABLE 18-3. Suggested Workup of the Fallen Patient Based on Site-Specific Injuries

Site of Injury	Type of Injury	Signs and Symptoms of Injury	Evaluation and Management Options
Head	Traumatic brain injury (concussion, subdural hematoma) Stroke	Altered consciousness, Acute/subacute confusion, Headache, Light-headedness, Visual changes, Focal neurologic deficit	Stop anticoagulation If anticoagulated and bleeding, consider administration of vitamin K Mental status assessment Neurology, Neurosurgery consult Perform neurologic assessments every 2 h for 24–48 h Imaging
Spinal Column	Cord injury Vertebral fracture	Absence of sensation Inability to move Localized pain	Immediate stabilization of spine and immobilization with backboard, rigid cervical collar, lateral head supports Palpate entire spine Consult spine surgery for assessment Imaging with x-rays, CT scan
Skin	Laceration	Bleeding Visible alteration of skin integrity	Hemostasis with pressure, ice cleansing, sterilization Suturing, stapling Pain management
Extremities	Ecchymoses	Discoloration	Ice Pain management
Abdominal and Pelvic Injuries	Fracture Dislocation	Pain Limb, joint deformity Inability to bear weight	Visualize injury site Check neurovasular integrity distal to injury site Splint site Consult orthopedics or reduce dislocation
	Blunt trauma Pelvic fracture	Pain	Physical exam X-ray/CT

Source: Reproduced, with permission, from McKean S, Ross JJ, Dressler DD, Scheurer DB, eds. *Principles and Practice of Hospital Medicine*, 2nd ed. www.accessmedicine.com.

CHAPTER 19 PALLIATIVE CARE

OVERVIEW OF HIGH-YIELD TOPICS IN PALLIATIVE CARE

INTRODUCTION

General facts

Palliative care and **hospice** are similar, but they are not the same. The following defines both in detail.

Hospice

- **Definition:** Hospice is a way of providing care directed at improving the quality of life when someone is in their last days, weeks, or months of life and has decided not to pursue further curative or life-prolonging therapies.
- **Location:** It can be provided in a variety of locations, including home, nursing homes, dedicated hospice facilities, and the inpatient setting.
- **Insurance:** It is also an insurance benefit paid for by the Medicare Hospice Benefit, Medicaid Hospice Benefit, and most private insurers. In order to qualify, a physician must document an anticipated prognosis of less than 6 months.

Palliative Care

- **Definition:** Palliative care, and the medical subspecialty of palliative medicine, is specialized medical care for people living with serious illness. It focuses on providing relief from the symptoms and stress of a serious illness. The goal is to improve quality of life for both the patient and the family. It is appropriate at any age and at any stage in a serious illness and can be provided along with curative treatment.
- **Location:** Primarily available in inpatient settings and outpatient clinics. There is growing availability of palliative care in patients' homes and in nursing homes.
- **Team approach:** Palliative care is provided by a team of doctors, nurses, social workers, and others who work together with a patient's other clinicians to provide an extra layer of support. (See Figure 19-1.)
- **How to explain palliative care to patients and families:** "Palliative care is a team that helps care for people living with serious illness, and can help in a few different ways: management of symptoms, help you think through medical decisions, and make sure the right supports are in place. We've asked them to come by to help you with...." It is important to note that most of the general public does not know what palliative care is.
- **Reasons to consult specialty-level palliative care:**
- Refractory symptom management.
- Complex goals of care (conflicting treatment decisions, complicated family dynamics, or team distress).

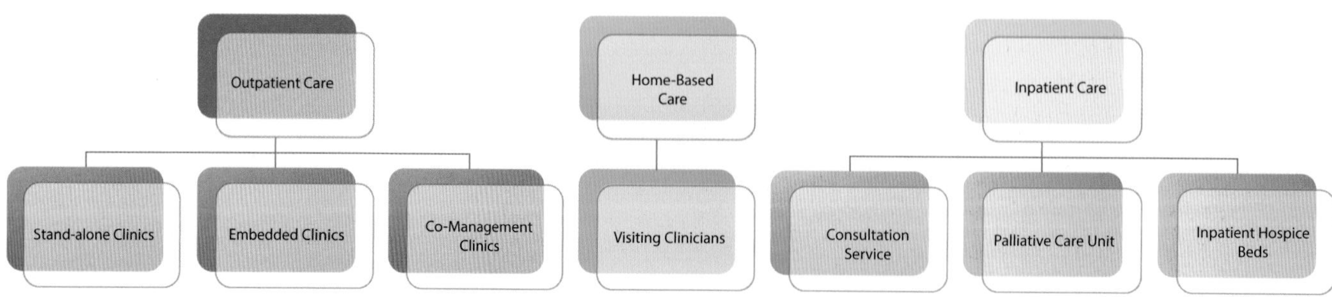

FIGURE 19-1. Locations Where Palliative Care Can Be Provided

- Psychological and spiritual support for significant existential distress.
- Other patients who may benefit: Those with frequent hospitalizations or emergency department (ED) visits, prolonged intensive care unit (ICU) stay, or multiple ICU visits during the same admission, as well as overall decline in functional status.
- **Core elements of palliative care:** Given the increasing burden of chronic and serious illness and an aging population, there will never be enough palliative care specialists to see all people living with serious illness. It is imperative that all clinicians learn the core elements of palliative care:
  - Basic symptom management.
  - Basic communication skills.
  - Fundamentals of end-of-life care.

Symptom Management

Regardless of prognosis, the same general approach to management of both pain and non-pain symptoms applies. The following discusses the 3 most common symptoms in patients with serious illness: **pain, dyspnea, and nausea.**

General Approach to Symptoms

- **Assessment:** Thorough history and physical exam.
- **Find cause:** Conceptualize likely underlying causes.
- **Treat** reversible underlying causes (when goal-concordant) using both:
  - Pharmacologic.
  - Nonpharmacologic management.
- **Reassess** at appropriate intervals and adjust treatment accordingly.
- **Education:** Provide ongoing education and support to the patient and their family.

PAIN MANAGEMENT

Pain Assessment

In pain assessment, it is important to remember to truly delineate and understand the patient's pain, as this will better allow you to treat their pain. You can do this by remembering your OPQRST questions and adding a **U** to the mnemonic–How does it affect your daily life?

Onset "When did it start?"
Palliative + Provocative "What makes it better? What makes it worse?"
Quality "How would you describe it?"
Radiation "Where is the pain? Does it go anywhere else?"
Severity "On a scale of 0 to 10, what number would you give it right now? What's the highest it's been today? The lowest?"
Timing "Is it there all the time, or does it come and go?"
yo**U** "How does it affect your daily life?"

> CONQUER THE **WARDS!**
>
> Set pain management goals. "Knowing that we can't often get pain to a 0, what is a number that will allow you to do the things you want to do?"

Causes of Pain

Pain is categorized into **acute** and **chronic pain** based on its duration. And within those 2 categories the cause of the pain can be **nociceptive** (direct stimulation of nociceptors that are present throughout the body) and **neuropathic** (damage to the nervous system) (see Tables 19-1 and 19-2).

TABLE 19-1. Acute vs. Chronic/Persistent Pain

	Acute	Chronic/Persistent
Cause	■ Generally known ■ Protective	■ Generally unknown ■ Function unknown
Duration	■ Less than 3 months ■ Relieved when healing is complete	■ Greater than 3 months ■ Can persist after healing is complete or be due to persistent pathology
Examples	■ Clear injury or disease ■ Appendicitis ■ Postprocedural pain	■ Back pain ■ Arthropathies

TABLE 19-2. Nociceptive vs. Neuropathic Causes of Pain

	Etiology	Location	Descriptors
Nociceptive–Somatic	Direct stimulation from tissue injury of intact nociceptors with transmission along undamaged nerves	Inflammation of: ■ Bone ■ Joints ■ Skeletal muscle	Easier to describe and localize: ■ Aching ■ Stabbing ■ Throbbing
Nociceptive–Visceral		Inflammation of: ■ Internal organs ■ Smooth muscle	More difficult to describe and localize: ■ Gnawing ■ Cramping ■ Colicky
Neuropathic	Damage caused by compression, transection, infiltration, ischemia, or metabolic injury of peripheral or central nerves	Injury of: ■ Peripheral or central nerves	Easier to describe and localize: ■ Numbness ■ Burning ■ Tingling ■ Shocklike

Treatment

The ability to assess the cause of the pain from history and physical is extremely important because treatment is based on the pain type the patient is experiencing.

- **Acute nociceptive pain**: Modified WHO Pain Ladder (Figure 19-2).

The following reviews the treatment of pain, but it is also important to remember to continuously evaluate whether the underlying cause of pain is reversible and if opioid pain medication can be reduced.

Mild Pain

Initial treatment of pain always starts with nonopioid medications such as acetaminophen and ibuprofen.

Moderate to Severe Pain

This is where opioids are added to the pain regimen. Before starting opioids, it is also important to know a patient's kidney and liver function. (Table 19-3 describes which medications should be avoided or reduced based on the patient's liver and kidney functions.) Here are also the typical starting doses for commonly used opioids.

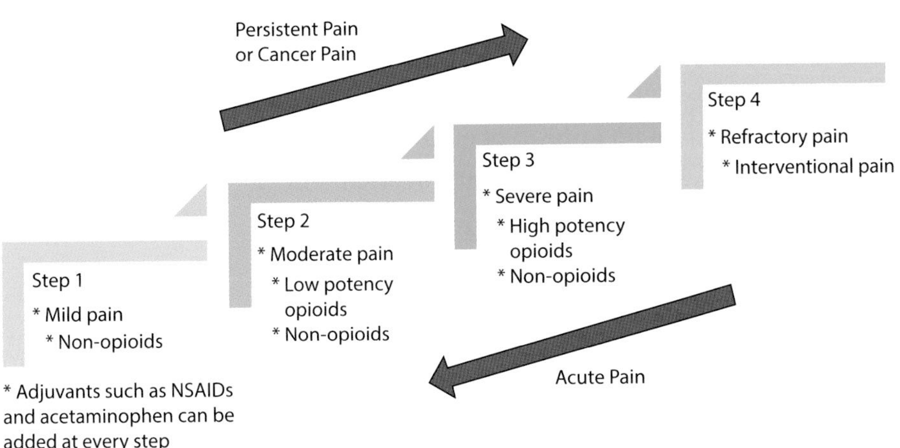

FIGURE 19-2. World Health Organization Pain Ladder. (Source: https://www.who.int/cancer/palliative/painladder/en/.)

TABLE 19-3. Opioid Medication Adjustment for Patients with Kidney and Liver Disease

	Kidney Disease			Liver Disease	
	eGFR 30–90	eGFR <30	Dialysis	Stable Cirrhosis	Severe Disease
Morphine	Caution*	**Do not use**	**Do not use**	Caution*	**Do not use**
Oxycodone	Caution*	Caution*	Caution*	Caution*	Caution*
Hydromorphone	Caution*	Caution*	Caution*	Caution*	Caution*
Fentanyl	Preferred	Preferred	Preferred	Preferred	Preferred
Codeine	Do not use	Do not use	Do not use	Do not use	Do not use
Methadone	Preferred**	Preferred**	Preferred**	Preferred**	Preferred**

eGFR, estimated glomerular filtration rate.
*Reduce dose and frequency.
**Consult with an experienced clinician before initiating or adjusting dose of methadone.

- For **moderate pain**, sample starting doses are as follows:
  - **Average-sized adult:**
    - Oral morphine immediate-release 7.5 mg.
    - Oral oxycodone immediate-release 5 mg.
    - Oral hydromorphone immediate-release 4 mg.
  - **Frail, older adults or adults with kidney or liver disease** (see Table 19-3):
    - Oral morphine immediate-release 5 mg.
    - Oral oxycodone immediate-release 2.5 mg.
    - Oral hydromorphone immediate-release 2 mg.
- For **severe pain**, sample starting doses are as follows:
  - **Average-sized adult:**
    - Intravenous morphine 4 mg.
    - Intravenous hydromorphone 0.4 mg.
  - **Frail, older adult:**
    - Intravenous morphine 2 mg.
    - Intravenous hydromorphone 0.2 mg.

Dose Finding

After initial intravenous (IV) dose, wait about 15 minutes (time to peak effect) and reassess pain severity.

- Severe pain: Repeat up to 100% of original dose.
- Moderate pain: Administer up to 50% of original dose.
- Mild pain: You're done.

  (It is important to manage expectations prior to treatment that 0 out of 10 pain is not always possible.)

  * Repeat until patient is in mild or tolerable amount of pain (50% reduction), add up total amount of opioid administered, and that is the new dose.

After controlling their pain initially, it's important to now think about how to control their pain over the next several days. First decide whether the pain is intermittent or constant.

- **For intermittent pain:**
  - Dose for time to peak effect.
  - Dose short-acting opioids as needed.
  - IV: q30min to q1h PRN (q2h PRN in older adult/liver/renal insufficiency).
  - Oral: q2h PRN.
- **For constant pain:**
  - Dose for duration of effect.
  - Schedule short acting opioids every 4 hours (every 6 hours in older adults or patients with liver or renal insufficiency).

After tracking the patient's pain and how much pain medications the patient is receiving, the next step is to think about **breakthrough pain**, which is transitory exacerbations of severe pain over a baseline of mild to moderate pain. Add up the patient's total 24-hour dose of opioids, and 10% of that will equal the patient's breakthrough pain dose. The frequency will be based on the time-to-peak effect of the opioid you are using.

Example: If the scheduled dose is **morphine 4 mg IV q4h around the clock**, then add up the 24-hour total (of scheduled opioids): 4 mg × 6 = 24 mg IV morphine × 10% = 2.4 mg, or about **2 mg IV morphine q1h PRN.**

Opioid Side Effects

Opioids are effective for nociceptive pain, but there are common side effects that can be managed. It is also important to warn patients about side effects and to educate them on which side effects patients develop tolerance for and which they do not. Tolerance is a change in the dose–response relationship induced by exposure to the drug and manifests as a need for a higher dose to maintain an effect. Time to tolerance for each opioid side effect is listed and compared next:

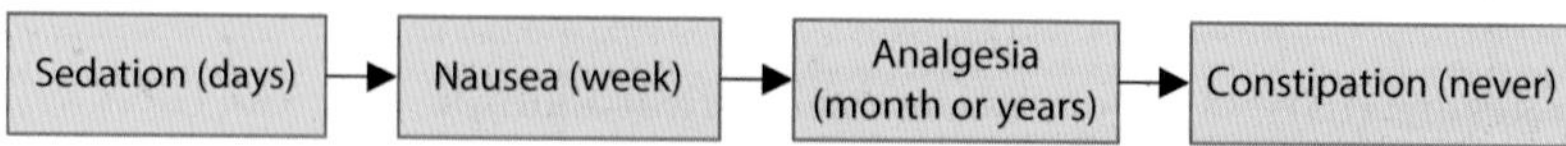

- **Constipation**: Common;
  - Tolerance does not develop for this side effect.
  - Always start a bowel regimen alongside opioid pain medication to prevent constipation.
  - Common regimen: Senna or polyethylene glycol powder.

TABLE 19-4. Equianalgesic Equivalency chart

Opioid	IV/SC/IM (mg)	PO (mg)	Duration of Effect*	Time to Peak Effect
Morphine	5	15	4 hours	IV: 10–15 min SC: 20–40 min PO: 30–90 min
Long-acting morphine		15	12 hours	
Oxycodone		10	4 hours	PO: 30–90 min
Long-acting oxycodone		10	12 hours	
Hydromorphone	0.8	4	4 hours	IV: 10–15 min SC: 20–40 min PO: 30–90 min

IM, intramuscularly; *IV*, intravenously; *PO*, by mouth; *SC*, subcutaneously.

* Approximate.

- **Nausea** – Common:
  - Tolerance develops within 7 days, so treat through and let the patient know that this side effect will likely pass.
  - Common antiemetics: Prochlorperazine, ondansetron, or metoclopramide.
- **Sedation** – Common:
  - Tolerance often develops within 1 to 3 days of initiation or dose escalation.
  - Because of this tolerance, it is important to counsel the patient and family.
- **Other** (for these consider opioid rotation):
  - Respiratory depression (for this consider naloxone administration).
  - Pruritis.
  - Dry mouth.
  - Delirium.
  - Urinary retention.
  - Delirium.
  - Myoclonus/seizures (rare).

Opioid Conversion

After reaching a steady state with pain medications, it often becomes necessary to convert IV opioids to oral or switch to another type of opioid. Following are the steps to converting opioid medications.

HIGH-YIELD LITERATURE

Gammaitoni AR, Fine P, Alvarez N, et al. Clinical application of opioid equianalgesic data. *Clin J Pain*. 2003;19:286-297.

- Thoroughly assess pain using OPQRSTU.
- Determine the total opioid usage in the past 24 hours.
- Choose a new opioid medication and route of administration, and set up a ratio using an equianalgesic equivalence chart (See Table 19-4).

- After calculating the dose, do the following:
  - If using the same opioid (e.g., converting from IV morphine to PO morphine).
    - No need to reduce for incomplete cross-tolerance.
  - If switching to a different opioid:
    - Pain controlled: Reduce by 50% for incomplete cross-tolerance.
    - Pain not controlled: Reduce by 25% or less.
- Reassess frequently and adjust regimen as needed.

Persistent/Chronic Nociceptive Pain

Chronic pain benefits from a multidisciplinary approach, as its pathophysiology and development are complex and multifactorial. Persistent pain can be due to chronic activation of C-peripheral nerve fibers causing changes that lower the threshold for pain signals. Additionally, alterations in brain structure or function, as well as dopaminergic dysfunction (linked to depression and insomnia), are thought to be related to chronic pain syndromes. It initially starts with pharmacotherapy, as outlined earlier under acute pain, but it's important to also involve nonpharmacologic interventions such as physical therapy (PT), psychosocial evaluation and support, and integrative modalities.

Acute and Chronic Neuropathic Pain

Neuropathic pain requires a different set of medications:

- **First-line:**
- Anticonvulsants (e.g., gabapentin, pregabalin).
- Serotonin-norepinephrine reuptake inhibitor (SNRI) (e.g., duloxetine, venlafaxine).
- Tricyclic antidepressants (TCAs) (e.g., amitriptyline, nortriptyline).

- **Second-line:**
- Topical capsaicin.
- Topical lidocaine.

- **Third-line** (or with neuropathic agents during an acute crisis):
- Opioids may be used along with neuropathic agents during an acute crisis.

DYSPNEA

General Facts

Definition: A *subjective* experience of breathing discomfort (not tachypnea, respiratory distress, or hypoxemia).

Treatment

First requires investigating the cause of dyspnea and trying to optimize the underlying disease, being mindful of prognosis and overall goals of care. For example:

- Nebulizers/steroids for bronchospasm.
- Thoracentesis for pleural effusion.
- Diuresis for pulmonary edema.
- Cancer-directed treatment for increased tumor burden.
- Blood transfusion for symptomatic anemia.

If the patient is optimized, consider both nonpharmacologic and pharmacologic treatments.

Management

Nonpharmacologic Management

- Is just as important as pharmacologic treatment along with educating patients and family.
- Create a relaxing environment (limit number of people, optimize temperature, reduce noise, window bed is ideal with clear line of sight to outside).
- Educate on behavioral techniques (relaxation, guided meditation, breathing exercises).
- Eliminate irritants such as strong-smelling perfume or cleaning agents.
- Reposition (elevate the head of the bed, support with pillows).
- Bedside fan.
- Supplemental O_2 if hypoxic.

Pharmacologic Management

- **Low-dose opioids** can reduce the sensation of air hunger. Mechanism is not known, but thought to be centrally mediated. Possible regiments are as follows:
  - Morphine immediate-release (MSIR) 2 to 5 mg PO and hydromorphone 1 to 2 mg PO.
  - Morphine 1 to 2 mg IV, hydromorphone 0.2 to 0.4 mg IV.
- **Anxiolytics** can be used if dyspnea is worsened by or causes anxiety. However, avoid combining opioids and benzodiazepines, as this increases the risk of respiratory depression.

CONQUER THE **WARDS!**

If the patient is not hypoxic, a bedside fan is equally effective to supplemental oxygen in relieving dyspnea.

NAUSEA

General Facts

Definition:

1. **Nausea** is subjective sensation of needing to vomit.
2. **Vomiting** is a neuromuscular reflex, involuntary contractions of the abdominal, thoracic, and gastrointestinal (GI) muscles leading to forceful expulsion of stomach contents from the mouth.

Causes

There are 4 emetic pathways:

- **Chemoreceptor trigger zone** (CTZ):
  - Predominantly mediated and stimulated by dopamine (D2), serotonin (5-HT3 and 5-HT4), and neurokinin (NK1).
  - **Common causes:**
    - Metabolic abnormalities.
    - Sepsis.
    - Medications such as prochlorperazine and ondansetron are commonly used for chemotherapy-induced nausea.
- **GI tract:** Anything that irritates, obstructs, or slows the GI tract.
  - Predominantly mediated by dopamine (D2) and serotonin (5-HT3 and 5-HT4).
  - **Common Causes:**
    - Delayed gastric emptying.
    - Constipation/bowel obstruction.

- Gastric compression/distension.
- Inflammation (e.g., gastritis, esophagitis).

- **Vestibular tract:**
  - Predominantly mediated by histamine (H1) and acetylcholine (ACH).
  - **Common causes:**
    - Motion sickness.
    - Inflammation (e.g., vestibular neuritis).
- **Cerebral cortex:**
  - Predominantly mediated by gamma-aminobutyric acid (GABA) and histamine (H1).
  - **Common causes:**
    - Unpleasant sights, smells, and tastes.
    - Anxiety.
    - Increased intracranial pressure.
    - Meningeal irritation.

Treatment

Treatment of nausea should be based on the emetic pathway that is causing it. Table 19-5 describes the different classes of antiemetic medications.

TABLE 19-5. Classes of Antiemetic Medications

Class	Action	Examples	Side Effects	Cost
Dopamine receptor antagonists	■ CTZ ■ GI tract	■ Prochlorperazine ■ Haloperidol ■ Olanzapine ■ Metoclopramide (also prokinetic)	■ Extrapyramidal ■ Sedation ■ Increased QTc	■ Low
Serotonin receptor antagonists	■ CTZ ■ GI tract	■ Ondansetron ■ Granisetron ■ Dolasetron ■ Tropisetron ■ Palonosetron	■ Constipation ■ Headache ■ Increased QTc	■ High
Antihistamines	■ Vestibular tract ■ Cerebral cortex	■ Diphenhydramine ■ Meclizine ■ Hydroxyzine ■ Doxepin	■ Sedation ■ Constipation ■ Delirium ■ Dry mouth	■ Low
Anticholinergics	■ Vestibular tract	■ Scopolamine	■ Delirium ■ Urinary retention ■ Dry mouth	■ Low
Neurokinin receptor antagonists	■ CTZ	■ Aprepitant ■ Fosaprepitant	■ Sedation ■ Constipation ■ Hiccups	■ High
Anxiolytics	■ Cerebral cortex	■ Lorazepam ■ Diazepam	■ Sedation ■ Delirium	■ Low
Corticosteroids	■ May relieve cancer-associated nausea by reducing inflammation (GI, intracranial)	■ Dexamethasone ■ Prednisone	■ Delirium, mood swings ■ Insomnia ■ Weight gain ■ Fluid retention ■ Osteoporosis	■ Low

CTZ, chemoreceptor zone; *GI*, gastrointestinal.

COMMUNICATION

Quality communication in patients with serious illness can be challenging and emotionally charged. As a result, many clinicians facing these types of conversations feel unprepared and uncomfortable. The good news is that patient-centered communication is a learnable skill. The following are some helpful tips for you to navigate these conversations.

NONVERBAL COMMUNICATION

Most interpersonal communication is nonverbal. It can be expressed by tone of voice, eye contact, facial expressions, and body position (distance, posture, and touch).

Tips for nonverbal communication:

- Sit at eye level with the patient or slightly lower.
- Sit in a relaxed position with an open body posture.
- Lean toward the patient (and keep an appropriate distance).
- Maintain eye contact.
- Use silence to allow the patient to share his or her thoughts first.
  Note: The average physician interrupts patients after only 11 seconds.

NURSE STATEMENTS FOR ARTICULATING EMPATHY

Emotions are commonly experienced during serious illness. When engaging in serious illness discussions, it is important to remember that:

- **Emotion happens faster than rational thought.**
- **Emotion is involuntary and unstoppable.**
- **Unacknowledged, emotion can derail the conversation.**

Responding to emotions can help build rapport and trust with patients and their families, help find out important goals and priorities for patients, and help patients move forward in difficult conversations. A mnemonic that is useful in responding to emotions is NURSE. Each technique described in Table 19-6 is one way to respond to a patient's emotion—all are considered empathic continuers. They acknowledge what the patient is experiencing and allow the patient to then expand upon their emotion. This is a toolbox and is not meant to be used in a particular order. Different statements may be helpful in different situations.

HELPFUL MNEMONICS

There are 3 common conversations around serious illness:

- Communicating serious news.
- Addressing goals of care early in the disease trajectory.
- Addressing goals of care late in the disease trajectory.

Following are some helpful mnemonics and tips to having these conversations incorporating the NURSE mnemonic. These conversations are challenging, and as a medical student, you likely will not be having these conversations alone. However, watch as your teams or palliative care teams use these techniques,

TABLE 19-6. NURSE Menomnic for Responding to Emotional Cues and please move this up to where it is referenced

	Example	Notes
Name	*"You seem upset…"* *"This is a frustrating situation…"*	■ Acknowledge the emotion by suggesting the emotion that the patient may be experiencing. ■ In general, turn down the intensity a notch when you name the emotion, or just name the situation.
Understand	*"I can't imagine what you are going through."* *"I can only imagine…"*	■ Think of this as another kind of acknowledgement, but stop short of suggesting you understand everything (you don't).
Respect	*"I can see you really care about your mother."*	■ Expression of praise or gratitude about the things they are doing. ■ This can be especially helpful when there is conflict.
Support	*"We will do everything we can to support you through this process."*	■ A good way to express nonabandonment. ■ Making this kind of commitment is a powerful statement.
Explore	*"Can you tell me more about…"*	■ When a question comes after serious news, it may be an emotion cue. ■ Exploring can help you understand their reasoning or actions.

and begin to incorporate them into your communication style. It is never too early to practice these techniques.

COMMUNICATING SERIOUS NEWS—SPIKES

The SPIKES protocol or talking map is one of the most commonly taught and commonly used in palliative care for communicating serious news. (See Table 19-7.)

ADDRESSING GOALS OF CARE

Shared decision-making is the dominant model for communication in caring for patients with serious illness. Experts define shared decision-making as an "interpersonal, interdependent process in which health care providers and the patient relate to and influence each other as they collaborate in making decisions about the patient's health care." Clinicians contribute to the conversation by sharing medical knowledge, including prognosis and risks/benefits of treatments. Patients and their families contribute to the conversation by sharing values and goals that are relevant to the medical context. The ultimate goal of this process is for patients to receive goal-concordant care. There are 2 types of serious illness conversations in palliative care: The early goals of care conversation (similar to advance care planning) and the late goals of care conversation.

PREMAP—ADDRESSING GOALS OF CARE (EARLY IN DISEASE TRAJECTORY)

Early goals of care conversations should take place at the point of diagnosis of a serious illness. These often occur in the outpatient setting or when patients

TABLE 19-7. SPIKES Mnemonic for Communicating Serious News

Task	Context	Language	Description
Setting and Setup	Prepare before you share the news		■ Review pertinent medical facts (in health record and with the medical team) ■ Ensure that key stakeholders are present (for patient and medical team) ■ Provide a quiet, private location ■ Minimize distractions (silence pagers and cell phones) ■ If going in as a group, create an agenda and make sure everyone is on the same page; negotiate roles with others
Perception	Assess how the patient views the medical situation	"Just so we are on the same page, what have the doctors told you about your illness?" "What do you know so far about your mother's health"	■ Decide who to ask if multiple family members are present ■ You may need to have follow-up questions to clarify their understanding ■ AVOID: "What's your understanding" or "what's your perception"
Invitation	Ask permission to talk about the news	"Would it be okay if we talked about the results of the CT scan?" "Would it be okay if we talked about something, I am worried about?"	■ Invitation is important to assess readiness ■ If not ready, must address other issues before moving forward ■ Even if they say yes, it may be a "no"
Knowledge	Share the medical facts	Labeling News: "I have difficult news to share" Headline: "The CT scan showed that the cancer is worse and this means that the chemotherapy is no longer working"	■ Give a headline: 1–2 sentences that summarize the information and share the meaning/impact it has for the patient ■ Fifth-grade reading level; avoid jargon ■ You may need to label the news as "difficult" or "bad" ■ Say the news and then stop
Empathy	Attend to patient's emotions	NURSE statements	■ May take more than a few statements ■ Ask permission before moving forward
Summarize and Strategize	Discuss next steps and a follow-up plan	CHECK UNDERSTANDING *"To make sure I did a good job giving you the information, tell me what you will tell your spouse about our conversation."* *"Who are you going to call when we finish this meeting? What will you plan on saying?"* EMOTIONAL CHECK *"How are you doing with that information?"*	■ Beware of the pull toward a plan ■ Check in before moving forward, particularly if there was not much emotion ■ Make a follow-up plan: • Details of plan • Timeline (clear timeline, set goals with deadlines) • Clarify your role in future medical care

are not necessarily hospitalized in a crisis. The key elements that should be addressed in this conversation include:

- Understanding of prognosis.
- Decision-making and information preferences.
- Prognostic information.
- Patient goals.

Even before having the conversation, you may need to introduce the conversation to the patient. This not only introduces the purpose of the conversation, but also helps to assess the patient's readiness for the conversation.

"I'd like to talk with you about what is ahead with your illness and what is most important to you, so that I can make sure we provide you with care that matches your values. Is this okay?"

The rest of the conversation can be followed as presented in Table 19-8. The below table lists the tasks and helpful language to use during these conversations. During an ideal conversation, the tasks are listed in chronological order but in

TABLE 19-8. Tasks During Goals of Care Discussions Early in Disease Trajectory

Task	Description	Language
Share Prognosis	■ Assess patient's understanding of prognosis, as well as their information preferences ■ Share the prognosis in 3 ways • Time based • Function based • Uncertain Note: Most of the time the resident or attending will be sharing the prognosis; you can assist by understanding what the patient knows about his or her health and help cater the prognosis sharing.	■ **Understanding**: *"What is your understanding of your illness?"* ■ **Information Preferences**: *"How much information about what to expect with your illness would be helpful for you?"* ■ **Readiness**: *"Would it be okay if I share my understanding of what lies ahead with your illness…"* ■ **Time:** *"I am worried that you may get sicker and return to the hospital in the next few months to a year."* ■ **Function**: *"I am worried that this may be as strong as you feel, and things are likely to get worse over time."* ■ **Uncertain**: *"I hope you will continue to live well for a long time. I am also worried that you could get sick quickly or unexpectedly."*
Expect Emotion	Emotions mean that the patient/family heard the headline/ prognosis. They may express this as ■ Nonverbal ■ Verbal ■ Emotion masked as a cognitive question (e.g., isn't there anything you can do?)	■ NURSE statements
Map Out What's Important	■ A focus on a broad array of goals that persons have for their life aids the clinician in creating a personalize care plan for the patient. ■ There is usually more than one thing that is important to patients; make sure that you continue to ask "what else" ■ Avoid questions that ask about treatment preferences (e.g., Would you want to be resuscitated? Would you want a breathing tube?), as these can narrow the focus of treatment plans	■ *"When thinking about the future of your health, what is most important to you?"* ■ *"If your health situation worsens, what would worry you?"* ■ *"What would be an unacceptable quality of life for you or a life worse than death?"*
Align with Goals	■ Aligning helps to make sure you got their values right ■ It also shows that you are listening ■ You can align after every goal or at the end of asking about goals	■ *"As I listen, it sounds like what's important is your family and being at home."* ■ *"Sounds like continuing to work is very important to you."*
Propose a Plan and Share the Plan with Others	■ Before a plan is proposed, you can make sure the patient is ready for it by asking permission ■ Recommend a plan based off of the patient's goals and explain why you are proposing that plan ■ Once you have proposed the plan, check in with the patient to make sure you have it right ■ Make sure that this conversation is documented and shared with others • Include the patient's surrogate decision-makers • Include other clinicians who may need to know about the goals and values Note: Most of the time the resident or attending will be proposing these plans; you can assist by understanding the patient's values and describing them to the team	■ *"Would it be okay if I make a recommendation regarding next steps?"* ■ *"Because you said that continuing to work, remaining active, interacting with people, and avoiding hospitalizations are important to you, I recommend that we continue your antibiotics and chemotherapy."* ■ *"How does that sound?"* ■ *"I recommend that we fill out a form called an advance directive that can document the values you just told me."* ■ *"I recommend that we bring in your health care agent to continue these discussions so that they know what is most important to you."*

practice, the order which these tasks are done change based on how the conversation is going. This is the art of palliative care.

REMAP—ADDRESSING GOALS OF CARE (LATE IN DISEASE TRAJECTORY)

Late goals of care conversations often occur in the hospital or when the serious illness is not responding to treatments. These conversations require helping patients reconfigure to a new normal with their disease and to reprioritize some of the goals. Older goals may not be possible anymore for patient's and/or their surrogate decision makers (see Table 19-9.) . The table below again lists the tasks in chronological order but in practice, but the order which these tasks are done change based on how the conversation is going.

TABLE 19-9. REMAP Menomnic for Addressing Goals of Care Late in Disease Trajectory

Task	Description	Language
Reframe the Situation	■ Examine why things are currently not proceeding as everyone hoped ■ Prior to sharing the context of the illness, it is important to learn about the patient's/family member's understanding of the illness ■ Sometimes you may have to label the news, especially if there is a gap between their understanding and yours ■ Share the news in a headline: • Summary of information (no more than 1–2 sentences) • Impact it has on patient's life Note: Most of the time the resident or attending will be sharing the prognosis; you can assist by understanding what the patient knows about their health and help cater the prognosis sharing	■ **Understanding:** *"What have you heard about how things are going with your cancer?"* ■ **Permission**: *"Would it be okay if I tell you what I know?"* ■ **Label News:** *"I have some difficult news to share."* ■ **Headline:** *"The CT scan results show that the cancer has worsened despite chemotherapy and we are concerned that more chemotherapy will no longer help treat your cancer."*
Expect Emotion	When a strong headline is **heard**, the patient will often respond with emotion.	■ NURSE statements
Map Out What's Important	■ Take a step back to explore the patient's values before discussing therapeutic choices ■ To map the patient's values, ask open-ended questions that are designed to help the patient think about the values that should guide treatment ■ When the patient cannot participate, ask the patient's surrogate decision-maker to participate	■ *"After hearing this news, what is most important to you?"* ■ *"Given the situation, what worries you ?"* ■ *"As you think about the future, what would you like to be doing?"* ■ *"What would your dad say is most important to him if he were sitting right here with us?"*
Align with Goals	■ Aligning helps to make sure you got their values right ■ It also shows that you are listening ■ You can align after every goal or at the end of asking about goals	■ *"It sounds like being at home, being with family, and communicating with her loved ones are important to your mother."*
Propose a Plan That Matches the Patient's Values	■ Before a plan is proposed, you can make sure the patient is ready for it by asking permission ■ Recommend a plan based off of the patient's goals and explain why you are proposing that plan ■ Focus on what can be achieved before what cannot ■ Once you have proposed the plan, check in with the patient to make sure you have it right. Note: Most of the time the resident or attending will be proposing these plans; you can assist by understanding the patient's values and describing them to the team	■ *"Would it be okay if I make a recommendation regarding next steps?"* ■ *"Because you said that being at home, being with family, and communicating with her loved ones are important, I recommend that we create a discharge plan that honors these values."* ■ *"I also recommend that at the time that her heart stops, we allow her to die naturally, as I don't think resuscitation will help her meet her goals."* ■ *"How does that sound?"*

CARE OF THE DYING PATIENT

During your medicine rotation, you will likely see a patient who dies. The majority of patients go through similar symptoms and signs in the days prior to their death. This time frame and pattern are often referred to as "actively dying." See Table 19-10.

COMMON SYMPTOMS AT THE END OF LIFE

- **Dyspnea:**
  - One of the most distressing symptoms at the end of life (prevalence 20% to 60%).
  - **Goal** for treatment is to help relax respiratory effort (decrease use of accessory muscles, nasal flaring); the goal is not to lower the respiratory rate.
  - **Management** is similar to dyspnea during serious illness (see earlier sections):
    - **Medications**: Opioids (e.g., morphine) or benzodiazepines (e.g., Ativan).
    - **Promote airflow**: Think about opening a window, bringing a fan into the room and/or giving them oxygen.
    - **Relaxation techniques** or music.
    - **Repositioning** in bed can also help.
- **Pain:**
  - Not as common as people think (only 20% to 50% of patients experience pain).
  - Thought to decrease as a patient is closer to death.
  - **Management** is similar to pain during serious illness (see earlier sections):
    - Medications: Tylenol, ibuprofen, opioids:
      - Oral (often higher concentrations like morphine 20 mg/mL solution) or intravenous.
      - Continuous or as needed.
    - Other modalities: Massage, reiki, music therapy.
    - Bed positioning and repositioning.
- **Delirium:**
  - Terminal delirium is defined as delirium in the final days/weeks of life, where treatment of the underlying cause is impossible, impractical, or not consistent with the goals of care.

TABLE 19-10. Actively Dying Stages

Stage	Time Frame	General Signs/Symptoms
Early	Days	■ Mostly bedbound ■ Decreased appetite, decreased oral intake ■ More time sleeping, some delirium
Middle	Days to hours	■ No oral intake ■ Mental status decline: Slow to arouse, only brief periods of wakefulness
Late	Hours to minutes	■ Comatose ■ Pooled oral secretions (death rattle) ■ Cold and mottled extremities ■ Changes to respiratory patterns: Periods of apnea and/or irregular breathing

- Most prevalent symptom (as high as 88% for patients in final days).
- May be frightening to patients, "premature separation" for family.

- **Preventing and mitigating delirium:**
  - Reorientation of patient to time and place (e.g., today is Jan 31st at 2 p.m.):
    - Ask relatives/friends/familiar people to visit and reorient the patient to the medical situation.
  - Lights on during the day/lights off at night.
  - Avoid interrupting sleep (e.g., do not take vitals at 2 am) and reduce other outside noises.
  - Avoid restraints (e.g., catheters, IVs) if possible.
- **Medications:**
  - First-generation antipsychotics:
    - Haloperidol (Haldol) is most commonly used, since it can be administered through oral, subcutaneous, and parenteral routes.
      - Starting doses are 0.5 to 1 mg PO/SC/IV every 4 to 6 hours. Titration can occur every 1 hour as needed until a total daily requirement is established, which is then administered in daily or twice-daily doses.
      - IV or SC haloperidol may cause fewer extrapyramidal symptoms than oral but may cause more significant QTc prolongation.
    - Chlorpromazine (Thorazine) has more sedative effects than haloperidol for patients in whom sedation is desired.
      - Starting dose is 25 to 50 mg PO or IV every 4 to 6 hours. Titration can occur by 25 to 50 mg every 1 hour until a total daily requirement is established, which is then administered in daily or twice-daily doses.
      - Maximum dose is 2000 mg/day.
  - Second-generation antipsychotics: Also known as atypical antipsychotics; have less evidence in efficacy at the end of life. They are also often taken orally and do not work as fast as conventional antipsychotics. They are associated with fewer extrapyramidal side effects than first-generation antipsychotics and may be recommended in patients with a history of extrapyramidal reactions.
    - Olanzapine: Starting dose is 2.5 to 5 mg PO at bedtime. Orally disintegrating tablets are available.
    - Quetiapine: Starting dose is 25 mg PO once or twice a day, which can be increased by 25 to 50 mg per dose every 2 to 3 days. It is the antipsychotic of choice for patients with Parkinson disease or Lewy body dementia.
    - Risperidone: Starting dose is 1 to 2 mg PO at night and is gradually raised 1 mg every 2 to 3 days. It has minimal anticholinergic effects and does not cause orthostasis. It is the least sedating.
    - Aripiprazole: Starting dose is initially 2 mg daily PO every 4 to 6 hours. Least likely to prolong QTc and has less sedation and fewer extrapyramidal side effects.
  - Benzodiazepines: Can make delirium worse and are only used as a last resort. It can be used in the following settings:
    - Uncontrolled or severe agitation.
    - Benzodiazepines or alcohol withdrawal.
    - Having side effects from the other delirium medications.
- **Dry mouth/thirst:**
  - Dry mouth is one symptom that increases near the end of life–experienced by >60% of patients at end of life.

- Treatment:
  - Fluid intake:
    - If patient can tolerate sips of fluids and/or ice chips.
  - Mouth care:
    - Swabs of fluid to the mouth and lips.
    - Artificial saliva spray.
    - Saline nebulizer.
    - Make sure oxygen supplement is humidified.
  - Lip care:
    - Lip balm.
    - A+D ointment.

- **Increased oral secretions:**
  - Salivary/bronchial secretions that can't be expectorated due to weakness/fatigue (called the death rattle).
  - Common as death nears (high prevalence rates – 45% to 92% in the literature).
  - Can be disturbing to patient's loved ones.
- **Treatment:**
  - **Nonpharmacologic treatments:**
    - Reposition the patient on his or her side or in a semi-prone position to facilitate drainage.
    - Gentle oropharyngeal suctioning; although this can be ineffective when secretions are beyond the reach of the catheter. Note: Frequent suctioning can be disturbing to both the patient and his or her loved ones.
    - Reduction of fluid intake.
  - **Pharmacologic treatments**: Muscarinic receptor blockers (anticholinergic drugs) are the most commonly used class of medication for oral secretions at the end of life. All of these agents can cause varying degrees of blurred vision, sedation, confusion, delirium, restlessness, hallucinations, palpitations, constipation, and urinary retention. **All of the medications only prevent future secretions and do not eliminate current ones.**
    - Glycopyrrolate (Robinul): Starting dose is 0.2 mg q6–8h with quick onset of about 1 minute. It does not cross the blood–brain barrier and therefore is less likely to cause sedation or delirium.
    - Atropine sulfate (Atropine ophthalmic solution): 1 to 2 gtt sublingual q4–6h with onset of 30 minutes.
    - Scopolamine (Transderm Scop): 1.5 mg patch q72h. This can cause sedation, as it crosses the blood–brain barrier. Its onset is 12 h and steady state is about 24 h.
    - Hyoscyamine (Lev sin): 0.125 mg PO or SL with onset in 30 minutes. Can cause sedation.
- **Anxiety:**
  - Anxiety and fear occur commonly in the dying patient. However, disabling anxiety and/or panic is not a normal aspect of the dying process.
  - Terminally ill patients with chronic dyspnea may often worry about "suffocating to death."
  - Management:
    - Optimize medical management of symptoms like pain and nonpain symptoms (especially dyspnea).

   - Consider nonpharmacologic treatments: Music therapy, massage therapy, guided imagery, biofeedback.
   - Benzodiazepines: Lorazepam 0.5 mg every 4 to 6 hours as needed to start is commonly used, and you can also consider long-acting agents such as diazepam 1 mg q12h or clonazepam 0.25 mg q12h.

- **Anorexia:**
  - Extremely common.
  - It is NOT the same as starvation.
  - Caregivers have HUGE distress when a patient is not eating.
  - Treatment:
    - Medications for nausea/vomiting.
    - Help patient eat as tolerated.
    - Educate caregivers regarding normal progression of disease; help find other ways to express their care (e.g., mouth care).
- **Constipation:**
  - Constipation can happen patients who are bedbound and not eating.
  - Patients still need to have a bowel movement every 2 to 3 days for comfort.
  - Treatment:
    - Mobility if possible.
    - Medications are challenging, since patients are often not able to take oral medications.
      - Bisacodyl 10 mg suppository daily as needed.
      - Enema daily as needed.
- **Incontinence:**
  - Urinary and fecal incontinence may occur near the end.
  - Treatment:
    - Catheters may be needed (Foley catheter, rectal tube).
    - Frequent changing and turning are important to prevent pressure ulcers.

INDEX

Page numbers followed by an f indicate figure; page numbers followed by a t indicate tables. **Bold** indicates the start of the main discussion.

B

C

F

G

H

O

P

W

X

Y

Z